T0177728

Advance Praise for *Diseases in the District of Maine 1772–1820: The Unpublished Work of Jeremiah Barker, a Rural Physician in New England*

"A remarkable and previously unknown source of diseases and medicine in early America. With meticulous research and sensitive prose, Dr. Kahn has set this treasure in its social, cultural, and scientific context, making it accessible, informative, and engaging for everyone."

—Jacalyn Duffin, MD, PhD,
Professor Emerita Queen's University, Kingston, Canada

"After a publication delay of over 200 years, *Diseases in the District of Maine* is fully worth the wait. It offers a fascinating and at times dramatic immersion into medical practice in one part of the early American nation. Dr. Barker proves to be an earnest physician and amiable reporter; while Dr. Kahn ably helps out as a meticulous scholar and annotator."

—Steven J. Peitzman, MD, FACP, Office of Educational Affairs,
Drexel University College of Medicine, Philadelphia, PA, USA

"This immensely readable book is the result of Richard Kahn's determination to see Jeremiah Barker's notes and views on the practice of medicine in rural Maine 200 years ago recognized today. Barker's fifty years' journey shows his progression from apprentice to a master of his craft. Throughout, his case notes, with description of the patients and justification for his diagnoses and treatment, reveal an enlightened approach. He noted the characteristics of his patients and their habits along with detailing the local climate and geography to inform his thoughts, particularly with regard to consumption. Though access to up-to-date scholarship was not easy, particularly in his early years, he read widely and corresponded with other practitioners and later published papers. He believed himself to be a scientific physician and his epidemiological observations led to him addressing life-style changes. This methodology was not that far from that of today and he can be considered a pioneer."

—Dr. John W. K. Ward, FRCPEdin, FRCGP, Past-president of
both the Osler Club of London and the British Society for the
History of Medicine

"This is an extraordinary look at 'ordinary' Maine physician Jeremiah Barker and his attempt to practice medicine at the turn of the 19th century. We see Barker practicing and writing his ultimately unpublished *History of Diseases in the District of Maine* amidst the rise and fall of medical theories and practices, the birth of medical journals in this country, and the attempt of orthodox medical practitioners to establish a seemingly rational therapeutics. Complementing Laurel Thatcher Ulrich's contextualization of Maine midwife Martha Ballard in *A Midwife's Tale*, Kahn places Barker's own evolving theories, practices, and identity, along with the full and annotated transcript of Barker's *History of Diseases of the District of Maine* itself, into historical context. All that's missing is a direct consultation between Ballard and Barker; but these two remarkable lives have definitely been placed into conversation with one another."

—Scott Podolsky, MD, Professor of Global Health and Social Medicine, Harvard Medical School and Director, Center for the History of Medicine, Countway Medical Library, Boston, MA, USA

DISEASES IN THE DISTRICT OF MAINE

1772–1820

The Unpublished Work of
Jeremiah Barker,
a Rural Physician in New England

RICHARD J. KAHN

OXFORD
UNIVERSITY PRESS

OXFORD
UNIVERSITY PRESS

Oxford University Press is a department of the University of Oxford. It furthers
the University's objective of excellence in research, scholarship, and education
by publishing worldwide. Oxford is a registered trade mark of Oxford University
Press in the UK and certain other countries.

Published in the United States of America by Oxford University Press
198 Madison Avenue, New York, NY 10016, United States of America.

Library of Congress Cataloging-in-Publication Data
Names: Kahn, Richard J., author.
Title: Diseases in the district of Maine 1772–1820 : the unpublished
work of Jeremiah Barker, a rural physician in New England /
Richard J. Kahn.
Description: New York : Oxford University Press, [2020] |
Includes bibliographical references and index.
Identifiers: LCCN 2020009364 (print) | LCCN 2020009365 (ebook) |
ISBN 9780190053253 (hardback) | ISBN 9780190053277 (epub) |
ISBN 9780190053284 (online)
Subjects: MESH: Barker, Jeremiah, 1752-1835. | Physicians | History of
Medicine | Medical History Taking | Manuscripts, Medical as Topic |
History, 18th Century | History, 19th Century | Maine | Biobibliography
Classification: LCC R128.7 (print) | LCC R128.7 (ebook) | NLM WZ 100 |
DDC 610.974—dc23
LC record available at https://lccn.loc.gov/2020009364
LC ebook record available at https://lccn.loc.gov/2020009365

1 3 5 7 9 8 6 4 2
Printed by Integrated Books International, United States of America

To my wife, Patricia Gamble Kahn, without whom this book would not have been possible, and to our son and daughter, Ian Jonas Kahn and Gillian Kahn Hargreaves, who have accepted Jeremiah Barker as a member of the family for the past thirty years.

Contents

List of Illustrations

Foreword

"WHEN I HAD finished my studies," Jeremiah Barker wrote of his 1769–1772 apprenticeship to the physician Bela Lincoln in Hingham, Massachusetts, "he gave me a recommendation as being qualified to practice physic," adding that "as I had his shoulders to stand upon, he hoped I would study diligently, keep exact records of cases, as they should occur in practice, whether fatal or otherwise; open dead bodies, when permitted, note appearances, and labour to make improvements in Medical Science." And so Barker did for the next half century, leaving behind a remarkable compendium of the practice of a physician in rural New England. He intended to publish his *Diseases in the District of Maine* by subscription—advance pledges to purchase the published volume—but for reasons that remain uncertain that never happened. However, the unpublished manuscript eventually found a safe home in the Maine Historical Society. Transcribed and reproduced here, and made accessible to general, medical, and scholarly readers alike through the meticulous editing and annotations of Richard J. Kahn, M.D., it offers an extraordinary window into the medical world of one nonelite, nonurban physician in the Early Republic.

What emerges is not only a richly detailed record of shifting patterns of diseases and their management but also a rare account of the quotidian epistemology and diagnostic and therapeutic reasoning of a physician in rural practice. This is a collection of "interesting" or "extraordinary cases," not a complete record of day-to-day practice. Yet, it provides a much more textured portrait of workaday thinking and acting at the bedside than the daybooks or account books that more often than not are all we have from the few physicians who left behind written records of their practices. The sheer fact of the creation of Barker's manuscript and his ambition to publish it, along with more than a dozen articles he did publish in the first two American medical journals—the *Medical Repository* (f. 1797 in New York City) and the *Medical*

Museum (f. 1804 in Philadelphia)—must give us pause in regarding Barker as "ordinary," "average," or even "typical." But in fact, he was in many ways exemplary. Through Barker's account of his persistent and reflective search for medical information from other physicians and from all-too-scarce medical publications, we have here a history of the networks of medical knowledge as they operated outside urban centers like Philadelphia, New York, Boston, and Charleston.

Barker's medical world was at once quintessentially local and remarkably cosmopolitan. On the one hand, in sharp contrast to the programmatic placelessness of biomedicine today, medical knowledge was in many ways closely tied to the place where it was generated and used: it was in essence local knowledge. Both the character of diseases and their appropriate treatment varied according to local climates, seasons, and topography, as well as local diets, constitutions, habits, and dress, which is the reason that Barker pays such painstaking attention to these variables in recording his histories. Diseases and their appropriate treatment in one town, Barker noted of the practice he observed in Cape Elizabeth, Maine, differed from that "in other towns where the mode of living, fashions, customs and employments of people were different," and therefore medical precept suited to other regions of the country or to Europe ran the risk of being inappropriate or even dangerous if uncritically applied to the sick he met with in New England. Barker's solution was to draw on his own bedside observations and those of neighboring physicians to create a new medical literature tailored to his own region.

At the same time, his manuscript displays the cosmopolitan ambitions and reach of a medical practitioner in rural New England. While Barker practiced on the margins, he sought to participate in and contribute to the mainstream, and his manuscript offers a vivid depiction of the dynamics of the circulation and consumption of medical knowledge. He recorded not only his own experiences but also case histories and opinions that he actively solicited from other physicians in the region. He sought medical information by correspondence with his medical brethren within New England and leading medical figures of the day further afield, such as Benjamin Rush in Philadelphia. He cited cases from European as well as American practice and labored hard to place his hands on the medical literature that he found so hard to come by in Maine. "What does the world yet owe to American physicians and surgeons," a commentator in the *Edinburgh Review* famously and contemptuously asked in 1820,[1] a year in which Barker again announced his proposal and subscription bid for publishing his *History of Diseases of the District of Maine*. He counted himself as among what he tellingly referred to as the wider community of "scientific physicians in the republic of medicine."

Barker's own identity as a scientific physician was rooted in his standing as what he and others called a "regularly educated" practitioner at a time when preceptorship, not school, was at the core of medical training and an intellectual, social, and moral warrant for the doctor's profession, a qualification vouched for by the preceptor's recommendation. This involved a different sense of the term "profession" than in common usage today, when the M.D. degree, white coat ceremony, and licensing mark a student's induction into the medical profession. In late-colonial and early Republican America, one did not merely join a profession but *made* a profession. "Physic is not a trade," one New England physician asserted in 1834, the year before Barker died. "It is a profession made by its members, that is, a declaration, and assertion, that the candidate possesses knowledge, skill, and integrity, sufficient to entitle him to confidence."[2] Medicine was a solitary occupation, principally learned through individual precept and practiced in patients' homes, isolating in ways now hard to recapture in an age when training and practice alike more often than not involve teams. The networks of information exchange in which Barker participated were a source of knowledge, guidance, and reassurance, but also a sense of belonging.

His identity and experience of belonging as a scientific physician were also rooted in medical history, for the good doctor was also a good historian—and not just in the modern sense of a doctor who takes a good clinical history. "Regularly educated" physicians of Barker's day drew on medical history as a source of definition, legitimacy, and authority in the present, placing themselves in a reassuring lineage of ideas, practices, and values they proudly traced back to Hippocrates. They also frequently cited what Barker called "practical observations" from "distinguished physicians, among the Ancients . . . as they are replete with instruction" for explaining and managing disease in the present. Moreover—reflecting the fundamental unity between historical and contemporary medicine—the compilation of a history of diseases, climates, and peoples in a physician's local region, far from being an antiquarian exercise, constituted a scientific contribution to the medical forefront.

---

[1] [Sydney Smith], Review of *Statistical Annals of the United States of America*, by Adam Seybert, *Edinburgh Review* 33 (1820): 69–80, p. 79.

[2] "Medical Improvement," *Boston Medical and Surgical Journal* 9 (1834): 202–205, p. 203.

Yet active engagement with the past and allegiance to tradition did not imply stasis. Indeed, giving an account of the transformation over time in diseases and their appropriate treatment was a central undertaking in Barker's *History*. As Kahn deftly analyzes, it was Barker's embrace of alkaline therapy for various diseases that led him to report, "I was called 'a dangerous innovator.'" More than this, Barker carefully chronicled how not only epidemiological change but also new medical ideas and the availability of new medical literature catalyzed change in his own therapeutic practice, sometimes in ways that led him to lament his earlier errors.

Books, though hard for Barker to obtain, mattered. For example, around 1788, Barker recounts, the Edinburgh physician John Brown's *Elements of Medicine* "first appeared in Maine," a rationalistic system of pathology and therapeutics and an embodiment of the Enlightenment aspiration to give medicine the unifying power that Newton's law of gravity had brought to the physical sciences. A distinctive hallmark of the Brunonian system was the aggressive use of stimulating remedies, especially the therapeutic use of alcohol. Then around 1798, Barker reports, "Dr Rush's 'Inquiry into the causes & cure of Pulmonary Consumption,' printed in 1793, was brought to Portland and read by me, as well as by some of my Brunonian brethren," a medical system that urged instead a depleting therapeutic approach, most especially copious bloodletting. Seconded by experience at the bedside, Barker recalls, "these events induced us to think on our ways, and acknowledge our folly," unraveling what he calls the Brunonian "enchantment." Looking back on this episode, Barker admits that he was "sorry to say that I was not the only physician, who had been drawn into its fascinating and very dangerous vortex."

Also striking are Barker's conviction that autopsy was an important source of change in medical explanation and the place that he accorded to postmortem examination—what he sometimes simply called "inspecting dead bodies" or "dissection"—in his rural practice. "In the past centuries many things inexplicable for the want of post mortem examinations," he asserted, "have been, chiefly by these instructive aids, in the present century, clearly investigated, so that good success has attended scientific physicians." His manuscript is peppered with occasions in which he—sometimes assisted by colleagues or a pupil—"by permission" opened the bodies of deceased patients. In 1784, for example, confronted by multiple cases of women attacked with puerperal or childbed fever, Barker related that "the ill success which attended my practice induced me to write to several aged & experienced physicians in different portions of Mass. for advice as puerperal fever had never appeared among us." He also consulted British books on the subject yet remained unsure about appropriate treatment. But "soon after I was permitted to open two of my patients who died of this fever, and had an opportunity of seeing another inspected," stating that "these appearances convinced me that the disease was highly inflammatory in the outset, and that the lancet was eligible." According to his account, "it then appeared to me, that a mode of prevention might be attempted," reasoning from autopsy and his own bedside observations that early bloodletting and other depleting therapies could forestall a fatal outcome.

In reading Barker's manuscript as a vehicle for understanding the medical world that he and his patients inhabited, we should also listen carefully for the silences. Regularly educated physicians—American and European, present and past, all of them men—loom large in his account. And his manuscript is peopled with practitioners he regarded as irregular and denounced as "empirics," "imposters," or "Patent Doctors," most especially adherents of the botanic system of healing proselytized early in the nineteenth century by Samuel Thomson, dissenters from regular medicine whom Barker denounced as "dangerous members of society." Yet, all but invisible in Barker's writings are the women healers who performed the lion's share of health care. This is especially ironic given that another manuscript from Maine, the diary kept by the Maine midwife and healer Martha Ballard between 1785 and 1812, in the hands of historian Laurel Thatcher Ulrich has provided one of the richest sources we have into such "social healers" and their work, which encompassed health care far beyond attendance at childbirth. In Ballard's diary, as Ulrich notes, "it is doctors, not midwives, who seem marginal."[3] The writings left behind by Barker and Ballard work together in providing a fuller portrait of suffering and healing in rural New England.

Barker's manuscript, like Ballard's diary, is above all full of stories. It is a source that one longs to assign for a seminar, inviting students to investigate further the tantalizing stories that abound in the text and the larger themes they suggest. We encounter a merchant from Falmouth fallen "insane": in Boston, "meeting a physician, who did not bow to him, he knocked off his hat. The Doctor requested two strong men to hold him, while he drew a quart of blood from his arm, in the street," after which, Barker reports, he soon

[3] Laurel Thatcher Ulrich, *A Midwife's Tale: The Life of Martha Ballard, Based on Her Diary, 1785–1812* (New York: Vintage Books, 1990), p. 28. The term "social medicine," the work of "social healers," is one that Ulrich borrows from the well-established historical concept of social childbirth (p. 61).

became rational. We meet the Reverend Ephraim Clark of Cape Elizabeth, who, Barker informs us, always carried a lancet with him on his parochial visits, "as his people were in the habit of being bled, not only in sickness; but in health, as a preventive of disease, particularly in the spring months." We are told of Barker's medical apprentice "of a florid countenance" James Folsome: "This bright & promising young man had been reading the Medical Elements of Dr John Brown; and, like many others, both in Europe & America, was 'too much influenced by his imaginary theories,'" and he died two years after commencing his medical studies. And we hear of Barker's negotiations over several years with his patient Peter Thacher, a thirty-year-old lawyer who repeatedly refused Barker's therapeutic recommendations as well as his diagnosis of pulmonary consumption, but who borrowed medical books from the doctor so that he could chart his own course in managing his illness. He remained "irreconcilable to the lancet and to mercury," succumbing to the disease, but died, Barker tells us, "reconciled to the will of God." Richard Kahn, through his careful transcription and editing of the writings of one nonelite physician, has given us an accessible, engaging, and important source for exploring and reimagining the medical world of the Early Republic.

John Harley Warner
Avalon Professor of the History of Medicine
Yale University

Preface

THE BARKER MANUSCRIPT was brought to my attention in 1990 by Glenn B. Skillin, then curator at the Maine Historical Society in Portland, Maine. The Jeremiah Barker Papers consist of two manuscript boxes containing letters, medical casebooks of 1771–1796 and 1803–1818, and several books published from 1736–1818 with marginalia by Barker. Box 1 contains the manuscript of Barker's valuable study of diseases in Maine, which he planned to publish by subscription as a book in two volumes. The title page of each is a subscription paper:

> *A Proposal for publishing a History of Diseases in the District of Maine,*
> *commencing 1772 to the present time, with biographical sketches of learned*
> *physicians both in Europe and America as well as other promoters of med-*
> *ical science and to which is annexed an inquiry to the causes, natures,*
> *prevalency and treatment of consumption; which is maintained to be cur-*
> *able . . . written so as to be intelligible to those who are destitute of Medical*
> *Science . . . containing about 400 pages—price Two Dollars in Boards.*

Though Barker claims on the title page that "About 100 subscribers have been procured in Maine [and] other states in New England," the book was never printed.[1] Volume 1 describes mental illness and the dangers of spiritous liquors, various epidemics and diseases, diagnoses and treatments, changes in medical philosophy, and general comments on health and how to preserve it.

---

[1] Publication by subscription, meaning that a person promised to take a certain number of copies of a book when published, was not uncommon in the eighteenth and early nineteenth century. Barker sought subscribers in the leading Portland newspaper of the day, offering a free copy to any person "for procuring twelve subscribers." See "Proposal for Publishing a History of Disease of the District of Maine with Endorsement by J. G. Coffin," *Eastern Argus*, January 18, 1820. See also Donald Farren, "Subscription: A Study of the Eighteenth-Century American Trade" (Doctor of Library Science, Columbia University, 1982), 2, 184, and Elizabeth Lane

This is accomplished through case histories of at least one hundred of Barker's patients and cases contributed by his fellow physicians, with careful citation of appropriate medical literature to justify diagnosis and treatment. Volume 2 deals with consumption—its prevention, diagnosis, and treatment—with several excerpts from the contemporary literature.

Barker saw himself as a "scientific physician" in the late-eighteenth-century mode, a practitioner who was a careful observer and communicator of contemporary medical practice. He read and contributed to the first US medical journals, reporting on various diseases and epidemics seen in the District of Maine, and he encouraged other Maine physicians to do likewise. From the rural backwater of early Maine, he described how he handled difficult clinical situations by obtaining medical books and journals, by corresponding with learned colleagues, and by making "postgraduate" educational trips to meet and discuss medicine with other New England physicians.

My Introduction in five chapters begins with a description of Dr. Jeremiah Barker—his background, education, and writings.[2] Chapter 2 is a discussion of medicine, medical practice, and the difficulty of obtaining medical literature during the fifty years leading up to Maine Statehood in 1820. Chapter 3 describes the target audience for the manuscript as well as thoughts on why he wrote it and why it was not published. Chapter 4 considers Barker as an "innovator" interested in the new chemistry and willing to risk the scorn associated with his use of alkaline remedies in fevers. Chapter 5 offers some suggestions to help the twenty-first-century reader critically evaluate Barker's medical knowledge, therapy, and reasoning while avoiding the introduction of present-day ideas and perspectives into a two-hundred-year-old document.

Following the Introduction, Barker's manuscript is presented in its entirety with all his citations checked and annotated, adding terminology and context as well as a glossary to make the manuscript accessible to general readers today, or in Barker's own words, to "*be intelligible to those who are destitute of Medical Science.*" The manuscript opens up an extremely interesting window on American medical history, of health, diet, and disease in the Early Republic with a surprising flow and penetration of advanced ideas to a place

Furdell, *Publishing and Medicine in Early Modern England* (Rochester, NY: University of Rochester Press; Woodbridge: Boydell & Brewer, 2002), 120–21.

[2] Richard Kahn, "Barker, Jeremiah (1752–1835), Physician," in *American National Biography*, ed. John A. Garraty and Mark C. Carnes (Oxford University Press for the American Council of Learned Societies, 1999), 158–59.

like the District of Maine, far removed from urban intellectual centers. It will be published as Maine celebrates the Bicentennial of statehood in 2020, having separated from Massachusetts in 1820 as part of the resolution of the Missouri crisis.[3]

Imagine my excitement upon seeing this manuscript thirty years ago. I could not identify a comparable work from a rural practitioner two hundred years ago, much less one that focused on consulting and adding to the medical literature, noting changes in medical philosophy and communicating with colleagues near and far, with specific attention on diagnosis, treatment, outcomes, and dissections. The manuscript struck me as unique, and I quickly obtained permission from the Maine Historical Society to work on it with a view to getting it published.

I doubt they thought it would take me thirty years to do it—in the midst of my own busy medical practice—but finally after my retirement I've been able to finish the project. I've researched, presented, and discussed Barker's manuscript with medical historians, my patients, my friends and family, and anyone else who would listen. Barker's practice took place from 1772 to 1818, exactly two hundred years before my own from 1972 to 2018, and I share his interest in "the production, circulation, and consumption of medical knowledge," as well as the instability of that knowledge.[4] What are the similarities and differences with medicine and care as practiced today? How did the physician and patient handle uncertainty—a constant factor in medicine—and how did they negotiate therapeutic choices and decisions? When did medical philosophy and theories change?

And why should anyone be interested in medical history at all? We are all recipients of health care and should have some understanding of the knowledge base, reasoning, and practice of medicine. The study of medical history gives us insights into the causes and changing burdens of disease over decades and centuries. We learn nuanced ways to consider apparent efficacy; that is, why did patients and healthcare providers think a treatment worked? Quoting an 1870 textbook, historian George Rosen observed that medical

[3] The Missouri Compromise admitted Maine as a free state and Missouri as a slave state, thus maintaining the balance of power in Congress between northern and southern states. For more about this, see Charles E. Clark, *Maine: A Bicentennial History*, The States and the Nation Series (New York: Norton, 1977), 79–82; Ronald Banks, *Maine Becomes a State* (Middletown, CT: Wesleyan University Press, 1970).

[4] R. Aronowitz and J. A. Greene, "Contingent Knowledge and Looping Effects—a 66-Year-Old Man with PSA-Detected Prostate Cancer and Regrets," *New England Journal of Medicine* 381, no. 12 (2019): 1093–96.

history is "so commendable for the useful examples that it offers us, and even more instructive, perhaps, because of the errors that it teaches us to avoid than the precepts that it transmits."[5] It teaches us which methods have been useful in the past and which have led us astray, even those of the best minds of the period. This promotes intellectual modesty and tolerance that serve us well.[6] Thus we may conclude that a better understanding of medical history can help offer health care providers and the public "perspective, [and] humility, where overconfidence frequently exists, as well as openness to change,"[7] while remembering George Santayana's words: "Skepticism is the chastity of the intellect, and it is shameful to surrender it too soon or to the first comer."[8]

In a sense Jeremiah Barker's manuscript "offers to do for the scientific model of medicine what Martha Ballard's diary, in the reading of Laurel Ulrich, did for the folk model: give it a new, complex reality."[9] Of the estimated 3,500 medical practitioners in America in 1775, "all but a few hundred are names only; of that small number fewer than 50 are usually cited in any description of the profession in the eighteenth century."[10] This unusual two-hundred-year-old primary source documenting the life and practice of a rural New England physician will be of interest to academic historians of medicine, but also to an array of students and teachers, genealogists, physicians, and general readers. The dilemma is that the notes and commentary must speak to all of these readers. Something new and fascinating to the general reader may be painfully obvious to the historian. My hope is that all will enjoy this work for what it is, and that the scholar will use it to build on our understanding of medicine in the late eighteenth and early nineteenth century.

Richard J. Kahn, MD, MACP, April 2020

[5] G. Rosen, "The Place of History in Medical Education," *Bulletin of the History of Medicine* 22 (1948): 596.

[6] Frank Huisman and John Harley Warner, eds., *Locating Medical History: The Stories and Their Meanings* (Baltimore: Johns Hopkins University Press, 2004), 6.

[7] Paraphrasing D. S. Jones et al., "Making the Case for History in Medical Education," *Journal of the History of Medicine and Allied Sciences* (2014): 631, 633.

[8] George Santayana, *Scepticism and Animal Faith: Introduction to a System of Philosophy* (New York: C. Scribner's Sons, 1929), 69–70.

[9] Personal communication with Richard D'Abate, former executive director of the Maine Historical Society, January 20, 2004. Rather than "folk medicine," Ulrich might prefer the term "popular" or "social medicine." Laurel Thatcher Ulrich, *A Midwife's Tale: The Life of Martha Ballard, Based on Her Diary, 1785–1812* (Alfred A. Knopf, 1990), 61.

[10] Joseph M. Toner, *Contributions to the Annals of Medical Progress and Medical Education in the United States before and during the War of Independence* (Washington, DC: Government Printing Office, 1874), 105, 106; Whitfield J. Bell, *The Colonial Physician and Other Essays* (New York: Science History Publications, 1975), 6.

Acknowledgments

I THANK MY wife, Patricia Gamble Kahn, MS, for transcribing the Barker manuscript and for working with me on this project over the past thirty years. Thanks also to Ramona Connolly for transcription help with volume 1, chapter 1. The Maine Historical Society provided access to the document and continued support and encouragement, and I thank the staff past and present for their invaluable help: Glen Skillin, Richard D'Abate, Nicholas Noyes, Stephen Seames, William David Barry, Jamie Kingman Rice, and Steve Bromage. I could not have completed this book without years of willing assistance by Jack Eckert, Librarian at Harvard's Countway Library. Access to the libraries at Pen Bay Medical Center, Tufts University, and Maine Medical Center has helped immeasurably over the years. I'm also grateful for the comments and suggestions given me at my presentations to the following societies: American Association for the History of Medicine, American Osler Society, Wood Institute for the History of Medicine of the College of Physicians of Philadelphia, Colloquium on the History of Psychiatry and Medicine, Countway Library of Medicine, Harvard Medical School, Maine Medical Center, Maine Medical Association, and the Baxter Society of Maine. And special thanks for reviews by Jacalyn Duffin, John Harley Warner, Jeremy Greene, Scott Podolsky, Mindy Schwartz, Tom Frank, Liam Riordan, Kathleen Graf, Wendy Carr, Michael Stanley, and Suzanne Hamlin. Thanks also to Gregory Higby for his review of the definitions of medications in the glossary. I am grateful for the subvention provided by Maine Medical Association, Maine Medical Center, and several anonymous donors. Many thanks to Craig Panner, Editor in Chief, Oxford University Press, who has been supportive and helpful from the proposal of this book to its completion. Any errors, of course, are my own.

CHAPTER 1

Jeremiah Barker: Background, Education, and Writings

If the coldness of our climate, is any measure owing to our country being covered with thick and heavy forests. . . . We do not wish to part with the blessings we enjoy. . . . The people of the District of Maine, may, in a tedious winter, long for the soft breezes of Virginia and the Carolinas; but they would be very unwilling to take the fever and ague, and the other disorders incident to those States, with the gentle weather, in exchange for our northern snow banks. (James Sullivan, 1795)[1]

My present seat of residence is that part of Falmouth, called Stroudwater, two miles from Portland, where I spend the great part of my time in reading the literary productions of Medical men and scriving and correcting my medical observations, over the course of 35 years. The rest of my time is chiefly employed in the practice of physic. . . . Thus, I had opportunities of observing the habits, customs and manner of living among the first settlers of this part of the state [c1780]; for many of the interior towns were thinly inhabited at that time; Indeed some were unsettled. In many towns I noted these things, as well as medical occurrences, always carrying pen, ink, and paper; so that I have collected considerable historical facts in this way, which I think may be useful to my successors in Maine at least. . . . The first white inhabitants of Maine, being chiefly poor and illiterate, lived and conducted, for a time,

---

[1] James Sullivan (1744–1808), born in Berwick, Maine, and governor of Massachusetts from 1807 to 1808, points out that it was well known that geographical location, climate, and weather altered the frequency and nature of diseases and epidemics. James Sullivan, *The History of the District of Maine* (Boston: Printed by I. Thomas and E.T. Andrews, 1795), 8.

*in a very similar manner as the Indians did. Their exercise was great, their
food simple and wholesome, consisting chiefly of Indian corn and salted
pork, sometimes Bear. Rum could be procured only in small quantities; and
happy would it have been for them and their posterity had this continued
to be the case. . . . Of late years [c. 1806] neat cattle[2] have been reared in
abundance, and lavishly eaten in the interior towns. Rum too is conveyed
into the country towns, as it were, through aqueducts; but none is lost for
want of throats.[3]*

We learn a lot about Jeremiah Barker from this letter, written in 1806 to
Philadelphia's Benjamin Rush, elite physician, scientist, and signer of the
Declaration of Independence. From a small community in Maine, Barker
communicated with one of the "greats" in medicine of his era. He wrote
constantly and was determined to inform other physicians and contribute
to medical knowledge. He was a thoughtful observer of human nature, concerned with the conditions, habits, and foibles of the people in his community.
And he wrote in a lively and engaging manner.

Barker's manuscript is not simply a daybook of cases or a ledger keeping
track of fees and payment. Rather, it is a fifty-year record of reflections on
problems, diagnoses, treatments, and outcomes with an unusual effort to consult and cite the contemporary medical literature and other physicians in a
changing medical landscape. Together with his case books, correspondence,
and published articles, it presents a remarkable record of medicine as practiced in northern New England in Barker's time.

WHO WAS JEREMIAH BARKER?

Jeremiah Barker had deep roots in what is now Plymouth County,
Massachusetts, which extends seventy miles south from Boston along the
coast from Hingham to Sandwich, at the base of Cape Cod. The town of

---

[2] "Neat cattle" refers to domestic cattle. For more on the importance of domesticated
cattle in early New England as a source of food, tilling the soil, furnishing manure,
and harvesting wood for shipbuilding, see Virginia DeJohn Anderson, *Creatures of
Empire: How Domestic Animals Transformed Early America* (New York: Oxford University
Press, 2004), 141–71, 243–46.

[3] Jeremiah Barker, "Letter from Jeremiah Barker in Falmouth, Maine to Benjamin
Rush in Philadelphia, 22 September 1806," Historical Society of Pennsylvania, Rush
Manuscripts, 1806, vol. 2, 28.

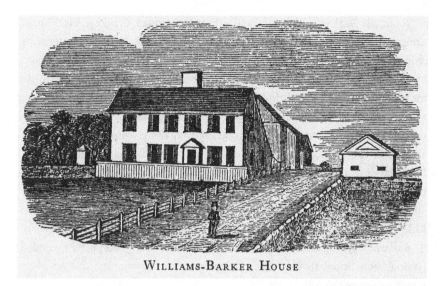

WILLIAMS-BARKER HOUSE

FIGURE 1.1. **Barker's birthplace, Scituate, Massachusetts.** The image is from the book *Old Scituate*, published by the Chief Justice Cushing Chapter, Daughters of the American Revolution, 1921. 2nd edition 1970, page 84. Courtesy of the Scituate Historical Society.

Plymouth (Plimouth or Plimoth), site of the colony founded in 1620 by the *Mayflower* Pilgrims, is where, in 1632, Jeremiah Barker's ancestor John Barker, Esq., married Anna, daughter of John Williams Sr. of Scituate. They settled in Kingston on the Jones River, named for *Mayflower* captain, Christopher Jones. In 1641 John Barker purchased the Jones River ferry, where he drowned in 1652. One of their children, also John Barker (1650–1729), moved around Plymouth County from Barnstable to Marshfield and finally to Scituate, where he married Desire Annable in 1677. Their son, Samuel Williams Barker (1686–1754), Jeremiah's grandfather, inherited what became known as the Barker Homestead and two hundred acres overlooking Scituate harbor.[4] In 1706 Samuel married Hannah Cushing of Scituate. Their third child, Capt. Samuel Barker (1707–1782), farmer, married Patience (Howland) Barker (1716–1802) of Bristol, Rhode Island in 1739.[5] On March 31, 1752, their son Jeremiah was born in Scituate. (See Figure 1.1.)

[4] Samuel Deane, *History of Scituate, Massachusetts, from Its First Settlement to 1831* (Boston: J. Loring, 1831), 216–17; Barker Newhall, *The Barker Family of Plymouth Colony and County* (Cleveland: F.W. Roberts, 1900), 75–80; Elizabeth Frye Barker, *Barker Genealogy* (New York: Frye Publishing Company, 1927), 231–41.

[5] Deane, *History of Scituate, Massachusetts*, 216–17; Newhall, *The Barker Family*, 75–81; James Alfred Spalding, *Jeremiah Barker, M.D., Gorham and Falmouth, Maine, 1752–1835* (Portland, ME: s.n., 1909), 1–2, 23–24.

Jeremiah Barker had a classical education under the Rev. Mr. Cutter, Congregational minister of Scituate, and served a medical apprenticeship from 1769 to 1772 under Dr. Bela Lincoln (1733/4–1774) of Hingham, Massachusetts. Preceptorship, or apprenticeship, was in Barker's time the most common form of training for American physicians who had any training at all, bearing in mind that one could simply hang out a shingle and declare oneself a physician, and also remembering that there were only two medical schools in the colonies at that time, neither of which was in New England.[6] Fortunately for Barker, Bela Lincoln had the best possible medical education. He was a 1754 graduate of Harvard College who then had a preceptorship under Ezekiel Hersey followed by training in London hospitals and an M.D. from King's College, Aberdeen, in 1765.[7] (See Figure 1.2.)

Barker began practice in Maine shortly after his preceptorship ended, having been asked to help with an epidemic in Newcastle, Maine,[8] about which he wrote the following:

[6] These two schools were the Medical Department of the University of Pennsylvania, which graduated its first student in 1768, and New York's Medical Department of Kings College (renamed Columbia University after the Revolutionary War) in 1769.

[7] King's College, Aberdeen, had a chair of medicine established in 1700. Hamilton points out that many established Scottish medical men requested a degree of M.D. later in life and that one could be obtained for a fee of £10 and one or two "testimonials to the doctor's skill from other practitioners." David Hamilton, *The Healers: A History of Medicine in Scotland* (Edinburgh: Canongate, 1981), 28–29, 53–54, 142–44. In 1860, the Marischal and King's Colleges merged to form the University of Aberdeen. "Bela Lincoln," in Clifford K. Shipton, *Biographical Sketches of Those Who Attended Harvard College in the Classes 1751–1755; Sibley's Harvard Graduates*, vol. 13 (Boston: Massachusetts Historical Society, 1965), 455–57. "Ezekiel Hersey," in Clifford K. Shipton, *Biographical Sketches of Those Who Attended Harvard College in the Classes 1726–30; Sibley's Harvard Graduates*, vol. 8 (Boston: Massachusetts Historical Society, 1951), 432–36. Bela Lincoln was a student of Dr. Ezekiel Hersey (1709–1770), whose bequest, with that of his brother Abner Hersey, would establish Harvard Medical School's professorship of anatomy and physic.

[8] It is a shortcut to refer to "Newcastle, Maine," in 1772, when Maine was still part of Massachusetts. The trouble brewing in seventeenth-century Britain between the Royalists and Puritans broke out in civil war in 1642. The various battles playing out in Maine and Massachusetts were finally resolved in 1691, when a new charter by William and Mary granted Massachusetts control of what is now Maine. All the land from New Brunswick, Canada, to Rhode Island, except for a small segment of New Hampshire that protruded to the sea, was under the control of Massachusetts. The 1755 map of "The Most Inhabited Part of New England" by Thomas Jefferys labels what is now Maine as the "Eastern Part of Massachusetts." Thus, as historian Ronald Banks stresses, "from 1691 to 1820 there was no political entity known as Maine . . . [though it was designated] the 'District of Maine of Massachusetts in 1778' [until Statehood in 1820]." Ronald Banks, *Maine Becomes a State* (Middletown, CT: Wesleyan University Press, 1970), 4. For a review of Maine history 1623–1820, see William David Barry,

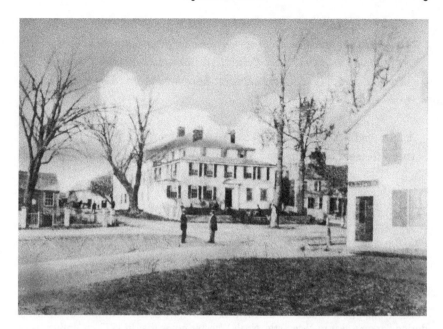

FIGURE 1.2. **Home of Bela Lincoln in Hingham, site of Barker's preceptorship.** Lincoln's house in Hingham, Massachusetts, is where Barker completed his preceptorship from 1769 to 1772. Courtesy of the Hingham Historical Society.

I repaired to the County of Lincoln, by invitation, on account of a malignant fever which appeared in Newcastle in the summer of 1772.—I tarried one year and had considerable practice. This fever evidently arose from tainted meat and damaged corn, brought into that town from Carolina.— It was confined to those families where these provisions were used.—It began in July and subsided in December.—Several Swine were invaded with disease, after being fed with this corn, and the offals of sick rooms.— They vomited, lost flesh, staggered as tho intoxicated, and died in about a week. In people, the fever generally terminated favorably or unfavorably in 9 or 10 days.—It was highly inflammatory in onset; a sense of heat in the stomach, oppression of the precordia, great pain in the head and thirst; pulse quick and hard, were the usual symptoms. A German physician, Dr. Shepard, had the chief of the practice. He employed the lancet successfully, and taught me the method of using the spring lancet [an instrument for bloodletting, venesection], which he preferred. One patient, a laboring man, died on the 9th day, and was covered with petechia after death. He was not bled. He died two days before I arrived at Newcastle. The efficacy of mercury in fevers was not well understood at that time, among us; so that very little was used.—The Bark was given in some cases,

*in the (remissions) of the fever; but it was found to be injurious, V.S. [ven-
esection] and common evacuants were the chief means employed and when
(reasonable) assistance was offered the disease generally ended favorably.
In no instance did the disease appear to be communicated from one person
to another.*[9]

Barker had hoped to practice in Gorham, Maine,[10] but, "finding the rumor
of the retirement of Dr. Stephen Swett,[11] of that place, premature, he returned

---

Maine: The Wilder Half of New England, 1st ed. (Gardiner, ME: Tilbury House, 2012),
17–78; Richard William Judd, Edwin A. Churchill, and Joel W. Eastman, *Maine: The
Pine Tree State from Prehistory to the Present*, 1st ed. (Orono: University of Maine
Press, 1995), 12–192; Charles E. Clark, *Maine: A Bicentennial History*, The States and
the Nation Series (New York: Norton, 1977), 1–90; James Sullivan, *The History of the
District of Maine* (Boston: Printed by I. Thomas and E.T. Andrews, 1795).

[9] Barker, "Letter from Jeremiah Barker in Falmouth, Maine to Benjamin Rush in
Philadelphia, 22 September 1806." There may also have been an outbreak of influenza
during Barker's year in Newcastle. Noah Webster notes that in 1772 an "Influenza or
Epidemic Catarrh" epidemic occurred in America "after an eruption of Vesuvius and
Heckla [a volcano in Southern Iceland], and a severe winter." Noah Webster, *A Brief
History of Epidemic and Pestilential Diseases with the Principal Phenomena of the Physical
World Which Precede and Accompany Them and Observations Deduced from Facts Stated*,
2 vols. (Hartford: Hudson and Goodwin, 1799), vol. 2, 32.

[10] The Gorhams were a prominent Massachusetts family, and Barker probably
benefited from his association with them. Nathanial Gorham (1738–1796), for ex-
ample, was a politician and merchant who was a delegate from Massachusetts to the
Continental Congress and presided over that body for six months. He also attended the
Constitutional Convention in Philadelphia and was a signer of the Constitution in 1787.
The town of Gorham, earlier Gorhamtown, was named after a relative, Captain John
Gorham, who had served in King Philip's War, 1675–1678. This refers to Metacomet, a
native American chief who adopted the name King Philip. The conflict, also known as
the Great Narragansett War, was a struggle between native Americans of New England
and the colonists. For details, see Jill Lepore, *The Name of War: King Philip's War and the
Origins of American Identity*, 1st ed. (New York: Knopf, 1998). Soldiers who took part in
this war were rewarded with land grants in New Hampshire and what would become the
District of Maine. These land grants were all thirty acres and were originally numbered;
Narragansett Number 7 was granted to Captain Gorham's company. Thus the Gorham
family owned land in the town from the first half of the eighteenth century. Hugh D. Mc
Lellan, *History of Gorham, Maine* (Portland: Smith and Sale, 1903), 516–23; a map of
Narragansett Number 7 is tipped in just before the Index; Donald G. Trayser, *Barnstable;
Three Centuries of a Cape Cod Town* (Hyannis, MA: F.B. & F.P. Goss, 1939), 118–19.

[11] Dr. Stephen Swett was born in Exeter, New Hampshire, in 1733 and moved to
Gorham, District of Maine, in 1770 with his wife and seven children. He was the town's
first physician, arriving six years after its incorporation; population 340. He served
as a surgeon in Colonel Phinney's 31st regiment, having enlisted May 7, 1775, and
discharged December 31, 1775. Swett practiced in Gorham for several more years, and
moved to Windham and later Otisfield, Maine, where he died in 1807. See Mc Lellan,
History of Gorham, Maine, 1903, 281, 339.

in the following year moving to Barnstable, Massachusetts."[12] He practiced
in Barnstable from 1773 to 1779 and, on October 12, 1775,[13] married Abigail
Gorham of Barnstable, daughter of Colonel David and Abigail (Sturgis) Gorham
and sister of Judge William Gorham. Their first child, Jeremiah Cushing
Gorham (born November 1, 1776, died at sea December 19, 1810), was born in
Barnstable. In 1779 Barker returned to Maine as part of the ill-fated Penobscot
Expedition,[14] about which he wrote the following: "Having been Surgeon to a
Ship in the memorable Penobscot expedition, I have saved a good assortment
of medicine from the flames of our Ships. This gave me some advantage, as
medicine was scarce and I soon commanded an extensive range of practice into
all the towns of the county, and into some of the adjacent counties."[15]

In 1780 he wrote, "Finding the air on Cape Cod injurious to my constitution and physicians being numerous, I removed to Gorham, Maine,"[16] a decision that was probably influenced by his wife and her brother, Judge William
Gorham. The Barkers built a large two-story house on an acre of land next
door to Judge Gorham.[17] There he practiced medicine from 1780 to 1789,

[12] James Alfred Spalding, "After Consulting Hours: Jeremiah Barker, M.D., Gorham
and Falmouth, Maine, 1752–1835," *Bulletin of the American Academy of Medicine* 10
(1909): 243. Spalding points out, "it was considered the height of impoliteness to settle
near" an established physician in a small town, thus dividing the business.

[13] Ninety miles away, in Concord and Lexington, the first battles of the Revolutionary
War had taken place in April 1775.

[14] Briefly, in June 1779 the British occupied Bagaduce (now Castine), causing
Massachusetts to send forty-five ships and fifteen hundred soldiers to Bagaduce
under the leadership of Commodore Dudley Saltonstall, General Solomon Lovell,
and commander-of-artillery Paul Revere. They delayed long enough that in August, a
British squadron came up the Penobscot River, driving the American fleet and men up
the river and destroying most of the fleet. It was an American naval disaster that led
historian William David Barry to call it "the worst American naval defeat until Pearl
Harbor." Judd, Churchill, and Eastman, *Maine: The Pine Tree State*, 156–59. Also Barry,
Maine: The Wilder Half, 51–53; James S. Leamon, *Revolution Downeast: The War for
American Independence in Maine* (Amherst: University of Massachusetts Press, 1993),
70–73; William Willis, *The History of Portland*, facsimile ed. 1972, (Somersworth: New
Hampshire Publishing Company and Maine Historical Society; Portland: Bailely &
Noyes, 1865), 516–22.

[15] Barker, "Letter from Jeremiah Barker in Falmouth, Maine to Benjamin Rush in
Philadelphia, 22 September 1806."

[16] Jeremiah Barker, "A History of Diseases in the District of Maine Commencing in
1735 and Continuing to the Present Time. . . . To This Is Annexed an Inquiry into the
Causes, Nature, Increasing Prevalency, and Treatment of Consumption," in *Jeremiah
Barker, Collection 13* (Portland: Maine Historical Society 1831), vol. 1, chap. 2, 2.

[17] To be more specific, the Barkers owned "an acre of land in the south corner of the
thirty acre lot, No. 112, on the north side of the Portland Road." Mc Lellan, *History of*

when, while Barker and his wife were visiting the Gorhams next door, their house "took fire and was consumed." Barker was alleged to have remarked to his wife, while the house was burning, "the money they had saved in the war was *going up* pretty fast." Undaunted, they immediately rebuilt the house around the old chimney.[18] (See Figure 1.3.)

Barker and his wife Abigail had four more children, all born in Gorham: Polly Gorham (born August 19, 1780; died August 30, 1780); Mary Gorham (born August 20, 1781; married in Stroudwater October 13, 1800, Daniel Johnson of Portland; died 1855); David Gorham (born March 7, 1784; married Deborah Josslyn of Pembroke, Maine; practiced medicine in Durham and Sedgwick; died April 15, 1830); and Elizabeth (born January 29, 1787; married Rev. Daniel A. Clark June 18, 1812; died July 1, 1864).

Abigail Barker died on June 29, 1790, and Barker married his second wife, Susanna Garrett of Barnstable (b. 1769), on December 17, 1790. Evidently at that time, the town of Gorham was not growing as anticipated, and in about 1792 the Barkers moved to Stroudwater, now a section of Portland (called Falmouth until 1786). The British had bombarded and burned Falmouth to the ground in the fall of 1775, but it was recovering, and by 1790 was Maine's largest settlement, with a population of 2,240, according to the 1790 US Census Report. Barker and Susanna had one daughter, Abigail, born July 1, 1793, who married John Johnson of Providence, Rhode Island, May 19, 1817.[19]

Barker's wife Susanna died on June 3, 1794, and in 1795 he married his third wife, Eunice Riggs of Capisic, part of Gorham, born in 1770. In 1799 he bought property in Stroudwater and built a foursquare, hip-roofed house with an ell[20]

Gorham, Maine, 396–98. But according to the Cumberland County Registry of Deeds, Barker bought almost nineteen acres of Lot 112 between July 18, 1780, and November 22, 1781. He sold the land and buildings to William Gorham, his brother-in-law, in 1786. Between 1780 and 1810 Barker bought six and sold eight parcels of land and buildings in Gorham and Stroudwater. (Thanks to S. T. Seames, then at the Maine Historical Society, for delving into the deeds.)

[18] Mc Lellan, *History of Gorham, Maine*, for moving the house, 397, and fire, 315. The Barker's house was sold in about 1792, moved "across the fields to the crossroads" and destroyed by fire in December 1889.

[19] Spalding, *Jeremiah Barker*, 24.

[20] An "ell" is an extension at right angles to the length of a building, creating an L-shaped outline. This term was first used in the 1770s.

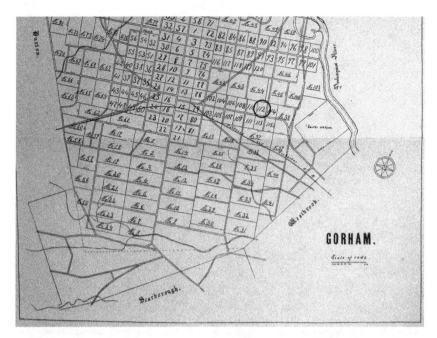

FIGURE 1.3. **Map of Barker's homesite in Gorham.** From the Land Grant—Grantees of Narragansett No.7—Gorham, Maine. Jeremiah Barker bought a one-acre lot on the south corner of Lot 112, on the North side of the Portland Road. The lot was probably purchased from John Goodspeed (or descendants) from Barnstable. The town of Gorham was born out of the Narragansett War, one of the seven townships granted by the General Court of Massachusetts to 840 people who either fought or were descendants of or closely allied to those who had fought. The Narragansett War was also called King Philip's War after the Wampanoag chief Metacom, later known as King Philip. McLellan explains "that a proclamation was made to the army in the name of the government, before they began their march against King Philip, that if they would . . . take the fort and drive the enemy out of the Narragansett country, they should have a gratuity of land besides their wages." All of the original lots granted were thirty acres in size. Barker's house was moved after he sold it, and it burned in 1889. No image of the house has been found. From McLellan, Hugh D. *History of Gorham, Me.* Portland: Smith and Sale, 1903.

and outbuildings, still standing, now called the Jeremiah Barker House.[21] (See Figure 1.4.)

Eunice Barker died on November 10, 1799, aged twenty-nine, and this time Barker did not remarry until 1802, when, on July 11, 1802, he published

[21] Also called the Barker/Hunt house. Barker would move back to Gorham in 1808 after marrying Judge Gorham's widow, Temperance. Dr. Jacob Hunt had been practicing in Stroudwater for six or seven years when, on June 25, 1815, he bought Barker's house for $1,000. M. K. Lovejoy, E. G. Shettleworth, and W. D. Barry, *This Was Stroudwater: 1727–1860* (National Society of Colonial Dames of America in the State of Maine, 1985), 199–200, and "Dr. Jeremiah Barker, a Man Who Had Five Wives," *The Deering News,* Saturday, April 23, 1898.

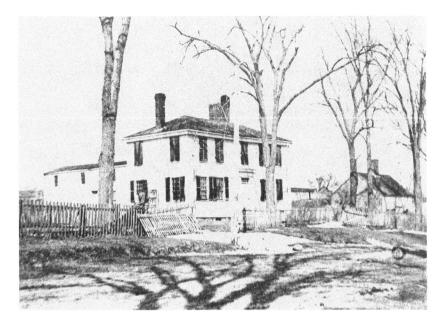

FIGURE 1.4. The Jeremiah Barker House in Stroudwater. Barker's house in Stroudwater, Maine was built in 1799. This image is from the early twentieth century. Courtesy of the Maine Historical Society.

to marry Mary Williams of Gorham. According to some records, they were married on July 11, 1802; the date of her death is unknown. At least three of Barker's wives died of consumption, and the progression of their illnesses is documented in his manuscript.

On November 17, 1808, Barker married his fifth and final wife, Temperance Garrett Gorham, widow of Judge William Gorham of Gorham, his first wife's brother. They moved back to the town of Gorham, where he practiced until 1818 and then, after retirement, continued work on his manuscript until at least 1830. He died on October 4, 1835, aged eighty-two, and his wife, Temperance, died in 1840.[22] The following maps of 1780 shows Barker's residences from birth to death; Boston is also marked. (See Figures 1.5, 1.6, and 1.7.)

[22] The genealogical data is derived from several sources that differ somewhat from each other. Newhall, *The Barker Family*, 80–81; Barker, *Barker Genealogy*, 240–41; Mc Lellan, *History of Gorham, Maine*, 396–98; Spalding, *Jeremiah Barker*, 23–24.

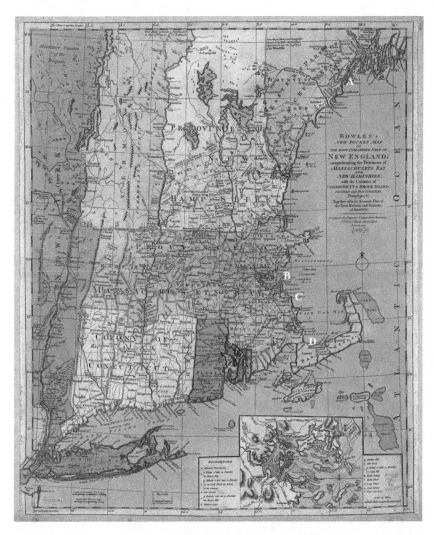

FIGURE 1.5. Bowles New Pocket Map of New England, 1780. "A" is Gorhamtown/ Falmouth (Portland), Maine; "B" is Boston, Massachusetts; "C" is Hingham & Scituate, Massachusetts; "D" is Barnstable, Massachusetts. Note that Maine is named the "Eastern Part of Massachusetts." It was not renamed "District of Maine of Massachusetts" until 1778, and this map has the earlier designation. Bowles, Carington. *Bowles's new pocket map of the most inhabited part of New England; comprehending the provinces of Massachusetts Bay and New Hampshire; with the colonies of Connecticut & Rhode Island; divided into their counties, townships, &c. together with an accurate plan of the town, harbour and environs of Boston.* [London], [1780]. Copy examined: https://www.loc.gov/item/74692147/. Thanks to Library of Congress, Geography and Map Division and Matthew Edney at the Osher Map Library in Portland, Maine, for help determining the variant of the map shown here.

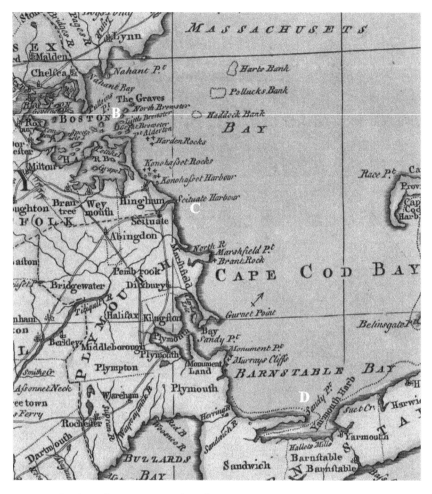

FIGURE 1.6. Massachusetts insert of Bowles Map shown in Figure 1.5.

PROVENANCE OF THE BARKER MANUSCRIPT

In 1909, Maine medical historian James Alfred Spalding (1846–1938), aware of Dr. Jeremiah Barker's published medical journal articles as well as his newspaper articles and advertisements, wrote that Barker had retired from practice in 1818 and devoted the rest of his life to studying and planning his *"History of Medicine and Epidemics in Maine from 1772–1819."*[23] According to Spalding,

---

[23] Here Spalding is referring to Barker's manuscript, the title of which is "*A History of Diseases in the District of Maine Commencing in 1772 and Continued to the Present Time . . . .*" Never having seen it, Spalding did not know its correct title. Barker's previously unpublished book appears at the end of these introductory chapters and is herein referred to as "the manuscript" or "Barker's manuscript."

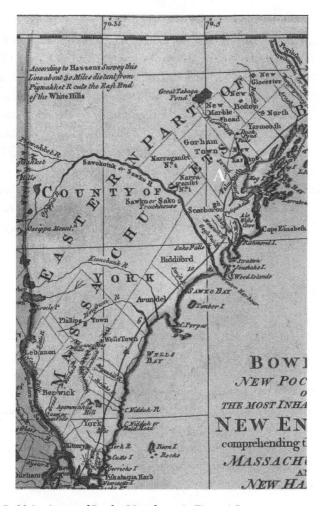

FIGURE 1.7. Maine insert of Bowles Map shown in Figure 1.5.

"This was to include personal cases as well as those handed in by friends and biographical notices of the physicians he has known. No copy of his work or even M.S.S. has ever been found and we must regret its disappearance for possessing excellent literary style, having seen so many patients, and having enjoyed so broad an acquaintance he was surely to have published a readable book. . . . [Barker was] a good old-fashioned general practitioner, and the pioneer medical writer of Maine."[24] Four years after Spalding's death in 1938, the "lost" manuscript was returned to Maine by Barker's great-grandson.

[24] Spalding, "After Consulting Hours," 260. Spalding also wrote, "No portrait of him [Barker] is extant, but an old citizen informs me that he was of medium height, firm of feature and clean shaven."

The provenance of the Barker manuscript appears to be clear: after Jeremiah Barker's death in 1835, his papers passed to his daughter Eliza and her husband, the Rev. Daniel Abraham Clark (1779–1840), an 1808 graduate of Princeton College. Their son, James Henry Clark, M.D. (1814–1869), graduated from Columbia Physicians and Surgeons in 1841 and settled in Newark, New Jersey.[25] Barker's papers then passed to his son, James Henry Clark Jr., M.D. (1856–1945), who, after Williams College, graduated from Columbia Physicians and Surgeons in 1881 and practiced in Newark, where he was police surgeon for thirty-four years. He donated the Barker collection to the Maine Historical Society on March 20, 1942, "through the interest of Hon. Percival P. Baxter."[26] It was duly cataloged and remained in the Maine Historical Society collection for forty-eight years until it was brought to the present author's attention in 1990.

DESCRIPTION OF THE BARKER MANUSCRIPT

The full title of Jeremiah Barker's manuscript printed on the subscription paper[27] is:

> A Proposal for publishing a History of Diseases in the District of Maine, commencing 1772 to the present time, containing also some account of diseases in New-Hampshire, and other parts of New-England, with biographical sketches of learned physicians both in Europe and America as well as other promoters of medical science and to which is annexed an inquiry to the causes, natures, prevalency and treatment of consumption; which is

[25] Dr. James Henry Clark wrote three books: *A History of Cholera as It Appeared in Newark in 1849, Medical Topography of Newark and Its Vicinity*, and in 1868 *Medical Men of New Jersey in the Essex District 1666–1866*.

[26] Accession Records. MHS 1942 #2671. Percival Baxter (1876–1969) was a graduate of Bowdoin College and Harvard Law School. He served as governor of Maine from 1921 to 1925 and is best known today for his part in obtaining Mount Katahdin and what would become Baxter State Park, the beginning or end of the Appalachian Trail. Barry, *Maine: The Wilder Half*, 166, 176.

[27] The printed subscription paper constitutes the first page of volume 1 of the manuscript. MHS Col. 13 box 1. Subscription papers are taken by individuals interested in the proposed publication. The title and brief description fill the upper half of the paper; the lower half has a place for subscriber's name and number of copies desired. Subscribers could procure others and receive a free book if they achieved a certain number of additional subscribers.

maintained to be curable if proper means are seasonably and duly employed. Containing about 400 pages—price two dollars in boards.[28] *Written so as to be intelligible to those who are destitute of Medical Science: by Jeremiah Barker, Esq. F.M.M.S. (See Figure 1.8.)*

Barker's manuscript is in two volumes. The first chapter of volume 1, examining mental illness and the dangers of spirituous liquors, was separated from chapters 2 through 9, which had been sewn together. This occurred as the result of a letter to Jeremiah Barker dated November 25, 1819, and found in the Barker papers: "Sir, if your History of diseases is to present anything on the subject of Insanity, I should be gratified by the loan of that part of your M.S. which shall be returned without delay. Respectfully, George Parkman." Barker sent his chapter 1 to Dr. Parkman in Boston as requested.[29] Parkman, a supporter of the moral treatment[30] of the mentally ill, knowing of Barker's

---

[28] "In boards" is a bookbinding term that refers to the rectangular pieces of strong pasteboard used for the covers of books. A book "in boards" has these covered only in paper (usually blue or gray); if covered in cloth the book is "in cloth boards"; if covered in leather or parchment it is "bound." Books were sold in boards to keep the price down and allow the purchaser to decide whether to have the book rebound more elaborately. (Also, note that Maine did not become a state until 1820, before which it was a known as the District of Maine of Massachusetts.)

[29] Dr. George Parkman (1790–1849), the son of a wealthy Boston merchant, was an 1809 graduate of Harvard College who then obtained a medical degree from Kings College, Aberdeen. His interest in mental illness led him to Paris, where he studied under Philippe Pinel (1745–1826) and Étienne Esquirol (1772–1840), pioneers in the humane treatment of the mentally ill. In 1814 he briefly managed a small private institution for the mentally ill, and he then encouraged the trustees of the Massachusetts General Hospital to include a psychiatric facility. That facility, first known as the "Asylum for the Insane," was founded on February 25, 1811, having been granted a charter by the Massachusetts Legislature for the "Massachusetts General Hospital Corporation." The Asylum opened October 1, 1818, and followed the principles of "moral treatment," as espoused by Pinel in France and William Tuke in England. It would later be renamed McLean Hospital.

[30] Pinel, in Paris, set out to change the medical and psychological assumptions about mental illness. He believed that insanity, rather than being a demonical possession, was associated with social and psychological stresses that should be treated with kindness, reason, and humanity instead of chains, bleeding, and corporal punishment. This was a 180-degree change from earlier thoughts. See Gerald N. Grob, *The Mad among Us: A History of the Care of America's Mentally Ill* (New York; Toronto: Free Press; Maxwell Macmillan Canada, 1994), 26–31, and Roy Porter, "The Eighteenth Century," in *The Western Medical Tradition: 800 B.C.–1800 A.D*, ed. Lawrence I. Conrad and Wellcome Institute for the History of Medicine (Cambridge; New York: Cambridge University Press, 1995), 425–29.

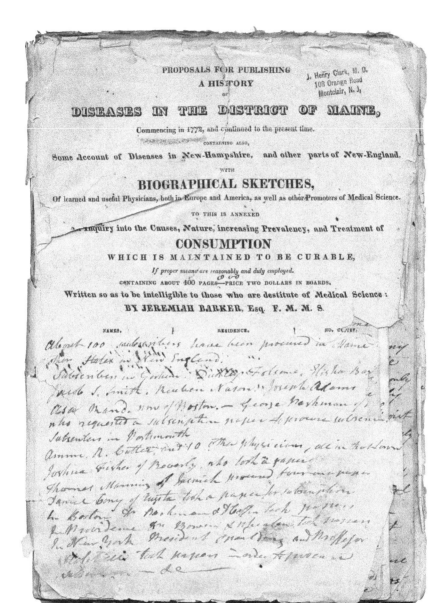

FIGURE 1.8. The subscription page that serves as the title page of Volume One. The first page of the Barker Manuscript is a supscription paper. It was bound with Chapters Two through Ten because Chapter One had been sent to George Parkman in Boston for his review, and was therefore found separate from the other chapters of Volume One. Courtesy of the Maine Historical Society.

work, requested and read the chapter, and returned it in 1819 with some of his own offprints on mental illness.[31]

The remainder of volume 1, chapters 2 to 9, consists of 146 neatly hand-written pages sewn together. In chapter 2, Barker introduced readers to Maine as he found it in 1780 and described other providers of medical care. These included the Rev. Thomas Smith, who had been minister of the First Parish Church of Falmouth (Portland) since 1727. Like other preacher-physicians, Smith tended to his parishioner's medical as well as ecclesiastical needs, re-cording occurrences of diseases and epidemics from the beginning of his ca-reer.[32] Barker was able to comment on epidemics and diseases from 1735–1780 by using Smith's diary, which was subsequently published in 1821.[33]

The remaining chapters of volume 1 are devoted to diseases such as ma-lignant fevers, pneumonia, childbed fever, apoplexy, dropsy, hydrophobia, cancer, and various epidemics. Barker noted in his manuscript, "they [the cases] will be related, in some order of time according to their occurrence, excepting consumptive cases, which will be reserved for the concluding part."[34]

Volume 2 is titled *An Inquiry into the causes, nature, increasing prevalency, and treatment of CONSUMPTION which is maintained to be curable if proper means are seasonably & duly employed*. Barker pointed out that in the late eighteenth and early nineteenth centuries several "learned & experienced physicians in North America have favoured us with truly valuable observations on Consumption,

---

[31] George Parkman, *Proposals for Establishing a Retreat for the Insane* (Boston: Printed by J. Eliot, 1814); George Parkman, *Management of Lunatics: With Illustrations of Insanity* (Boston: John Eliot, 1817); George Parkman, "Remarks on Insanity," *New England Journal of Medicine and Surgery* 7, no. 1 (1818): 117–30. The offprints are roughly sewn together with a copy of the letter dated November 25, 1819, as quoted earlier.

[32] The Reverend Thomas Smith (1702–1788) was born in Boston and graduated from Harvard College in 1720; sixteen of the twenty-one students in his class trained for the ministry. He was invited to minister to the Falmouth (Portland) settlement in 1726 and accepted the offer on January 23, 1727. Barker knew and cared for Smith and wrote in 1782, "I was consulted by him in case of sickness, and obtained much information, relative to his [Smith's] successful practice." See Barker MS pages **18** and MS **4** and **5**. Smith's diary (1720–1788) provided Barker with early Maine medical history otherwise unavailable. Reverend Smith died on May 25, 1795. For more on preacher-physicians, see Patricia A. Watson, *The Angelical Conjunction: The Preacher-Physicians of Colonial New England* (Knoxville: The University of Tennessee Press, 1991), 64–65.

[33] Samuel Freeman, *Extracts from the Journals Kept by the Reverend Thos Smith from the Year 1720 to the Year 1788, with an Appendix Containing a Variety of Other Matter Selected by Samuel Freeman* (Portland: T. Todd & Co., 1821).

[34] Barker, "Barker Manuscript," vol. 1, chap. 2, 5.

though chiefly in the middle & Southern States."[35] He wished to present his "inquiries & observations, relative to this disease, as it has appeared in the northern & eastern parts of the Union, having been pretty constantly engaged in the practice of Medicine for nearly half a century, both upon the sea coast and in the interior parts of the country."[36] Epidemics such as those of yellow fever appeared suddenly, devastated populations physically, socially, and economically, and then just as suddenly receded. But the leading known cause of death in North America during the colonial and early republic periods was consumption. Variously called consumption, phthisis, the Great White Plague, and since mid-nineteenth century, tuberculosis and TB, it behaved like a chronic disease with exacerbations and remissions.[37] Consumption was the leading known cause of death in four practices in Boston and New Hampshire in 1735–1820 at 18 percent, New York City in 1810–1815 at 25 percent, and Portland, Maine, in 1830 at 31 percent.[38]

---

[35] The principle of a generalizable, universal "specific" in therapeutics was not applicable during Barker's medical life, because treatment was specific to patient and environment, not just disease. See John Harley Warner, *The Therapeutic Perspective: Medical Practice, Knowledge, and Identity in America, 1820–85* (Cambridge, MA: Harvard University Press, 1986), 59. The preface of an English translation of a French textbook stipulates, "The Southern climate of the United States, seems to require more bold and decisive practice, than the Northern climate of Paris or London." He continues that the principles of physiology and pathology are universally applicable but the therapeutics may differ. F. J. V. Broussais and Thomas Cooper, *On Irritation and Insanity: A Work, Wherein the Relations of the Physical with the Moral Conditions of Man Are Established on the Basis of Physiological Medicine* (Columbia, SC: Printed by S. J. M'Morris, 1831), vi.

[36] Barker, "Barker Manuscript," vol. 2, MS7–8.

[37] Sheila M. Rothman, *Living in the Shadow of Death: Tuberculosis and the Social Experience of Illness in American History* (New York: BasicBooks, 1994), 13–25. Historical epidemiologists maintain that consumption accounted for "some 20 per cent of the deaths" (not including the plague years) in the London bills of mortality published in the seventeenth century. Note that the diagnosis of consumption does not necessarily equate exactly with what today is called tuberculosis. Helen Bynum, *Spitting Blood: The History of Tuberculosis* (Oxford: Oxford University Press, 2012), 40, and for an overview of phthisis or consumption from Hippocratic writings to the eighteenth century, 10–76. In 2019 "tuberculosis [still] kill[ed] more people [worldwide] than any other infection." Matthew J. Saunders and Carlton A. Evans, "Ending Tuberculosis through Prevention," *New England Journal of Medicine* 380, no. 11 (2019), 1073–74.

[38] J. Worth Estes, "Therapeutic Practice in Colonial New England," in *Medicine in Colonial Massachusetts, 1620–1820: A Conference Held 25 & 26 May 1978*, ed. Frederick S. Allis (Boston: The Colonial Society of Massachusetts, 1980), table 8, 308; J. Worth Estes, *The Changing Humors of Portsmouth: The Medical Biography of an American Town, 1623–1983* (Boston: The Francis A. Countway Library of Medicine, 1986), 7; John Duffy, *A History of Public Health in New York City 1625–1868* (New York: Russel Sage Foundation, 1968), 258; John F. Murray, "A Century of Tuberculosis," *American Journal of Respiratory and Critical Care Medicine* 169, no. 11 (2004): 203; "Deaths in Portland during the Year 1830," *Eastern Argus*, January 25, 1831, 2.

THE MEDICAL GEOGRAPHY OF THE DISTRICT OF MAINE, 1760–1830

The District of Maine was heavily forested but thinly settled by Euro-Americans, who first arrived along the southern coast and then up major river valleys. Recent scholarship suggests that Falmouth, before its destruction by the Royal Navy on October 18, 1775, had been a "boomtown" from 1760 to 1775, with a population approaching four to five thousand, of whom 44 percent of physically capable men were laborers (including transients), 16 percent craftsmen, 15 percent businessmen, 9 percent professionals, 8 percent ship and boat builders, and 8 percent master mariners (ship captains and officers). Before the Revolution, Falmouth had become extremely important to Britain through its trade of timber products, particularly the white pine necessary for the masts of His Majesty's war ships and merchant vessels.[39] Other than the merchants and professionals in the towns, most people depended on farming, livestock, and lumbering.[40] Gradually lumbering, wooden ship building, and fishing became more important sources of income.

Congregationalism was the most common religious affiliation of Falmouth in 1760,[41] but by 1775 there were at least seven hundred people who were Anglicans, or Episcopalians as they were called after the Revolution. The

[39] Charles P. M. Outwin, "Thriving and Elegant Town: Eighteenth-Century Portland as a Commercial Center," in *Creating Portland: History and Place in Northern New England*, ed. Joseph A. Conforti (Hanover, NH: University Press of New England, 2005), 20–43. See also Charles P. M. Outwin, "Thriving and Elegant, Flourishing and Populous: Falmouth in Casco Bay, 1760–1775" (University of Maine, unpublished PhD dissertation, 2009), 40–53. Outwin gathered data from numerous sources.

[40] By 1820, Cumberland county, which incorporates Portland, had 5,638 people working in agriculture, 632 in commerce, and 1,631 in manufacturing. Portland had almost twice the "relative worth or taxable property of the average individual" relative to the other towns in Maine. Moses Greenleaf, *A Survey of the State of Maine in Reference to Its Geographical Features, Statistics and Political Economy* reprint ed. (Augusta: Maine State Museum, 1970; Portland: Shirley & Hyde, 1829), 150, 456–59.

[41] By Ezra Stiles's calculations of membership in the various religious groups in New England in 1760: Congregationalists, 440,000; Baptists, 22,000; Friends, 16,000; Episcopalians, 12,600. Ezra Stiles, *A Discourse on the Christian Union: The Substance of Which Was Delivered before the Reverend Convention of the Congregational Clergy in the Colony of Rhode-Island Assembled at Bristol. April 23, 1760. By Ezra Stiles, A.M. Pastor of the Second Congregational Church in Newport. [Six Lines of Quotations]*, ed. Dan Merriam et al. (Brookfield, Massachusetts by Ebenezer and Dan Merriam, 1799), 144; James H. Cassedy, *Demography in Early America: Beginnings of the Statistical Mind, 1600–1800* (Cambridge, MA: Harvard University Press, 1969), 91–116.

Anglican affiliation tended to imply political solidarity with the British.[42] Maine historian Ronald Banks points out that following the War, newcomers arrived in Maine in large numbers with "attitudes and values which soon made the District a stronghold of Jeffersonian Democracy,"[43] that is, favoring rights of the common man and liberty over the commitment to hierarchy and social order of Federalists. He further maintains that the symbols of deference such as cloak and wig, used by the upper classes to maintain their control of local communities, soon began to disappear and "Congregational orthodoxy, an instrument of social control, eroded under the subversive influence of the Baptists and Methodists."[44]

The population was increasing and the economy improving. Most of Maine's agricultural, lumber, and fishing exports as well as travelers were transported by ship, though there were some major disruptions during Jefferson's embargo in 1807 and the War of 1812.[45] Roads were poor and there were many rivers to be crossed. The chief mode of land transportation was on horseback; even in the towns where chaises had been in use since roughly 1760, they were mainly used on Sundays or "gala days." The first accommodation stage[46] from Portland to Portsmouth, New Hampshire, began running regularly, three times a week, in 1818. Briefly there had been a line running during the War of 1812, as the British cruisers off the coast interrupted travel by sea.

---

[42] Outwin, "Thriving and Elegant," 55–56. As one moved inland and further North, the settlers tended to live without religion for a while, but gradually churches were established and by 1800 "two-thirds of mid-Maine communities had at least one church." Rather than Congregational, the new, more rural churches tended to be Calvinist Baptist, Methodist, and Freewill Baptists. Alan Taylor, *Liberty Men and Great Proprietors: The Revolutionary Settlement on the Maine Frontier, 1760–1820* (Chapel Hill: Published for the Institute of Early American History and Culture, Williamsburg, Virginia, by University of North Carolina Press, 1990), 131–53.

[43] Banks, *Maine Becomes a State*, 6.

[44] Banks, *Maine Becomes a State*, 6–7.

[45] Barry, *Maine: The Wilder Half*, 47–48, 57–78. See also Stephen J. Hornsby and Richard William Judd, "Historical Atlas of Maine" (Orono, ME: University Press of Maine, 2015), Part I plate 19 and Part II.

[46] An accommodation stage stops at nearly all of the stages on its route (OED); as late as 1840 this mode took two days from Portland to Boston with an overnight at Portsmouth, New Hampshire. One could travel by mail stage, leave Portland at 2 A.M. and, "if the roads were in good order . . . reach Boston by ten o'clock at night, with aching head and bones." Willis, *The History of Portland*, 587–92. By 1823, there was an accommodation stage leaving at 8 A.M. daily except Sunday and arriving in Boston at 5 P.M. Nathaniel G. Jewett, *The Portland Directory and Register* (Portland: Todd and Smith, 1823), 71.

Many physicians, even going back to Hippocrates, were aware of the fact that location and geography affected health and disease. Dr. Samuel Mitchill of New York City, for example, published an article on medical geography in 1798, pointing out that certain areas of England and the United States suffered "rare pestilential and febrile distempers. . . . The healthfulness of Oxfordshire [for example] is almost proverbial, and the judicious choice of King Alfred has long been commended for pitching upon so wholesome a spot as that where the beautiful city of Oxford stands, as a seat for the muses."[47] He then observed that the areas where calcareous material (limestone) prevails were generally the healthiest and that the tracts along the Atlantic from New York to Florida, especially New York and Philadelphia, were without significant calcareous earth and therefore were the sickly parts. He also noted that the "septic and other acids" of the Thames might be neutralized by the calcareous earth before reaching London, but the quality of the water there "will be, in a good degree, determined by the material furnished by the city."[48] This geography fits in with Mitchill's theory of septon and septic acids causing pestilential and febrile distempers, which is discussed in chapter 4 of this Introduction.

In 1828, Dr. James Thacher (1754–1844), a physician and historian well known to Barker for fifty years, wrote of Maine: "This district of Massachusetts, before separation [1820], possessed little claim to the merit of contributing to the improvement of medical science; a scattered settlement over an extended country affords no facilities of union and enterprise in scientific pursuits."[49] Most medical writing and authority in the Early Republic came from Europe and from the major American coastal cities further south whose climate, geography, and population density resulted in disease rates that were not comparable to those found in Maine.[50] This situation probably contributed to Barker's decision to write.

---

[47] Samuel Mitchill, "Outlines of Medical Geography," *Medical Repository* 2, no. 1 (1798): 41.

[48] Mitchill, "Outlines of Medical Geography," 43.

[49] James Thacher, *American Medical Biography: Or Memoirs of Eminent Physicians Who Have Flourished in America. To Which Is Prefixed a Succinct History of Medical Science in the United States, from the First Settlement of the Country* (Boston: Richardson & Lord and Cottons & Barnard, 1828), 45.

[50] Cassedy, *Demography in Early America, 1600–1800*, 275–77; James Roger Fleming, *Meteorology in America, 1800–1870* (Baltimore: Johns Hopkins University Press, 1990), 5–7; William Currie, *An Historical Account of the Climates and Diseases of the United States of America and of the Remedies and Methods of Treatment, Which Have Been Found Most Useful and Efficacious, Particularly in Those Diseases Which Depend on Climate and Situation*, reprint ed. (New York: Arno Press, 1972; Philadelphia: T. Dobson, 1792), Introduction 1–4, and "Accounts of Diseases Which Occur In The Several States of New-England," 1–40; Mark Harrison, *Contagion: How Commerce Has Spread Disease* (New Haven: Yale University Press, 2012), 16–20.

BARKER'S CONTRIBUTION TO THE MEDICAL LITERATURE
OF NORTHERN NEW ENGLAND

Until July 1797, the United States had produced no medical journals and
few textbooks. English books dominated the American market following the
Revolution. American printers could not keep up with the demand, nor could
they approach the quality of English books, argues John Hruschka, a historian of the American book trade.[51] The American copyright law of May 1790
protected American authors, but there was no US international copyright law
until 1891, and Americans "freely pirated English material."[52] As late as 1818,
a Boston book catalog[53] of "medical, botanical, and chemical books" lists 129
books, of which only 22, or 17 percent, were written by American authors.
However, many of the listed books were American imprints of English books,
not infrequently with an American author adding an introductory section.

   In addition to the constant difficulty in obtaining medical literature,
Barker and others like him were frustrated by the fact that much of the available literature was not necessarily appropriate to their locality. The types
and frequencies of diseases in Maine and New England, for example, clearly
differed from those of London and Paris, Virginia, and the Carolinas. As Barker
pointed out with regard to consumption, most North American authors who
were writing at all focused on the middle and southern states rather than the

---

[51] John Hruschka, *How Books Came to America: The Rise of the American Book Trade*
(University Park: The Pennsylvania State University Press, 2012), 49–60. James
N. Green, "The Rise of Book Publishing," in *An Extensive Republic: Print, Culture, and
Society in the New Nation, 1790–1840*, ed. Robert A. Gross and Mary Kelley (Chapel
Hill: Published in association with the American Antiquarian Society by the University
of North Carolina Press, 2010), 75–127; Hugh Amory, "The New England Book Trade,
1773–1790," in *The Colonial Book in the Atlantic World*, ed. Hugh Amory and David
D. Hall, A History of the Book in America (Cambridge, UK; New York; Worcester,
MA: Cambridge University Press; American Antiquarian Society, 2000).

[52] Hruschka, *How Books Came to America*, 52. The first US International copyright law
protecting foreign authors was passed in 1891. Robert A. Gross, "Introduction" to: An
Extensive Republic," in Gross and Kelley, eds., *An Extensive Republic*, 22–30.

[53] R. P. & C. Williams, "Catalogue of Medical, Botanical, and Chemical Books for Sale
by R. P. & C. Williams" (Boston: R. P. & C. Williams, 1818). The first formal cooperation among US booksellers and publishers took place in the form of book fairs in
Philadelphia in 1801 that led to "the first formal American trade bibliography" in the
United States in 1804. Green, "The Rise of Book Publishing," 91–94. For the books
on "Physic" in that 1804 catalog, see Adolph Growoll, *Book-Trade Bibliography in the
United States in the XIXth Century: To Which Is Added a Catalogue of All the Books Printed
in the United States with Prices, and Places Where Published, Annexed Published by the
Booksellers in Boston, January, 1804* (New York: Reprinted by Burt Franklin in 1939,
1898), 6–10.

northeastern ones. Thus, Barker was faced with the limitations of medical literature that did not apply to Northern New England, and his solution was to contribute to a new medical literature for his own region.

In documenting the diseases of his area, Jeremiah Barker became Maine's first medical historian. One other Northern New England state medical history was written during this period: *Sketches of Epidemic Diseases in the State of Vermont* by Joseph A. Gallup, published in 1815. The reviewer of Gallup's book, writing in the *New England Journal of Medicine and Surgery* that year, complained that "in the first period of practice . . . the writer [Gallup] imbibed a disrelish for books and laid them mostly aside."[54] Gallup's book is similar to a single author textbook of medicine about diseases rather than patients. His forty-one-page chapter on consumption, for example, includes only five patient narratives and two references to the medical literature. The Barker manuscript volume on consumption, in comparison, records at least sixty patient case histories, many from his own practice and some from other New England physicians, as well as case reports from the medical literature, citing at least forty-eight references to medical journals, books, and newspapers. Other American books devoted to diseases of particular regions include *An Account of the Weather and Diseases of South Carolina*, by Lionel Chalmers, 1776; *An Historical Account of the Climate and Diseases of the United States* by William Currie, 1792; and *Physical observations, and medical tracts and researches, on the topography and diseases of Louisiana* by Jabez W. Heustis, 1817.[55] The author is not aware of any similar treatise by a nonelite rural physician documenting a lifetime's case-based observations of life and death, healing and disease, nutrition, diagnosis and therapy in the period between 1772 and 1820.

---

[54] Joseph A. Gallup, *Sketches of Epidemic Diseases in the State of Vermont* (Boston: T. B. Wait & Sons, 1815). See also "Review. Sketches of Epidemic Diseases in the State of Vermont, from Its First Settlement to the Year 1815; with a Consideration of Their Causes, Phenomena, and Treatment. To Which Is Added, Remarks on Pulmonary Consumption. By Joseph A. Gallup, M.D. 1 Vol. 8vo. Boston, T. B. Wait & Sons, 1815," *New England Journal of Medicine and Surgery* 4 (1815): 357–72; the reviewer's comment is found on 371.

[55] George Rosen, *A History of Public Health* (Baltimore: The Johns Hopkins University Press, 1958 (1993 Edition), 154–55; Lionel Chalmers, *An Account of the Weather and Diseases of South-Carolina*, 2 vols. (London: Edward and Charles Dilly, 1776); Currie, *Historical Account of the Climates and Diseases of the United States*,1792. The two books just cited include meteorological correlations with diseases but almost no case reports or references. Jabez Wiggins Heustis, *Physical Observations, and Medical Tracts and Researches, on the Topography and Diseases of Louisiana* (New York: T. and J. Swords 1817); J. W. Heustis, "Art. II. Remark on the Endemic Diseases of Alabama," *American Journal of the Medical Sciences (1827–1924)* 2, no. 3 (1828).

Barker's manuscript has significance beyond the borders of the District of Maine because it documents the thought and practice of a physician in everyday practice, including his constant effort to use contemporary medical literature and personal communication to justify diagnosis and treatment. In 1967, medical historian Erwin Ackerknecht wrote, "the medical history we read and write today is still based mostly on the writings of elite of medical men. We are primarily students of scientific literature. Excellent as this may be, it teaches us relatively little concerning what this elite actually did, and even less, what the average physician or surgeon did."[56] And from historian Whitfield Bell: "[I]t is misleading to describe the [medical] profession in colonial America in terms of its most visible and articulate leaders."[57] Historians Eckland and Davis commented, "The relationship between British thought and American practice is even more difficult, largely because we know so little about the "average" practitioner, even "average" in the sense of being university educated but less famous, than say a founder of a medical school in Philadelphia or a signer of the Constitution. The spirit of doubt and inquiry that characterized the best of British medical thinking in both Edinburgh and London allowed the American physician to strike out on his own; it allowed the American environment and experience, as reflected in American social and intellectual practices, to mold and attenuate British and continental ideas to fit American situations."[58]

Although Barker displayed an unusually scholarly approach to medicine, demonstrated by his determined efforts to use, cite, and add to the medical literature, he may be considered an "average physician" in the sense that he had only preceptorship training, no college or medical school education, and did not practice in Boston, New York, or Philadelphia or teach at one of the

---

[56] Erwin H. Ackerknecht, "A Plea for a "Behaviorist Approach in Writing History of Medicine," *Journal of the History of Medicine Allied Sciences* 22, no. 3 (1967): 211–14. He was one of the leading medical historians at The Institute of the History of Medicine in Zurich as well as the Institute for the History of Medicine at Johns Hopkins University and the University of Wisconsin. See also John C. Burnham, *What Is Medical History?* (Cambridge, UK; Malden, MA: Polity, 2005), 28–30.

[57] Whitfield J. Bell, *The Colonial Physician and Other Essays* (New York: Science History Publications, 1975), 7.

[58] J. B. Eklund and A. B. Davis, "Some Thoughts on the Influence of British Medicine on American Medicine in the 18th Century," *Proceedings XXIII Congress of the History of Medicine* (1972). And on the French influence on American medicine, John Harley Warner, *Against the Spirit of System: The French Impulse in Nineteenth-Century American Medicine* (Princeton, NJ: Princeton University Press, 1998), 3–16.

few medical schools of the period. Until well into the nineteenth century the vast majority of American physicians with any training at all were, like Barker, trained by preceptorship, a form of apprenticeship.[59] Most medical records available from the period are account or ledger books consisting of the patient's name, "meds given" (frequently not named specifically), and fee. In 1980 J. Worth Estes studied the account books of four physicians practicing in New Hampshire and Massachusetts from 1770 to 1795. Two were Harvard graduates, one had some hospital experience, and all were preceptorship trained. "No data pertaining to clinical diagnoses were included regularly in any of the ledgers."[60] Medical historian and clinician Jacalyn Duffin records the practice of James Miles Langstaff (1825–1889), who lived near Toronto and whose practice began nearly a century after Barker was born. She had access to Langstaff's records, contacts, remuneration, diagnostics, and his library, but she writes that her book is "a 'biography' of a practice not a person" and regrets the absence of "first person narratives by Langstaff, such as letters or a personal diary."[61] The thing that distinguishes Barker from many of his medical peers is the fact that he recorded and kept interesting case histories from the beginning of his practice, as well as noting the literature, letters, and philosophy that guided his diagnosis and treatment decisions.

Barker described his patient's complaints, physical findings, therapies, outcomes, and sometimes autopsies, with frequent reference to the medical

[59] It wasn't until 1871 that Harvard Medical School dropped apprenticeship as a formal requirement for an M.D. degree. Kenneth M. Ludmerer, *Learning to Heal: The Development of American Medical Education* (New York: Basic Books, 1985), 16, 113; William G. Rothstein, *American Medical Schools and the Practice of Medicine: A History* (New York: Oxford University Press, 1987), 25–27; William G. Rothstein, *American Physicians in the Nineteenth Century; from Sects to Science* (Baltimore: Johns Hopkins University Press, 1972), 34–35, 85–87; Ronald L. Numbers, *The Education of American Physicians: Historical Essays* (Berkeley: University of California Press, 1980), 7–12, in an essay by Martin Kaufman. Barker's preceptorship took place between 1769 and 1772. The first medical schools in what is now the United States were the Medical Department of the University of Pennsylvania, which opened its doors in 1765, the Medical Department of Kings College (Columbia University after the Revolutionary War) in 1767, and the Medical Department of Harvard College in 1782. See J. S. Billings, "Literature and Institutions," in *A Century of American Medicine: 1776–1876*, ed. Edward H. Clarke (Philadelphia: Henry C. Lea, 1876), 355–59.

[60] Estes, "Therapeutic Practice in Colonial New England," 291.

[61] Jacalyn Duffin, *Langstaff: A Nineteenth-Century Medical Life* (Toronto; Buffalo: University of Toronto Press, 1993), 5–6.

literature that justified his choice of treatment. Furthermore, he published some of his findings and thoughts in the earliest medical journals in the United States.[62] Like many eighteenth- and early-nineteenth-century physicians, Barker was also interested in and recorded climatic conditions to correlate with epidemic disease.[63] In volume 1, he cites Noah Webster's *A Brief History of Epidemic and Pestilential Diseases* (1799), in which Webster went into great detail about disease associated with weather condition and climate.[64] Following the latest scientific literature regarding chemistry and medicine, Barker risked patient and peer disapproval as a clinical "innovator" by using alkaline therapy for various fevers and diseases. When his articles and those of others appeared in the *Medical Repository* in 1798, he was partially vindicated, as discussed in chapter 4. An announcement of Barker's forthcoming book appeared in the *Medical Repository* in 1797, and he went on to publish at least twelve articles in that journal between 1797 and 1818, most describing prevalent diseases and treatment in Cumberland County, District of Maine, during the prior year. It is worth noting that the case books, manuscript, and published articles reflect each other closely. (See Figures 1.9 and 1.10.)

[62] S. J. Reiser, "The Clinical Record in Medicine. Part 1: Learning from Cases," *Annals Internal Medicine* 114, no. 10 (1991): 902–907. Also Volker Hess and J. Andrew Mendelsohn, "Case and Series: Medical Knowledge and Paper Technology, 1600–1900," *History of Science* 48 (2010): 287–312. The *Medical Repository*, New York City, 1797–1824, was the first US medical journal; the second was the *Philadelphia Medical Museum*, 1804–1811. R. J. Kahn and P. G. Kahn, "The Medical Repository—the First U. S. Medical Journal (1797–1824)," *New England Journal of Medicine* 337 (1997): 1926–30.

[63] In 1806 Barker placed the following request in the *Portland Gazette*: "The subscriber would be obliged to any gentleman for Thermometrical and Meteorological observations made in the District of Maine previously to 1790. For those satisfactory compensation would be made." Jeremiah Barker, "Request for Thermometrical and Meteorological Observations before 1790," *Portland Gazette*, Monday September 29, 1806, p. 3 col. 4. In an 1806 letter to Benjamin Rush in Philadelphia: "Dr. Deane, and the Hon. Wm. Tyng have furnished me with accurate thermometrical and meteorological observations for many years past. Of late years I have noted them myself," from Barker, "Letter from Jeremiah Barker in Falmouth, Maine to Benjamin Rush in Philadelphia, 22 September 1806." From Hippocratic times health was thought to be a balance between the organism and the environment. Sun, temperature, wind, water, and topography all played a part. For Massachusetts, see Currie, *Historical Account of the Climates and Diseases of the United States*, 13–31; Fleming, *Meteorology in America*, 5–7.

[64] Webster, *A Brief History of Epidemic and Pestilential Diseases*.

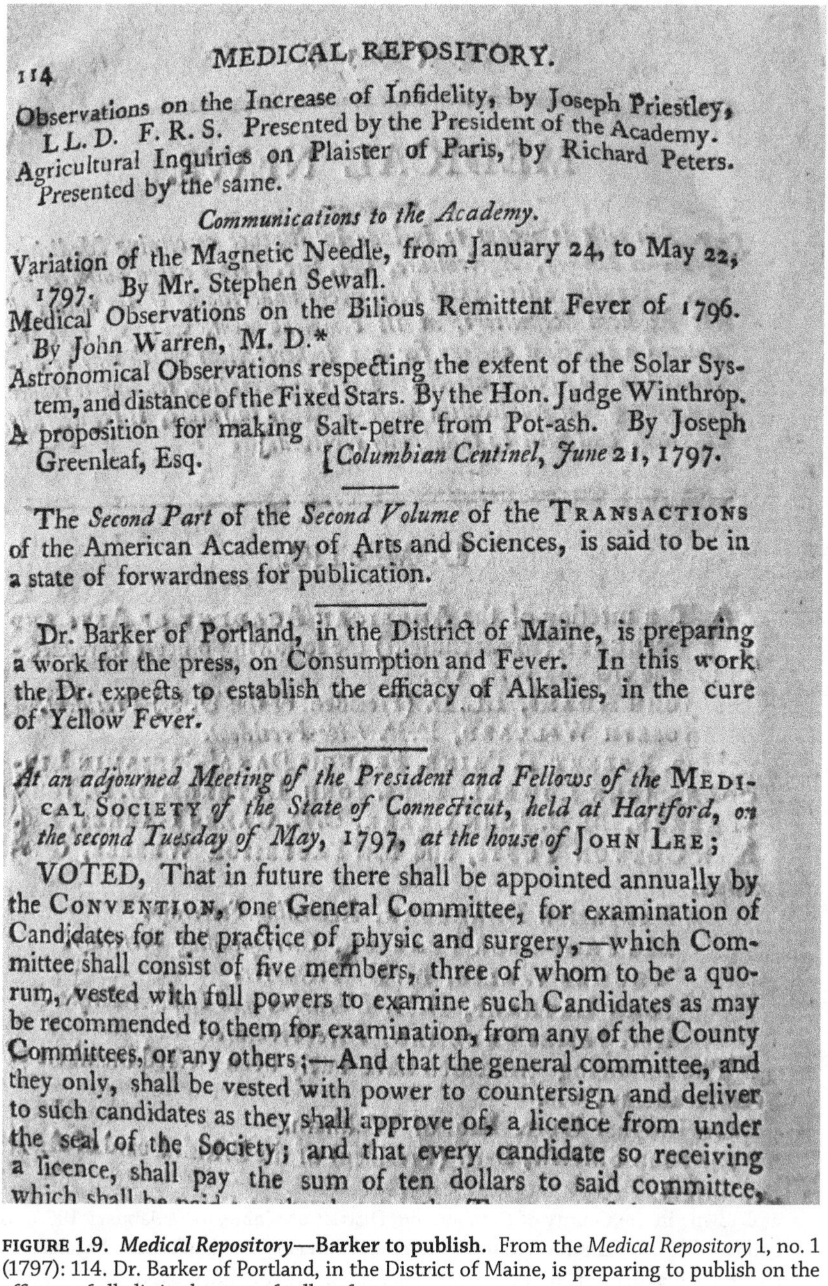

Observations on the Increase of Infidelity, by Joseph Priestley, LL.D. F. R. S. Presented by the President of the Academy. Agricultural Inquiries on Plaister of Paris, by Richard Peters. Presented by the same.

Communications to the Academy.

Variation of the Magnetic Needle, from January 24, to May 22, 1797. By Mr. Stephen Sewall.
Medical Observations on the Bilious Remittent Fever of 1796. By John Warren, M. D.*
Astronomical Observations respecting the extent of the Solar System, and distance of the Fixed Stars. By the Hon. Judge Winthrop.
A proposition for making Salt-petre from Pot-ash. By Joseph Greenleaf, Esq.   [*Columbian Centinel, June* 21, 1797.

The *Second Part* of the *Second Volume* of the TRANSACTIONS of the American Academy of Arts and Sciences, is said to be in a state of forwardness for publication.

Dr. Barker of Portland, in the District of Maine, is preparing a work for the press, on Consumption and Fever. In this work the Dr. expects to establish the efficacy of Alkalies, in the cure of Yellow Fever.

At an adjourned Meeting of the President and Fellows of the MEDICAL SOCIETY *of the State of Connecticut, held at Hartford, on the second Tuesday of May,* 1797, *at the house of* JOHN LEE;

VOTED, That in future there shall be appointed annually by the CONVENTION, one General Committee, for examination of Candidates for the practice of physic and surgery,—which Committee shall consist of five members, three of whom to be a quorum, vested with full powers to examine such Candidates as may be recommended to them for examination, from any of the County Committees, or any others;—And that the general committee, and they only, shall be vested with power to countersign and deliver to such candidates as they shall approve of, a licence from under the seal of the Society; and that every candidate so receiving a licence, shall pay the sum of ten dollars to said committee, which shall be paid

FIGURE 1.9. *Medical Repository*—**Barker to publish.** From the *Medical Repository* 1, no. 1 (1797): 114. Dr. Barker of Portland, in the District of Maine, is preparing to publish on the efficacy of alkalis in the cure of yellow fever.

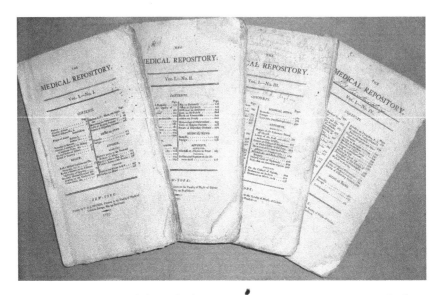

FIGURE 1.10. First year of the *Medical Repository*, 1797–1798. The four issues of Volume 1 of the *Medical Repository*, 1797–1798. This image shows how the journal issues were sent to subscribers, ready to be bound (or not) by the purchaser.

ARTICLES PUBLISHED BY JEREMIAH BARKER

In the *Medical Repository*

Vol. I (1797) p. 114: Dr. Barker of Portland, in the District of Maine, is preparing a work for the press, on Consumption and Fever. In this work the Dr. expects to establish the efficacy of Alkalies, in the cure of Yellow Fever.

Vol. II, No. 2 (1798) pp. 147–52: On the febrifuge Virtue of Lime, Magnesia and Alkaline Salts in Dysentery, Yellow-Fever and Scarlatina Anginosa. In a Letter from Dr. Jeremiah Barker, of Portland, (Maine) dated May 30, 1798.

Vol. III, No. 4 (1800) pp. 364–68: An Account of Febrile Diseases, as they have appeared in the County of Cumberland, District of Maine, from July 1798, to March 1800: Communicated in a Letter from Dr. Jeremiah Barker, of Portland, to Dr. Mitchill.

pp. 412–13: Obstinate Eruption over the whole Surface of the Body cured by Chalk (Alkaline Earth, or Carbonate of Lime).

Vol. IV (1801) pp. 415–16: Use of Alkalies in Cancer. Extract from a Letter of Dr. J. Barker to Dr. Mitchill, dated Portland (Maine), March 12, 1801.

Vol. V (1802) pp. 144–52: An Account of Febrile Diseases, as they have appeared in several Towns in the County of Cumberland, District of Maine, from January 1800, to January 1801: Communicated by Dr. Jeremiah Barker of Portland, to Dr. Mitchill.

pp. 220–21: Beneficial effects of alkalies in consumption of the lungs[65]

---

[65] Lyman Spalding and Jeremiah Barker, "Beneficial Effects of Alkalis in Consumption of the Lungs," *Medical Repository* 5, no. 2 (1802): 220–21. This brief communication by Spalding was about Jeremiah Barker's apparent success in the use of alkalis in patients with consumption. Spalding was a lifelong friend of Nathan Smith, an early American

pp. 267–72: An Account of Bilious Colics, as they appeared in several Towns in the County of Cumberland, District of Maine, in the Months of May, June, and July 1801; and of the surprising Relief obtained therein by Alkaline Remedies. By Dr. Jeremiah Barker, of Portland.

Vol. VI (1802) pp. 18–24: An Account of Febrile Diseases, as they appeared in Portland and its Vicinity, in August and September 1801. By Jeremiah Barker, M.D.

Second Hexade Vol. I (1804) pp. 125–34: An Account of the Measles, and some other Distempers, as they appeared in several Towns in the District of Maine, from January 1802 to January 1803. Communicated by Dr. Jeremiah Barker, of Portland.

Second Hexade Vol. III (1805) pp. 132–40: An Account of Diseases as they appeared in several Parts of the District of Maine, from January 1803 to January 1804: Communicated in a Letter from Dr. Jeremiah Barker to Dr. Mitchill.

Second Hexade Vol IV (1807) pp. 137–40: An Account of the Weather and Diseases in the County of Cumberland, District of Maine, from January 1804 to January 1805: Communicated in a Letter from Jeremiah Barker, M.D. of Portland, to Dr. Mitchill.

pp. 237–40: A Case of Tetanus, consequent upon an Injury done to one of the Great Toes, and ceasing after Amputation of the wounded Parts, and the Use of Opium and Alkohol: In a Communication from Dr. Jeremiah Barker, of Portland, to Dr. Mitchill.

New Series Vol. 19, No. 3 (1818): pp. 286–90: An account of a malignant fever, sporadically formed, in Falmouth, County of Cumberland, District of Maine

In the *Philadelphia Medical Museum*

Vol. III (1807) pp. cxlii–cxliii: Of the Efficacy of Blood-letting in Parturition, and of a Salivation in the Pulmonary Consumption. Extracted from a letter of Dr. Jeremiah Barker, of Falmouth in the District of Maine, to Dr. Benjamin Rush, dated September 22d.

YELLOW FEVER IN THE DISTRICT OF MAINE?

Barker's first published articles in the *Medical Repository*, and indeed the pro-spectus for his book, include the words "yellow fever" in their titles, which is interesting considering the fact that there had been no epidemics of yellow fever in Maine to our knowledge. Yellow fever epidemics along the Atlantic coast from the seventeenth through the nineteenth centuries commanded

medical educator and teacher at Dartmouth Medical School, University of Vermont College of Medicine, Yale School of Medicine, and the Medical School of Maine, who would conceive of and direct the first US Pharmacopeia, 1817–1820. Martin Kaufman, Stuart Galishoff, and Todd Lee Savitt, *Dictionary of American Medical Biography*, 2 vols. (Westport, CT: Greenwood Press, 1984), vol. 2, 709.

a great deal of attention, fear, and dread.[66] Of the epidemics occurring in America during the colonial and early republic periods, the frequently fatal yellow fever and smallpox aroused the most attention.[67] Other diseases such as consumption and diarrheal diseases might kill more people in a given year, but the fear and impact of yellow fever was out of proportion because of the concentration of deaths over a short period and the associated disruption of society.[68]

Dr. William Bean, internist and medical historian (1909–1989) succinctly described yellow fever during Barker's time as a "disease of unknown cause, curious almost haphazard spread, short duration, and often a high fatality rate. It died out soon after a frost and did not appear in cool climates or high elevations. Some thought filth caused its spread, that is, it arose in the fetid, reeking decay around docks. Others believed it to be imported, by ships from tropical lands. . . . The very mystery increased the sickening fear it created. It

[66] Thomas A. Apel, *Feverish Bodies, Enlightened Minds: Science and the Yellow Fever Controversy in the Early American Republic* (Stanford, CA: Stanford University Press, 2016); Margaret Humphreys, *Yellow Fever and the South* (Baltimore: The Johns Hopkins University Press, 1992), 1–2; J. Worth Estes, "Introduction: The Yellow Fever Syndrome and Its Treatment in Philadelphia, 1793," in *A Melancholy Scene of Devastation: The Public Response to the 1793 Philadelphia Yellow Fever Epidemic,* ed. J. Worth Estes and Billy G. Smith (USA, Canton, MA: Science History Publications, 1997), 1– 17; William Coleman, *Yellow Fever in the North: The Methods of Early Epidemiology* (Madison: University of Wisconsin Press, 1987), 3–13; J. H. Powell, *Bring Out Your Dead: The Great Plague of Yellow Fever in Philadelphia in 1793,* Studies in Health, Illness, and Caregiving (Philadelphia: University of Pennsylvania Press, 1993).

[67] John Duffy, *The Sanitarians: A History of American Public Health* (Chicago: University of Illinois Press, 1992), 23. Yellow fever was a major focus for health reformers even in the middle-Atlantic and New England states during 1790s; see Duffy, *A History of Public Health in New York City 1625–1868,* 101–23, and John B. Blake, *Public Health in the Town of Boston 1630–1822* (Cambridge, MA: Harvard University Press, 1959), 151–76. And for an excellent study on trans-Atlantic views and controversies on yellow fever, see Katherine Arner, "Making Yellow Fever American: The Early American Republic, the British Empire and the Geopolitics of Disease in the Atlantic World," *Atlantic Studies* 7, no. 4 (2010), 447–71.

[68] "True epidemic [in this case, yellow fever] is an event, not a trend. It elicits imme- diate and widespread response" by mobilizing communities as determined by social values and modes of understanding of the disease. Humphreys, *Yellow Fever and the South,* 2. Charles E. Rosenberg, *Explaining Epidemics and Other Studies in the History of Medicine* (New York: Cambridge University Press, 1992), 293–94. See also J. H. Powell, *Bring Out Your Dead,* reprint ed. (Philadelphia: University of Pennsylvania Press, 1993), 265, where the author points out, "it is not deaths that make a plague, it is the fear and hopelessness in people." Estes and Smith, *A Melancholy Scene of Devastation,* includes a series of essays on the social and political effects of the 1793 Philadelphia epidemic.

brought business to a halt. People fled from it if they could."[69] The generally accepted explanations of yellow fever epidemics in the mid-nineteenth century included miasmata or noxious vapors arising from marshlands or from decaying organic matter, epidemic constitution,[70] or transmission after importation by ships.[71]

One such epidemic took place in 1793 in Philadelphia, which was at that time the seat of the US Government (1790–1800). Of 25,000 inhabitants, 4,041 died, with 150 deaths per day at one point. Yellow fever recurred in Philadelphia from 1794 to 1798, and other coastal cities from Boston south were frequently attacked in the next decades. "It became the most thoroughly written-about disease in medicine."[72] There were apparently only a few cases and no epidemics of yellow fever in Maine: Augustin's tome on yellow fever lists cases in Portland in 1801 and 1839 and in Eastport in 1902, but without "diffusion of the disease."[73] But the fear of yellow fever was still very much present, and Barker wrote about it as an epidemic disease with high mortality attacking coastal cities of his country during his years of practice.

Historian Margaret Humphreys concludes that by the mid-nineteenth century, yellow fever was considered a distinct disease (like smallpox) that could

[69] W. B. Bean, "Landmark Perspective: Walter Reed and Yellow Fever," *Journal of the American Medical Association* 250, no. 5 (1983): 659.

[70] Epidemic constitution refers to a physical environment that might influence the development of an epidemic such as climate, temperature, and other weather conditions. Rosenberg, *Explaining Epidemics*, 135; Warner, *The Therapeutic Perspective*, 69.

[71] We now know that yellow fever is hemorrhagic fever caused by a single-stranded RNA flavivirus and transmitted by mosquitoes, the *Aedes aegypti* in Africa, and *Haemagogus* species in the Americas, a short-winged mosquito that breeds in standing water. Yellow fever is characterized clinically by fever, viremia, jaundice, and in its fulminant form by prostration, hemorrhage, shock, and variable organ damage involving mainly the liver, kidneys, and heart. Urban yellow fever generally is epidemic and is associated with domestic and peridomestic water sources. C. S. Bryan, S. W. Moss, and R. J. Kahn, "Yellow Fever in the Americas," *Infectious Disease Clinics of North America* 18, no. 2 (2004): 275–92; "Yellow Fever Vaccine," *Morbidity and Mortality Weekly Report* 39, no. RR-6 (1990): 1–6. The last epidemic of yellow fever in the United States occurred in 1905. See Humphreys, *Yellow Fever and the South*, 1–16; P. L. J. Bres, "A Century of Progress in Combating Yellow Fever," *Bulletin of the World Health Organization* 64 (1986): 775–86; and K. David Patterson, "Yellow Fever Epidemics and Mortality in the United States, 1693–1905," *Social Science and Medicine* 34, no. 8 (1992): 855–65.

[72] Powell, *Bring Out Your Dead*, 283.

[73] George Augustin, *History of Yellow Fever* (New Orleans: Searcy & Pfaff Ltd., 1909), 915–16. Augustin's reference to the 1801 outbreak is Jeremiah Barker, "An Account of Febrile Diseases, as They Appeared in Portland and Its Vicinity, in August and September, 1801. By Jeremiah Barker, M. D.," *Medical Repository* 6 (1802): 144–52.

be transported, requiring sanitation and quarantine for its prevention. The proof of transmission by *the Aedes aegypti* mosquito would be reported in 1901 and the viral etiology established in 1927.[74]

CONCLUSION

Jeremiah Barker was the product of his time and place, trained by apprenticeship, devoted to his quest for information, connected to the changing ideas of his profession. He was responsive to the concerns of his peers and patients, whether a rare dreaded outbreak of childbed fever or disease thought to be yellow fever. He believed in the idea of "medical geography" and was determined to contribute to the medical literature of his region. His published articles and unpublished book give us a rare glimpse into the reality of everyday practice in late-eighteenth- and early-nineteenth-century New England.

[74] Bryan, Moss, and Kahn, "Yellow Fever in the Americas," 287–88.

CHAPTER 2

Obtaining and Sharing Medical Literature, 1780–1820

I n a letter dated September 16, 1783, Dr. Benjamin Rush of Philadelphia wrote to Dr. William Cullen, one of his teachers in Edinburgh, "What has physic to do with taxation or independence? . . . One of the severest taxes paid by our profession during the war was occasioned by the want of a regular supply of books from Europe, by which means we are eight years behind you in everything."[1] If Rush in Philadelphia had difficulty obtaining European medical literature, it must have been nearly impossible for an average physician such as Jeremiah Barker, hungry for scarce available medical literature and information, to keep up to date. One of the most interesting aspects of Barker's manuscript is his constant struggle to obtain medical information, use it in his practice, document its use, share it with other physicians, and add to it with his own writings. Why was this process so difficult?

MEDICAL INFORMATION BY MAIL

It is difficult to imagine, in our age of easy access, that in Barker's time the post was essential for the exchange of information. Physicians who couldn't get their hands on the literature mailed information to each other, laboriously copying out whole sections of books and journals. Postal regulations didn't

---

[1] Benjamin Rush, *Letters. Edited by L. H. Butterfield*, 2 vols. (Princeton: Princeton University Press, 1951), vol. 1, 310.

help with this situation: starting in 1792, letters, packets, and newspapers were recognized by the US postal system as mail matter, and magazines were accepted in 1799, but not until 1825 were unbound journals allowed, and bound books could not be sent by mail until 1851.[2]

Thus on February 17, 1799, Dr. Benjamin Vaughn of Hallowell, District of Maine, wrote to Dr. Rush asking for the latest edition of "your [Rush's] Medical Inquiries,"[3] Dr. [Samuel] Mitchill on Contagion, Dr. [David] Hosack's account of fever, and other American works on the subject of modern fever. "What is sent to me will, by me, be communicated through the neighborhood. Though the post be shut to us, we must employ the stages in private channels. . . . If it will save you trouble, I will gladly pay the expense of amanuensis[4] for your own remarks, which probably will not be very long."[5]

On December 6, 1800, Dr. John G. Coffin of Boston wrote to Dr. Barker in Portland, "I only regret, at present, that I am not in possession of the [Medical] Repository, as I wish more fully to be acquainted with your theory and practice."[6] Coffin is another good example of an elite physician bemoaning the difficulty of obtaining current medical literature. Born in New Buxton, Maine, Coffin practiced in Boston, was one of the board of managers of the Boston Dispensary, and in 1805 would become the first secretary of the Boston Medical Library. In 1823 he would found and edit the *Boston Medical Intelligencer*, a precursor to the *Boston Medical and Surgical Journal*, which became the *New England Journal of Medicine*.[7] Though he did not have access to the *Medical Repository* on December 6, 1800, Coffin did send Barker a four-page letter with

---

[2] Richard B. Kielbowicz, "Mere Merchandise or Vessels of Culture? Books in the Mail, 1792–1942," *Papers of the Bibliographical Society of America* 82, no. 2 (1988): 169–200.

[3] Vaughn is probably referring to Rush's *Medical Inquiries and Observations* (Philadelphia: Thomas Dobson, 1794–98). Austin, Robert B. Early American Medical Imprints: 1668–1820. (Arlington, MA: The Printers' Devil, 1961), 175.

[4] An amanuensis is a literary assistant who takes dictation or copies manuscripts.

[5] Benjamin Vaughan, "Letter from Benjamin Vaughan to Benjamin Rush," in *Manuscript Correspondence of Benjamin Rush UV18*, ed. Historical Society of Pennsylvania (1799), MSS 42 February 17.

[6] Letter from J. G. Coffin to J. Barker. M.H.S. Coll.13, Box 1/1.

[7] Joseph E. Garland, *The Centennial History of the Boston Medical Library, 1875–1975* (Boston: Boston Medical Library in the Francis A. Countway Library of Medicine, 1975), 6–7, 9, 89. *The New England Journal of Medicine and Surgery and the Collateral Branches of Science*, begun by John Collins Warren and James Jackson in 1812, became the *Boston Medical and Surgical Journal* in 1828 when the five-year-old *Boston Medical Intelligencer* was purchased from J. G. Coffin.

excerpts from Edward Jenner's new (1798) book and the latest Boston news on vaccinating with cowpox to prevent smallpox.

This was cutting-edge information for physicians in the United States. Inoculation with live smallpox, in order to prevent a later attack of the disease, had been introduced in Boston in 1721, and Barker himself was inoculated there by Isaac Rand in 1774.[8] Dr. Edward Jenner's book describing his discovery of vaccinating with cowpox instead of live smallpox was published in London in 1798 and announced in American "newspapers and in the *Medical Repository* of New York of that year."[9] In the fall of 1798 John Coakley Lettsom of London wrote to Benjamin Waterhouse in Boston about Jenner's new

---

[8] Dr. Isaac Rand would become president of the Massachusetts Medical Society from 1798 to 1804. Barker wrote that in order to be inoculated in 1774, he "sailed from Boston to Charlestown and then to Cambridge," as there were no bridges yet (1774 Casebook, Col 13, Box 1/2). There had been a private toll ferry service between Boston and Charlestown since 1631, but in 1640 the Massachusetts General Court granted the ferry to Harvard College. The first bridge at the site was opened in June 1786, with two hundred pounds a year going to Harvard College for forty years to pay for the loss of ferry income. Boston Transit Commission Boston. Transit Commission, *The Ferry, the Charles-River Bridge and the Charles-Town Bridge. Historical Statement Prepared for the Boston Transit Commission by Its Chairman [G. G. Crocker] and Submitted at the Opening of the New Bridge November 27, 1899*, ed. George G. Crocker (Boston: Rockwell and Churchill Press, 1899), 3–5. This early process of inoculation was introduced from Turkey by Lady Mary Wortley Montague (1689–1762). For details on and her place in the development of smallpox inoculation, see B. A. Cunha, "Smallpox and Measles: Historical Aspects and Clinical Differentiation," *Infectious Disease Clinics of North America* 18, no. 1 (2004): 84–87; and W. F. Bynum, "Placing Diseases," in *Science and the Practice of Medicine in the Nineteenth Century*, Cambridge History of Medicine (Cambridge; New York: Cambridge University Press, 1994), 20–24. Stephen Coss, *The Fever of 1721* (New York: Simon & Schuster, 2016), 74–96. Historian Genevieve Miller points out that "inoculation [for smallpox] was the chief medical contribution of the Enlightenment, at least in the opinion of the age itself." Genevieve Miller, *The Adoption of Inoculation for Smallpox in England and France* (Philadelphia: University of Pennsylvania Press, 1957), 195.

[9] "Article I. The Following Important Account of a New Publication in Great-Britain, by Dr. Jenner, Entitled 'a Inquiry into the Causes and Effects of the Variolae Vaccinae, or Cow Pox,' Is Extracted from the Analytical Review for July, 1798," *Medical Repository* 2, no. 2 (1798): 255–58. James Thacher, *American Modern Practice* (Boston: Ezra Read, 1817), 25–26. Coffin's letter mentions Drs. Jenner, Waterhouse, Woodville, and Pea(r)son. Dr. Edward Jenner published his discovery, *An Inquiry into the Causes and Effects of the Variole Vaccinae, a Disease discovered in some of the Western Counties of England, particularly Gloucestershire, and known by the name of the cow-pox* (London), in 1798. Dr. Woodville of London supplied Dr. James Jackson with "matter" later in 1800 and wrote *Observations on the Cow-pox* (London) in 1800. Dr. Pearson of London supplied Dr. Miller in New York with the cowpox matter. Physicians were providing each other with matter; Barker asks John G. Coffin (Boston) for smallpox matter in 1800 and Lyman Spalding (Portsmouth, New Hampshire) in 1806–1807. James Alfred Spalding, *Spalding Collection 1487*, ed. Maine Historical Society (unpublished and unpaginated, 1846–1938). Box 2/1.

book.[10] Waterhouse obtained and read the book in 1799 and wrote an article on it for *The Colombian Centinel* of March 12, 1799.[11] He received some cowpox "matter" from John Haygarth in Bath, England, in June 1800 and promptly vaccinated his son and two servants,[12] thus introducing the actual procedure to Boston and the rest of the United States.[13]

Personal communication from London to Boston from 1798 to 1800 is what kept Waterhouse up to date in the absence of the indexes and other sources we have today. The Coffin/Barker letter of December 6, 1800, represents the same sharing of hand-written excerpts of books and medical news and information. We know that Barker was inoculating patients with cowpox (also called kine pox) by January 1803 as per a receipt from John Quinby to Jeremiah Barker,[14] but it's quite possible that he began inoculating with cowpox much sooner.

THE FIRST US MEDICAL JOURNALS AND MEDICAL NATIONALISM

From the 1806 Barker casebook, the daily record of his encounters with patients, comes this "Copy of a letter to Dr. Rush: Dear Sir, The *Philadelphia*

[10] Edward Jenner, Edward Pearce, and William Skelton, *An Inquiry into the Causes and Effects of the Variolae Vaccinae: A Disease Discovered in Some of the Western Counties of England, Particularly Gloucestershire, and Known by the Name of the Cow Pox* (London: Printed, for the author, by Sampson Low, no. 7, Berwick Street, Soho: and sold by Law, Ave-Maria Lane; and Murray and Highley, Fleet Street, 1798).

[11] William K. Beatty and Virginia L. Beatty, "Sources of Medical Information," *Journal of the American Medical Association* 236 (1976): 78–82. For more details on Waterhouse and the introduction of vaccination to the United States, see Philip Cash, *Dr. Benjamin Waterhouse: A Life in Medicine and Public Service (1754–1846)* (Sagamore Beach, MA: Science History Publications/USA, 2006), 111–98.

[12] John H. Talbott, *A Biographical History of Medicine* (New York: Grune & Stratton, 1970), 445–48. For more extensive review of the introduction of vaccination into the United States, see Cash, *Dr. Benjamin Waterhouse*, 111–98.

[13] Lloyd E. Hawes and J. Worth Estes, *Benjamin Waterhouse, MD; First Professor of the Theory and Practice of Physics at Harvard and Introducer of Cowpox Vaccination into America . . . Including a Concordance of Dr. Waterhouse's Hortus Siccus*, Boston Medical Library Studies, 1 (Boston: Francis A. Countway Library of Medicine, 1974), 37. Cash, *Dr. Benjamin Waterhouse*, 124.

[14] The Quinby receipt was found at Countway Library of Medicine, B MS misc Barker, Jeremiah 1800–1806. Kine, the archaic plural of cow, refers to cowpox or vaccinia, a term in use before 1803, per OED; that is, vaccination using vaccinia (kine- or cowpox) to prevent smallpox. The Great Pox was syphilis. The Lesser Pox originally included rubella, chickenpox, and smallpox, but came to mean only smallpox. In the late eighteenth century, smallpox was one of the leading causes of death and disability.

Medical Museum[15] has of late arrived at the Portland Book Store, which I readily purchased, and think it my duty to promote its circulation in Maine with as much assiduity as I have the New York *Med' Repository*."[16] Barker demonstrated a lifelong attention to his own medical education and that of his fellow physicians and the community, continuing after his retirement in 1818.

The first article in the January 1813 issue of the *New England Journal of Medicine and Surgery* is titled the "Historical Outline of the Progress of Medical Science During the Last Three Years." The author complained that "slow and precarious receipt of European publications in this country, and the limited circulation of such copies as are received, constitute very considerable obstacles to the early dissemination of medical information from foreign sources."[17] There seems to have been a bit of War of 1812 hostility in addition to the medical literature transfer problem. In a *New England Journal of Medicine and Surgery* article dated July 1, 1813: " 'America,' said the learned editors of the *London Medical Review*, 'seems to be the country of epidemics, as much as swamps, woods, and savannahs.' England, we might say in return, seems to be a country of scrophula and consumption, as much as it is of fogs and vapours. Such observations are at least injudicious, not to say incorrect."[18] The first 1814 issue of *New England Journal of Medicine and Surgery* noted difficulties due to the "interrupted intercourse between this country and Europe, an evil which is far from being diminished . . . a few works of some importance have reached us from England and France."[19] War with Britain was again interfering with transfer of medical information, and these comments are examples of medical nationalism. In 1789 Noah Webster wrote that we must establish a "national language, as well as a national government. . . . As an independent people, our reputation abroad demands that, in all things, we should be federal; be

---

[15] The *Philadelphia Medical Museum* (1804–1811) was the second medical journal published in the United States. See J. S. Billings, "Literature and Institutions," in *A Century of American Medicine: 1776–1876*, ed. Edward H. Clarke (Philadelphia: Henry C. Lea, 1876), 332.

[16] Jeremiah Barker, "1806 Casebook," in *Maine Historical Society, Barker Collection 13, Box 1/5* (Portland, Maine, 1806), unpaginated.

[17] "Historical Outline of the Progress of Medical Science during the Past Three Years," *New England Journal of Medicine and Surgery* 2, no. 1 (1813): 1.

[18] "Some Account of the Disease, Which Was Epidemic in Some Parts of New-York and New-England, in the Winter of 1812–13," *New England Journal of Medicine, Surgery and Collateral Branches of Science* 2, no. 3 (1813): 241–52.

[19] "Historical Outline of the Progress of Medical Science during the Past Three Years," 1–6; "Some Historical Account of the Progress of Medical Science during the Last Year," *New England Journal of Medicine and Surgery* 3, no. 1 (1814): 5–11.

national; for if we do not respect ourselves, we may be assured that other nations will not respect us . . . we may expect success, in attempting changes favorable to language, science and government."[20] Webster, who would subsequently publish twenty-five letters and two books on medical topics between 1796 and 1799, might well have added medicine to his list.[21]

Nationalism and national identity were issues in American medicine, as they were in politics. Paraphrasing comments by historian Robert A. Gross, our young nation did not have "ingredients deemed necessary for a respectable state in the Old World."[22] We had no ancient traditions, no Oxford or Cambridge Universities, no medical centers like Leiden, Edinburgh, London, Paris, or Montpelier. Though the United States was a federal republic overseen by a central government, most of its citizens saw themselves as New Englanders or Virginians rather than identifying as Americans.[23]

In 1817, writing about topography and diseases in Louisiana, Jabez W. Heustis wrote, "Many of us have too long been led astray by the delusion of Britannic greatness. Nature is there exhibited but on a slender scale. To use an observation of the learned Dr. [Samuel] Mitchill, if we wish to see anything great, new, wonderful, excellent, or strange, we must turn our backs upon the European world, and direct our attention to the contemplation of our own country. . . . If young physicians, instead of crossing the Atlantic, to complete their education in the European schools, would but take the same pains to

[20] Noah Webster, *Dissertations on the English Language: With Notes, Historical and Critical to Which Is Added by Way of an Appendix, an Essay on a Reformed Mode of Spelling, with Dr. Franklin's Arguments on That Subject* (Boston: Isaiah Thomas and Company, 1789), 405–406.

[21] Noah Webster, *A Collection of Papers on the Subject of Bilious Fevers Prevalent in the United States for a Few Years Past* (New York: Hopkins, Webb & Co., 1796); Noah Webster, *A Brief History of Epidemic and Pestilential Diseases with the Principal Phenomena of the Physical World Which Precede and Accompany Them and Observations Deduced from Facts Stated*, 2 vols. (Hartford: Hudson and Goodwin, 1799); Benjamin Spector, "Noah Webster: Letters on Yellow Fever Addressed to Dr. William Currie. An Introductory Essay," in *Supplements to the Bulletin of the History of Medicine (No. 9)*, ed. Henry E. Siegerist and Genevieve Miller (Baltimore: The Johns Hopkins Press, 1947); Thomas Apel, "The Thucydidean Moment: History, Science, and the Yellow-Fever Controversy, 1793–1805," *Journal of the Early Republic* 34, no. 3 (2014), 315–47; Thomas A. Apel, *Feverish Bodies, Enlightened Minds: Science and the Yellow Fever Controversy in the Early American Republic* (Stanford, CA: Stanford University Press, 2016), 35–64.

[22] Robert A. Gross, "Introduction," in *An Extensive Republic: Print, Culture, and Society in the New Nation, 1790–1840*, ed. Robert A. Gross and Mary Kelley (Chapel Hill: Published in association with the American Antiquarian Society by the University of North Carolina Press, 2010), 11.

[23] Gross, "Introduction" in *An Extensive Republic*, 11–50.

visit, with an attentive eye, the different parts of our extensive Republic, I am inclined to think, they would be much better qualified for the exercise of their profession."[24] Certainly, American physicians were following the British and French literature, but Barker and others were emphasizing and adding new American contributions as well.[25]

Barker arrived in Maine more than eighty years before Oliver Wendell Holmes would write, "the Boston State-House is the hub of the solar system."[26] Though Barker was a New Englander who knew and corresponded with a number of physicians in Boston and surrounding towns, the "hub" of his medical world was Philadelphia and New York City. Boston was older than Philadelphia, but by 1790 Philadelphia was wealthier and had almost twice the population of Boston. Pennsylvania Hospital had begun in 1752 and a medical school at the College of Philadelphia in 1765 (the University of Pennsylvania after 1791), and hospital training had become an integrated part of medical education in Philadelphia. Barker and many American physicians were influenced by Dr. Benjamin Rush, who, having trained in Edinburgh, taught medicine in Philadelphia and wrote several influential books on medicine, epidemics, and diseases of the mind. With the hospital, medical school, Rush, and other authors, Philadelphia became a center of medical book and journal publication in the late eighteenth and early nineteenth centuries.[27] King's College in New York City organized a medical faculty in 1767, closed in

[24] Jabez Wiggins Heustis, *Physical Observations, and Medical Tracts and Researches, on the Topography and Diseases of Louisiana* (New York: T. and J. Swords, 1817). 163–64. Jabez Heustis (1784–1841) was born in St. John, New Brunswick, received his medical education at the College of Physicians and Surgeons in New York, served as a surgeon in the US Navy and later in the Army, and finally lived and, in 1841, died in Alabama. Howard A. Kelly and Walter L. Burrage, *American Medical Biographies* (Baltimore: The Norman, Remington Company, 1920), 522–23.

[25] Americans were reading British and French literature, and some of the elite physicians were taking part of their training in Britain and France. C. Helen Brock, "The Influence of Europe on Colonial Massachusetts Medicine," in *Medicine in Colonial Massachusetts 1620–1820*, ed. J. Worth Estes, Philip Cash, and Eric H. Christianson (Boston: The Colonial Society of Massachusetts distributed by the University of Virginia Press, 1980), 101–43; John Harley Warner, *Against the Spirit of System: The French Impulse in Nineteenth-Century American Medicine* (Princeton, NJ: Princeton University Press, 1998), 17–31.

[26] Oliver Wendell Holmes, *The Autocrat of the Breakfast Table* (Boston: Houghton, Mifflin, 1881), 143. (Originally published in 1858.)

[27] Using Austin, one can make a rough estimate of the relative number of books and pamphlets published between 1668 and 1820. Of a total of 2,016 publications recorded, 1,047 were published in Philadelphia and 338 in Boston. Robert B. Austin, *Early American Medical Imprints: 1668–1820* (Arlington, MA: The Printers' Devil, 1961).

1775, and reopened as Columbia College in 1784. The Medical Institution at Harvard College[28] began in 1782 and was in Cambridge, a small village across the Charles River from Boston and connected only by ferryboat until a bridge was built in 1793. More importantly, there was no hospital in Boston until the opening of the Massachusetts General Hospital in 1821.[29] All of these developments contributed to the sense of nationalism. At last the "ideal education" could be obtained in the new republic.

PROBLEMS ENCOUNTERED BY EARLY MEDICAL JOURNALS

The *Medical Repository* (New York, 1797–1824) was the only US medical journal published before 1800 and was the first attempt to present the relation between science and practice in a serial format that allowed response and communication. Six journals were added before 1809, and ten between 1810 and 1820, but many were short-lived, with an average lifespan of only 5.4 years. Many succumbed to competition, costs of printing and postage, and loss of institutional support and dedicated editors.

Internationally, financial shenanigans contributed to the delay in transmitting information, in addition to the mails and war. The following note is found in the second American medical journal, the *Philadelphia Medical Museum* in 1807:

> *Important Information to Booksellers.*
> *Dr. [Lyman] Spalding, of Portsmouth, New Hampshire, complains that not a single volume of this Journal [*The Medical and Physical Journal (London)*], later than the 13th, is to be found in America, and ascribes the circumstance to some inattention on the part of our Publisher. On inquiry we find, however, that the bad faith and the bad credit of the American booksellers, are the causes why very few good books are exported from England to the United States. The merchants are not paid for one half they*

---

[28] Of the first three professors at the Harvard Medical Institution, Aaron Dexter, John Warren, and Benjamin Waterhouse, only Waterhouse had any formal medical training beyond preceptorship, having studied in Europe.

[29] Whitfield J. Bell, "Medicine in Boston and Philadelphia: Comparisons and Contrasts, 1750–1820," in *Medicine in Colonial Massachusetts 1620–1820* (Boston: The Colonial Society of Massachusetts, 1980), 162, 165–66, 176; Francis R. Packard, *Some Account of the Pennsylvania Hospital from Its First Rise to the Beginning of the Year 1938* (Philadelphia: Engle Press, 1938), 1–8, 97–106; William G. Rothstein, *American Medical Schools and the Practice of Medicine: A History* (New York: Oxford University Press, 1987), 28–29.

send, consequently they seldom export any books for America, except such as they can purchase at the price of waste paper. Our publisher says he sent quantities of this Journal to New York, with little or no return, for several years; and that he has not yet received from his Agents a tenth of the sum due to him. The complaint of Dr. Spalding has frequently been made to us by other American Correspondents, and we embrace this opportunity of explaining the origin of the evil, conceiving that it may be easily removed by the establishment and support of some Bookselling House in America, of unquestionable punctuality and credit.

Med. and Phys. Jour[30]

Finally, from James Thacher's *American Modern Practice* of 1817:

The Medical Repository *is not now our only medium of medical intelligence. Many others of real merit have since been introduced; among which are Dr. Barton's* "Philadelphia Medical and Philosophical Journal" *and the* "Medical and Philosophical Register," *a respectable work, by Dr. Hosack of New York; Dr. Coxe's valuable* "Medical Museum" *is discontinued. The* "New-England Journal of Medicine and Surgery" *commenced in Boston with the year 1812. It is edited by gentlemen of professional eminence and evinces the talents and ardour for medical improvement which distinguish the faculty of Massachusetts. In addition to many valuable original essays, it exhibits to the American student and physician the earliest information of whatever is new, ingenious or useful in foreign publications, connected with the science of medicine.*[31]

Thacher did not mention that Barton's journal had also ceased publication in 1808–1809; so much for "keeping up with the literature."[32]

---

[30] The *Medical and Physical Journal* (London) is printed in the *Medical and Philosophical Register* section in the *Philadelphia Medical Museum* 3 (1807): ccxxxii. Spalding had complained that "not a single volume of this Journal [*Medical and Physical Journal*, London], later than the 13th is to be found in America." Volume 13 was January to June 1805; two years earlier.

[31] Thacher, *American Modern Practice*, 61.

[32] The *Philadelphia Medical and Physical Journal* was published irregularly between 1804 and 1809 by Benjamin Smith Barton. See Billings, "Literature and Institutions," 332, and M. Ebert, "The Rise and Development of the American Medical Periodical 1797–1850," *Bulletin of the Medical Library Association* 40, no. 3 (1952): 248.

NEWSPAPERS AS A SOURCE OF MEDICAL INFORMATION

Much of the medical information acquired by physicians in the period from 1780 to 1820 came from sources other than medical books, journals, and personal communication filled with original observations and excerpts copied from books and journals. "Newspapers [also] provided a major source of medical information for the practitioners of medicine. Between 1704 (*The Boston News-letter*) and September 1785, two hundred different newspapers had appeared in the colonies; of 250,000 pages, there were 10,000 articles of medical interest, many aimed at the practitioner. A large proportion of writing [by physicians] was intended to influence the lay public rather than to advance knowledge."[33]

One example of a Maine newspaper as a source of medical information for the public and physicians can be found in *The Falmouth Gazette*, Maine's first newspaper, which began publication on January 1, 1785.[34] In the February 12, 1785, issue a controversy between Dr. Jeremiah Barker of Gorham and Dr. Nathaniel Coffin of Portland on the prevention and cure of puerperal sepsis (childbed fever) arose, and it continued in the next four issues. In an article focusing on midwifery and mortality, historian Laurel Thatcher Ulrich devotes four pages to this series of newspaper articles and the Barker manuscript. She concludes that this exchange is "a clear example of the way in which medical literature in combination with local experience came to define a practice."[35]

This public argument in a newspaper serves to inform us on several levels. Nathanial Coffin Jr. was born in Falmouth in 1744 and trained under his father, an established physician in the community. At age twenty, he went to London for further training at Guys under John Hunter and also studied at St. Thomas' Hospital.[36] Barker, at the time of the newspaper debate, had been preceptorship trained and had moved to Gorham only five years earlier.

---

[33] Beatty and Beatty, "Sources of Medical Information."

[34] Ronald Banks, *Maine Becomes a State* (Middletown, CT: Wesleyan University Press, 1970), 13.

[35] "[Controversy between Dr. Barker of Gorham and Dr. Nathaniel Coffin of Portland on the Prevention and Cure of Puerperal Fever]," *The Falmouth Gazette and Weekly Advertiser*, February 12, 19, 26, and March 5, 12, 1785. Laurel Thatcher Ulrich, "'The Living Mother of a Living Child': Midwifery and Mortality in Post-Revolutionary New England," *The William and Mary Quarterly* 46, no. 1 (1989): 40–45.

[36] James Alfred Spalding, *Maine Physicians of 1820; a Record of the Members of the Massachusetts Medical Society Practicing in the District of Maine at the Date of Separation* (Lewiston: Lewiston Print Shop, 1928), 8–11; James Thacher, *American Medical*

Barker opened the argument, pointing out that no man "can be unaffected with the mortality among child-bed women." He claimed to be "taking the opinion of the [then four-year-old] Massachusetts Medical Society respecting the cause, prevention and method of relief in the epidemic disorder." Barker gave reasons the stomach and intestine should be cleared of the "bilious fomes"[37] and believed that bleeding be used only very early in the course if at all. Coffin stated that bleeding should be used freely.

Coffin saw childbed fever as inflammation or gangrene of the uterus, but Barker reported that he had observed a woman at dissection (autopsy) with the same symptoms, whose uterus, "was entirely free from inflammation or gangrene but the intestines, mesentery, and omentum were inflamed." Furthermore, Barker appears to have made a connection between the childbed fever outbreak and a larger epidemic of unusually virulent infections, which he said was a disorder "not only to child-bed women, but others from different and more immediate causes." When Barker later described the epidemic of childbed fever in his manuscript, it was in a paragraph immediately following a discussion of men at the same time dying from normally trivial injuries leading to gangrene and death.

Clearly Coffin did not appreciate the fact that Barker mentioned cases in Portland and Falmouth: he wrote that Barker should "not overlook that [mortality] of Gorham where he resides, and where he has had *more* opportunities of making observations in these particular cases." Coffin then wrote that Barker was "awakening fear and apprehension among women." Barker replied that he was "complying with the request of members of the faculty [presumably physicians dealing with the epidemic] who are not properly furnished with medical authors." Barker also pointed out that Coffin's response referred to "authors who are obsolete;" that is, Coffin was not keeping up with the medical literature. Coffin's authority came from his position as a second-generation local physician with training in London. Barker, in Maine for only five years, supported his arguments by referring to the latest medical literature on the subject and calling on recent Medical Society opinion.

The September 15 and 22, 1806, issues of the *Portland Gazette and Maine Advertiser* included an article of nearly six full columns by Jeremiah Barker

---

Biography: Or Memoirs of Eminent Physicians Who Have Flourished in America. To Which Is Prefixed a Succinct History of Medical Science in the United States, from the First Settlement of the Country (Boston: Richardson & Lord and Cottons & Barnard, 1828), 229–34.

[37] Morbific matter, meaning disease-causing material.

regarding the efficacy of alkalies in the treatment of fevers and the fumigation of rooms and ships. He included the names of at least thirty-three
philosophers and physicians, as well as references to journal articles and
books, to bolster his arguments. Barker claimed that he wished to "aid the
efforts of the Massachusetts Medical Society in eradicating medical prejudices
and disseminating useful knowledge and . . . exposing & suppressing empirical
impositions, which rapidly increase; finally, in rendering the science of medicine more respectable and important in the view of mankind."[38]

Barker's manuscript was in progress by 1797, as evidenced by the announcement in the *Medical Repository* of that year: "Dr. Barker of Portland,
in the District of Maine, is preparing a work for the press, on Consumption
and Fever. In this work the Dr. expects to establish the efficacy of Alkalies,
in the cure of Yellow Fever."[39] He also advertised heavily in newspapers, with
a number of announcements and articles regarding his book over the next
three decades. One such article appeared in *The Eastern Argus* of January 13,
1820, entitled *Proposal for Publishing a History of Diseases in the District of
Maine*. "Subscription papers are left at the *Gazette* (Portland) office, and with
Messrs. Isaac Adams, and William Hyde Booksellers in Portland. Gentlemen
holding subscription papers, in the District of Maine, are requested to return
them to Mr. Arthur Shirley, printer in Portland, at any convenient time, in
May 1820, and they will be entitled to 1 volume when printed, for procuring
twelve subscribers. Gorham Dec. 1819 . . . Subscription received at this office
(*Eastern Argus*)."[40] And in the *Christian Mirror* of February 22, 1828, Barker
wrote that regarding "my M.S. History of Disease of Maine, I have been induced to select a part of my first chapter, which treats of the use and abuse of
ardent spirits . . . any suggestions to render it more perfect, will be gladly received."[41] Thus, newspapers were a frequent conduit for medical information,
and Barker's story serves to illustrate the fluid boundaries between medical
and lay journalism in the early nineteenth century.

---

[38] Jeremiah Barker, "Medical by Jeremiah Barker," *Portland Gazette and Maine Advertiser*, September 15 and 22, 1806, 1.

[39] Jeremiah Barker, "Dr. Barker of Portland, in the District of Maine, Is Preparing a Work for the Press, on Consumption and Fever. In This Work the Dr. Expects to Establish the Efficacy of Alkalies, in the Cure of Yellow Fever," *Medical Repository* 1, no. 1 (1797), 114.

[40] *Eastern Argus*, January 13, 1820, p. 2 col 3.

[41] *Christian Mirror*, February 22, 1828; p.3 col 4.

AND LAST BUT NOT LEAST, BOOKS

"Books were read, re-read, and handed down to younger men."[42] Sometime between 1811 and 1824, Barker wrote, "as the *Medical Museum* as well as the *Medical Repository* are rare books [referring here to volumes of journals bound by year] in Maine, and the former discontinued [in 1811], I have been requested to extract some of the most interesting cases of consumption, from these voluminous works, which cannot conveniently be purchased, by young physicians."[43] As we have seen, most medical texts in Barker's time came from Europe and were obtained with difficulty. They were expensive to purchase and to transport. And once owned, they were rarely replaced with newer editions.

Barker's own library, with its books, journals, ledgers, and financial records, was said in 1909 by Maine medical historian James Spalding to have contained "nearly two thousand volumes at his death." Many books had marginalia such as "Now Dr. Rush, I cannot agree with you there."[44] Unfortunately this library has disappeared. Probate records from Cumberland county of 1835 were destroyed in a Portland fire. Libraries in Maine, Massachusetts, Rhode Island, New York, and New Jersey, book sales, and the 1945 probate records of Barker's great-grandson J. Henry Clark, who donated the Barker collection to the Maine Historical Society in 1942, have yielded no trace of Barker's books.

CONCLUSION

The quest for medical literature, both new and old, was a concern for elite as well as rural physicians in the early days of the nation, as much a problem for Benjamin Rush of Philadelphia and Samuel Mitchill of New York as for Jeremiah Barker of Portland, Maine. It was the focus of correspondence, the topic of newspaper articles, and the inspiration for new medical journals and books. Obtaining and sharing medical books and journals was heavily

[42] B. Riznik, "The Professional Lives of Early Nineteenth-Century New England Doctors," *Journal of the History of Medicine and Allied Sciences* 19 (1964), 1–16.

[43] The first line of volume 2, chapter 8, MS **C225C. The *Medical Repository* was published from 1797 to 1824 and the *Medical Museum* from 1804 to 1811.

[44] Kelly and Burrage, *American Medical Biographies*, 63; and James Alfred Spalding, *Jeremiah Barker, M.D., Gorham and Falmouth, Maine, 1752–1835* (Portland, ME: s.n., 1909), 20.

supplemented by both personal correspondence and by newspapers for dissemination of medical information to the public as well as to professionals. At a time when medicine was undergoing profound change, Jeremiah Barker constantly documented his own efforts to keep up with and contribute to the medical literature of the new nation.

CHAPTER 3

The Old Medicine and the New: Why Did Barker Write This Manuscript, for Whom Was It Written, and Why Was It Not Published?

In 1772, [having completed my studies] Dr. Bela Lincoln . . . gave me a recommendation as being qualified to practice physic. But, at parting, he observed that the Science of Medicine was, as yet, involved in great obscurity, and that many things were unknown, in the healing art, particularly concerning the nature and treatment of Consumption & hectic fever, which needed to be discovered; and that as I had his shoulders to stand upon, he hoped I would study diligently, keep exact records of cases, as they should occur in practice, whether fatal or otherwise; open dead bodies, when permitted, note appearances, and labour to make improvements in Medical Science.[1]

THE IMPORTANCE OF OBSERVATION AND RECORDING

Barker included this quotation from Benjamin Rush in his manuscript:[2] " 'Did all our young physicians record the history of the diseases they met with, and the effects of the remedies on them, they would find their Journals and

[1] Jeremiah Barker, "A History of Diseases in the District of Maine Commencing in 1735 and Continuing to the Present Time . . . To This Is Annexed an Inquiry into the Causes, Nature, Increasing Prevalency, and Treatment of Consumption," in *Jeremiah Barker, Collection 13,* ed. Maine Historical Society (Portland, ME, 1831), vol. 2, 62–63.

[2] Benjamin Rush (1745–1813) studied medicine with John Redman, graduated from the College of New Jersey (later Princeton), and studied in Liverpool, London, and Edinburgh. He then practiced medicine and taught chemistry and later clinical practice at the College of Philadelphia, which would soon become the University of Pennsylvania.

common place books, more useful to them, in the evening of life, than any of the books which belong to their libraries.' RUSH"[3]

From the days of his preceptorship, 1769–1772, Barker recorded his medical cases in case books and commonplace books and subsequently transferred many of them to his manuscript, *A History of Diseases of the District in Maine,*[4] which contains over 100 case reports, with Barker's findings, treatments and outcomes, a few autopsies, and observations on matters of diet and public health. He often included his thoughts about accepted medical philosophies and ideas on various illnesses and epidemics, and described changes as he saw them. He cited cases from contemporary medical texts, letters, and medical journals including the *Medical Repository,*[5] to which he contributed at least twelve articles between 1797 and 1818. Barker documented his constant efforts to use the contemporary medical literature to support his therapies, trying always to be a "scientific physician" at a time of great changes in medicine. Thus, his manuscript is an unusually complete example of the day-to-day

[3] Barker, "Barker Manuscript," vol. 2, 4.

[4] Barker, "Barker Manuscript." Collection 13 includes several of Jeremiah Barker's case books, abstracts of several medical texts from 1765 to 1814, commonplace books, letters, offprints, and books. For example, his "Abstract from Brooke's Practice of Physic particularly a relation of symptoms" is dated 1771; see R. Brookes, *The General Practice of Physic: Extracted Chiefly from the Writings of the Most Celebrated Practical Physicians, and the Medical Essays, Transactions, Journals, and Literary Correspondence of the Learned Societies in Europe: To Which Is Prefixed, an Introduction, Containing the Distinction of Similar Diseases, the Use of the Non-Naturals, an Account of the Pulse, the Consent of the Nervous Parts, and a Sketch of the Animal Œconomy* (London: Printed for J. Newbery, 1765). The cases recorded at the bedside in case books are accurately represented in the manuscript. For more on the background of commonplace books see: Ann Blair, *Too Much to Know: Managing Scholarly Information before the Modern Age* (New Haven, CT: Yale University Press, 2010), 131–32.

[5] For more on the *Medical Repository*, see Catherine O'Donnell Kaplan, *Men of Letters in the Early Republic Cultivating Forums of Citizenship* (Chapel Hill, NC: Published for the Omohundro Institute of Early American History and Culture, Williamsburg, Virginia, by the University of North Carolina Press, 2008), 87–113; R. J. Kahn and P. G. Kahn, "The Medical Repository—the First U.S. Medical Journal (1797–1824)," *New England Journal of Medicine* 337 (1997), 1926–30. Though Barker cites many sources with extracts, he should be considered the "author" of his book and not a merely a "compiler." Around the year AD 1250, Bonaventure at the University of Paris wrote: "Fourfold is the manner of making a book. For one who writes another's [words], by adding or changing nothing; he is called merely a scribe [scriptor]. Another writes another's words by adding, but not from his own; and that one is called a compiler. Another writes both his own words and another's but the other's as the principal ones and his own as those annexed for evidence; and that one is called a commentator, not an author. Another writes both his own words and another's but his own as the principal ones, the other's as things annexed for conformation; and such ought to be called an author." See Blair, *Too Much to Know*, 175–76.

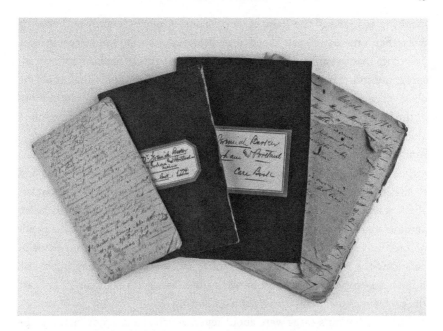

FIGURE 3.1. Barker's case books. Barker used material from his case books from as early as 1772 to write his *History of Diseases* manuscript. Careful checking reveals that his cases were accurately described, without change or embellishment. Courtesy of the Maine Historical Society.

practice of an ordinary rural physician, a man unaffiliated with a university, hospital, or medical school, a person whose scholarly efforts were entirely of his own making. As such, it should further expand our understanding of medicine, disease, and public health in the new republic. (See Figure 3.1.)

BASICS OF GREEK MEDICINE AND FEVER

The big changes in medicine began in the eighteenth century and were well underway by Barker's time, but the influence of the ancients, especially Hippocrates and Galen, was still strong. Part of Barker's compulsion to observe and record information stemmed from his efforts to understand and explain the huge changes he saw in the everyday practice of medicine.

Barker would surely have read about the science of the ancient Greeks, which included the four ultimate elements (substances)—air, water, fire, and earth, and the four primary qualities—dry, moist, hot, and cold. These were coupled with the primary four humors—blood, *sanguis* (air); phlegm, *flegma* (water); yellow bile, *chole* (fire); and black bile, *melanchole* (earth). Greek medicine as found in the "Hippocratic corpus," almost certainly authored by more than one man, "systemized a medical outlook that had largely broken free of its magical and religious sources . . . [and] encouraged disciplined observation and experiment."[6] The theory involved body fluids that could be observed, and disease was defined as disproportionate amounts of one or more of the humors.[7] Illness was thought to be caused by imbalance of the humors altered by various forces including air, water, and places, the patient's environment. Historian Helen Bynum points out "there were diseased individuals rather than diseases" and treatment involved "rebalancing the humours and regulating the six non-naturals: air (surrounding atmosphere), diet, exercise, sleep, wastes (excretions), and emotions."[8] Health was considered to be an agreeable balance of the four humors, and restoration of health was the result of a return to the natural balance of these humors. This ancient medicine of balancing the four humors sounds peculiar and unworkable today, but it still influenced everyday practice in Barker's time. Two good examples of this are the problem of fever and the use of bloodletting.

Many of Barker's cases were about fever, which was a major factor of life and death in the Early Republic.[9] Body temperature and fever (*pyretos*) have been monitored for more than two millennia as a means of differentiating

---

[6] David J. Rothman, Steven Marcus, and Stephanie A. Kiceluk, *Medicine and Western Civilization* (New Brunswick, NJ: Rutgers University Press, 1995), 43.

[7] The subject of Greek medical theory is far more complicated and involves solid organs as well as fluids. See V. Nutton, "Medicine in the Greek World, 800–50 BC," in *The Western Medical Tradition: 800 BC–1800 AD*, ed. Lawrence I. Conrad and Wellcome Institute for the History of Medicine (Cambridge, UK; New York: Cambridge University Press, 1995), 11–38. For further study, see Henry E. Sigerist, *A History of Medicine: Vol. 2: Early Greek, Hindu, and Persian Medicine* (New York: Oxford University Press, 1961), 317–35; *The Genuine Works of Hippocrates*, ed. Francis Adams (Baltimore: Williams and Wilkins, 1939); Lester S. King, *The Road to Medical Enlightenment, 1650–1695*, History of Science Library (Cambridge) (London: MacDonald, 1970), 18–21; Lester S. King, *The Philosophy of Medicine: The Early Eighteenth Century* (Cambridge, MA: Harvard University Press, 1978), 189–95; Lawrence I. Conrad and Wellcome Institute for the History of Medicine, *The Western Medical Tradition: 800 BC to AD 1800* (Cambridge, UK; New York: Cambridge University Press, 1995), 60–70, 480–82; Jacalyn Duffin, *History of Medicine: A Scandalously Short Introduction* (Toronto: University of Toronto Press, 1999), 43–46, 70–77.

[8] Helen Bynum, *Spitting Blood: The History of Tuberculosis* (Oxford: Oxford University Press, 2012), 11, and 1–22 for an overview of the Ancients' view of disease.

[9] Christopher Hamlin, *More Than Hot: A Short History of Fever*, Johns Hopkins Biographies of Disease (Baltimore: Johns Hopkins University Press, 2014), 1. Hamlin quotes Gerard van Swieten (1700–1772), who said that fever was a normal part of life that "ended most lives—an exaggeration, but not by so great a stretch."

health from disease. Hippocrates of Cos (c. 450–370 BCE)[10] considered fever an imbalance of the humors that was determined by touch (skin warmer than normal) and an accelerated pulse.[11] Claudius Galen of Pergamum (c. 131–201 CE), however, thought fever itself was a disease rather than a sign of disease. Galen believed that the yellow bile, black bile, and phlegm were pathological humors that are there "to preserve the balance" and if there is too much of them, fever results. He described several kinds of fever. Ephemeral fever is due to temporary overheating of the body and the doctor's task is to cool it. Inflammatory fevers are more difficult, and bloodletting may be necessary. If putrefaction of the humors has taken place, the problem is even more difficult, and in addition, the body must rid itself of the residues; hence the need for laxatives, cathartics, and medication to treat suppressed menses.[12] Barker, who would have begun his practice in 1772 following the ideas of the ancients, was by 1797 talking about a revolution in the practice of medicine that included his own new ideas about using alkaline therapy for fever, rather than "emptying the intestines of this *mischievous liquor*" called acrid bile.[13]

---

[10] Sometimes referred to as "the Hippocratic corpus," the name Hippocrates actually refers to "a heterogenous collection of works by an unknown number of different writers compiled over a period of up to two centuries." Ian Johnston, *Galen on Diseases and Symptoms* (Cambridge, New York: Cambridge University Press, 2006), 86.

[11] Hippocrates "directs us to observe the Pulse . . . [and that] the pulse 'tis vehement in inflamed Parts . . . And in the fourth book of Epidemics he calls the pulse in high Fevers quick and great." John Floyer, *The Physician's Pulse-Watch; or, an Essay to Explain the Old Art of Feeling the Pulse, and to Improve It by the Help of a Pulse-Watch. In Three Parts. I. The Old Galenic Art of Feeling the Pulse Is Describ'd, and Many of Its Errors Corrected: The True Use of the Pulses, and Their Causes, Differences and Prognostications by Them, Are Fully Explain'd, and Directions Given for Feeling the Pulse by the Pulse-Watch, or Minute-Glass. II. A New Mechanical Method Is Propos'd for Preserving Health, and Prolonging Life, and for Curing Diseases by the Help of the Pulse-Watch, Which Shews the Pulses When They Exceed or Are Deficient from the Natural. III. The Chinese Art of Feeling the Pulse Is Describ'd; and the Imitation of Their Practice of Physick, Which Is Grounded on the Observation of the Pulse, Is Recommended. To Which Is Added, an Extract out of Andrew Cleyer, Concerning the Chinese Art of Feeling the Pulse. By Sir John Floyer, Knight* (London: printed for Sam. Smith and Benj. Walford, at the Prince's-Arms in St. Paul's Church-Yard, 1707), Monograph, 1–2.

[12] Johnston, *Galen on Diseases and Symptoms*, 114, 160–63; W. F. Wright and P. A. Mackowiak, "Origin, Evolution and Clinical Application of the Thermometer," *American Journal of the Medical Sciences* 351, no. 5 (2016): 526. For more on Galen and diagnosis and prognosis, see Luis Garcia Ballester, "Galen as a Medical Practitioner: Problems in Diagnosis," in *Galen: Problems and Prospects*, ed. V. Nutton (London: The Wellcome Institute for the History of Medicine, 1981), 13–46.

[13] Jeremiah Barker, "On Febrifuge Virtues of Lime, Magnesia and Alkaline Salts in Dysentery, Yellow-Fever and Scarlatina Angiosa. In a Letter from Dr. Jeremiah Barker, of Portland, (Maine) Dated May 30, 1798," *Medical Repository* 2, no. 2 (1798). This is discussed further in chapter 4 of the Introduction.

BLOODLETTING: THE BLOOD WAS "SIZY AND BUFFY"

One of the most accepted healing procedures "firmly imbedded in Greek hu-moral pathology" was bloodletting (venesection), which was used to treat var-ious disease states including acute inflammations, pneumonia, and orthopnea (shortness of breath when lying flat). Historian Guenter Risse notes that therapeutic "bleeding reached new levels of popularity and intensity both in Europe and America in the early nineteenth century."[14] Thus on June 21, 1801, Dr. Benjamin Vaughan of Hallowell, Maine, wrote to Benjamin Rush in Philadelphia: "Bleeding is now in such repute in our town, that our patients send to the doctor not for his advice, but to be blooded."[15]

Barker frequently prescribed bloodletting and often described the patient's blood as being normal or "sizy and buffy." What does this mean? In 1921, Robin Fåhraeus[16] explained that in humoral or "Grecian hematology" a sample of the patient's blood removed therapeutically and placed in a vessel soon divides into components of black bile on the bottom of the "blood cake," with yellow bile above it (serum), and a thin layer of "phlegm" on top. A thick "phlegm" layer, called a buffy coat, is seen in diseases such as pneumonia; in the humoral system of the ancient physicians, expectoration would represent dissolved sizy material or "phlegm." In studying the suspension-stability of blood, Fåhraeus noted, as had earlier researchers, that the red blood cells fall faster in patients with inflammatory diseases and that the thick "fibrin coagula," is strongest "in the case of a deadly disease [that] gives rise to a thick buffy coat."[17] Fåhraeus

---

[14] Guenter B. Risse, "The Renaissance of Bloodletting: A Chapter in Modern Therapeutics," *Journal of the History of Medicine and Allied Sciences* 34, no. 1 (1979): 3–22; Heinrich Stern, *Theory and Practice of Bloodletting* (New York: Rebman Company, 1915), 3–43; Robin Fåhraeus, *The Suspension-Stability of the Blood* (Stockholm: Norstedt, 1921), 3–44; Robin Fåhraeus, "The Suspension Stability of the Blood," *Physiological Reviews* 9, no. 2 (1929), 241–74.

[15] Benjamin Vaughan, "Letter from Benjamin Vaughn to Benjamin Rush, 21 June 1801," in *Manuscript Correspondence of Benjamin Rush UV 18, MSS 55*, ed. Historical Society of Pennsylvania (1801).

[16] Robin Fåhraeus (1888–1968) was a Swedish hematologist, pathologist, and medical historian whose studies formed some of the basic works developing hemorheology, the study of flow properties of blood, plasma, and cells; viscosity.

[17] In the first two chapters of his 1921 book, Fåhraeus discusses the history of the buffy coat in blood, as drawn from patients and not treated with an anticoagulant; the remainder of the book discusses later works and his research on blood. Very briefly, he explains that in chronically ill/febrile patients, the red corpuscles sink so rapidly that they form a sediment before the blood clots, therefore making "a more or less thick fibrinous layer which does not form in the blood of a healthy person, in whom the corpuscles sink comparatively slowly." Fåhraeus, "The Suspension Stability of the

concluded that "in the works of Galeus we find the earliest description of the buffy coat which has been preserved up to our times."[18] This evaluation of the buffy coat, as described, may represent a precursor of the first laboratory tests, though observation of urine and stool had also been part of the diagnostic process. It is safe to assume that Barker, observing the "buffy coat," would consider this additional evidence that an inflammatory process was taking place, and that his treatment should be altered accordingly.

Blood," 241. Other names for the buffy coat include *crusta pseudomembranacea* and *crusta inflammatoria* and in a more specific case, *crusta pleuritica*. Here we are interested in his extensive review of the buffy coat as reported by Hippocrates, Galen, von Helmont, Malpighi, Harvey, Sydenham, Boerhaave, Gaubius, John Hunter, Cullen, Piorry, Rokitansky, van Swieten, Deewes, and Denis. Fåhraeus points out that before the use of microscopes, laboratory chemistry, and bacteriology, careful macroscopical observation of the buffy coat provided a rich source of data for the physician. Some thought the buffy coat was phlegm (the fibrin layer looks like phlegm) and part of the disease-causing process, whereas others, such as Paracelsus (1493–1541), thought that changes in the various layers of drawn blood were the result of disease (p. 15). In Sydenham's discussion of pleurisy (seventeenth century), he describes a buffy coat that "looks like melted tallow . . . the top resembles true pus." Thomas Sydenham, Samuel Johnson, and John Swan, *The Entire Works of Dr. Thomas Sydenham, Newly Made English from the Originals: Wherein the History of Acute and Chronic Diseases, and the Safest and Most Effectual Methods of Treating Them, Are Faithfully, Clearly, and Accurately Delivered. To Which Are Added, Explanatory and Practical Notes, from the Best Medicinal Writers* (London: Printed for Edward Cave, at St. John's Gate, 1742), 231. He believed the two signs of inflammation are the buffy coat and fever. The studies of suspension-stability by Fåhraeus form part of our current understanding of a test still in use today, the erythrocyte sedimentation rate (ESR). Fåhraeus credits Biernacki as being the first to call attention to the clinical use of the sedimentation speed of blood cells using anticoagulated blood (pp. 62–68). It is a test of acute-phase reactants (certain proteins) and viscosity in the evaluation of acute or chronic inflammation. In recent years the test has largely been replaced by another test, the C-reactive protein (CRP). Fåhraeus, *The Suspension-Stability of the Blood*, 3–68.

[18] Fåhraeus, *The Suspension-Stability of the Blood*, 13, with a footnote citing Kühn's translation of Galen, 1821: Galen, and Karl Gottlob Kühn. *Klaudiou Galenou Hapanta = Claudii Galeni Opera Omnia. Medicorum Graecorum Opera Quae Exstant.* 20 vols. Lipsiae: Cnoblochii, 1821, vol. 1, p. 496. Maxwell M. Wintrobe, *Blood, Pure and Eloquent: A Story of Discovery, of People, and of Ideas* (New York: McGraw-Hill, 1980), 1–4; John Harley Warner, *The Therapeutic Perspective: Medical Practice, Knowledge, and Identity in America, 1820–85* (Cambridge, MA: Harvard University Press, 1986), 131–32; Duffin, *History of Medicine: A Scandalously Short Introduction*, 178. For more on buffy coat, see William Heberden, "Is the Sizy Covering Which Is Often Seen Upon Blood of Any Use in Directing the Method of Cure?," *Medical Tansactions of the Royal College of Physicians of London*. 2 (1772): 499–505; John Hunter, *A Treatise on the Blood, Inflammation, and Gun-Shot Wounds*, 2 vols. (Philadelphia: Thomas Bradford, 1796); John Hunter and James F. Palmer, *The Works of John Hunter, Frs: With Notes*, 4 vols., vol. 1 (London: Longman, 1835); H. C. Gram, "On the Causes of the Variations in the Sedimentation of the Corpuscles and the Formation of the Crusta Phlogistica (Size, Buffy Coat) on the Blood. Blood Sedimentation Mechanism," *Archives of Internal Medicine*. 28 (1921): 312–30.

A rational basis for managing disease could be made by balancing the humors by diet, exercise, and other means, such as bloodletting, and by making a sound prognosis. The works and comments of Hippocrates and later Galen would continue to influence medicine for more than fifteen hundred years. Eventually changes in the philosophy of science, the enlightenment, and the study of chemistry, physiology, anatomy, and pathology would bring us to the eighteenth century.[19] This is where Barker practiced and struggled with the changes that were taking place.

"SCIENTIFIC DOCTORS" AND THE "EMPIRICS"

For millennia and through the eighteenth century, religion taught that illness and death were the will of God and should be accepted humbly and submissively as God's judgment. The healing arts were often practiced by ministers, as illustrated in the Barker manuscript, and by self-taught or minimally trained "empirical" doctors. Regular physicians often used "empirics" as a derogatory term for anyone who was content with his direct experience, that is, satisfied with "facts which are real and inescapable, and do not depend for their force on any theoretical consideration. It was not necessary to have general premises, deductions, or inferences."[20] Nor was it necessary to read about current medical theory.

It is important to remember that in the colonial period and early nineteenth century, most communities were too small and too poor to support full-time physicians. Therefore, except in major cities and towns, the practice of medicine was often a part-time job, with physicians who also worked as teachers, farmers, or shopkeepers. These were among the "empirics" who were seen as dangerous rivals to the emergence of medicine as a learned profession.[21] The elite, "regular," or "scientific" physicians and their students, however, had

[19] For details, see Conrad and Wellcome Institute, *The Western Medical Tradition: 800 BC to AD 1800*, 19–31, 58–70. See also King, *The Philosophy of Medicine: The Early Eighteenth Century*, 190–232; Duffin, *History of Medicine: A Scandalously Short Introduction*, 11–89.

[20] Lester S. King, *The Medical World of the Eighteenth Century* (Huntington, NY: Robert E. Krieger Publishing Co. Inc. [reprint 1971], 1958), 40–41; Warner, *The Therapeutic Perspective*, 43–46.

[21] William G. Rothstein, *American Physicians in the Nineteenth Century; from Sects to Science* (Baltimore: Johns Hopkins University Press, 1972), 34–36; Guenter B. Risse, "Introduction," in *Medicine without Doctors: Home Health Care in American History*, ed. Judith Walzer Leavitt, Ronald L. Numbers, and Guenter B. Risse (New York: Science History Publications, 1977), 1–8; Ronald L. Numbers, "Do-It-Yourself the Sectarian Way," in *Medicine without Doctors: Home Health Care in American History*, ed. Judith

difficulty showing the superiority of their diagnosis and treatment to those of the so-called empirics.[22] In addition to diagnosis and therapy, "scientific physicians" were expected to name the disease, understand its causes, and offer a prognosis, but the truth is that at that time there were few treatments that were properly understood and genuinely effective. However, the work of Sir Isaac Newton had created "a single mathematical system that provided orderly explanation for terrestrial and celestial phenomena"; might not medicine improve health of society with the right systems/science and information in place?[23]

In its efforts to promote "scientific medicine," the Massachusetts Medical Society and Harvard Medical School hoped to bring the healing arts in Massachusetts up to European standards. Possession of a regular medical education, that is, a preceptorship by a preceptorship-trained physician, with or without didactic lectures at a medical school, continued to be one mark of a regular physician and gradually increased the prestige that physicians gained in society as medicine became a true profession.[24] This tension and

Walzer Leavitt, Ronald L. Numbers, and Guenter B. Risse (New York: Science History Publications, 1977), 49–72.

[22] With a few exceptions, "science made little impact on medicine until the end of the nineteenth century . . . [but] physicians employed the rhetoric of science in their search for professional legitimation." S. E. D. Shortt, "Physicians, Science, and Status: Issues in the Professionalization of Anglo-American Medicine in the Nineteenth Century," *Medical History* 27, no. 1 (1983): 52, 62. But what is science? I. Bernard Cohen points out that in the eighteenth century, "without a qualifier [it] could imply knowledge in general." I. Bernard Cohen, *Science and the Founding Fathers: Science in the Political Thought of Jefferson, Franklin, Adams and Madison*, 1st ed. (New York: W.W. Norton, 1995), 238. Thomas Kuhn notes that science "owes its success to the ability of scientists regularly to select problems that can be solved with conceptual and instrumental techniques close to those already in existence." Thomas S. Kuhn, *The Structure of Scientific Revolutions*, 3rd ed. (Chicago: The University of Chicago Press, 1996), 96. See also the OED definitions of the word "science." There are 379 medical titles from 1665 to 1799 in Margaret Batschelet, *Early American Scientific and Technical Literature: An Annotated Bibliography of Books, Pamphlets, and Broadsides* (Metuchen, NJ: Scarecrow Press, 1990). All of this is not to say that medicine is not useful, as Jacalyn Duffin comments in a personal communication: providing comfort, naming, giving a prognosis, a number of surgical procedures, and some medications still in use today used the less technical definition of "science" in the eighteenth-century sense of the word.

[23] Lester S. King, *Transformations in American Medicine: From Benjamin Rush to William Osler* (Baltimore: Johns Hopkins University Press, 1991), 13, 22.

[24] John Harley Warner, *Against the Spirit of System: The French Impulse in Nineteenth-Century American Medicine* (Princeton, NJ: Princeton University Press, 1998), 20. Augmentation of knowledge and skills or professional improvement, "enhanced professional standing, chances to win recognition and esteem from other physicians, and improve prospects for recruiting affluent patients." Warner also points out that a physician's professional identity was based more on practice and "not as it became

competition between the self-taught or slightly trained "empirical" doctors and others, and the learned or "scientific" practitioners continued through the nineteenth century. Barker claimed that his principal aim in writing his book was "to aid the efforts of my medical brethren, in eradicating medical prejudices & disseminating useful knowledge; in engaging the mind to greater solicitude for the enjoyment of life & health; in exposing & suppressing empirical impositions, which rapidly increase; and finally in rendering the Science of Medicine more respectable & important in the view of mankind."[25]

MORE COMPETITION: DOMESTIC AND SECTARIAN MEDICINE

Self-help or domestic medicine as a familial or communal activity dates back to ancient times. Mothers and grandmothers were, and still are, frequently the first consulted when illness struck the family. Their recipe or "receipt" books included instructions for curing hemorrhoids and infected fingers as well as cooking and preserving food and dyeing homespun fabrics. Increasing literacy and decreasing cost of paper and printing encouraged numerous self-help books, such as William Buchan's *Domestic Medicine*, first published in Edinburgh in 1769.[26] Historian Guenter Risse attributes the motivation concerning domestic medicine or self-help to feelings of self-reliance, scarcity of medical professionals (particularly in rural areas), inability to pay for such care, and for some, a general distrust of the medical profession.[27] A doctor was more likely to be called for severe disease, major trauma, arterial bleeds, fractures, and during epidemics than for ordinary everyday ailments.

Often the first call, after mothers and grandmothers, was to the female (and sometimes male) healer, one of many who moved in and out of the community's sick rooms as friends and neighbors with a local reputation for care-giving based on experience—watching at the bedside, delivering babies, laying out the dead. They are often difficult to identify in contemporary accounts, lacking "Doctor" before their names. Although there were no laws

to a large extent after the late nineteenth century, upon a claim of special knowledge." Warner, *The Therapeutic Perspective*,1986, 13.

[25] Barker, "Barker Manuscript," vol. 2, 8.

[26] William M. D. Buchan, *Domestic Medicine; or, the Family Physician . . . Chiefly Calculated to Recommend a Proper Attention to Regimen and Simple Medicines* (Edinburgh: Balfour, Auld & Smellie, 1769); Paul Starr, *The Social Transformation of American Medicine* (New York: Basic Books, 1982), 32–35.

[27] Risse, "Introduction to Medicine without Doctors," 1–8.

preventing them from drawing blood or administering strong drugs such as calomel (a mercury preparation), they generally did not do so, and they sometimes called in the physician for difficult or possibly lethal cases. The terms "domestic," "folk," "popular," "indigenous," "traditional," "herbal," "lay," or "social medicine" bring with them different connotations for these women. Historian Laurel Thatcher Ulrich tells us that some physicians resented them,[28] but Barker makes scant mention of these healers and does not include them in his denunciations of empirics and others. This is interesting, because we know that they were everywhere, and he must have encountered them often in his practice. He complains bitterly and frequently about the empirics, sectarians, and the followers of Brown, discussed later, but not about the domestic healers who also provided competition for his practice. The implication is, perhaps, that he considered their ministrations to be helpful and useful, whereas he disagreed strongly with some of the other so-called physicians of his day.

Jeremiah Barker and Martha Ballard, the midwife in A Midwife's Tale, were both caring for patients during the same years and their practices were only sixty miles apart in Maine. They both worked very hard—Barker, for example, wrote in a casebook that in the influenza epidemic in 1807, "For two entire months I did not spend a single day in my own home, and seldom slept more than three hours out of the twenty-four." He must have spent most of his time reading and writing when not directly caring for patients. Martha Ballard's diary records her treatment of patients but also her many other womanly activities such as washing clothes, gardening, helping neighbors with other work. "There is no evidence in the diary of borrowing [books]—she never mentions reading a medical book—yet Ballard's remedies obviously rested on a long accumulation of English remedies."[29] And many of her "folk" medicines were used by the regular physicians of her time. Thus, we see the two sides of medical knowledge—word of mouth and recipe books on one hand, and the transmitted written word found in books, journals, and letters, on the other—overlapping and both practicing the art of medicine.

Part of Barker's purpose in writing was to make a strong case for regular medicine at a time of increasingly stiff competition from an array of medical sectarians. The term "sectarian" refers to "botanics and eclectics, homeopaths and hydropaths, movement-curists and mind-curists, and others

---

[28] Laurel Thatcher Ulrich, A Midwife's Tale: The Life of Martha Ballard, Based on Her Diary, 1785–1812 (Alfred A. Knopf, 1990), 60–61, 65.

[29] Ulrich, A Midwife's Tale: The Life of Martha Ballard, Based on Her Diary, 1785–1812, 51.

too numerous to mention" who "arose in the nineteenth century to chal-
lenge the heroic therapy of the regulars with their seemingly endless rounds
of bleedings, blisterings, and purgings."[30] These included the Thomsonians
led by leader Samuel Thomson, a farmer interested in botanic medicine. His
was a movement that began in 1806 and was waning by the 1840s. Thomson
believed that all illnesses were cold and therefore needed heat in the form of
steam, pepper, and lobelia as an emetic. He sold individual and family rights
to practice his system, and his book, *Every Man His Own Physician*, allowed
people to have a less costly way of providing family care and avoiding the regular physicians. Another sect, homeopathy, began in Germany and appeared
in the United States in 1825. Homeopathic pills did not cause puking, purging,
or salivation, and the bleeding still being used by regular physicians was
strictly forbidden. Hydropathy or the "water cure" arrived in the United States
from Silesia, now Poland, in the mid-1840s and became popular throughout
the nineteenth century.[31]

Thomsonians and homeopaths gradually increased their numbers as the
"therapeutic impotence of the regular practitioners became obvious."[32] As
medical sociologist William Rothstein concludes, the relative causal effects of
scientific and economic forces are difficult to quantify.[33] However, although
there were few remedies that actually worked at this time as viewed by the
twenty-first-century reader, the regular physician versed in science gradually
gained an advantage as science became an increasing element of middle-class
discourse, allowing physicians to achieve "social legitimacy." [34] The development of medical societies and medical schools provided prestige and, with
some regulation of economic competition, helped regular physicians compete
with empirics, sectarians, and others. Physicians "gained stature not because

[30] Numbers, "Do-It-Yourself the Sectarian Way," 49.

[31] Numbers, "Do-It-Yourself the Sectarian Way," 49–72, and Rothstein, *American Physicians in the Nineteenth Century; from Sects to Science*, 125–174. Starr, *The Social Transformation of American Medicine*, 30–54.

[32] Shortt, "Physicians, Science, and Status: Issues in the Professionalization of Anglo-American Medicine in the Nineteenth Century," 55; John Duffy, *The Healers: A History of American Medicine*, Illini books ed. (Urbana, IL: University of Illinois Press, 1979), 109–28.

[33] Rothstein, *American Physicians in the Nineteenth Century; from Sects to Science*, 5, 15.

[34] Rothstein, *American Physicians in the Nineteenth Century; from Sects to Science*, 4–10, 26–37.

they could always act effectively, but because only they could name, describe and explain."[35]

SCIENCE, INSTITUTIONS, EDUCATION, FRAMING DISEASE, AND CULTURAL AUTHORITY

Though Barker wrote about his discussions with "scientific physicians," medicine in his day was not a science in the sense of searching for general truths or universal laws of nature. Science as we know it requires controlling the variables, and most of the variables of disease and illness cannot be controlled in the individual patient. Medicine has since been defined by ethicist Kathryn Montgomery Hunter as "a science-using, judgement-based practice committed to the knowledge and care of human illness,"[36] and more recently, as the "systematic work of observation, data collection, theorizing about natural causes, or experimental production of knowledge."[37] But historian of science Lorraine Daston points out the period before 1850, when the word "science" referred to different disciplines and practices than the current restrictive usage: "that practices now considered unambiguously scientific (e.g., systematic observation of astro-meteorological phenomena) were pursued by people who had nothing to do with the university professors usually singled out as the past counterparts of modern scientists."[38]

The elite physicians, their students, and the existing medical institutions of the eighteenth century gradually gained strength following the Revolutionary

[35] Shortt, "Physicians, Science, and Status: Issues in the Professionalization of Anglo-American Medicine in the Nineteenth Century," 63; Charles E. Rosenberg, Janet Lynne Golden, and Francis Clark Wood Institute for the History of Medicine, *Framing Disease: Studies in Cultural History*, Health and Medicine in American Society (New Brunswick, NJ: Rutgers University Press, 1997), xvi–xviii; Warner, *The Therapeutic Perspective*, 17–23. For more on medical pluralism internationally, see Robert Jütte and Institut für Geschichte der Medizin Robert Bosch Stiftung, *Medical Pluralism: Past, Present, Future* (Stuttgart: Franz Steiner Verlag, 2013).

[36] Kathryn Montgomery Hunter, *Doctors' Stories: The Narrative Structure of Medical Knowledge* (Princeton, NJ: Princeton University Press, 1991), 47. Cohen, *Science and the Founding Fathers: Science in the Political Thought of Jefferson, Franklin, Adams and Madison*, 52–53. Brooke Hindle, "The Doctors: Naturalists and Physicians," in *The Pursuit of Science in Revolutionary America 1735–1789* (Chapel Hill: The University of North Carolina Press, 1956), 36–58.

[37] Bolton Conevery Valencius et al., "Science in Early America: Print Culture and the Sciences of Territoriality," *Journal of the Early Republic* 36, no. 1 (2016): 82.

[38] Lorraine Daston, "The History of Science and the History of Knowledge," *KNOW: A Journal on the Formation of Knowledge* 1, no. 1 (2017): 140.

War through politics, the support of learned societies, and emulation of British institutions held in high esteem.[39] Again, this occurred even though the merits of scientific medicine "were open to reasonable doubt" until after the mid-nineteenth century.[40] Barker was elected a Fellow of the Massachusetts Medical Society in June of 1803. A year later he, Nathaniel Coffin, and four other Maine physicians petitioned the Council of the Massachusetts Medical Society to allow a District of Maine Medical Society with meetings to be held in Portland.[41]

As we have seen, little formal training was required to practice medicine in America through the first half of the nineteenth century. So why would an American physician "voluntarily labor for advanced education" in a society that did not require nor "reward superior professional knowledge?"[42] In the late eighteenth and early nineteenth century, the core program for an American who aspired to a regular medical practice consisted of a three-year preceptorship (apprenticeship) that might be supplemented with didactic

[39] Ralph Samuel Bates, *Scientific Societies in the United States*, 3rd ed. (Cambridge: MIT Press, 1965), 16–21, 237–41. Bates points out that "more men in the colonies were devoting their time to study and practice the healing arts than to any other field of scientific endeavor . . . [and the physicians] had banded together for the advancement of their knowledge and to protect and further the interest of their profession." By 1820 there were at least twenty-one Learned and Medical Societies in the colonies and early Republic. John C. Greene, "The Boston Medical Comunity and Emerging Science, 1780–1820," in *Medicine in Colonial Massachusetts 1620–1820* (Boston: The Colonial Society of Massachusetts, 1980), 187–97.

[40] Richard D. Brown, "The Healing Arts in Colonial and Revolutionary Massachusetts: The Context for Scientific Medicine," in *Medicine in Colonial Massachusetts, 1620–1820: A Conference Held 25 & 26 May 1978*, ed. Philip Cash, Eric H. Christianson, and J. Worth Estes (Boston: The Colonial Society of Massachusetts, 1980), 36–47. Warner, *The Therapeutic Perspective*, 37–57.

[41] Jeremiah Barker, "Letter to Dr. Joseph Whipple of Boston Thanking Him for Notifying Barker of His Election a Fellow of the Massachusetts Medical-Society," in *Barker, Jeremiah*, ed. Countway Library Harvard (1803), B MS c 75.2. Nathaniel Coffin, Jeremiah Barker, Shirley Ervin, Dudley Folsom, Stephen Thomas, Aaron Kinsman, "Letter to the the Massachusetts Medical-Society Requesting Permission to Allow a District of Maine Medical Society," in *Coffin, Nathaniel*, ed. Countway Library Harvard (Portland, Maine, 1804). Dr. Samuel Emerson of Kennebunk, District of Maine, placed a notice in the *Eastern Argus* on December 19, 1819, calling for members of the Massachusetts Medical Society living in Maine to form a Maine Medical Society. The meeting was held in 1820 and the Society was legally incorporated in 1821; Dr. Nathaniel Coffin of Portland was elected president. See James Alfred Spalding, *Maine Physicians of 1820; a Record of the Members of the Massachusetts Medical Society Practicing in the District of Maine at the Date of Separation* (Lewiston: Lewiston Print Shop, 1928), 5–10.

[42] Warner, *Against the Spirit of System: The French Impulse in Nineteenth-Century American Medicine*, 17–22.

lectures at a medical school. This three- to four-month lecture series, repeated twice, gradually became the norm during the second quarter of the nineteenth century, and attendance at medical school increased as more schools joined the two that existed during Barker's training.[43]

The professionalization of medicine in America was developing within and without state and local medical societies, and "regular medicine" would form "an emerging group [coalescing] around a particular configuration of knowledge."[44] Thus, when Barker wrote about "scientific physicians," he was referring to "learned or regular" physicians who read the same books and articles on medicine and science that he read and interacted with those of similar education and reading. The term "regular physician" cannot be defined precisely, but medical historian Whitfield Bell maintains that it "connotes a combination of formal preparation, ethical conduct, and a demonstrated success in practice."[45]

Sociologist Paul Starr points out that cultural authority[46] for physicians to interpret signs and symptoms in the diagnosis, prognosis, and treatment of illness involves "shaping the patients' understanding of their own experience . . . to create the conditions under which [the physician's] advice seems appropriate."[47] Historian Charles Rosenberg concludes that "Both physician

---

[43] J. S. Billings, "Literature and Institutions," in *A Century of American Medicine: 1776–1876*, ed. Edward H. Clarke (Philadelphia: Henry C. Lea, 1876), 355–59; William G. Rothstein, *American Medical Schools and the Practice of Medicine: A History* (New York: Oxford University Press, 1987), 25–36.

[44] Shortt, "Physicians, Science, and Status: Issues in the Professionalization of Anglo-American Medicine in the Nineteenth Century," 52. Philip Cash, "Professionalization of Boston Medicine, 1760–1803," in *Medicine in Colonial Massachusetts, 1620–1820*, ed. Philip Cash, Eric H. Christianson, and J. Worth Estes (Boston: The Colonial Society of Massachusetts, 1980), 69–100. Warner, *Against the Spirit of System: The French Impulse in Nineteenth-Century American Medicine*, 17–31.

[45] Whitfield J. Bell, *The Colonial Physician and Other Essays* (New York: Science History Publications, 1975), 9. Regarding "success in practice," Warner notes that for most of the nineteenth century many practitioners "enjoyed the public's high esteem at a time when the profession as a whole was in a degraded position." Warner, *The Therapeutic Perspective*, 15–16.

[46] Cultural authority is the power to influence action, opinion, or belief. OED.

[47] Starr, *The Social Transformation of American Medicine*, 14. Bynum stresses that cultural authority in the eighteenth century came from the patient in a patient-dominated environment, whereas in the nineteenth century that cultural authority would shift to "hospitals, localistic pathology, and esoteric vocabulary (crucial characteristics of modern medicine) to dominate their patients." W. F. Bynum, "Health, Disease and Medical Care," in *The Ferment of Knowledge: Studies in the Historiography of Eighteenth-Century Science*, ed. G. S. Rousseau and Roy Porter (Cambridge: Cambridge University Press, 1980), 212. Historian Michael Worboys concludes that localized or "localistic"

and patient must share a compatible—though not necessarily identical—framework of explanation."[48] One of the responsibilities of the scientific or regular physician was naming the disease and giving it a regular context that would be understood by all. Today we call this framing the disease, and it is done in a way that reflects the social, moral, and religious attitudes of the time.

Illness is the unhealthy condition of not feeling well, but the disease must be given a name. How we frame a disease has great implications as to what kinds of treatment might be considered, what resources society is willing to expend, and how much sympathy the patient might deserve.[49] For historian John Burnham, disease has been defined as "a biological, a generation-specific repertoire of verbal constructs reflecting medicine's intellectual and institutional history, an occasion for and potential legitimation of public policy."[50] Our definitions of disease change over time with discoveries of biopathological mechanisms such as germ theory in the second half of the nineteenth century and genetic diseases in the twentieth century, but they are always influenced by societal attitudes and values at any point in time. Was consumption (tuberculosis) truly influenced by place of residence, demographics, personal behavior choices, inappropriate clothing, poverty, and/or poor nutrition? Are drug addiction, alcoholism, and HIV/AIDS diseases or results of willful immorality? The answers have significant influence on how medicine and society judge the victim and how much care and funding should be provided. Certainly, in

pathology was the "key conceptual revolution of the first half of the nineteenth century." The opportunities offered by hospitals allowed physicians to see many more patients and to compare and contrast symptoms with anatomical changes in organs and tissues found at dissection. The physicians could show that a particular symptom was associated with a particular pathological change and is "sometimes referred to as solidism" as contrasted with humoralism or fluidism. Michael Worboys, *Spreading Germs: Disease Theories and Medical Practice in Britain, 1865–1900* (Cambridge, UK; New York: Cambridge University Press, 2000), 28.

[48] Charles E. Rosenberg, "The Therapeutic Revolution: Medicine, Meaning, and Social Change in Nineteenth-Century America," *Perspectives in Biology and Medicine* 20, no. 4 (1977): 486; Charles E. Rosenberg, *Explaining Epidemics and Other Studies in the History of Medicine* (New York: Cambridge University Press, 1992), 9–31.

[49] Rosenberg, Golden, and Francis Clark Wood Institute, *Framing Disease: Studies in Cultural History*, xiii–xxvi. See also John C. Burnham, *What Is Medical History?* (Cambridge, UK; Malden, MA: Polity, 2005), 55–79; Joseph E. Davis and Ana Marta Gonzalez, eds., *To Fix or to Heal: Patient Care, Public Health, and the Limits of Biomedicine* (New York: New York University Press, 2016), 42–45.

[50] Burnham, *What Is Medical History?*, 56–58. See also Charles Rosenberg in Rosenberg, *Explaining Epidemics*, 305–18; Rosenberg, Golden, and Francis Clark Wood Institute, *Framing Disease: Studies in Cultural History*, xiii–xxvi.

Barker's time the increasingly complex language of medicine contributed to the growing influence of the regular physician. This shift in cultural authority began just at the time of Barker's practice, as formal education for physicians increasingly became the norm, and therefore more highly valued.

Barker apparently realized this when he wrote in his 1806 casebook that he carried medical books with him during his "attendance upon the sick, when engaged in extraordinary & difficult cases. . . . I have been induced to adopt this mode of conduct from observing that most learned & experienced Lawyers and even Judges, have recourse to books and notes when deciding upon intricate and important cases. Yet I have been told by some that it savours of ignorance for a physician to read after he has acquired an establishment in business!" Barker added that the lack of reading by physicians is a major reason for the "hostility with which improvements in medicine have been pursued by empirics."[51] He would show his patients that he was following the leading medical authorities in his choice of therapeutics. Bringing books to the bedside may also have conveyed Barker's self-image as a scholar/scientist/physician for, as historian Whitfield Bell tells us, "The practice of medicine in colonial America did not rank with law or the ministry in the intellectual endowments it required or, therefore, in the social rank it conferred."[52]

The importance of science in American intellectual life of seventeenth- and eighteenth-century colonial elites was accompanied by secularization[53] that emerged with the separation of church and state in the New Republic. In medicine, this resulted in a loss of religious authority (this illness is the will of God) and gain of medical authority (this illness can be treated).[54] Gradually the cultural authority of the regular physician became "based in the scientific profession of medicine rather than any person who claimed to be a doctor,

---

[51] Jeremiah Barker, "1806 Casebook," in *Maine Historical Society, Barker Collection 13, Box 1/5* (Portland, Maine, 1806), unpaginated.

[52] Bell, *The Colonial Physician and Other Essays*, 16. Warner concludes that "a physician looked to his profession for much of his identity but derived little of his status from that source." Warner, *The Therapeutic Perspective*, 15. Doctors in colonial America took the English as a model, though England had a much more hierarchical society. There physicians were a small, elite group of Oxford and Cambridge graduates, a learned profession, separate from the lower orders of surgeons and apothecaries. Starr, *The Social Transformation of American Medicine*, 37–40.

[53] Secularization is the transformation of a society away from close identification with religious values and institutions.

[54] Charles E. Rosenberg, *No Other Gods: On Science and American Social Thought* (Baltimore: The Johns Hopkins University Press, 1997), 2–3.

or any type of healing based on other theories."[55] As always in times of great change, society took two steps forward and one back. For example, medical licensure, in which the state grants exclusive privileges to physicians who meet certain qualifications, was encouraged by medical societies and medical schools after the 1760s, but these laws were weak and poorly enforced throughout the years of Barker's practice. A rising desire for an earlier simpler way of life and the critique of a professional aristocracy during the Jacksonian period led to repeal of many licensing laws during the 1820s and 1830s.[56]

Though there were only four medical schools in the United States in 1800, there were twenty-two by 1830.[57] Learned societies and medical journals also began to proliferate during the first three decades of the nineteenth century,[58] and there was an increasing competition for patients, particularly those of the middle and upper classes. Eighteenth-century enlightenment writers used medicine as a model of their new philosophy, conveying the hope of the promotion of health among the middle and upper class readers. The embrace of

---

[55] B. A. Pescosolido and J. K. Martin, "Cultural Authority and the Sovereignty of American Medicine: The Role of Networks, Class, and Community," *Journal of Health Politics, Policy and Law* 29, no. 4–5 (2004): 735. See also Gordon Gauchat, "The Cultural Authority of Science: Public Trust and Acceptance of Organized Science," *Public Understanding of Science* 20, no. 6 (2011), 752–70; Starr, *The Social Transformation of American Medicine*, 9–21.

[56] Warner, *Against the Spirit of System: The French Impulse in Nineteenth-Century American Medicine*, 203–204; Rothstein, *American Physicians in the Nineteenth Century; from Sects to Science*, 70–80. Also Richard Harrison Shryock, *Medical Licensing in America, 1650–1965* (Baltimore: Johns Hopkins Press, 1967), 3–42. Historian James Mohr points out that the 10th Amendment to the Constitution gave the power to regulate health to the States, but with "regulars" and the various sects having different views, "lawmakers had no objective criteria upon which to justify such [medical] licenses." James C. Mohr, *Licensed to Practice: The Supreme Court Defines the American Medical Profession* (Baltimore: Johns Hopkins University Press, 2013), 9, 10, 12, 18. Sociologist Paul Starr concludes that attempts by the American medical professional societies to set boundaries, standards, educational requirements "were rapidly eroded by competition, dissention, and contempt." Starr, *The Social Transformation of American Medicine*, 37.

[57] Rothstein, *American Medical Schools and the Practice of Medicine: A History*, 49. The number of graduates from US medical schools increased from 221 students for the period 1769–1799, to 4,338 in the decade from 1820 to 1829. Billings, "Literature and Institutions," 359.

[58] Kaufman, Martin. "American Medical Education" in *The Education of American Physicians: Historical Essays*, edited by Ronald L. Numbers, Berkeley: University of California Press, 1980, 7–12. See also Rothstein, *American Medical Schools and the Practice of Medicine: A History*, 15–36. Bates, *Scientific Societies in the United States*, 237–41.

science by the medical profession gradually increased the complexity of medi-cine, so that it would require explanation by an "expert" working and reading in the field regularly.[59] Barker practiced just at the cusp of this period of re-lentless change.

CASE REPORTS AND THE CLINICAL EXAM 1800

Barker used many case reports of his patients to teach and to illustrate and justify his diagnoses and treatments. The case report enabled him to describe the problem, inspire possible diagnoses on the part of his readers, and then relate his own diagnosis and treatment.[60] The patient's "history" or story was in Barker's era, as it is today, the most important part of the diagnostic pro-cess,[61] and diseases in the late eighteenth and early nineteenth century were classified based on the subjective feelings of sickness, called symptoms, expe-rienced by the patient. In 1837, Pierre Louis in Paris, who had become a major influence on American medicine during the first third of the nineteenth cen-tury,[62] wrote of the great advances in chemistry over the prior forty years and connected those advances to medicine. He believed in the necessity of exact-ness in medicine: "Medicine is a science of observation" and a "rigid method" is needed if medicine is to grow as chemistry had. "The history of symptoms"

[59] Pescosolido and Martin, "Cultural Authority and the Sovereignty of American Medicine: The Role of Networks, Class, and Community," 735–56; Starr, *The Social Transformation of American Medicine*, 3–29.

[60] Hunter, *Doctors' Stories: The Narrative Structure of Medical Knowledge*, 6, 28. In 1919, Richard Cabot of Harvard Medical School wrote, "Each case should lead us to arrange before the mind's eye a selected group of reasonably probable causes for the symptoms complained of and for the signs discovered." Richard C. Cabot, *Differential Diagnosis*, 4th ed., vol. 1 (Philadelphia and London: W. B. Saunders company, 1919), 18.

[61] In studies from 1975 to 2000, the correct diagnosis was made on history alone in 76–90 percent of patients in a primary care setting. M. C. Peterson et al., "Contributions of the History, Physical Examination, and Laboratory Investigation in Making Medical Diagnoses," *Western Journal of Medicine* 156, no. 2 (1992), 163–65. J. R. Hampton et al., "Relative Contributions of History-Taking, Physical Examination, and Laboratory Investigation to Diagnosis and Management of Medical Outpatients," *British Medical Journal* 2, no. 5969 (1975): 486–89.

[62] Warner, *Against the Spirit of System: The French Impulse in Nineteenth-Century American Medicine*, 127–31; Kenneth M. Ludmerer, *Learning to Heal: The Development of American Medical Education* (New York: Basic Books, 1985), 30; Russel C. Maulitz, "Pathology," in *The Education of American Physicians: Historical Essays*, ed. Ronald L. Numbers (Berkeley: University of California Press, 1980), 131–32, 149.

is crucial and "if one proceeds in an inaccurate or too rapid manner, neither diagnosis, prognosis, nor therapeutics, can to a certain degree, be possible."[63]

We can imagine a fairly clear picture of Barker's examination, which would begin with questions about the duration of symptoms, severity and character, location and radiation, the pace of illness, and any associated additional symptoms, correlating the responses with the patient's age, gender, occupation, and environment. He would then observe the patient for physical signs such as skin lesions, color, and warmth, the rate, irregularity, and force of the pulse, and excreta such as bloody stool and dark or bloody urine. He might draw blood and note whether it was sizy or buffy.[64] Palpation, or the examination by touch, would reveal irregularities such as a mass or tumor. He would listen to the patient's breathing to note wheezing, for example, or the cough of croup. The stethoscope did not come into being until a year after Barker's retirement in 1818,[65] but he might have listened to sounds of the heart, lungs, or abdomen with his ear against the chest or abdomen. This procedure dates back to the time of Hippocrates, but was rarely used except, perhaps, for certain unusual diseases.[66] A book on use of percussion, that is, tapping the chest or abdomen with the examiner's finger, was first published in 1761, but the

---

[63] P. C. A. Louis, "Memoir on the Proper Method of Examining a Patient, and of Arriving at Facts of a General Nature," in *Dunglison's American Medical Library: Medical and Surgical Monographs*, ed. Robley Dunglison and G. Andral (Philadelphia: Waldie, 1838), 150, 156.

[64] See Introductory chapter 2.

[65] R. T. H. Laennec, *De L'auscultation Médiate, Ou, Traité Du Diagnostic Des Maladies Des Poumons et Du Coeur: Fondé Principalement Sur Ce Nouveau Moyen D'exploration* (Paris: Chez J.-A. Brosson et J.-S. Chaudé, Libraires, 1819). Jacalyn Duffin, *To See with a Better Eye: A Life of R.T.H. Laennec* (Princeton, NJ: Princeton University Press, 1998), 27. Duffin points out that medical students were required to memorize various nosological classifications that took various symptoms and signs and then classify each group as a disease. Acceptance of these nosologies was beginning to fall away during the first decades of the nineteenth century and the influence of the French school. Warner, *Against the Spirit of System: The French Impulse in Nineteenth-Century American Medicine*, 4–5, 220–21.

[66] Historian Jacalyn Duffin, an authority on Laennec and the introduction of the stethoscope, points out that there were random reports of the use of immediate auscultation (ear against the chest or abdomen) before Laennec. Personal communication and Duffin, *To See with a Better Eye: A Life of R.T.H. Laennec*, 122–23. Victor McKusick refers to its use in Hippocratic writings "successful in demonstrating what is now referred to the Hippocratic succession splash of hydropneumothorax (fluid and air between the lung and inside of the chest wall)." He also refers to other types of sounds such as pleural friction rub (a creak like new leather). Victor A. McKusick, *Cardiovascular Sound in Health and Disease* (Baltimore: Williams & Wilkins, 1958), 3. A number of other authors refer to immediate auscultation, but they all seem to indicate the procedure "has been used scantily for many hundreds of years," as Paul Dudley White commented. Paul Dudley White, *Heart Disease*, Macmillan Medical Monographs (New York: The Macmillan Company, 1931), 83.

method was not yet in general clinical use during Barker's years of practice.[67] The common clinical use of laboratory tests was decades away and the discovery of X-rays would not occur until the end of the nineteenth century. Thus, the case history, that is, the patient's story as discovered by examination and narrated by the physician, was clearly the most important part of the process that would then lead to the patient's diagnosis, treatment, and prognosis.

RECORDING CASES, OBSERVATIONS, AND THE NUMERICAL METHOD

A good physical examination is important, but unless the information is captured, the value of the examination is lost. We know that Barker always took pen, ink, and paper to the bedside, recording "exact records of cases" as instructed in his preceptorship. He probably intended from the beginning to bring his case reports together into a published work, so for that reason they may be more complete than most. They are especially valuable to us today because of his constant efforts to include reference to the medical literature that guided him.

Recording patient's medical case histories and observations is almost as old as medicine itself. How this data was collected, sorted, compared, and used to generate knowledge has recently been studied by several authors, but particularly by Hess and Mendelsohn in Europe.[68] The use of "commonplace books" for recording information was facilitated by developments in the technology

---

[67] Leopold Auenbrugger, *Inventum Novum Ex Percussione Thoracis Humani Ut Signo Abstrusos Interni Pectoris Morbos Detegendi* (Vindobonae: Typis Joannis Thomae Trattner, 1761). After twenty years of studying percussion, Jean-Nicholas Corvisart popularized it after 1810 in Paris. It was brought the United States by those reading his books and by a growing number of Paris-trained American physicians. Duffin, *History of Medicine: A Scandalously Short Introduction*, 77, 194. Stanley Joel Reiser, *Medicine and the Reign of Technology* (Cambridge; New York: Cambridge University Press, 1978), 20–22.

[68] Volker Hess and J. Andrew Mendelsohn, "Case and Series: Medical Knowledge and Paper Technology, 1600–1900," *History of Science* 48 (2010): 287–314; Ann Blair, "Humanist Methods in Natural Philosophy: The Commonplace Book," *Journal of the History of Ideas* 53, no. 4 (1992), 541–51; Ann Blair, "Reading Strategies for Coping with Information Overload ca. 1550–1700," *Journal of the History of Ideas* 64, no. 1 (2003), 11–28; Lucia Dacome, "Noting the Mind: Commonplace Books and Pursuit of Self in Eighteenth-Century Britain," *Journal of the History of Ideas* 65, no. 4 (2004), 603–25; John Harley Warner, "Grand Narrative and Its Discontents: Medical History and the Social Transformation of American Medicine," *Journal of Health Politics, Policy and Law* 29, no. 4 (2004): 757–80; Lauren Kassell, "Casebooks in Early Modern England: Medicine, Astrology, and Written Records," *Bulletin of the History of Medicine* 88, no. 4 (2014): 595–625; J. Andrew Mendelsohn and Annemarie Kinzelbach, "Common Knowledge: Bodies, Evidence, and Expertise in Early Modern Germany," *Isis* 108, no. 2 (2017): 259–79.

of paper and printing in the seventeenth century. These books, with indexing and alphabetizing to allow for case clustering, provided a great improvement in the ability to compare and contrast cases.

Numerical methods were introduced in the eighteenth century with procedures such as recording the use of smallpox inoculation by Zabdiel Boylston in Boston, 1721–1722.[69] Medical interventions were very gradually subjected to more sophisticated data evaluation, from single case studies to case series such as Barker's, organized by disease but "controlled, in essence, by unqualified past experience," and slowly to increasingly sophisticated controlled studies from the mid nineteenth century to the present.[70]

Although John Graunt had used numerical approaches to study mortality in seventeenth-century London,[71] the use of numerical methods to study medical therapeutics did not often occur until the eighteenth century. Francis Clifton, for example, published *Tabular observations recommended, as the plainest and surest way of practising and improving physic* in 1731 and *The state of physick, ancient and modern, briefly consider'd: with a plan for the improvement of it* the following year.[72] In the later book, after reviewing medicine from the earliest ages of the Greeks, he wrote, "the reader is convinced, I hope, of the insignificance of *hypothesis* and the importance of *observation*." Observation

---

[69] John B. Blake, *Public Health in the Town of Boston 1630–1822* (Cambridge, MA: Harvard University Press, 1959), The innoculation controversy: 1721–1722; 52–73; Zabdiel Boylston, *An Historical Account of the Small-Pox Inoculated in New England, Upon All Sorts of Persons, Etc* (London: S. Chandler, 1726). Sixty years later William Black decried the fact that "none of the systematick medical authors to the present day . . . having ever converted it [arithmetical medical analysis] to the advantage of their profession, and of the community, medicinally. William Black, *An Arithmetical and Medical Analysis of the Diseases and Mortality of the Human Species*, 2nd ed. (London: The Author etc., 1789), introduction.

[70] Annick Opinel et al., "Commentary: The Evolution of Methods to Assess the Effects of Treatments, Illustrated by the Development of Treatments for Diphtheria, 1825–1918," *International Journal of Epidemiology* 42, no. 3 (2013): 662. This article gives a detailed review of numerical methods in the eighteenth century.

[71] John Graunt, *Natural and Political Observations Mentioned in a Following Index, and Made upon the Bills of Mortality*, 3rd ed. (London: John Martyn and James Allestry, Printers to the Royal Society, 1665).

[72] Francis Clifton, *Tabular Observations Recommended, as the Plainest and Surest Way of Practising and Improving Physick; in a Letter to a Friend* (London: Printed for J. Brindley, and sold by the booksellers of London and Westminster, 1731); Francis Clifton, *The State of Physick, Ancient and Modern, Briefly Consider'd: With a Plan for the Improvement of It* (London: J. Nourse, 1732).

was essential, "especially as the *Materia Medica* is so vastly improved to what it was among the *Ancients*." He then suggested that to improve Physick "three or four persons of proper qualifications should be employed in the *Hospitals* . . . to set down cases of the patients there from day to day, *candidly* and *judiciously*, without any regard to private opinions or public systems" and publish the facts at the end of the year. Such would provide information of the nature of diseases more useful "than all the books of *Theories*." He continued, should that be too great an undertaking, "only every *uncommon* case should be obliged to be recorded in the *College of Physicians*, or *Surgeons Hall*." Finally, an additional reason to carefully observe and record cases is to "suppress those *idle* pieces, [written by pretenders] that come out from year to year, to the scandal of Physick, and shame of Physicians." [73] He did suggest that physicians should communicate their observations using a table. [74]

The more common practice of "numerical culture," established in Britain during the eighteenth century, and France and Germany by the beginning of the nineteenth century, would reach America during the first third of the nineteenth century. Gradually the evaluation of therapies would require the support by numerical statements. [75] Barker's manuscript was written during this early American period of the change in medical information-gathering. Compared with institutional records, the usefulness of case records from private practice was limited by having fewer cases and a shorter time frame, though Barker practiced in the same community for forty years and did his

---

[73] Clifton, *The State of Physick, Ancient and Modern, Briefly Consider'd: With a Plan for the Improvement of It*, 166–73.

[74] Clifton, *The State of Physick, Ancient and Modern, Briefly Consider'd: With a Plan for the Improvement of It*, 174–75.

[75] Ulrich Tröhler, "The Introduction of Numerical Methods to Assess the Effects of Medical Interventions during the 18th Century: A Brief History," *Journal of the Royal Society of Medicine* 104, no. 11 (2011): 465–74. The *Medical Repository*, which began in New York in 1797, encouraged "systematic fact-finding" and published mortality and hospital statistics. See James H. Cassedy, *American Medicine and Statistical Thinking, 1800–1860* (Cambridge, MA: Harvard University Press, 1984), 1–24; W. F. Bynum, *Science and the Practice of Medicine in the Nineteenth Century*, Cambridge History of Medicine (Cambridge; New York: Cambridge University Press, 1994), 42–44. For numerical methods not described in the evaluation of drugs in the medieval and early modern periods, see E. Leong and A. Rankin, "Testing Drugs and Trying Cures: Experiment and Medicine in Medieval and Early Modern Europe," *Bulletin of the History of Medicine* 91, no. 2 (2017), 157–82; Evan R. Ragland, "Experimental Clinical Medicine and Drug Action in Mid-Seventeenth-Century Leiden," *Bulletin of the History of Medicine* 91, no. 2 (2017), 331–61; Jeremy A. Greene, "Therapeutic Proofs and Medical Truths: The Enduring Legacy of Early Modern Drug Trials," *Bulletin of the History of Medicine* 91, no. 2 (2017), 420–29.

best to get follow-up information on the patients he had treated.[76] He recorded case histories and epidemics and read the contemporary medical literature, but did not tabulate the information in what would gradually become the
preferred method of data collection. However, the recording and publication
of individual cases from practice continued, and in 1828, the *Boston Medical
and Surgical Journal* was encouraging "Reports of Cases in Private Practice: . . .
There seems no reason why reports of cases occurring in their ordinary rounds
of practice should not be as useful and improving to physicians, as hospital
reports are to surgeons," pointing out that ordinary cases throw light on
everyday practice much more than rare ones.[77]

An attempt to help physicians collate their cases was made by Allen &
Ticknor, Boston, in 1832 when they published *The Physician's Case Book*,[78] with
a review appearing in the *Medical Magazine*, Boston, 1833.[79] The book has a
full-page foldout template for systematic recording of a history and physical
examination. At the bottom of the page are thirteen questions such as "What
function is deranged," "What organ is affected," and "What are the grounds
for the diagnosis?" There is a small index section for names and/or diseases
and then 100 pages, one per patient, to record Name/Number, Age, Abode,
Occupation, History and Probable Cause, Reports, and Treatment. The 1833
review states, "every scientific and thinking physician does or ought to have
this Case Book."[80] From antiquity, physicians have been urged to record their
cases. Hippocrates, Thomas Sydenham, Benjamin Rush, William Osler, and in
the twentieth century, Lawrence Weed—all discuss keeping accurate records
of cases seen. Medical historian S. J. Reiser concludes the reasons to record
cases include: to recall observations, inform others, to instruct students, to
gain knowledge, to monitor performance, and to justify interventions.[81]

---

[76] G. B. Risse and J. H. Warner, "Reconstructing Clinical Activities: Patient Records in
Medical History," *Social History of Medicine* 5, no. 2 (1992): 188.

[77] "Reports of Cases in Private Practice," *Boston Medical and Surgical Journal* 1
(1828): 426–29. It is interesting that this article is preceded by an eight-page article
titled "Abstract of Lectures on Medical Statistics, Delivered at the College of Physicians
(London) by Dr. Bisset Hawkins" on pages 418–26.

[78] The bookseller and publisher Allen & Ticknor was the forerunner of Ticknor & Fields,
later to become Houghton Mifflin. *The Physician's Case Book* was their first publication.
Warren Stenson Tryon and William Charvat, *The Cost Books of Ticknor and Fields, and
Their Predecessors, 1832–1858*, Bibliographical Society of America Monograph Series
(New York: Bibliographical Society of America, 1949), 3.

[79] "Art. 7. The Physicians' Case Book," *The Medical Magazine* 1 (1833): 298–99.

[80] "Art. 7.The Physicians' Case Book," 298–99.

[81] S. J. Reiser, "The Clinical Record in Medicine. Part 1: Learning from Cases," *Annals of
Internal Medicine* 114, no. 10 (1991): 902–907.

"THUS SAYETH GALEN" MEETS CULLEN, RUSH, AND BROWN

For centuries preceding 1800, if an observation refuting ancient teaching arose, the argument might have been settled with: "Thus sayeth Galen," end of the discussion. In the early nineteenth century some leaders and future leaders of American medicine returned from study in France under Pierre Louis, Jean-Nicholas Corvisart, Rene Laennec, and others with new ideas about clinical observation, getting away from the *isms* such as Cullinism, Brownism, Broussaisism, "and all the host of other so-called rational *isms*."[82] All those *isms* represented hypothetical explanations of diseases transformed into systems with therapeutic implications. Henceforth, these would be subjected to severe scrutiny.

William Cullen (1710–1790), who taught in Glasgow and later Edinburgh, published his most famous work, *First Lines of the Practice of Physic*, in successive volumes beginning in 1776. Leiden's Herman Boerhaave (1668–1738), a highly regarded medical professor in the Western world, had emphasized the importance of blood vessels, but Cullen focused on the nervous system. For example, Cullen maintained that fever or pyrexiae had a neurotic origin, in the obsolete sense of the word, "acting on nerves" (OED). He defined fever as having "the following appearances: After beginning with some degree of cold shivering, they show some increase of heat, and an increased frequency of pulse, with some interruption and disorder of several functions, particularly some diminution of strength in animal functions."[83] So fever was diagnosed by quizzing and observing the patient. Although crude thermometers had existed from the sixteenth century, a practical, clinically useful thermometer

---

[82] Warner, *Against the Spirit of System: The French Impulse in Nineteenth-Century American Medicine*, 175–77. Warner was referring to the 1840s work of Elisha Bartlett, who called all the "isms" "hypothetical explanations of, and not legitimate deductions from them." Warner, *Against the Spirit of System: The French Impulse in Nineteenth-Century American Medicine*, 176 and footnote #50. Elisha Bartlett, *An Essay on the Philosophy of Medical Science* (Philadelphia: Lea & Blanchard, 1844). See also Risse and Warner, "Reconstructing Clinical Activities: Patient Records in Medical History"; Warner, *The Therapeutic Perspective*; Warner, "Grand Narrative," 757–80. David Hosack (1769–1835) of New York City, educated at Columbia, Princeton, University of Pennsylvania, and Edinburgh Medical Schools, was a physician, educator, and botanist. He tried to make sense out of many of the systems and published David Hosack, *A System of Practical Nosology; to Which Is Prefixed, a Synopsis of the Systems of Sauvages, Linnaeus, Vogel, Sagar, Macbride, Cullen, Darwin, Crichton, Pinel, Parr, Swediaur, Young, and Good, with References to the Best Authors on Each Disease* (New York: Van Winkle, 1821).

[83] William Cullen, *First Lines of the Practice of Physic with Supplementary Notes, Including More Recent Improvements in the Practice of Medicine by Peter Reid*, two volumes in one (Brookfield: E. Mirriam & Co. for Isaiah Thomas, 1807), 25.

did not come into use until the last third of the nineteenth century.[84] Cullen's system was based on symptoms and physiology rather than anatomy, saying "almost the whole of the diseases of the human body might be called Nervous."[85] Cullen's student Benjamin Rush (1746–1813) would develop a similar system, though with a focus on tension in the arteries rather than the nerves; depletive means such as bloodletting was his treatment of choice, with calomel as an additional favorite. Rush had a major influence on American medicine in general and on Barker in particular through correspondence and readings.

John Brown (1735–1788), another of Cullen's students, believed that all disease could be characterized by what he called "excitability," too much of which he deemed "sthenic" and too little, "asthenic." Opium and alcohol were his favorite treatments for "asthenic" conditions and bloodletting, emetics, and cathartics for the "sthenic" conditions. It was simple: one or the other and a suggested therapy would be clear.[86] At one point Barker embraced

---

[84] W. F. Bynum, "Cullen and the Study of Fevers in Britain, 1760–1820," *Medical History* 25, no. S1 (1981): 135–47; Reiser, *Medicine and the Reign of Technology*, 110–21; Joel D. Howell, *Technology and American Medical Practice, 1880–1930: An Anthology of Sources*, Medical Care in the United States (New York: Garland Pub., 1988). Austin Flint, "Remarks on the use of the thermometer in diagnosis and prognosis," *New York Medical Journal* 4, November, 81–93; William F. Wright, "Early Evolution of the Thermometer and Application to Clinical Medicine," *Journal of Thermal Biology* 56 (2016), 18–30; Wright and Mackowiak, "Origin, Evolution and Clinical Application of the Thermometer," 526–34. Wunderlich's research over eighteen years and thousands of patients provided the data that allowed him "to put it [clinical thermometry] on a scientific basis." C. A. Wunderlich, *Das Verhalten Der Eigenwärme in Krankheiten (the Course of Temperature in Diseases)* (Leipzig: Wigand, 1868); Philip A. Mackowiak, "History of Clinical Thermometry," in *Fever: Basic Mechanisms and Management*, ed. Philip A. Mackowiak (Philadelphia: Lippincott-Raven Publishers, 1997), 9.

[85] Cullen, *First Lines of the Practice of Physic*, 387; King, *Transformations in American Medicine: From Benjamin Rush to William Osler*, 18–35.

[86] Bynum, *Science and the Practice of Medicine in the Nineteenth Century*, 1–32; W. F. Bynum, "Cullen and the Study of Fevers in Britain, 1760–1820," in *Theories of Fever from Antiquity to the Enlightenment*, ed. W. F. Bynum and V. Nutton (London: Wellcome Institute for the History of Medicine; Medical History, Supplement No. 1, 1981), 135–47; King, *Transformations in American Medicine: From Benjamin Rush to William Osler*, 19–27. Risse discusses the tension between the Cullen and Brown systems and the developing French establishment of disease entities based on clinical and pathological observations. G. B. Risse, "The Quest for Certainty in Medicine: John Brown's System of Medicine in France," *Bulletin of the History of Medicine* 45, no. 1 (1971): 1–12. Brown came from a poor family, was very bright, and was taught and helped by Cullen and others in Edinburgh. Brown's theory and treatment with laudanum (opium) and alcohol led him to lose support in Edinburgh, where he may also have become addicted to opium and alcohol used to treat his gout. His reputation faded in Edinburgh and then in London, where he subsequently moved and died in 1788. Historian David

Brownism, but later rejected the system and its frequent use of alcohol as therapy.[87] Barker, in fact, became active in the Temperance Movement,[88] writing to Benjamin Rush in 1806, "Rum could be procured [in Maine] only in small quantities [c 1780]; and happy would it have been for them and their posterity had this continued to be the case."[89]

There was a change in attitude from the late seventeenth century to the end of the eighteenth century. Alcohol as a beverage and a medicine in the form of hard cider, wine, and beer, and drinking, but not drunkenness, were accepted. The use of "ardent spirits," (distilled alcohol) became the problem in the late-eighteenth and early-nineteenth centuries, perhaps in part because of the "need for sober laborers to operate machinery."[90] In 1812, the Rev. Edward Payson of Portland organized a group, sometimes referred to as the Tythingmen, "for the suppression of vice and immorality," which gradually

Hamilton maintains that "In Europe and America, the humble origins of Brown and his iconoclasm harmonized well with the revolutionary atmosphere, and enthusiastic supporters appeared there also." David Hamilton, *The Healers: A History of Medicine in Scotland* (Edinburgh: Canongate, 1981), 137–38.

[87] Barker mentions Brown several times in his manuscript. The following example is found in volume 2 (Consumption) on MS page **C** 140, and refers to a young physician who dies in 1795: "This bright & promising young man had been reading the Medical Elements of Dr John Brown; and, like many others, both in Europe & America, was 'too much influenced by his imaginary theories.' myself not excepted," (Barker's underlining).

[88] The American Temperance Movement began in the early nineteenth century as a reaction against ungodly and unscrupulous behavior which, it was thought, would damage the New Republic. Temperance advocates urged others to reduce and even eliminate their consumption of alcohol.

[89] Jeremiah Barker, "Letter from Jeremiah Barker in Falmouth, Maine to Benjamin Rush in Philadelphia, 22 September 1806" (Historical Society of Pennsylvania, Rush Manuscripts, 1806). Rush published many editions of *An Inquiry into the Effects of Ardent Spirits upon the Human Body and Mind: With an Account of the Means of Preventing and of the Remedies for Curing Them* since circa 1784 and also in the numerous editions of his collected works such as Benjamin Rush, *Medical Inquiries and Observations*, 4th ed., 4 vols. (Philadelphia: Johnson & Warner, 1815), vol. 1. For the various editions, see Robert B. Austin, *Early American Medical Imprints: 1668–1820* (Arlington, MA: The Printers' Devil, 1961), 173–76. Rush discussed the immediate effects of ardent spirits/drunkenness such as unusual garrulity or silence, disposition to quarrel, profanity, disclosing secrets, rude and immodest actions, fighting, and temporary fits of madness. He also related the chronic effects of ardent spirits such as obstruction of the liver, jaundice, and dropsy, diabetes, skin eruptions, belching, epilepsy, gout, and madness.

[90] Ruth Clifford Engs, *Clean Living Movements: American Cycles of Health Reform* (Westport, CT: Praeger, 2000), 36–42.

became more and more associated with the Temperance Movement. As one of the sixty-nine people who attended its first meeting at the Friends' Chapel in Portland, Barker became a member of the "Sixty-niner(s) Society" of circa 1816, the first organized Temperance meeting in Maine.[91] The purpose of the meeting was to prohibit the drinking on the premises of rum and other hard liquors sold in pubs and bars in Portland.[92]

In 1817 James Thacher, physician, historian, and colleague of Barker's, wrote, "Cullen is now in decline."[93] An article on medical statistics published in the *Boston Medical and Surgical Journal* in 1828 states that it was more than probable that "if the doctrines of Brown had been subjected to the test of statistics, they would never have obtained so baneful an influence over the practice of continental Europe [and the United States]."[94] A reaction was developing to previously accepted medical philosophical generalization and speculations,

[91] "This little germ [temperance] was planted in 1816, at the Quaker's Meeting House. Sixty-nine names were pledged for its support. Hence its name [Sixty-Niners]." Issac Weston, *Our Pastor: Or, Reminiscences of Rev. Edward Payson, D.D., Pastor of the Second Congregational Church in Portland, Me* (Boston: Tappan & Whittemore, 1855), 325, footnote.

Anti-Sixty-Niner leagues were formed and, in the tradition of broadside balladry:

Thus the bottle we'll visit at noon in a trice
And only just call it "Suppression of Vice,":
Then drive out the tipplers tho' dry as a pine,
To yield to the pious, the brave Sixty-Nine.
                    (sung to the tune of "Derry Down, an old English ballad
                    popular in late eighteenth-century United States) Donald A. Sears,
                    "Folk Poetry in Longfellow's Boyhood," *The New England Quarterly* 45,
                    no. 1 (1972), 96–105; related ballad on pp. 101–102.

[92] Howard A. Kelly and Walter L. Burrage, *American Medical Biographies* (Baltimore: The Norman, Remington Company, 1920), 62–63; Hugh D. Mc Lellan, *History of Gorham, Maine* (Portland: Smith and Sale, 1903), 398; Neal Dow, *The Reminiscences of Neal Dow: Recollections of Eighty Years* (Portland, ME: The Evening Express Publishing Company, 1898), 184–91. For a general review of the early temperance movement: Jack S. Blocker, *American Temperance Movements: Cycles of Reform* (Boston: Twayne Publishers, 1989), 1–10; Katherine Chavigny, "Reforming Drunkards in Nineteenth-Century America," in *Altering American Consciouness: The History of Alcohol and Drug Use in the United States, 1800–2000*, ed. Sarah W. Tracy, Acker, Caroline Jean (Amherst, MA: University of Massachusetts Press, 2004), 108–13.

[93] James Thacher, *American Modern Practice* (Boston: Ezra Read, 1817), iii.

[94] Dr. Bisset Hawkins, "From the Med. Gazette. Abstract of Lectures on Medical Statistics, Delivered at the College of Physicians," *Boston Medical and Surgical Journal* 1 (1828): 418–26.

many dating back hundreds if not thousands of years. The method of authority was giving way to the method of observation and inquiry.[95]

"INTELLIGIBLE TO THOSE WHO ARE DESTITUTE OF MEDICAL SCIENCE"

Barker's printed subscription paper,[96] which served as a title page for the manuscript, declared that the book was "Written so as to be intelligible to those who are destitute of Medical Science." His intended audience included nonphysicians such as ministers, some of whom practiced medicine,[97] and educators, lawyers, merchants, and anyone else who was literate and interested. This was not unusual at that time; the first subscription list (1797–1798) of the *Medical Repository* included 269 people, of whom 75 (28 percent) were nonphysicians.[98] Writing about the medical world in Britain a century before Barker's book, historian Mary Fissell studied the vernacular medical literature, i.e., medical literature in English (not Latin) that allowed ordinary people to "understand the symptoms, nature and true cause of their own illnesses."[99] She pointed out that "arguably the most market-oriented group of vernacular medical books . . . were those that promoted the author or his (rarely her) remedies."[100] Barker's book was aimed at a broad cross-section of

[95] Paraphrasing Dr. Thayer's 1916 comment in William Sydney Thayer and William Osler, *Osler and Other Papers* (Baltimore: Johns Hopkins University Press; London: H. Milford; Oxford University Press, 1931), 191.

[96] Subscription papers are taken by people interested in the proposed publication. The title and brief description fill the upper half of the paper; the lower half has a place for the subscriber's name and number of copies desired. Subscribers could sign up others and would receive a free copy of the book if they reached a certain number of additional subscribers.

[97] The diary of the Reverend Thomas Smith (17021–795; Harvard College 1720) of the First Parish Church in Falmouth (Portland) was used by Barker to report on diseases and epidemics occurring in Maine before Barker arrived in 1780. Like many ministers at that time, Smith tended to the medical as well as spiritual needs of his congregation. Patricia A. Watson, *The Angelical Conjunction: The Preacher-Physicians of Colonial New England* (Knoxville: The University of Tennessee Press, 1991), 64. Also Bell, *The Colonial Physician and Other Essays*, 12–14.

[98] Elihu Hubbard Smith, Samuel L. Mitchill, and Edward Miller, "List of Subscribers," *Medical Repository* 2, no. 1: unpaginated addition. July 31, 1798.

[99] Mary E. Fissell, "The Marketplace of Print," in *Medicine and the Market in England and Its Colonies, C.1450–C.1850*, ed. Mark S. R. Jenner and Patrick Wallis (Basingstoke, UK: Palgrave Macmillan, 2007), 111.

[100] Fissell, "The Marketplace of Print," 120.

readers, and his promotion of alkali therapy, which was not tied to any commercial interest, does not appear to have been promoting anything other than his erudition.

The list of physicians who had already taken out subscription papers, suggests considerable interest in Barker's book. Many of those names were leaders of American medicine in 1800–1820:

> *About 100 subscribers have been procured in Maine [and]*
> *other states in New England.*
> *Subscribers in Gorham: Dudley Folsome, Elisha Bax[ter],*
> *Jacob S. Smith, Reuben Nason, Joseph Adams,*
> *Asa Rand, now of Boston.*[101] *–George Parkman of [Boston]*[102]
> *who requested a subscription paper to procure subs[cribers.]*
> *Subscribers in Portsmouth.*

---

[101] Dr. Dudley Folsom[e] moved to Gorham circa 1797. He left to become a military surgeon in the War of 1812, returned to Gorham, practiced for years, and died there in 1836. Dr. Elisha Bax[ter] is almost certainly Dr. Elihu Baxter, born April 10, 1781, in Norwich, Vermont. He studied at Dartmouth in Hanover and practiced in Lemington, Vermont, where in April of 1806, his wife of six weeks set off on horseback and broke through the ice and drowned when crossing a river. He then moved to Alna (New Milford), Maine (1810 census), Wayne, and then to Gorham in 1812 (1820 census). In 1832 he moved to Stillwater, now Orono, and finally to Portland in 1840, where he died on January 3, 1863. His youngest child was historian James Phiney Baxter, and his grandson, Maine Governor Percival P. Baxter. See Mc Lellan, *History of Gorham, Maine*, 282, 398–99; Alfred Johnson, "Hon. James Phinney Baxter, A.M., Litt.D.," *The New England Historical and Geneological Register* 75 (July 1921), 163–74; Neil Rolde, *The Baxters of Maine* (Gardiner, Maine: Tilsbury House, 1997), 14–23. Jacob S[heaff] Smith, a lawyer, came to Gorham circa 1808, practiced twenty-five years, and died in Brooklyn, New York, in 1880. Mc Lellan, *History of Gorham, Maine*, 286. Rev. Ruben Nasson served as preceptor of the Gorham Academy from 1806–1810. Mc Lellan, *History of Gorham, Maine*, 231–39. Joseph Adams, a lawyer, was born in Wayland (Sudbury), Massachusetts, graduated from Harvard College in 1805, and a few years later began practice in Gorham. He moved to Portland in 1821, suggesting that this list of subscribers began before 1821. Mc Lellan, *History of Gorham, Maine*, 286. The Rev. Asa Rand, from Rindge, New Hampshire, an 1806 graduate of Dartmouth College, was ordained in Gorham in 1809 and served there until 1822, when he move to Portland (1822–1825) and then Boston (1826–1831). Mc Lellan, *History of Gorham, Maine*, 193, and Chapman, George T. *Sketches of the Alumni of Dartmouth College, from the First Graduation in 1771 to the Present Time, with a Brief History of the Institution.* Cambridge: Riverside Press, 1867, 129.

[102] George Parkman (1790–1849) graduated from Harvard Medical School in 1813, practiced medicine in Boston, and maintained a strong interest in the plight of the insane. As noted earlier, Parkman wrote to Jeremiah Barker asking if he could read his chapter on mental illness, promising to return it promptly. The details of Parkman's 1849 murder at the hands Harvard Chemistry Professor John Webster, though fascinating, are not relevant to this work, but from *The Boston Medical and Surgical Journal*: "Never

Ammi R. Cutter,[103] *and 10 other physicians, all in that town.*

Joshua Fisher of Beverly, who took a paper.[104]

Thomas Manning of Ipswich procured four on a paper.[105]

Daniel Cony of Augusta took a paper for subscription.[106]

In Boston, Dr Parkman & Dr Coffin took papers.[107]

has this community had a severer shock than is now agitating it. Geo. Parkman, M.D., a very wealthy and well-known physician of this city, was unaccountably missing after Friday, November 23d." "Suspected Murder of George Parkman, M.D.," *Boston Medical and Surgical Journal* 41 (1849): 366–67. The identification of Parkman's body was made in part by forensic dentistry.

[103] Ammi Ruhamah Cutter (1735–1820) was born in North Yarmouth, Maine, and graduated from Harvard College in 1752. After apprenticeship training, he practiced medicine in Portsmouth, New Hampshire, and was a charter member of the New Hampshire Medical Society in 1791. Cutter was active in politics and was still practicing in 1792, when he was awarded an honorary M.D. by Harvard University. John A. Garraty and Mark C. Carnes, *American National Biography* (New York: Oxford University Press, 1999), vol. 5, 938–39; and see J. Worth Estes, *The Changing Humors of Portsmouth: The Medical Biography of an American Town, 1623–1983* (Boston: The Francis A. Countway Library of Medicine, 1986), 15.

[104] Joshua Fisher (1748–1833) was born in Dedham, Massachusetts, and graduated from Harvard College in 1766. After teaching for two years, he studied medicine under Bela Lincoln (Harvard College and M.D. from Aberdeen). Fisher's preceptorship with Bela Lincoln overlapped Barker's from 1769 to 1772. Fisher joined the Massachusetts Medical Society in 1782 and was its president from 1815 to 1823. Walter L. Burrage, *A History of the Massachusetts Medical Society* (Norwood, MA: Plimpton Press, 1923), 104–105.

[105] Thomas Manning of Ipswich became a Fellow of the Massachusetts Medical Society in 1805 and retired in 1836. See Massachusetts Medical Society, *Fellows of the Massachusetts Medical Society.* (Boston: Printed by John Wilson, 21 School Street; 1850).

[106] Daniel Cony was born in Tewksbury, Massachusetts, and studied medicine under Dr. Curtis of Marlborough, Massachusetts. He moved to Hallowell circa 1789 and then relocated to Augusta, just north of Hallowell. A member of the Massachusetts Medical Society (1792), he was one of the founders of the Maine Medical Society in 1820. After twenty years of practice he delved into politics and became a Judge of Probate for Kennebec County. He died in 1842. Spalding, *Maine Physicians of 1820*, 61–64.

[107] John Gorham Coffin (1769–1829) was born in New Buxton, Maine, and apprenticed with his uncle, Charles Coffin of Newburyport, Massachusetts. He practiced in Boston, was an attending physician at the Boston Dispensary, and founded and edited the *Boston Medical Intelligencer*, a precursor to the *Boston Medical and Surgical Journal* and later the *New England Journal of Medicine.* He was also a founder and first secretary of what would become the Boston Medical Library, now part of the Countway Medical Library at Harvard Medical School. He wrote about medical education in 1822. Joseph E. Garland, "Medical Journalism in New England 1788–1924," *Boston Medical and Surgical Journal* 190 (1924): 865–79; Joseph E. Garland, *The Centennial History of the Boston Medical Library, 1875–1975* (Boston: Boston Medical Library in the Francis A. Countway Library of Medicine, 1975), 6–7, 89.

In Providence Drs Bowen & Wheaton took papers.[108]
In New York President [of the College of Physicians and
Surgeons of the Western District of New of the College of
Physicians and Surgeons of the Western District of New
York] Spalding and Professor Mitchill [Professor of
Chemistry at Columbia University] took papers in order to
procure subscriptions[109]

---

[108] Levi Wheaton (1761–1851) practiced medicine in Providence, Rhode Island, was professor of theory and practice of medicine at the medical school at Brown University from 1815 to 1828, and was one of the founders of the Rhode Island Medical Society. Kelly and Burrage, *American Medical Biographies*, 1222. See also *Historical Catalogue of Brown University* (Providence: The University, 1905). William Bowen (1747–1832) graduated from Yale College in 1766, practiced in Providence, and was one of the original Fellows of the Rhode Island Medical Society. He was a preceptor to Levi Wheaton.

[109] Lyman Spalding (1775–1821) A letter dated March 21, 1820, from Jeremiah Barker to Lyman Spalding was written on a Subscription Paper titled "Proposals for Publishing a History of Diseases in the District of Maine," by Jeremiah Barker of Gorham, Maine. A Subscription Paper, probably identical to the one sent to Dr. Spalding, constitutes the first page of volume 1, chapter 2 of the Barker manuscript. Barker's letter to Spalding is interesting for several reasons. Six days earlier, on March 15, 1820, the District of Maine had entered the Union as the twenty-third state after nearly forty years of agitation; see Ronald Banks, *Maine Becomes a State* (Middletown, CT: Wesleyan University Press, 1970), 3. Barker thanks Spalding for his contribution of cases that are found in volume 2 and then asks, "Will you, my Dear Sir, afford me your assistance? [in procuring subscribers] . . . Please dispose of them [the subscription papers] as you may judge proper." See James Alfred Spalding, *Dr. Lyman Spalding* (Boston: W. M. Leonard, 1916), 315–16. Dr. Spalding had a distinguished career as a physician and educator, culminating in 1817 with his proposal for a national pharmacopoeia. Under Spalding's guidance, the first United States Pharmacopoeia was published in December 1820 and represented a "nationwide professional consensus" on the uniform preparation of drugs proven to be useful. See J. Worth Estes, "Lyman Spalding," in *Dictionary of American Medical Biography*, ed. Martin Kaufman, Stuart Galishoff, and Todd L. Savitt (Westport, CT: Greenwood Press, 1984), vol. 2, 709. Samuel Latham Mitchill (1764–1831) was born in North Hempstead, Long Island, New York, apprenticed to Dr. Samuel Bard 1781–1783, and studied medicine in Edinburgh from 1783 to 1787. Mitchill helped found the College of Physicians and Surgeons at Columbia University and became professor of chemistry, natural history, and agriculture at Columbia College. He taught the chemical theories of Lavoisier and was at or near the center of the controversy concerning the changing theories of chemistry and medicine at the beginning of the nineteenth century. In 1797, with Elihu Hubbard Smith and Edward Miller, Mitchill founded, and for twenty-three years edited, the first medical journal in the United States, the *Medical Repository*, which was sometimes referred to as *Mitchill's Repository*. See Kahn and Kahn, "The Medical Repository—the First U.S. Medical Journal (1797–1824," and Kelly and Burrage, *American Medical Biographies*, 806–807. For a more comprehensive examination of Mitchill's life, see Courtney Robert Hall, *A Scientist in the Early Republic: Samuel Latham Mitchill, 1764–1831* (New York: Columbia University Press, 1934).

WHY WAS BARKER'S MANUSCRIPT NEVER PUBLISHED?

We can only hypothesize why the Barker manuscript was never published. The reason may have been financial, if there were not enough subscribers and Barker did not want to publish the book using his own savings. Publication by subscription was a frequent but "by no means dominant factor in the eighteenth-century American book trade."[110] It was more commonly used in regions composed of small towns and villages without a major center of cultural and economic life, because the printer/bookseller could not undertake to produce a book unless it was one that could reasonably guarantee a large readership.[111] It is also possible that Barker never considered his manuscript finished, or that he became infirm before it was finished.[112] Barker's manuscript includes dates up to 1829, citing references at least as late as 1824. And in an 1828 newspaper article, his quotations from the first chapter of the book differ from material written before 1819 and sent to Dr. George Parkman for review.[113]

Perhaps Barker worried that the Northern New England market was saturated with such books. Dr. James Thacher, born in Barnstable, Massachusetts, was visited by Barker on several of his "post-graduate tours."[114] In 1817 Thacher published the 744-page *American Modern Practice; or a simple method of Prevention and Cure of Disease* that begins with a sixty-three-page "Historical Sketch of Medical Science."[115] Then in 1828 Thacher published a 280-page

---

[110] Donald Farren, "Subscription: A Study of the Eighteenth-Century Amerian Trade" (Doctor of Library Science, Columbia University, 1982), 184.

[111] Farren, "Subscription: A Study of the Eighteenth-Century Amerian Trade," 181–85; Elizabeth Lane Furdell, *Publishing and Medicine in Early Modern England* (Rochester, NY: University of Rochester Press; Woodbridge: Boydell & Brewer, 2002), 120–21; Rollo G. Silver, *The American Printer, 1787–1825* (Charlottesville: Published for the Bibliographical Society of the University of Virginia by the University Press of Virginia, 1967), 97–113.

[112] Tuchman suggests, "One must stop conducting research before one has finished; otherwise, one will never stop and never finish." Barbara W. Tuchman, *Practicing History: Selected Essays*, 1st ed. (New York: Knopf, 1981), 20.

[113] "History of Disease in Maine," *Christian Mirror*, February 22, 1828, 3 col. 4.

[114] Thacher's preceptor was Abner Hersey. Barker's preceptor, Bela Lincoln, studied under Ezekiel Hersey, Abner's brother, in Hingham, Massachusetts.

[115] Thacher, *American Modern Practice*, 3–66. An announcement of the publication of this book was printed in *The Eastern Argus* (Portland) by Mussey & Whitman on October 28, 1817, page 3 column 5. The advertisement concludes, "This [book] should be in the possession of every physician and will be useful in families." He also published James Thacher, *The American New Dispensatory Containing General Principles*

American Medical Biography . . . to which is prefixed a Succinct History of Medical Science in the United States that includes one page on the "State of Maine."[116] Other medical books from New England authors include Noah Webster's 1799 volume, *A Brief History of Epidemic and Pestilential Diseases* published in Hartford, Connecticut, Joseph Gallup's *Sketches of Epidemic Diseases in the State of Vermont* in 1815, Jacob Bigelow's *American Medical Botany* in 1817, and in 1822, his *Treatise on the materia medica. Intended as a sequel to the Pharmacopoeia of the United States* in Boston.[117] These books were published during the years that Barker was writing and revising his manuscript and were among the 105 medical books being offered by a Boston bookseller in 1818.[118]

Barker wrote in the plea for subscribers to *Diseases in the District of Maine* that the book was to contain "about 400 pages—price two dollars in boards."[119] Was the cost of Barker's book a deterrent to its publication? "Books averaged

of *Pharmaceutic Chemistry . . . The Whole Compiled from the Most Approved Authors, Both European and American* (Boston: T. B. Wait and Co., 1810); James Thacher, *The American New Dispensatory Containing General Principles of Pharmaceutic Chemistry . . . With an Appendix, Containing an Account of Mineral Waters . . . And the Method of Preparing Opium . . . The Whole Compiled from the Most Approved Authors, Both European and American*, 3rd ed. (Boston: Thomas B. Wait, 1817).

[116] James Thacher, *American Medical Biography: Or Memoirs of Eminent Physicians Who Have Flourished in America. To Which Is Prefixed a Succinct History of Medical Science in the United States, from the First Settlement of the Country* (Boston: Richardson & Lord and Cottons & Barnard, 1828), 45.

[117] Noah Webster, *A Brief History of Epidemic and Pestilential Diseases with the Principal Phenomena of the Physical World Which Precede and Accompany Them and Observations Deduced from Facts Stated*, 2 vols. (Hartford: Hudson and Goodwin, 1799); Joseph A. Gallup, *Sketches of Epidemic Diseases in the State of Vermont* (Boston: T. B. Wait & Sons, 1815); Jacob Bigelow, *American Medical Botany: Being a Collection of the Native Medicinal Plants of the United States, Containing Their Botanical History and Chemical Analysis, and Properties and Uses in Medicine, Diet and the Arts, with Coloured Engravings*, 3 vols. (Boston: Published by Cummings and Hilliard, at the Boston Bookstore, no. 1, Cornhill, 1817); Jacob Bigelow, *A Treatise on the Materia Medica. Intended as a Sequel to the Pharmacopoeia of the United States* (Boston: Charles Ewer, 1822).

[118] R. P. & C. Williams, "Catalogue of Medical, Botanical, and Chemical Books for Sale by R. P. & C. Williams" (Boston: R. P. & C. Williams, 1818). Of first and later editions of books printed in the United States from 1810 to 1829, 163 were written by American authors while 246 were written by European authors. Billings, "Literature and Institutions," 294.

[119] The amount of $2.00 in 1820 has an approximate purchasing power of $43 in 2018, although there are different ways to calculate this. "In boards" is a bookbinding term referring to the rectangular pieces of strong pasteboard used for book covers. A book "in boards" had these covered only in paper; more costly bindings were covered in cloth, leather, parchment, etc. One who bought a book in boards could decide whether to have it rebound to order.

about $2.00 in the 1820s";[120] a Boston and a New York bookseller's catalogs from 1818–1819 show prices ranging from $2.75–$5.00 for four identical medical books.[121] The *Physician's case book, or a guide for taking cases*, printed in Boston in 1832, had a trade price of $1.75.[122] So the proposed price of Barker's book seems to have been reasonable, making this an unlikely reason for not publishing.

Could the general reader afford this book? In 1830, the average daily wage of a Massachusetts laborer was $0.83, a mason $1.22, and a printer $1.25; a yard of cotton cost $0.21, a bushel of apples $0.44, and a pair of boots $4.75,[123] so perhaps there was no "spending money" available for this book for many people.

Could physicians afford this book? Historian Ben Mutschler, writing about eighteenth-century Massachusetts, maintains that a medical "social credit" rather than a "money" economy functioned in farming communities, and many rural physicians practiced only part-time. People helped their neighbors, and physicians were expected to help the sick. "Interdependence was the norm in farm society; scarcities in labor and material resources meant only through exchange could the needs of the farm be met."[124] The "poor were the responsibility of the town in which they had legal settlement," and physicians frequently made special arrangements "accepting payment in goods and labor" and forgiving charges to the town.[125] Thus it is difficult to know how much

[120] James J. Barnes, *Authors, Publishers, and Politicians: The Quest for an Anglo-American Copyright Agreement, 1815–1854* (Columbus: Ohio State University Press, 1974), 4.

[121] James Eastburn, *A Catalogue of Books for 1818* (New York: The Proprietors, 1819); Williams, "Catalogue of Medical, Botanical, and Chemical Books for Sale by R. P. & C. Williams."

[122] The *Physician's Case Book, or a Guide for Taking Cases* was published by Allen & Ticknor in 1832, the first book printed by what shortly became Ticknor and Fields. It was a guide to help physicians take notes and organize their case histories. Tryon and Charvat, *The Cost Books of Ticknor and Fields, and Their Predecessors, 1832–1858*, 3.

[123] Massachusetts and Carroll Davidson Wright, *Comparative Wages, Prices, and Cost of Living: (from the Sixteenth Annual Report of the Massachusetts Bureau of Statistics of Labor, for 1885)* (Boston: Wright & Potter Printing Co., 1889), 194–96.

[124] Ben Mutschler, "Illness in the 'Social Credit' and 'Money' Economies of Eighteenth-Century New England," in *Medicine and the Market in England and Its Colonies, C.1450–C.1850*, ed. Mark S. R. Jenner and Patrick Wallis (Basingstoke, UK: Palgrave Macmillan, 2007), 178.

[125] Mutschler, "Illness in the 'Social Credit' and 'Money' Economies of Eighteenth-Century New England," 187.

money rural physicians of the period earned, and more specifically, how much was available to purchase medical books. The Boston Medical Society established a fee schedule in 1780, and its successor, the Boston Medical Association, in 1806.[126] The Portland Medical Association published a fee schedule beginning in 1833: $1.00 for a visit, $1.50 for venesection, and $2.00 for passing a catheter.[127] But that doesn't tell us how many visits and procedures were performed in a day or whether bills were paid.[128] We do know that a price of $2.00 fell well within the normal range for a medical book, so the proposed cost of Barker's book was not prohibitive.

RAPIDLY CHANGING MEDICAL THEORY AND PHILOSOPHY: NOAH WEBSTER

As he absorbed the contemporary medical literature during the first three decades of the nineteenth century, Barker would have seen cultural changes in medical theory and philosophy that required frequent revisions, and therefore publication delays. A good example of this problem involves Noah Webster. During the same years that Barker was writing and revising his manuscript, Webster, best known as a lexicographer and orthographer, ventured into medical writing. Between 1796 and 1799 he published two books and a series of

---

[126] For a detailed study of fee schedules, see Mark S. Blumberg, "Medical Society Regulation of Fees in Boston 1780–1820," *Journal of the History of Medicine and Allied Sciences* 39, no. 3 (1984): 303–38.

[127] Portland Medical Association, "Constitution of the Portland Medical Association Together with the Rules and Regulations of the Police and Practice Adopted June 28, 1833," ed. Portland Medical Association (Portland, Maine: J. & W. E. Edwards, 1833), 11. Portland is in Cumberland county and a year earlier the following had been written: "Gratuitous services to the poor are by no means prohibited. The characteristical beneficence of the profession is inconsistent with the sordid views and avaricious rapacity. The poor of every description should be the objects of our peculiar care. Dr. Boerhave [sic] used to say they were his because God was their paymaster." Cumberland District Medical Society, "Bylaws of the System of Police of the Cumberland District Medical Society," ed. Cumberland District Medical Society (Portland, Maine: Arthur Shirley, printer, 1832), 18.

[128] One bill for Dr. Barker's care in 1803 included "inoculation for the kinepox," $1.00, examining and dressing son's gunshot wounds over fourteen days $11.75, and for elixir Paregoric, $1.75. Mr. John Quinby to Jeremiah Barker, paid in full in 1805. Countway Library of Medicine: Barker, Jeremiah 3MS. D.s.: [n.p.] 1800–1806 3 s. (6 p.). For comparison, a fee bill from New Haven, Connecticut, February 15, 1803, reports "inoculating for the kine pox" at $3.00 and in the 1806 Boston Fee bill, $3.00. Blumberg, "Medical Society Regulation of Fees in Boston 1780–1820," 321.

twenty-five letters in two New York newspapers on yellow fever epidemics and public health, and his medical observations led directly to the founding of the nation's first medical journal, so important to Barker, the *Medical Repository* (1797–1824).[129] Webster's book, *A Brief History of Epidemic and Pestilential Disease* was published in 1799.[130]

Almost certainly due to the epidemic of Asiatic cholera 1831–1832, Webster began to revise his 1799 book to make it acceptable in 1832,[131] but found so many needed changes that he never did finish it. His "Second Edition review by the author" with corrections and revisions in his own hand, circa

---

[129] Noah Webster, *A Collection of Papers on the Subject of Bilious Fevers Prevalent in the United States for a Few Years Past* (New York: Hopkins, Webb & Co., 1796); Webster, *A Brief History of Epidemic and Pestilential Diseases* (Hartford, 1799). The "Letters to Dr. William Currie" were published in the October, November, and December issues of the (New York) *Commercial Advertiser* and *The Spectator*, and they have been reprinted with comments in Benjamin Spector, "Noah Webster: Letters on Yellow Fever Addressed to Dr. William Currie. An Introductory Essay," in *Supplements to the Bulletin of the History of Medicine (No. 9)*, ed. Henry E. Siegerist and Genevieve Miller (Baltimore: The Johns Hopkins Press, 1947), 1–17. See Emily Ellsworth Ford Skeel, *A Bibliography of the Writings of Noah Webster*, ed. Edwin H. Carpenter Jr. (New York: The New York Public Library, 1958), 413–16. Webster was the catalyst for the first US medical journal, *Medical Repository*. In *A Collection of Papers on the Subject of Bilious Fevers*, on page v, dated July 1, 1796, he wrote, "I have neither the inclination nor leisure to devote much time to this object [writing a book on epidemic disease]." Six weeks later, on August 11, 1796, a young New York City physician, Elihu Hubbard Smith, wrote in his diary, "I think, as Mr. Webster has relinquished his plan of continuing his collection [book on epidemic disease], of taking it up myself . . . & publishing an annual volume; the principal object of which will be the preserving & collecting of the materials for a History of the Diseases of America, as they appear in the several seasons." The first edition of the *Medical Repository*, a quarterly, was published in July 1797 and E. H. Smith was one of the three editors. J. E. Cronin, *The Diary of Elihu Hubbard Smith (1771–1798)* (Philadelphia: American Philosophical Society, 1973), 201; Kahn and Kahn, "The Medical Repository—the First U.S. Medical Journal (1797–1824)." Though Webster had written that he had "neither the inclination nor leisure," he did continue his research and, in 1799, published *A Brief History of Epidemic and Pestilential Diseases*.

[130] Webster, *A Brief History of Epidemic and Pestilential Diseases* (Hartford, 1799); C. E. A. Winslow, "The Epidemiology of Noah Webster," *Transactions of the Connecticut Academy of Arts and Sciences* 32 (1934): 102–103; and C. E. Winslow, *The Conquest of Epidemic Disease: A Chapter in the History of Ideas*, University of Wisconsin Reprint (1980) ed. (Princeton: Princeton University Press, 1943), 215. George Rosen, "Noah Webster—Historical Epidemiologist," *Journal of the History of Medicine and Allied Sciences* 65 (1965): 113.

[131] There is a "Proposal for publishing [a revised edition of *A Brief History of Epidemic and Pestilential Diseases*] by subscription . . . L.H. Young. New Haven, June 1832." Skeel, *A Bibliography of the Writings of Noah Webster*, 348. Also a "Proposal for Publishing by Subscription the History of Epidemic and Pestilential Diseases by Noah Webster, Ll.D.," *Connecticut Herald*, July 10, 1832. An Asiatic cholera epidemic in eastern and western Europe had arrived in Montreal and New York City in June 1832. Charles

1832, is in the Rare Books and Manuscripts Department of the New York
Public Library.[132] Webster made several types of revisions, but most involved
changes in theory/philosophy such as the effect of electricity on climate and
pestilence. He deleted almost all references to electricity, crossing out, for example: "Morbid matter floats in the air, but the principal stimulating power
consists in the electricity of the atmosphere."[133] He also deleted reference to
"septic acid, conveyed to the blood," a controversial theory in some repute
in 1799.[134] In 1799 Webster had agreed with some comments on the proximate cause of bilious plague (yellow fever) found in Brown's *Elements of
Medicine,* but he deleted four paragraphs referring to Brown's theories in his
"Correction Copy."[135] He also crossed out the final seventy pages of volume
2.[136] He discarded some of his earlier theories after thirty years of new data

E. Rosenberg, *The Cholera Years: The United States in 1832. 1849, and 1866,* reprint, 1987
ed. (Chicago: The University of Chicago Press, 1962), 23–39.

[132] Skeel, *A Bibliography of the Writings of Noah Webster,* 345–49; note 8 led me to pursue
the existence of Webster's manuscript correction copy. As of 1999 the printed copy
of *Brief History . . .* with MS corrections did not appear in CATNYP (Catalogue of the
New York Public Library) or in their Rare Book Catalogue. Its existence was confirmed
in the old printed catalog cards that had been photocopied, bound, and preserved, and
the book was, in fact, on the shelf. Personal communication with librarians at NYPL.
An interesting story about the 1800 London edition of Webster's book is not relevant
to this book (unpublished research).

[133] Webster, *A Brief History of Epidemic and Pestilential Diseases (Hartford, 1799),* vol. 2,
222. For a later reference to electricity and epidemics see William Craig, *On the Influence
of Electric Tension as a Remote Cause of Epidemic and Other Diseases* (London: John
Churchill, 1859).

[134] Webster, *A Brief History of Epidemic and Pestilential Diseases (Hartford, 1799),* vol. 2,
222. The *Medical Repository* had numerous articles on septic acid and disease, many by
one of its editors, Samuel L. Mitchill. Jeremiah Barker researched and published on
this topic; see Barker, "On Febrifuge Virtues of Lime, Magnesia and Alkaline Salts in
Dysentery, Yellow-Fever and Scarlatina Angiosa. In a Letter from Dr. Jeremiah Barker,
of Portland, (Maine) Dated May 30, 1798"; Jeremiah Barker, "Beneficial Effects of
Alkalies in Consumption of the Lungs," *Medical Repository* 5 (1802), 220–21. This topic
is discussed further in this Introduction, chapter 4.

[135] Webster, *A Brief History of Epidemic and Pestilential Diseases (Hartford, 1799),* vol.
2, 219–22. Numerous editions of Brown's work were published during his life (1735–
1788) and following his death; one example of this popular text is John Brown, *The
Elements of Medicine; or a Translation of the Elementa Medicinae Brunonis* (London: J.
Johnson, 1788). By the 1820s, Brown's "simplified construct" of the unity of fever was
losing its popularity in the United States, as was the system of Rush, though some of
his ideas persisted. See Cassedy, *American Medicine and Statistical Thinking, 1800–1860,*
21–22; and Warner, *The Therapeutic Perspective,* 46.

[136] Webster, *A Brief History of Epidemic and Pestilential Diseases (Hartford, 1799),* vol. 2,
282–352. Webster also discarded many of the proposed spelling innovations he had
made during the last two decades of the eighteenth century. He began work on the

and ideas on the origin and prevention of pestilential disease.[137] Webster finally abandoned the idea of a revised edition, possibly because the extent of required changes was overwhelming. It seems quite possible that Barker made a similar decision about final revisions to his manuscript.

Perhaps Barker was never quite satisfied with his own book in a changing world of medicine; was it to be a "history" or narrative explaining current practice?[138] Timing may also have been an issue. After retiring from practice in 1818, Barker continued to work on his book for over ten years and, in 1831, asked Dr. Emerson of Kennebunk to review it.[139] Meanwhile, Asiatic cholera had invaded Europe in 1831–1832 and its westward expansion was being followed closely by the American public and its physicians; it reached Canada and the United States in 1832. Barker had only briefly mentioned "cholera" in 1784 and 1795.[140] Though the world was thinking, worrying, writing, and

dictionary that bears his name in 1800 and completed it by 1828. In his 1832 correction copy of *A Brief History of Epidemic and Pestilential Disease* he crossed out many of his spelling changes that had not been accepted.

[137] A historian writing about Webster's dictionary and orthography pointed out that "Webster often changed his opinions, not only on matters relating to language, but also in politics and religion . . . [and was] willing to acknowledge that his earlier views were mistaken." So it was with his thoughts on medical theory and epidemiology. David Micklethwait, *Noah Webster and the American Dictionary* (Jefferson, NC: McFarland & Company, Inc., 2000), 11.

[138] Allan M. Brandt, "Emerging Themes in the History of Medicine," *Millbank Quarterly* 69, no. 2 (1991): 200. In 1991, medical historian Brandt observed, "Prior to [the late-nineteenth century] . . . the study of medical history could not be distinguished from the study of medicine."

[139] Dr. Samuel Emerson (1765–1851) of Kennebunk, Maine, was a 1785 graduate of Harvard College, practiced medicine from circa 1790, and helped form and was elected first chairman of the Maine Medical Society on its founding in 1820, the year of Maine statehood. Spalding, *Maine Physicians of 1820*, 6–8. Emerson did review Barker's manuscript in 1831 and wrote the following to Barker, "I have carefully perused your manuscript with great pleasure, particularly relating to consumption [volume 2]." His letter is found on the first page of volume 2 of the Barker manuscript. Jeremiah Barker, "A History of Diseases in the District of Maine Commencing in 1735 and Continuing to the Present Time. . . . To This Is Annexed an Inquiry into the Causes, Nature, Increasing Prevalency, and Treatment of Consumption," in Jeremiah Barker, Collection 13, ed. Maine Historical Society (Portland, Maine, 1831) of the book in manuscript. The letter from Emerson to Barker is pasted in and is marked by me as page 1 of volume 2.

[140] Epidemic Asiatic cholera first appeared in the United States in 1832. In 1784 and 1795 "cholera" generally defined as "an excessive vomiting and purging." John Redman Coxe, *The Philadelphia Medical Dictionary*, 2nd ed. (Philadelphia: Thomas Dobson, 1817), 129.

talking about epidemic Asiatic cholera, it was a disease that had not been an issue in America during Barker's years of medical practice.

CONCLUSION

During the first third of the nineteenth century, the works of Cullen and Rush, so important to Barker, were become increasingly criticized and marginalized. As medical historian Charles Rosenberg argues, "By the 1830s, criticism of traditional therapeutics had become a cliché in sophisticated medical circles: physicians of any pretension spoke of self-limited diseases, of skepticism in regard to the physician's ability to intervene and change the course of most diseases, of respect for the healing powers of nature."[141] During the 1820s, at the same time that Jacksonian democracy and medical pluralism were accelerating, physicians were questioning their own previously held doctrines and "medical truths." All of these factors may have contributed to the fact that Barker's revisions were never finished, and his manuscript never published.

[141] Rosenberg, "The Therapeutic Revolution: Medicine, Meaning, and Social Change in Nineteenth-Century America," 497. Eighteenth- to nineteenth-century medical theory and practice is the focus of King, *Transformations in American Medicine: From Benjamin Rush to William Osler*. For an extensive study of nineteenth-century therapy, see Warner, *The Therapeutic Perspective*.

CHAPTER 4

"Alkaline Doctor" and "A Dangerous Innovator"

Dr. Barker, of Portland, in the District of Maine, is preparing a work for the press, on Consumption and Fever. In this work the Doctor expects to establish the efficacy of Alkalies in the cure of Yellow Fever.[1]

LAVOISIER AND THE NEW CHEMISTRY

The summer of 1795 found Jeremiah Barker reading "M. Lavoisier's chemical Works,"[2] and two years later, when the announcement of Barker's proposed

---

[1] Jeremiah Barker, "Dr. Barker of Portland, in the District of Maine, Is Preparing a Work for the Press, on Consumption and Fever. In This Work the Dr. Expects to Establish the Efficacy of Alkalies, in the Cure of Yellow Fever," *Medical Repository* 1, no. 1 (1797): 114. The volumes of the *Medical Repository* ran from July to July, meaning that when the year's issues were bound, the title page of the bound Volume 1 would be dated 1798 or later, as there were several reprints of the first several years of this journal.

[2] Jeremiah Barker, "1806 Casebook," in *Maine Historical Society, Barker Collection 13, Box 1/5* (Portland, Maine, 1806), unpaginated. "Lavoisier had done for chemistry what Newton had done for mechanics a century earlier in his immortal Principia." See Douglas McKie, "Introduction to the Dover Edition," in *Elements of Chemistry by Antoine Lavoisier (1789)*, trans. Robert Kerr (New York: Dover Publications, 1965), xxvii. This is a reprint of the Kerr translation (Edinburgh: William Creech, 1790); see also Douglas McKie, *Antoine Lavoisier: Scientist, Economist, Social Reformer* (London: Constable, 1952). Other biographies include Arthur Dovovan, *Antoine Lavoisier: Science, Administration, and Revolution* (Oxford: Blackwell, 1993); Madison Smartt Bell, *Lavoisier in the Year One: The Birth of a New Science in an Age of Revolution*, 1st ed., Great Discoveries (New York: W.W. Norton, 2005).

book (see epigraph) appeared in the first issue of the *Medical Repository*, he specifically included "Alkalies" in his proposal. His reading had inspired him to perform experiments on tainted meats made edible by soaking in alkalis, and he had begun to use alkaline therapy such as limewater[3] for several diseases, including what were then termed dysentery, consumption, scarlatina angiosa, and yellow fever. His first article on the use of alkaline therapy in treatment of the "septic acid" of epidemic fever appeared in the *Medical Repository* in 1798.[4]

The use of alkalies for febrile disease had fallen into disrepute and was not accepted therapy in Barker's time,[5] but over the next decade several of his published articles in the *Medical Repository* (New York) and *Medical Museum* (Philadelphia) described the use of alkaline therapy in the treatment of prevailing epidemics and febrile disease in Maine. He wrote to Samuel Mitchill and later Benjamin Rush that he had been called "a dangerous innovator" by his fellow physicians until his articles on alkaline therapy and those of others were published in the *Medical Repository*.[6]

---

[3] Limewater (*aqua calcis*) is made from water and quicklime, or calcium oxide made from the thermal decomposition of limestone. The solution is alkaline and in dilute concentrations is an antacid; some common antacids today such as Tums consist of calcium oxide. Lye can be sodium or potassium hydroxide as they were not clearly distinguished historically. It is a very strong alkali made from quicklime (lime) and soda ash, and is clearly not to be taken internally unless in dilute forms. J. Worth Estes, *Dictionary of Protopharmacology* (Canton, MA: Science History Publications, 1990), 34, 161; Andrew Duncan, *The Edinburgh New Dispensatory*, 1st Worcester ed. (Worcester: Press of Isaiah Thomas, 1805), 413–15; Daniel A. Goldstein, *The Historical Apothecary Compendium: A Guide to Terms and Symbols* (Atglen, PA: Schiffer Publishing Ltd., 2015), 184.

[4] Jeremiah Barker, "On Febrifuge Virtues of Lime, Magnesia and Alkaline Salts in Dysentery, Yellow-Fever and Scarlatina Angiosa. In a Letter from Dr. Jeremiah Barker, of Portland, (Maine) Dated May 30, 1798," *Medical Repository* 2, no. 2 (1798): 147–52.

[5] For a review of pre-eighteenth-century medical chemistry, see Allen G. Debus, *Chemistry and Medical Debate: Van Helmont to Boerhaave* (Canton, MA: Science History, 2001), and H. J. Cook, "Sir John Colbatch and Augustan Medicine: Exerimentalism, Character and Entrepreneurialism," *Annals of Science* 47, no. 5 (1990): 475–505.

[6] The *Medical Repository* (1797–1824), as previously stated, was the first medical journal published in the United States. The editors included Dr. Elihu H. Smith, a Yale College graduate who studied medicine under his father and a course in Philadelphia; Dr. Edward Miller, a graduate of the Medical Department of the University of Pennsylvania; and Dr. Samuel Latham Mitchill, who studied under Dr. Bard, graduated from the University of Edinburgh, and was professor of chemistry and natural history at Columbia College. Published in New York, The *Medical Repository* was the major source for medical, agricultural, and scientific information in the United States until 1804, when the *Medical Museum* (1804–1810) began publication in Philadelphia with John Redman Coxe as editor. See J. S. Billings, "Literature and Institutions," in *A Century of American Medicine: 1776–1876*, ed. Edward H. Clarke (Philadelphia: Henry C. Lea,

The interesting revelations of Barker's manuscript include his openness to experimentation and his determination to make his findings known. His manuscript, casebooks, and letters reveal him to be a regular physician practicing standard therapy in a relatively remote region of New England while experimenting with, trying to make sense of, and incorporating into his practice the new chemistry of Lavoisier, Black, Priestley, and Mitchill.[7] Medicine was beginning to accept the chemical laboratory as a source of cultural authority as experimenters analyzed fermentation and other physiologic processes.[8] But why was Barker, in the rural setting of his own practice, willing to risk his professional reputation in order to employ a "new" mode of therapy using the latest chemical explanations? Was his use of alkaline therapy "following the development of scientific ideas . . . in medicine as a source of

1876), 328–32, and R. J. Kahn and P. G. Kahn, "The Medical Repository—the First U.S. Medical Journal (1797–1824)," *New England Journal of Medicine* 337 (1997): 1926–30.

[7] For an overview of the chemical revolution in the eighteenth century, see Maurice Crosland, "Chemistry and the Chemical Revolution," in *The Ferment of Knowledge: Studies in the Historiography of Eighteenth-Century Science*, ed. G. S. Rousseau and Roy Porter (New York: Cambridge University Press, 1980). For a very concise history and description of the eighteenth-century chemical terminology, see Frederic H. Holmes, "Appendix: Names, Substances, and Apparatus in Eighteenth-Century Chemistry," in *Antoine Lavoisier: Or the Sources of His Quantitative Method in Chemistry* (Princeton: Princeton University Press, 1998), 153–55. Joseph Black (1728–1799), see J. R. Partington, *A History of Chemistry*, 3 vols. (London: Macmillan & Co., 1964), vol. 3, 130–43, and Jon B. Ecklund and Audrey B. Davis, "Joseph Black Matriculates: Medicine and Magnesia Alba," *Journal of the History of Medicine and Allied Sciences* 27, no. 4 (1972), 396–417. Joseph Priestley (1733–1804), see Partington, *A History of Chemistry*, vol. 3, 237–97; F. W. Gibbs, *Joseph Priestley: Adventurer in Science and Champion of Truth* (London: Thomas Nelson and Sons Ltd, 1965); and J. W. Severinghaus, "Fire-Air and Dephlogistication: Revisionisms of Oxygen's Discovery," *Advances in Experimental Medicine and Biology* 543 (2003), 7–19. Antoine Lavoisier (1734–94), see McKie, *Antoine Lavoisier: Scientist, Economist, Social Reformer*; McKie, "Introduction to the Dover Edition," v–xxxi; and Dovovan, *Antoine Lavoisier*. Samuel Latham Mitchill (1764–1831), see Courtney Robert Hall, *A Scientist in the Early Republic: Samuel Latham Mitchill, 1764–1831* (New York: Columbia University Press, 1934).

[8] In his *Elements of Chemistry*, Lavoisier devotes three chapters to fermentation; see Antoine Lavoisier, *Elements of Chemistry in a New Systematic Order, Containing All the Modern Discoveries*, trans. Robert Kerr (New York: Dover, 1965; Edinburgh: William Creech, 1790), 129–48. Rosenberg maintains that fermentation had been providing a "basis for metaphors explaining epidemic disease." Charles E. Rosenberg, *Explaining Epidemics and Other Studies in the History of Medicine* (New York: Cambridge University Press, 1992), 311. The utility of chemistry at the beginning of the eighteenth century was predominately restricted to medicine, but by the end of the century applications in industry, agriculture, and warfare developed. Crosland, "Chemistry and the Chemical Revolution," 142.

authority and legitimacy, or as a means of professional advancement" to be exploited, as historians Amsterdamska and Hiddinga suggest?[9]

THE ACID/ALKALI DEBATES OF THE SEVENTEENTH AND EIGHTEENTH CENTURIES

During the last decades of the seventeenth century, physicians demonstrated a continuing and growing interest in chemistry.[10] Medicinal alchemists had been distilling herbs and performing various chemical procedures for centuries.[11] Physician and chemist Jean Baptiste van Helmont (1579–1644) emphasized the importance of chemistry in understanding how the body functions, including digestion as a form of fermentation involving acid and alkali, "the acid/alkali theory."[12] Otto Tachenius (fl. 1644–1699), a pharmacist and physician, drew further attention to the acid/alkali theory.[13] Robert Boyle (1627–1691), an Anglo-Irish natural philosopher, physicist and chemist, became interested in the acid/alkali theory as early as 1675 but did not discuss its relationship to medicine.[14]

---

[9] Olga Amsterdamska and Anja Hiddinga, "Trading Zones or Citadels? Professionalization and Intellectual Change in the History of Medicine," in *Locating Medical History: The Stories and Their Meanings*, ed. Frank Huisman and John Harley Warner (Baltimore: The Johns Hopkins University Press, 2004), 238.

[10] Chemical medicines were increasingly accepted by the mid-seventeenth century, and more medical schools were establishing appointments in chemistry. See Allen G. Debus, *The Chemical Promise: Experiment and Mysticism in the Chemical Philosophy, 1550–1800: Selected Essays of Allen G. Debus* (Sagamore Beach, MA: Science History Publications, 2006), 502.

[11] Bruce T. Moran, *Distilling Knowledge: Alchemy, Chemistry, and the Scientific Revolution* (Cambridge, MA: Harvard Univeristy Press, 2005), 13.

[12] Moran, *Distilling Knowledge*, 89, 116. This was the main theory of the Iatrochemical School, that is, "the functions of the living organisms were mainly determined by chemical activities ('effervescences'), particularly the acidic or alkaline character of certain, often imaginary constituents." See Partington, *A History of Chemistry*, vol. 2, 283–84. Van Helmont rejected the Galenic system of digestion and replaced it with a six-stage process "understood largely in chemical terms to include acids, alkalies, salts, and ferments." Debus, *Chemistry and Medical Debate*, 46–47.

[13] Debus, *Chemistry and Medical Debate*, 114–18.

[14] Robert Boyle, *Experiments, Notes, &C. About the Mechanical Origine or Production of Divers Particular Qualities: Among Which Is Inserted a Discourse of the Imperfection of the Chymist's Doctrine of Qualities; Together with Some Reflections Upon the Hypothesis of Alcali and Acidum*. The Second Edition. (London: Printed and sold by Sam. Smith at the Prince's Arms in St. Paul's Church-yard, 1690). Early English Books, 1641–1700; Permalink: https://lib.ugent.be/catalog/rug01:001578158. [581] p. in various pagings.

A debate over the place of alkaline therapy arose almost a century before Barker's consideration of the topic. Late seventeenth-century theory and practice included the use of alkaline therapy, particularly on the Continent.[15] John Colbatch, trained as an apothecary, became a licentiate of the London College of Physicians in 1696,[16] and that year he published a book, *A Physico Medical Essay Concerning Alkaly and Acid so far as They Have Relation to the Cause or Cure of Distempers: . . .* The preface includes the following:

> *It is scarce possible for a man to converse with a Person that is ill, let the Distemper be what it will, especially those, who have a smattering of Physick, which most people now a days have, but that they presently tell you, that their blood is so very acid, that unless that acidity can be corrected, it is impossible for them to be well: And accordingly they presently flye to the use of Alkalious Medicines as Powder of Pearle, Corral, Crab eyes or something of the same nature, and if they send for a Physician, which few people do, till they have first used vast Farrago of Alkalious Medicines.*[17]

Colbatch was criticized for use of the acid/alkali theory and for his selection of alkali rather than acid as a cause for disease by Richard Boulton, an

---

See section "Reflections upon the hypothesis of alkali and acidum," 3–38. Boyle was less than enthusiastic about the theory, and on page 4 wrote, "but consideration of them [acid and alkali] may frequently enough be of good use, (especially to Spagyrists [alchemists], and Physitians) when they are conversant about the secondary and (if I may so call them) Chemical Causes and Operations of divers mixed bodies." See also Debus, *Chemistry and Medical Debate*, 119.

[15] See Cook, "John Colbatch and Augustan Medicine," 489–94, for more details on the contemporary debates. At Leiden, earlier in the century, iatrochemist F. Sylvius de le Boë (1614–1672) claimed that disease was caused by "acridity" produced by either acid or alkali and the treatment was to be chemical of the opposite class. See Partington, *A History of Chemistry*, vol. 2, 283–84.

[16] For more on Colbatch, see Cook, "John Colbatch and Augustan Medicine," and Debus, *Chemistry and Medical Debate*, 126–32.

[17] John Colbatch, "A Physico Medical Essay Concerning Alkaly and Acid so Far as They Have Relation to the Cause or Cure of Distempers: Wherein Is Endeavoured to Be Proved That Acids Are Not (as Is Generally and Erroneously Supposed) the Cause of All or Most Distempers, but That Alkalies Are: Together with an Account of Some Distempers and the Medicines with Their Preparations Proper to Be Used in the Cure of Them: As Also a Short Digression Concerning Specifick Remedies," Printed for Dan. Browne, http://gateway.proquest.com/openurl?ctx_ver=Z39.88-2003&res_id=xri:eebo&rft_val_fmt=&rft_id=xri:eebo:image:42743, online book, preface. "Farrago" is a confused mixture; from the Latin farragin, mixed fodder, mixture.

editor of Boyle's work. He opined that Boyle had already shown the acid-alkali explanations were unsatisfactory.[18] Harold J. Cook (1990) and Allen J. Debus (2001) have extensively reviewed the debate.[19]

Hermann Boerhaave (1669–1738) held various teaching positions at the University Leiden beginning in 1701 and became professor of chemistry in 1718.[20] His inaugural address in 1718 had the somewhat inflammatory title, "On Chemistry Purging Itself of Its Own Errors."[21] He discussed therapeutics in the section "Uses of Chemistry in Medicine" in the 1727 English translation of *A New Method of Chemistry*.

> *. . . all the genuine indications of it [therapeutics] are fetched from chemistry alone. When a patient is seized with a burning fever, chemistry immediately informs us, that, from the additional heat, the salts of the blood become sharper; and, as the heat increases, are rendered alkaline, and the oils more volatile, and exhalable. Whence we infer, that acids ought to be prescribed, to prevent the putrefaction that is bringing upon the juices: and this indication could be fetched from nothing but chemistry.*[22]

[18] Debus, *Chemistry and Medical Debate*, 137.

[19] Cook, "John Colbatch and Augustan Medicine"; and Debus, *Chemistry and Medical Debate*.

[20] Boerhaave may have been "the first to introduce biochemistry in the education of students." See Gerrit Arie Lindeboom, "Medical Education in the Netherlands 1575–1750," in *The History of Medical Education: An International Symposium Held February 5–9, 1968*, ed. C. D. O'Malley (Los Angeles: University of California Press, 1970), 211. His chemical teachings had great influence, as "over 700 English-speaking students" studied under Boerhaave and many held important positions in the major centers such as Edinburgh, London, and Dublin. See Edgar Ashworth Underwood, *Boerhaave's Men at Leyden and After* (Edinburgh: Edinburgh University Press, 1977), 1–14. See also Gerrit Arie Lindeboom, *Herman Boerhaave: The Man and His Work* (London: Methuen, 1968), and Partington, *A History of Chemistry*, vol. 2, 740–59.

[21] Lindeboom, *Herman Boerhaave: The Man and His Work*,1968, 113–16; Debus, *Chemistry and Medical Debate*, 193.

[22] Herman Boerhaave, *New Method of Chemistry; Including the Theory and Practice of That Art . . . .To Which Is Prefix'd a Critical History of Chemistry and Chemists . . . Translated from the Printed Edition . . .* trans. P. Shaw, E. Chambers (London: J. Osborn and T. Longman, 1727), 197. Boerhaave also mentioned Sydenham's successful use of "small beer acidulated with spirit of vitriol" during a smallpox epidemic (pp. 197–198). Boerhaave was an eclectic with regard to the Iatrophysical and Iatrochemical Schools. He was concerned, apparently, that "adherents of the iatrochemical doctrine were very one-sided, since they explained nearly all normal and pathological processes by the antagonism between acids and alkalis, by effervescence and by putrefaction." See Lindeboom, *Herman Boerhaave: The Man and His Work*, 272–73.

The various editions of Boerhaave's chemistry books, beginning with the *Institutiones et experimenta chemiae* in 1724, became "the standard work[s] on chemistry in the middle decades of the eighteenth century."[23]

In his 1771 paper "Some Experiments on Putrefaction," F. L. F. Crell added to the debate:

> . . . the volatile alkali is essential to, or at least always present in putrefac-
> tion, it seems to follow, that the alcalies never can be used in living bodies,
> as antiseptics, for laying aside their stimulating quality, which must pre-
> vent their use in most of the putrid diseases, they would increase the mor-
> bific matter . . . and the most celebrated physicians agree in the good effect
> they have observed from acids in putrid diseases and recommend them
> strongly.[24]

Barker's clinical application of alkali occurred during a chemical revolution in which phlogiston[25] was being replaced by oxygen. The phlogiston theory of Johann Joachim Becher, further developed by George Ernst Stahl in the early eighteenth century, continued to be defended by Joseph Priestley, but by the 1790s it was losing favor.[26] By the mid-eighteenth century, William Cullen and his student Joseph Black in Scotland were hard at work developing chemistry as an academic discipline.[27] In the 1750s, Joseph Black, known for his work in pneumatic chemistry, had planned to study limewater but instead studied

---

[23] Debus, *Chemistry and Medical Debate*, 199. Another historian writes, the book [*Elementia chemiae*] exerted a great influence for at least sixty years." Underwood, *Boerhaave's Men at Leyden and After*, 9. Herman Boerhaave, *Elementa Chemiae*, 2 vols. (Lugduni Batavorum: apud I. Severinum, 1732). See also Partington, *A History of Chemistry*, vol. 2, 743–45.

[24] F. L. F. Crell, "Some Experiments on Putrefaction: By F.L.F. Crell, M.D. And Professor of Chemistry at Brunswick," *Philosophical Transactions (1683–1775)* 61 (1771): 338–39. Crell followed and refuted experiments by others who had refuted his conclusions.

[25] Phlogiston was thought to be a material substance present in all combustible substances and released in combustion. Thomas S. Kuhn, *The Structure of Scientific Revolutions*, 3rd ed. (Chicago: The University of Chicago Press, 1996), 52–57; Frederic H. Holmes, "The 'Revolution in Chemistry and Physics,'" *Isis* 91, no. 4 (2000); and Dovovan, *Antoine Lavoisier*, 133–87.

[26] Partington, *A History of Chemistry*, vol. 2, 637–686, vol. 3, 237–301.

[27] Partington, *A History of Chemistry*, vol. 2, 128–43. Jan Golinski, *Science as a Public Culture: Chemisty and Enlightenment in Britain, 1760–1820* (New York: Cambridge University Press, 1992), 11–49. Medical practice would soon be influenced by the study of the phenomena of heat, pneumatics, and electricity, the improved instrumentation of the second half of the eighteenth century in Scotland, and the work of researchers such as Priestley and Lavoisier.

magnesia alba (magnesium carbonate), hoping that an aqueous solution of *magnesia alba* would be an alkaline therapy more potent than limewater (calcium hydroxide).[28] In New York, Samuel Mitchill, who had studied under Cullen and Black in Edinburgh, introduced the new chemical nomenclature to the United States as early as 1792.[29]

Cavendish, Priestley, and others were studying combustion and pneumatic chemistry. Antoine Lavoisier[30] (1734–1794), whose work began in the 1760s, found that metals gained rather than lost weight during calcination; his quantitative studies made the phlogiston theory untenable.[31] Lavoisier's new theory of combustion and calcination, the composition of air and water, and

[28] The title of Black's medical thesis of 1754 was "On the Acid Humor Arising from Food and on Magnesia Alba." Ecklund and Davis, "Joseph Black Matriculates: Medicine and Magnesia Alba"; Audrey B. Davis and Jon B. Ecklund, "Magnesia Alba before Black," *Pharmacy in History* 14, no. 4 (1972), 139–46. For more on magnesia alba, see Duncan, *The Edinburgh New Dispensatory*, 419–21.

[29] Thomas A. Apel, *Feverish Bodies, Enlightened Minds: Science and the Yellow Fever Controversy in the Early American Republic* (Stanford, CA: Stanford University Press, 2016), 65–93. D. Duveen and H. Klickstein, "The Introduction of Lavoisier's Chemical Nomenclature into America," *Isis* 45 (1954): 285, and Dennis Duveen and Herbert S. Klickstein, "The Introduction of Lavoisier's Chemical Nomenclature into America: Part 2," *Isis* 45, no. 4 (1954). Mitchill was unsuccessful in trying to find a compromise between the phlogistonists, with Priestley as the major protagonist, and antiphlogistonists such as John Maclean at Princeton and James Woodhouse at the University of Pennsylvania. See Robert Siegfried, "An Attempt in the United States to Resolve the Differences between the Oxygen and Phlogiston Theories," *Isis* 46, no. 4 (1955); and Samuel Mitchill, "An Attempt to Accomodate the Dispute among the Chemists Concerning Phlogiston. In a Letter from Dr. Mitchill to Dr. Priestley, Dated 14th Nov. 1797," *Medical Repository* 1, no. 4 (1798): 504–11. Mitchill's letter to Priestly failed, as reflected in Priestley's response two months later: Joseph Priestley, "A Letter to Dr. Mitchill, in Reply to the Proceding [Mitchill's Letter Attempting to Accomodate the Dispute on Phogiston], by Joseph Priestley," *Medical (The) Repository* 1, no. 4 (1798): 511–12.

[30] Marie-Anne Paulze Lavoisier (1758–1836) participated in her husband's research in many ways. She translated important English books and documents on chemistry, such as those of Cavendish and Priestley, into French. She also assisted in the laboratory and her watercolor sketches of the instruments became the plates illustrating their experiments. Roald Hoffmann, "Mme. Lavoisier," *American Scientist* 90, no. 1 (2002), 22. See also the entry for Marie-Anne Lavoisier in D. Millar, *The Cambridge Dictionary of Scientists*, 2nd ed. (Cambridge, UK: Cambridge University Press, 2002).

[31] Lavoisier's chemical revolution began at the same time as the American Revolution; his research, writing, and life ended with his beheading at the hands of the French revolutionists in 1794. Working with his wife, he overturned the ancient chemistry, altered the understanding of combustion, and established the weight gain of metals on oxidation with one-fifth of the atmosphere. The other four-fifths of atmospheric air was later called nitrogen. Priestly had isolated oxygen in 1774, but the Lavoisiers observed that it was absorbed during oxidation. Their new chemistry listed thirty-three elements. McKie, "Introduction to the Dover Edition," v–xxxi; John H. Talbott,

fermentation slowly gained adherents from the 1780s onward.[32] His *Traité élémentaire de chimie*, published in 1789, was translated into English a year later.[33] The third through sixth editions (1791–1801) of the *Edinburgh New Dispensatory* included a section on the "new chemical doctrines published by Mr. Lavoisier."[34] By 1796 there were two American imprints of the *Edinburgh New Dispensatory* containing Lavoisier's doctrines, making them even more accessible to American physicians and pharmacists,[35] and by the end of the eighteenth century most of those studying and teaching chemistry were using the French nomenclature.[36]

BARKER, MITCHILL, SEPTON, AND THE *MEDICAL REPOSITORY*

In January 1796, Barker sent the results of his observations on fevers to William Payne, secretary of the Humane Society in New York, a man formerly

---

A Biographical History of Medicine (New York: Grune & Stratton, 1970), 278–80, for a brief introduction to their contributions to chemistry and physiology.

[32] Black was teaching it to students in Edinburgh before 1784. McKie, "Introduction to the Dover Edition," v–xxxi, see xxv. See also Robert Siegfried, "The Chemical Revolution in the Histroy of Chemistry," *Osiris* 2nd Series, Vol. 4 (1988): 34–50.

[33] Antoine Lavoisier, *Traité Élémentaire De Chimie* (Paris: Gaspard-Joseph Cuchet, 1789); and Lavoisier, *Elements of Chemistry in a New Systematic Order, Containing All the Modern Discoveries*.

[34] David L. Cowen, *The Edinburgh Dispensatories* ([s.l.]: Bibliographical Society of America, 1951), 12; and David L. Cowen, *Pharmacopoeias and Related Literature in Britain and America, 1618–1847* (Burlington, VT: Ashgate, 2001), 69, 75.

[35] Cowen, *The Edinburgh Dispensatories*; and Duveen and Klickstein, "The Introduction of Lavoisier's Chemical Nomenclature into America." The first dispensatory authored by an American was not published until 1806. See John Redman Coxe, *The American Dispensatory . . . Illustrated and Explained, According to the Principles of Modern Chemistry: Comprehending Improvements on Dr. Duncan's Second Edition* (Philadelphia: Thomas Dobson, 1806). Cowen credits James Thacher for the first dispensatory based "to any extent" on an American "pharmacopeia." James Thacher, *The American New Dispensatory Containing General Principles of Pharmaceutic Chemistry . . . The Whole Compiled from the Most Approved Authors, Both European and American* (Boston: T. B. Wait and Co., 1810). See David L. Cowen, *America's Pre-Pharmacopoeial Literature* (Madison, WI: American Institute of the History of Pharmacy, 1961), 25.

[36] By 1797, Mitchill wrote that he "adopts the Antiphlogistic System." Samuel Mitchill, *The Present State of Medical Learning in the City of New York* (New York: T. and J. Swords, 1797), 6, and Samuel L. Mitchill, *Explanation of the Synopsis of Chemical Nomenclature and Arangement: Containing Several Important Alterations of the Plan Originally Reported by French Academicians* (New York: T. and J. Swords, 1801). And at Dartmouth College: Lyman Spalding, *A New Nomenclature of Chemistry Proposed by De Morveau, Lavoisier, Bertholet and Fourcroy* (Hanover, NH: Moses Davis, 1799).

from Massachusetts and Barker's only acquaintance in the middle states at that time.[37] Mr. Payne conveyed Barker's ideas to Samuel Latham Mitchill, physician, chair of natural history, and professor of economics and chemistry at Columbia College.[38] Mitchill was at the forefront of the introduction of the new chemistry in the United States and in 1797 would found the first United States medical journal, the *Medical Repository*, an outlet for his chemical theory and teaching.[39]

[37] The Constitution of the Humane Society of the State of New York, dated July 12, 1794, records William Payne as secretary and Drs. Samuel Mitchill and Elihu H. Smith as medical counselors of the society. *To the Public with a View of Promoting the Interests of Humanity, a Number of Respectable Citizens Have Associated under the Name of "the Humane Society of the State of New-York," and Have Agreed to the Following Constitution*, Variation: Early American Imprints.; 1st Series; No. 47079. References: Bristol; B8701; Shipton & Mooney; 47079 (s.n.; United States; New York; New York., 1794), book, Internet resource; and *The Constitution of the Humane Society of the State of New-York: To Which Are Subjoined the Address of the Medical Counsellors to the Citizens* (New-York: Printed by J. Buel, 1795).

[38] In 1792 Mitchill was appointed professor of economics at Columbia College, which in 1794 was also called the College of New York. "Economics" at the time referred to the science "relating to the development and regulation of the material resources of a community or nation" (OED). The course provided "facts which form the basis of medicine, agriculture, and other useful arts, as well as manufactures." Chemistry was an important part of the course, and that year he published "an edition of the New Nomenclature of Chemistry, in French, German, and English." Samuel L. Mitchill, *The Present State of Learning in the College of New York (Columbia)* (New York: T. and J. Swords, 1794). See also Hall, *A Scientist in the Early Republic*, 19–30.

[39] David Ramsey's 1800 review of medicine in the eighteenth-century names three American chemistry professors, Mitchill, Maclean, and Woodhouse, who "can bear a comparison of the same in the oldest seminaries of Europe." He also mentions Joseph Priestley's move from Britain to Pennsylvania. "Art. II. A Review of the Improvements, Progress, and State of Medicine in the 18th Century. Read on the First Day of the 19th Century, before the Medical Society of South-Carolina, in Pursuance of Their Vote, and Published at Their Request. By David Ramsay, M.D. 8vo. Pp. 47. Charleston. Young," *Medical Repository* 4, no. 4 (1800–1801): 390–99. See also Hall, *A Scientist in the Early Republic*, 35–36; and James Whorton, "Chemistry," in *The Education of American Physicians: Historical Essays*, ed. Ronald Numbers (Berkley: University of California Press, 1980), 72–80. John Maclean, educated in Glasgow, Paris, and in Edinburgh under Joseph Black, was professor of chemistry at the College of New Jersey (later Princeton University) from 1795–1812. John A. Garraty and Mark C. Carnes, *American National Biography* (New York: Oxford University Press, 1999), vol. 14, 267–68. James Woodhouse studied under Benjamin Rush and followed him as professor of chemistry at the University of Pennsylvania from 1795 until 1809; Garraty and Carnes, *American National Biography*, vol. 23, 796–97. Aaron Dexter, the first professor of chemistry and materia medica at Harvard Medical school, taught from 1783 to 1816; Garraty and Carnes, *American National Biography*, vol. 6, 531–32.

In the summer of 1796 Mitchill sent Barker his 1795 treatise on contagion and fever,[40] with the following note: "Dr. Mitchill's compliments to Dr. Barker, and is happy to find that there is such a coincidence of sentiment between them on the subject of distempers occasioned by a combination of the principle of acidity with a septic base."[41] Thus we see revealed the late-eighteenth century lines of communication that furthered the development of medical thought: Barker sent observations to his friend Payne, who had moved to New York. Payne sent Barker's information to Mitchill, who took the time to write to Barker and send him his own article. How delighted Barker must have been, given the difficulty in obtaining medical information, to receive that article from Mitchill, and to know that he had established a personal connection with a prominent New York physician and professor of chemistry.

Mitchill's "Remarks on the gaseous oxyd of azote [septon] or of nitrogene," published in 1795, begins with a discussion of oxygen, the "principle of acidity," and the fact that the French declared "acidity as one of the early signs of animal putrefaction."[42] Mitchill believed that gaseous oxyd of nitrogene was being released in the process of putrefaction in the streets, sewers, and docks, and that, when breathed or ingested, it could produce or encourage febrile

---

[40] Samuel L. Mitchill, *Remarks on the Gaseous Oxyd of Azote or of Nitrogene, and on the Effects It Produces When Generated in the Stomach, Inhaled into the Lungs, and Applied to the Skin: Being an Attempt to Ascertain the True Nature of Contagion, and to Explain Thereupon the Phenomena of Fever / by Samuel Latham Mitchell, M.D. F.R.S.E. Professor of Chemistry, Natural History and Agriculture in the College of New-York* (New York: T. and J. Swords, 1795).

[41] Jeremiah Barker, "Letter from Jeremiah Barker in Falmouth, Maine to Benjamin Rush in Philadelphia, 22 September 1806" (Historical Society of Pennsylvania, Rush Manuscripts, 1806).

[42] Mitchill, *Remarks on the Gaseous Oxyd of Azote or of Nitrogene, and on the Effects It Produces When Generated in the Stomach, Inhaled into the Lungs, and Applied to the Skin: Being an Attempt to Ascertain the True Nature of Contagion, and to Explain Thereupon the Phenomena of Fever / by Samuel Latham Mitchell, M.D. F.R.S.E. Professor of Chemistry, Natural History and Agriculture in the College of New-York*, 6–11. In 1796 Mitchill wrote that the "establishment of the new nomenclature in France, in 1787, may be considered as forming a new epoch in science." For the first effort by the French to standardize the language of the new chemistry, see Louis Bernard Guyton de Morveau et al., *Méthode De Nomenclature Chimique* (A Paris: Chez Cuchet, libraire, rue & hôtel Serpente, 1787). Samuel Mitchill's preface to Erasmus Darwin, *Zoonomia, or the Laws of Organic Life*, Vol. 1 (New York: T. and J. Swords, 1796), xxvi. One hundred-sixty years later Thomas S. Kuhn, historian and philosopher of science, would agree that the oxygen theory of combustion was "the keystone for the reformulation of chemistry so vast that it is usually called the chemical revolution." Kuhn, *The Structure of Scientific Revolutions*, 56.

diseases.[43] Barker admitted he did not completely understand the precise nature of this acid, and its chemical combination with azote or septon (Mitchill's
theoretical septic principle).

From 1795 to 1800, Samuel L. Mitchill wrote numerous articles on septon[44]
that relate the new chemistry to agriculture and medicine. The November
1796 issue of *New-York Magazine, or Literary Repository* carried an article
whose title reads in part "[S]epton (azote) . . . operates on plants as food, and
animals as poison."[45] Septon from animal decomposition was thought to be
taken up by plants and oxygen and then discharged in large quantities in cities
and into wells, producing "septic vapours" that explained in part why "great
cities are the graves of the human species." Mitchill speculated that combining
septic acid with lime would neutralize the septon and make it a safe and a valuable manure.[46] A letter to Thomas Percival dated January 17, 1797, is titled
"Concerning the Use of Alkaline Remedies in Fevers, and the Analogy between
Septic Acid and Other Poisons." It was published in the lay press and would
soon be republished in the nascent *Medical Repository*.[47]

---

[43] Mitchill, *Remarks on the Gaseous Oxyd of Azote or of Nitrogene, and on the Effects
It Produces When Generated in the Stomach, Inhaled into the Lungs, and Applied to the
Skin: Being an Attempt to Ascertain the True Nature of Contagion, and to Explain Thereupon
the Phenomena of Fever / by Samuel Latham Mitchell, M.D. F.R.S.E. Professor of Chemistry,
Natural History and Agriculture in the College of New-York*, 14–43. Mitchill's paper was
used by others attempting to use contemporary chemistry to explain pestilential
diseases.

[44] "Septon," like "sepsis," is from the Greek work for rot or decay.

[45] Samuel Mitchill, "Operations of Septon on Plants and Animals for the 'New-York
Magazine.' On Septon (Azote) and Its Compounds, as the Operate on Plants as Food,
and Animals as Poison: Intended as a Supplement to Mr. Kirwin's 'Pamphlet on
Manures.' In a Letter to the Rev. Dr. Henry Muhlenberg, of Lancaster, Pennsylvania
from Mr. Mitchill, on New-York, Dated October 24, 1796," *The New York Magazine, or
Literary Repository*, November 1796.

[46] Mitchill, "Operations of Septon on Plants and Animals for the 'New-York Magazine.'
On Septon (Azote) and Its Compounds, as the Operate on Plants as Food, and Animals
as Poison: Intended as a Supplement to Mr. Kirwin's 'Pamphlet on Manures.' In a Letter
to the Rev. Dr. Henry Muhlenberg, of Lancaster, Pennsylvania from Mr. Mitchill, on
New-York, Dated October 24, 1796." One of the meanings under the word "manure" is
"a chemical or treated fertilizer." The OED definition of manure includes a reference
to R. Kirwan in 1794: "The substances principally used as manures, are chalk, lime,
gypsum, etc." in Transactions of the Royal Irish Academy 5 Science 137.

[47] Samuel Mitchill, "Concerning the Use of Alkaline Remedies in Fevers, and the
Analogy between Septic Acid and Other Poisons; in a Letter to Thomas Percival M. D.
&C of Manchester, from Dr. Mitchill, Dated New-York, January 17, 1797," *The New York
Magazine, or Literary Repository*, April 1797. Samuel L. Mitchill, "Concerning the Use of
Alkaline Remedies in Fevers, and the Analogy between Septic Acid and Other Poisons;

The *Medical Repository* would bring together the seemingly disparate topics of fermentation, farming, and physic. A "Circular Address" proposing the publication of the *Medical Repository* is dated November 15, 1796. In addition to medicine there were to be articles on disease among domestic animals, accounts of insects, the progress and condition of vegetation and farming, and information about the state of the atmosphere.[48] Several articles were about the risks and benefits of manure; indeed the second article in the first issue of the *Medical Repository* was written by Samuel L. Mitchill and is titled "On Manures: . . . It Will Be Seen How Nearly Physic and Farming are A'lied to Each Other."[49] Mitchill made the point that lime and alkalis overcome and neutralize the septic acids, thus disagreeing with the experiments and philosophy of John Pringle one-half century earlier.[50] Detractors of medical practice would surely enjoy the juxtaposition of medicine and manure.

BARKER'S USE OF ALKALINE THERAPY

In his casebook of 1806, Barker wrote that in 1795, after reading "M. Lavoisier's chemical works . . . [I performed some] . . . experiments on putrid animal

in a Letter to Thomas Percival M. D. &C of Manchester, from Dr. Mitchill, Dated New-York, January 17, 1797," *Medical Repository* 1 (3rd ed.), no. 2 (1798).

[48] "Circular Address," *Medical Repository* 1, no. 1 (1797), vii–xii.

[49] Samuel Mitchill, "Remarks on Manures: Wherein, by an Inquiry into the Nature of Septon, (Azote) and Its Relations to Other Bodies, It Will Be Seen How Nearly Physic and Farming Are A'lied to Each Other. Intended as a Sequel to Judge Peter's Agricultural Inquiries on Plaister of Paris," *Medical (The) Repository* 1 (3rd ed., 1804), no. 1 (1797), 32–55. Samuel Mitchill, "Affinities of Septic Fluids to Other Bodies. Affinities and Relations of Septic (Nitric) or Pestilential Fluids to Other Bodies. In a Letter from Dr. Mitchill, F.R.S.E. Professor of Chemisty, Agriculture and Medicine, in the College of New-York, to Sir John Sinclair, Bart. M.P. President of the Board of Agriculture, Etc. Dated New-York, the 28th of November, 1796. Intended as an Additional Article Proposed Report of the British Board of Agriculture on the Subject of Manures," *The New York Magazine, or Literary Repository*. January 1797, 9–17.

[50] John Pringle, "Further Experiments on Substances Resisting Putrefaction; with Experiments Upon the Means of Hastening and Promoting It," *Philosophical Transactions (1683–1775)* 46 (1749–1750): 56, where he reports that "corruption [decay] not only went sooner, but went higher" when chalk was added to flesh and water. Pringle's two earlier papers were more confusing; see John Pringle, "Some Experiments on Substances Resisting Putrefaction," *Philosophical Transactions (1683–1775)* 46 (1749–1750), 480–88, and John Pringle, "A Continuation of the Experiments on Substances Resisting Putrefacton," *Philosophical Transactions (1683–1775)* 46 (1749–1750), 525–34.

matter.[51] [It occurred to me that] azotic air[52] entered into the composition of pestilential fluids; and that the exciting cause of fever was a virulent acid often generated by the stomach from substances undergoing putrid fermentation . . . the precise nature of this acid I did not pretend to understand."[53]

Barker's first "experiments" are described in volume one of his manuscript:

> On the 6th of August 1795, a quarter of veal was brought to my house, from some distance, which had been tied up in a bag, 24 hours, and exposed to the heat of the sun the preceding day. On examining the meat, it was found highly tainted, and to smell very sour. I then directed it to be put into some brine of common salt, in a cask, to see if it could be purified. But, through mistake, it was thrown into a barrel containing soft soap,[54] where it remained till the next day, when it was taken out, washed in cold water, and found to be entirely free from sourness & fœtor. It was then roasted and eaten with palatableness.[55] This accidental experiment was repeated with

[51] It is interesting to note that Dr. Elihu Hubbard Smith of New York, a coeditor of the *Medical Repository*, began reading "Lavoisier's Elements Chemistry" on Sunday, September 18, 1796, a year after Barker read it. See J. E. Cronin, *The Diary of Elihu Hubbard Smith (1771–1798)* (Philadelphia: American Philosophical Society, 1973), 221.

[52] Lavoisier, *Elements of Chemistry in a New Systematic Order, Containing All the Modern Discoveries*, table opposite 179, 185. Azotic air refers to "A name in the new chemistry for the basis of atmospheric air, and of ammonia, nitrous acid, etc, azotic gas, mephitic or phlogisticated air, nitrogene." Azotic air: of pertaining to or chemically combined with azote (nitrogen). Azote was the name given by Lavoisier for its inability to support life (OED). "Azote combined with oxygen . . . form powerful acids . . . [and] with hydrogen forms ammonia." Thacher, *The American New Dispensatory*, 27.

[53] Barker, "1806 Casebook," unpaginated. A medical dictionary of 1817 defines acid as "the combination of oxygen, or the base of vital air, with certain elementary substances." John Redman Coxe, *The Philadelphia Medical Dictionary*, 2nd ed. (Philadelphia: Thomas Dobson, 1817). Acids "are distinguished by their sour, styptic taste; by their greater or less causticity." Thacher, *The American New Dispensatory*, 26–27. The OED definition of acid: "Popularly, A sour substance. Chem. A substance belonging to a class of which the commonest and most typical members are sour, and have the property of neutralizing alkalis, and of changing vegetable blues to red; all of which are compounds of hydrogen with another element or elements (oxygen being generally the third element)." Lavoisier thought oxygen was the principle of acidity, though Humphry Davey would later show that acids such as muriatic (hydrochloric acid) might not have any oxygen at all. See Siegfried, "The Chemical Revolution in the Histroy of Chemistry," 35.

[54] "A smeary semi-fluid soap, made with potash lye [potassium carbonate, pearl-ash]." "Oxford English Dictionary, 2nd Edition, Online," Oxford University Press, 1989.

[55] Preserving meats by curing, drying, salting, smoking, fermenting, and pickling had been done since ancient times, but how does one deal with tainted, foul-smelling meat? C. Anne Wilson refers to the *Art of Cookery*, circa 1770, by Hannah Glasse: "Twelve hours' immersion in meare sauce would also disguise the flavour of tainted venison,

some variation. I procured a tainted quarter of veal, which had a very sim-
ilar smell, and was condemned in the market. This I immersed in an aqueous
solution of pearl ash [potassium carbonate],[56] which restored it to sweet-
ness. . . . Now, it appeared to me, highly probable, that if these materials
had remained much longer unalkalized, the extricated azotic air, would have
acquired such a degree of virulent acidity as to produce pestilential & malig-
nant fevers; and that alkalines were proper remedies.[57]

so that it could be baked in a pastry." Meare sauce is made of vinegar, small drink, and salt to which herbs could be added. Thus, some apparently did eat masked tainted meat. In her section "How to choose butcher's meat," Glasse wrote about lamb, "if it be azure blue it is new and good, but if greenish or yellowish; it is near tainting, if not tainted already." C. Anne Wilson, *Food and Drink in Britain: From the Stone Age to the 19th Century*, ed. C. Anne Wilson (Chicago: Academy Chicago Publishers 1991), 109–10; Hannah Glasse et al., *The Art of Cookery, Made Plain and Easy: Which Far Exceeds Any Thing of the Kind yet Published, Containing . . . To Which Are Added, One Hundred and Fifty New and Useful Receipts, and a Copious Index* (London: Printed for a Company of Booksellers, and sold by L. Wangford, in Fleet-Street, and all other booksellers in Great Britain and Ireland, 1770), 245–46. In the summer of 1801, Barker commented on the relationship between tainted meat, fish, and dysentery. In 1806 he wrote of an experience in 1772, an "account of a malignant fever which appeared in Newcastle [Maine] in the summer of 1772. . . . This fever evidently arose from tainted meat and damaged corn, brought into that town from Carolina.——It was confined to those families where these provisions were used." Barker, "Letter from Jeremiah Barker in Falmouth, Maine to Benjamin Rush in Philadelphia, 22 September 1806." In 1801 Barker was called to a neighboring town by a young man suffering "with a burning pain in his bowels, and vomiting . . . [Barker] took a half a day's journey in order to obtain an accurate statement of these facts [and found the man had eaten fish] rather damaged by being conveyed a considerable distance into the country." Jeremiah Barker, "An Account of Bilious Colics, as They Appeared in Several Towns in the County of Cumberland, District of Maine, in the Months of May, June, and July, 1801; and of the Surprising Relief Obtained Therein by Alkaline Remedies. By Dr. Jeremiah Barker, of Portland," *Medical Repository* 5 (1802): 267–77, quotation on p. 71. We can assume that in 1795 Barker knew that fever and dysentery can be caused by ingesting tainted meats. And from Boston in 1817, Thacher wrote that dysentery is "produced by the use of unwholesome and putrid foods, [adding] and by noxious exhalations and vapours . . . most prevalent in autumn, and is frequently of a contagious nature, and in some particular conditions of the atmosphere it prevails epidemically." James Thacher, *American Modern Practice* (Boston: Ezra Read, 1817), 587.

[56] Pearl Ash is impure carbonate of potash, a fixed vegetable alkali. Thacher, *The American New Dispensatory*, 94. Also called "lixivium or lixivia; see Estes, *Dictionary of Protopharmacology*, 117–18.

[57] Jeremiah Barker, "A History of Diseases in the District of Maine Commencing in 1735 and Continuing to the Present Time . . . To This Is Annexed an Inquiry into the Causes, Nature, Increasing Prevalency, and Treatment of Consumption," in *Jeremiah Barker, Collection 13*, ed. Maine Historical Society (Portland, Maine, 1831), vol. 1, mss., 140.

Barker soon began treating his patients with alkaline therapy. The following is an abbreviated account this treatment of one family found in his casebook and manuscript:

> *About the middle of August 1795, William Knight, a seaman, was attacked with fever in Philadelphia, and took passage for Falmouth, Maine, his native place, where he arrived on the 23ᵈ day. He was lodged in a decayed house, containing nine in family. He died on the 11ᵗʰ of September, attended with black stools and a yellow skin. Two weeks after his death, a sister aged 13 years, was seized with vomiting, pain in the head &c. succeeded by low delirium . . . During her sickness, a brother aged 7 years was attacked with fever. A hemorrhage from the nose, took place, in the 2ᵈ week, with black stools, he died on the 14ᵗʰ day. A sister aged 18 years was seized with fever and died in 8 days. . . . A profuse hemorrhage from the bowels, took place two hours before death. . . . The mother, aged 49 years, was then seized and died the 9ᵗʰ day, attended with black stools. . . . Three days before the death of the mother, a daughter, aged 25 years, was seized with fever. I was called on the 6ᵗʰ day, when her eyes were suffused with redness; skin of a pale yellow; stools loose, bottle green and very fœtid, pulse low & frequent, tongue dry & dark colored, unable to sit up. . . . I then made a liberal use of aqua calcis [limewater], and volatile alkaline salts.⁵⁸ In four days, the fœtor was removed, and the stools became natural. She soon recovered, without any other means. Soon after a youth sickened with fever. I was called on the 3ᵈ day. He complained of nausea, head ach, & thirst, bowels rather loose, stools greenish, pulse 90. . . . I directed lime water and pearl ash. His complaints were removed in one week, and he recovered. The sick rooms were then washed with soap suds and the walls were whitewashed with lime.*

---

[58] Aqua calcis (lime-water) is a "powerful antacid" that neutralizes acids and also treats diarrhea, scrofula, and worms. Coxe, *The American Dispensatory . . . Illustrated and Explained, According to the Principles of Modern Chemistry: Comprehending Improvements on Dr. Duncan's Second Edition*. Limewater is an alkaline water solution of calcium hydroxide and is used as an antacid. See also Thacher, *The American New Dispensatory*, 269; and Duncan, *The Edinburgh New Dispensatory*, 413–15. Duncan describes the preparations for limewater in Edinburgh, London, and Dublin. Volatile alkaline salts refer to carbonate of ammonia made by combining calcium carbonate with sal ammoniac. See Duncan, *The Edinburgh New Dispensatory*, 402–405, and Mitchill, "Concerning the Use of Alkaline Remedies in Fevers, and the Analogy between Septic Acid and Other Poisons; in a Letter to Thomas Percival M. D. &C of Manchester, from Dr. Mitchill, Dated New-York, January 17, 1797," 184.

Three of the family escaped the fever, and none of their visitors, which were numerous, were invaded.

After suitable depleting and evacuating means, I made a liberal use of al-kaline salts & lime water, which were found congenial to the stomach, and to remove the fœtor of the stools; so that the intestinal discharges soon became natural. But when alkaline remedies were neglected or too sparingly used, the putrefactive process, in the alimentary canal increased and the disease proved fatal, tho other means were used.[59]

Barker claimed that he was accused, presumably by unnamed local physicians, of using alkalines in putrid fevers, which had been considered by some physicians "as tending to promote putrefaction and dissolve blood."[60] He later recalled in an 1806 letter: "At this time [1795–96] I subjoined [added] alkaline salts & lime, to the usual remedies, tho amidst great opposition, to the damage of my interest; for I was called 'a dangerous innovator [Barker's underlining].'"[61] Alkaline salts had been an accepted therapy for fevers a cen-tury earlier but had lost favor and, for more than seventy-five years, had been replaced by the use of dilute acids.[62] Though alkaline salts and lime-water continued to be used for years as antacids and absorbents as well as lithonotriptic (drugs that dissolve lithic, i.e., uric acid stones), their use in putrid fevers was at issue.[63] Elixir vitriol (dilute sulfuric acid) did, however,

---

[59] Barker, "Barker Manuscript," MS, vol. 1, chap. 9, 141–43. Curious, although aware of the risk of retrospective diagnosis, I sent this narrative of a "mini-epidemic" to Dr. Scott Halstead, an expert on arboviruses, of which yellow fever and dengue are examples. Arbovirus is an informal name used to refer to any viruses that are transmitted by ar-thropod vectors (*Aedes aegypti* mosquitoes in this case); it is an acronym (ARthropod-BOrne virus). In a personal communication November 30, 2018, he concluded that the narrative suggested yellow fever, not dengue, and that a rain barrel may have allowed a few of these mosquitos to propagate locally. He also remarked that the ships at the time were "floating mosquito factories." Again, there have been no definite community epidemics as far north as Portland, Maine.

[60] Barker, "1806 Casebook," unpaginated. Putrid fevers include fevers associated with diseases such as typhus, gangrenous pharyngitis, and diphtheria.

[61] Barker, "Letter from Jeremiah Barker in Falmouth, Maine to Benjamin Rush in Philadelphia, 22 September 1806."

[62] See Debus, *Chemistry and Medical Debate*, 103–37, Cook, "John Colbatch and Augustan Medicine," and Boerhaave, *New Method of Chemistry; Including the Theory and Practice of That Art . . . To Which Is Prefix'd a Critical History of Chemistry and Chemists . . . Translated from the Printed Edition . . . By P. Shaw*, 197. The fall and rise of alkaline is discussed in more detail later in this chapter.

[63] William Cullen, *First Lines of the Practice of Physic with Supplementary Notes, Including More Recent Improvements in the Practice of Medicine by Peter Reid*, two volumes in one

seem to be an accepted treatment for fever at the time.[64] J. Worth Estes, historian of pharmacology, studied the drugs prescribed by four New England physicians, evaluating 3,336 drugs administered into the 1790s. Three of the four physicians prescribed vitriol (dilute sulfuric acid) as a tonic, but none recorded the use of aqua calcis or limewater, though two did use sal carbonas calcis (calcium carbonate).[65]

In a letter dated January 12, 1797, Barker thanked William Payne for sending him a "valuable collection of books" including Mitchill's theory on fever and contagion, which he shared with his "medical brethren" in Portland. The material helped Barker think and write about fevers; he would add practical remarks on therapy to Mitchill's theories and promised to hold himself responsible for a "faithful narrative."[66] Barker claimed, in 1806, that he "had to pursue the alkaline method of practice in fevers with increasing opposition till Jan'y 1797, when Dr. Mitchill, in his letter to Dr. Percival, recommended alkalines. This [the publication of Mitchill's letter] served to reconcile some of my opponents to their use [of alkali] in fevers."[67]

(Brookfield: E. Mirriam & Co. for Isaiah Thomas, 1807), 426. J. Worth Estes, "Therapeutic Practice in Colonial New England," in *Medicine in Colonial Massachusetts, 1620–1820: A Conference Held 25 & 26 May 1978*, ed. Frederick S. Allis (Boston: The Colonial Society of Massachusetts, 1980), table XI. Guenter B. Risse, *Hospital Life in Enlightenment Scotland: Care and Teaching at the Royal Infirmary of Edinburgh* (Cambridge: Cambridge University Press, 1986), 200. Duncan, *The Edinburgh New Dispensatory*, 414. For help with terminology, see Estes, *Dictionary of Protopharmacology*.

[64] See Cullen, *First Lines of the Practice of Physic*, 161. Elixir vitriol was given to 15.4 percent of sixty-five patients the Royal Infirmary in 1795. See Risse, *Hospital Life in Enlightenment Scotland: Care and Teaching at the Royal Infirmary of Edinburgh*, 354. The practices of four New England physicians (1751–1795) studied by Estes used elixir vitriol. Estes, "Therapeutic Practice in Colonial New England," table XI. "From its refrigerent and antiseptic properties, it [elixir vitriol] is a valuable medicine in many febrile diseases, especially those called putrid." Duncan, *The Edinburgh New Dispensatory*, 125. The previous quotation is published verbatim in Thacher, *The American New Dispensatory*, 71.

[65] Estes, "Therapeutic Practice in Colonial New England," Table XI, 316–29.

[66] Letter from Jeremiah Barker, of Portland to William Payne of New York, dated January 12, 1797, in the Jeremiah Barker Papers, Collection 13, Maine Historical Society, Portland, Maine. Barker mentions that he has already written a hundred pages of his book on "cause, cure, and increasing prevalency of consumption" in Maine and that he would now add febrile diseases to his topics. Barker includes some remarks on William Cullen and John Brown's thoughts on the danger of acids in food. Finally, he states that "Dr. [John] Brown's sentiments concerning food and acid are generally adhered to by physicians in this state."

[67] Barker, "Letter from Jeremiah Barker in Falmouth, Maine to Benjamin Rush in Philadelphia, 22 September 1806." Mitchill's letter to Percival, dated January 17, 1797, was not published until April; see Mitchill, "Concerning the Use of Alkaline Remedies

In a letter to Thomas Percival dated January 17, 1797, and published in the *New-York Magazine; or, Literary Repository* (1790–1797) in April 1797 and in the *Medical Repository* in November 1797, Mitchill commented on the state of chemical knowledge: "The discordant opinions of physiologists and physicians, two of whom can scarcely be found to agree . . . [on the causes of fever]."[68] In the same letter Mitchill wrote that, like Joseph Black and Richard Kirwan, he had changed from the phlogistonist to the antiphlogistonist theory; he also opined that "septic acids," particularly those of nitrogen, were intimately involved with pestilential diseases, alkaline remedies were recommended.[69]

The 1795 article that Mitchill had sent to Barker, "Remarks on the Gaseous Oxyd of Azote or of Nitrogene . . . Being an Attempt to Ascertain the True Nature of Contagion and to Explain Thereupon the Phenomena of Fever" was purely theoretical.[70] Years later, Barker wrote in his manuscript, "that Professor [Mitchill] had closed his treatise without entering into the practical

in Fevers, and the Analogy between Septic Acid and Other Poisons; in a Letter to Thomas Percival M. D. &C of Manchester, from Dr. Mitchill, Dated New-York, January 17, 1797." The same letter was subsequently published in the *Medical Repository* (vol. 1, no. 2, pp. 253–67) on November 9, 1797. Barker, writing to Rush in 1806, used the date of the letter in the title of the article rather than when the journal appeared in Maine. Cronin, *The Diary of Elihu Hubbard Smith*, 338.

[68] Mitchill, "Concerning the Use of Alkaline Remedies in Fevers, and the Analogy between Septic Acid and Other Poisons; in a Letter to Thomas Percival M. D. &C of Manchester, from Dr. Mitchill, Dated New-York, January 17, 1797." Mitchill, "Concerning the Use of Alkaline Remedies in Fevers, and the Analogy between Septic Acid and Other Poisons; in a Letter to Thomas Percival M. D. &C of Manchester, from Dr. Mitchill, Dated New-York, January 17, 1797," 255.

[69] Mitchill, "Concerning the Use of Alkaline Remedies in Fevers, and the Analogy between Septic Acid and Other Poisons; in a Letter to Thomas Percival M. D. &C of Manchester, from Dr. Mitchill, Dated New-York, January 17, 1797," 251–54, and Mitchill, "Concerning the Use of Alkaline Remedies in Fevers, and the Analogy between Septic Acid and Other Poisons; in a Letter to Thomas Percival M. D. &C of Manchester, from Dr. Mitchill, Dated New-York, January 17, 1797." See also Crosland, "Chemistry and the Chemical Revolution," 389–416; Dovovan, *Antoine Lavoisier*, 133–86; Holmes, "The 'Revolution in Chemistry and Physics,'" and Seymour Mauskopf, "Richard Kirwan's Phlogiston Theory: Its Success and Fate," *Ambix* 49, Part 3 (2002), 185–205. By 1789 Black had accepted Lavoisier's theory. See Golinski, *Science as a Public Culture*, 134. Actually by 1794 Mitchill had already turned away from phlogiston: "After the explosion of the delusive and fallacious hypothesis of Stahl, phlogiston and its derivatives." See Samuel L. Mitchill, *Nomenclature of the New Chemistry* (New-York: T. and J. Swords, 1794), microform, 4.

[70] Mitchill, *Remarks on the Gaseous Oxyd of Azote or of Nitrogene, and on the Effects It Produces When Generated in the Stomach, Inhaled into the Lungs, and Applied to the Skin: Being an Attempt to Ascertain the True Nature of Contagion, and to Explain Thereupon the Phenomena of Fever. / by Samuel Latham Mitchell, M.D. F.R.S.E. Professor of Chemistry, Natural History and Agriculture in the College of New-York.*

consideration."[71] In 1798, Barker published an article in the *Medical Repository* on the therapeutic use of alkaline remedies titled, "On Febrifuge Virtues of Lime, Magnesia and Alkaline Salts in Dysentery, Yellow-Fever and Scarlatina Angiosa." He began, "There are some among us who still consider the phenomena of fever to depend upon redundant quantity or acrid quality of bile. Therefore, their views are chiefly directed to emptying the intestines of this mischievous liquor, as they term it." This suggests he is beginning to turn away from the humoral explanation, "redundant quantity or acrid quality of bile," in favor of a chemical explanation of fever. Barker presented "thirty severe cases" of epidemic fever manifested by prostration, nausea, vomiting, abdominal pain, and diarrhea, at times bloody. He used standard remedies such as ipecac and rhubarb but "depended upon . . . alkaline salts and earths" to cure, and reported that he lost only one adult and two children. He had been using alkaline therapy for almost three years at this point and was confident of its usefulness. Barker was convinced that "the ravages made in the stomach, intestines, throat, or other parts, must be due to the septic acid."[72]

In 1800, Dr. David Hosack (1769–1835), New York physician and Professor of Materia Medica at Columbia College, published an article in the *Medical Repository*: "Dr. Hosack writes warmly in favour of lime-water.[73] . . . [L]ime-water, in that species of black-vomiting in which the matter discharged resembles coffee-grounds . . . that [lime-water] have operated by neutralizing the corrosive acid. "[He added that Jeremiah Barker's article, "On Febrifuge Virtues of Lime,"[74] "had been received by the editors, and read publicly to

---

[71] Barker, "Barker Manuscript," MS, 146. Mitchill actually ends his paper with a comment that he had planned to discuss practical considerations, but his manuscript was already too long. Mitchill, *Remarks on the Gaseous Oxyd of Azote or of Nitrogene, and on the Effects It Produces When Generated in the Stomach, Inhaled into the Lungs, and Applied to the Skin: Being an Attempt to Ascertain the True Nature of Contagion, and to Explain Thereupon the Phenomena of Fever / by Samuel Latham Mitchell, M.D. F.R.S.E. Professor of Chemistry, Natural History and Agriculture in the College of New-York*, 43.

[72] Barker, "On Febrifuge Virtues of Lime, Magnesia and Alkaline Salts in Dysentery, Yellow-Fever and Scarlatina Angiosa. In a Letter from Dr. Jeremiah Barker, of Portland, (Maine) Dated May 30, 1798," *Medical Repository* 2, (1798): 147–52.

[73] David Hosack, "Dr. Hosack Writes Warmly in Favour of Lime-Water," *Medical Repository* 3 (1800): 404–406.

[74] Barker, "On Febrifuge Virtues of Lime, Magnesia and Alkaline Salts in Dysentery, Yellow-Fever and Scarlatina Angiosa. In a Letter from Dr. Jeremiah Barker, of Portland, (Maine) Dated May 30, 1798."

the students of physic in the New-York Hospital, early in the season of 1798."[75]

Mitchill's "Doctrine of Septon" was embraced by others who were attempting to use contemporary chemistry to explain and treat pestilential diseases.[76] Numerous letters referring to septon/azote appeared in the *Medical Repository* from 1797–1800. Inaugural dissertations by Mitchill's students formed one group who would be expected to approve of their professor's theory of septon.[77] British physician Colin Chisholm (1755–1825) wrote on epidemic diseases and subscribed to Mitchill's theory, but with

---

[75] For biographical material on David Hosack see Howard A. Kelly and Walter L. Burrage, *American Medical Biographies* (Baltimore: The Norman, Remington Company, 1920), 561–62; and Garraty and Carnes, *American National Biography*, 238–39.

[76] For a list of nineteen articles by Mitchill on septon, see "Article VIII. An Inaugural Dissertation, Showing in What Manner Pestilential Vapours Acquire Their Acid Quality, and How This Is Neutralized by Alkalis, . . . By Adolph C. Lent, Citizen of the State of New York. T. And J. Swords. 1798. 8vo. Pp. 54," *Medical Repository* 2, no. 1 (1799): 96–98. Mitchill's enthusiasm for his theory included the publication of an article within which is a four page poem, "The Doctrine of Septon: attempted after the manner of Dr. Darwin." Samuel L. Mitchill, "Further Facts Tending toward an Explanation of the True Operation of Alkalis and Lime Upon Other Substances. In a Letter from Dr. Mitchill to Thomas Beddoes, M.D., September 15, 1797," *Medical Repository* 1, no. 2 (1797): 178–87; and Erasmus Darwin, *The Botanic Garden. A Poem, in Two Parts. Part I. Containing the Economy of Vegetation. Part II. The Loves of the Plants. With Philosophical Notes*, 3rd ed. (London: J. Johnson, 1795). Citing the *Medical Repository* can be confusing. The journal began publication in July 1797, but the bound editions usually have the following year. If one looks at the individual issues of volume 1, the first two are dated 1797 and the second two 1798. Further complicating the situation is the fact that there was a second edition of the first and second volumes in 1800, and a third edition of the same volumes in 1804–1805. See Billings, "Literature and Institutions," 330.

[77] Examples include "Art. VI. An Inaugural Dissertation on the Operation of Pestilential Fluids Upon the Large Intestines Termed by Nosologists Dysentery. By William Bay, Citizen of the State of New-York. New-York. T. And J. Swords. 1797. 8vo. Pp. 109," *Medical Repository* 1 (3rd ed., 1804), no. 2 (1798): 232–38. "Article VIII. An Inaugural Dissertation, Showing in What Manner Pestilential Vapours Acquire Their Acid Quality, and How This Is Neutralized by Alkalis, . . . By Adolph C. Lent, Citizen of the State of New York. T. And J. Swords. 1798. 8vo. Pp. 54," 96–98; and Winthrop Saltonstall and Samuel L. Mitchill, *An Inaugural Dissertation on the Chemical and Medical History of Septon, Azote, or Nitrogene: And Its Combinations with the Matter of Heat and the Principle of Acidity* (New-York: T. and J. Swords, 1796). The reviewers of the Saltonstall dissertation in *The New-York Magazine* had some reservations about Mitchill's theory of septon, however, and wrote that they were inclined to "wait for the remaining evidence, before we pronounce sentence . . . and we are sincerely glad to see the philosophers of America at last attempting to make some return for the abundant chemical knowledge which they have received from Europe." "Review of Saltonstall's 'Dissertation on Septon, Azote, or Nitrogene,'" *The New-York Magazine, of Literary Repository* 2 (March 1797): 143–46.

some reservations.[78] He opined that the "yellow remittent fever" seen in the West Indies is "almost universally allowed not to be contagious" and is therefore different from the continued malignant and pestilential fever related to gaseous oxyd of azote.[79] Chisholm reported on an epidemic that broke out in "Demarara" [sic] in 1800, "Mitchill's gaseous oxyd of azote (septic acid vapour), proceeding from the decomposition of animal matter . . . produced, at first, a disease of a pure pestilential nature."[80] Another "pro-septon" writer was the Canadian physician Francois Blanchet (1776–1830), who left Québec to study under Mitchill at Columbia College from 1799 to 1800. In 1800 he published a book in New York City, in French, on the application of chemistry to medicine, agreeing with Mitchill's conviction that septic acid or its gas is the exciting cause of pestilential distempers.[81]

---

[78] See Lester S. King, *The Medical World of the Eighteenth Century* (Huntington, NY: Robert E. Krieger Publishing Co. Inc. [reprint 1971], (1958), 150–51; and Colin Chisholm, *An Essay on the Malignant Pestilential Fever, Introduced into the West Indian Islands from Boullam, on the Coast of Guinea, as It Appeared in 1793, 1794, 1795, and 1796. Interspersed with Observations and Facts, Tending to Prove That the Epidemic Existing at Philadelphia, New-York, &C. Was the Same Fever Introduced by Infection Imported from the West Indian Islands: And Illustrated by Evidences Found on the State of Those Islands, and Information of the Most Eminent Practitioners Residing on Them*, 2nd ed., 2 vols., vol. 1 (London: Mawman, 1801), 260–66, 70, 73n., 81–83.

[79] Chisholm, *An Essay on the Malignant Pestilential Fever*, 1, 270. He went on to suggest that the work of Hunter and Volta on the gaseous inflammable emanations in marshes may be the chemical reason for marsh fever. Chisholm, *An Essay on the Malignant Pestilential Fever, Introduced into the West Indian Islands from Boullam*, 1, 273.

[80] Demarara [sic] (Demerara), previously British Guiana and now Guyana in South America. See Colin Chisholm, "Intelligence from Dr. Chisholm since the Publication of the Second Edition of His Work on Fever," *Medical Repository* 5, no. 2 (1805): 228–34.

[81] François Blanchet, *Recherches Sur La Medecine, Ou L'application De La Chimie a La Medecine* (New York: De l'imprimerie de Parisot, Chatham-Street, 1800), microform, xxiij, [1], 246, [2] p.; 21 cm. (8vo); and, for a review of his book in the *Medical Repository*, see "Art. III. Recherches Sur La Medecine, Ou L'application De La Chimie a La Medecine. Par Francois Blanchet. A New-York. Parisot. 8vo. Pp. 246. 1800," *Medical Repository* 4, no. 2 (1801): 172–76. The review claimed that Blanchet "expresses his perfect conviction that septic acid, or its gas, according to Mitchill's doctrine, is the exciting cause of pestilential distempers (p. 75), yet he considers the azotic basis of this acid as having very little to do in the business." Blanchet also questioned the reason given by Mitchill and Citizen Guyton as to why azote and oxygen do not spontaneously combine in the atmosphere. See François Blanchet, "Article IX. To the Editors of the Medical Repository. Gentlemen, If the Following Observations Appear to Deserve a Place in Your Repository, in Insertion of Them Will Oblige Your Most Obedient, F. Blanchet. New-York, 24th August, 1800," *Medical Repository* 4, no. 4 (1801): 369–70. In an article on the use of alkali in embalming in Teneriffe and ancient Egypt Blanchet wrote, "oxygene, assisted by caloric, will connect itself with the septon (azote) of the substance, and engender or constitute the ACID OF PUTREFACTION [Blanchet's emphasis]." He then referred to six of Mitchill's articles as well as three others supporting

Not all agreed with Mitchill's theory, however. Dr. Joshua Fisher, a student with Barker under Bela Lincoln, practiced in Beverly, Massachusetts. In a letter dated May 5, 1797, Fisher replied to some questions from Barker. Fisher had not read of Mitchill's theory of fevers and wrote that he doubted that "quaffing copious potations of lime water will cure a fever when formed. . . . I shall always be happy assisting your enquiries after truth, but such is the passion for innovation in Religion, Government, & medicine & so absurd & whimsical the theories that they scarcely deserve serious consideration."[82]

There was further refutation of Mitchill's paper in "Remarks on the Gaseous Oxyd of Azote or of Nitrogene" (1795), which was reprinted in 1796 in the appendix of *Medical Cases and Speculations*, a book published in Britain by Thomas Beddoes and James Watt.[83] From 1793 to 1797, Beddoes and Watt in Bristol had been campaigning for therapeutic trials of pneumatic medicine, that is, the therapeutic use of artificially produced gases including oxygen and nitrous oxide.[84] Humphry Davy joined them and "quickly refuted Mitchill's claim that the gas [gaseous oxyd of azote] was poisonous."[85] The refutation was challenged by the editors of the *Medical Repository*, Mitchill and Edward Miller. After discussing the Medical Pneumatic Institute in Bristol, they reviewed H. Davy's book, *Researches, Chemical and Philosophical . . . 1800*.[86] The reviewer

the use of alkali. See François Blanchet, "Facts and Remarks on the Antiseptic Powers of Lixivial and Oleaginious Substances: Communicated by Mr. F. Blanchet, to Dr. Mitchill," *Medical Repository* 3, no. 2 (1800): 156.

[82] Letter from Joshua Fisher of Beverly, Massachusetts, to Jeremiah Barker of Falmouth, Maine, dated May 5, 1797, in Collection 13, Jeremiah Barker Papers at the Maine Historical Society, Portland, Maine. Fisher was vice president of the Massachusetts Medical Society from 1804 to 1814, and then president until 1823. See Walter L. Burrage, *A History of the Massachusetts Medical Society* (Norwood, MA: Plimpton Press, 1923), 462–63.

[83] Thomas Beddoes and James Watt, *Medical Cases and Speculations; Including Parts IV and V of Considerations on the Medicinal Power, and the Production of Factitious Airs*, 3rd ed., 2 vols., vol. 2 (Bristol: Bulgin & Rosser, 1796), 41–69. Beddoes mentioned the use of acids and alkalis (nitre) in consumption, but was not enthusiastic about either mode of therapy in that disease. See Thomas Beddoes, *Observations on the Nature and Cure of Calculus, Sea Scurvy, Consumption, Catarrah, and Fever* (Philadelphia: T. Dobson, 1797), 134–35.

[84] Julian M. Leigh, "Early Treatment with Oxygen: The Pneumatic Institute and Panaceal Literature of the Nineteenth Century," *Anesthesia* 29, no. 2 (1974): 194–208.

[85] Beddoes and Watt, *Medical Cases and Speculations; Including Parts IV and V of Considerations on the Medicinal Power, and the Production of Factitious Airs*, 2. Appendix No. 1, 56; and Golinski, *Science as a Public Culture*, 166–67.

[86] "Medical and Philsophical News. Domestic. Progress of Pneumatic Medicine," *Medical Repository* 4, no. 2 (1800–1801): 183–89. Humphry Davy, *Researches, Chemical*

pointed out that Davy's investigation was stimulated by "Dr. Mitchill's attempt to explain the phenomena of contagion; in which the Doctor originally conjectured that some of the symptoms of endemic distempers were induced by this modification of azote exhaling from corrupting substances, and infecting the atmosphere."[87]

Mitchill had been influenced by the experiments of Priestley and others in 1795, but in the following five years he did not write a second edition of his book, though it had been requested.[88] Thus it appears that Mitchill gradually shed his enthusiasm for the "Doctrine of Septon" and oxyd of azote as the key to understanding pestilential disease. He may have begun to agree with Davy and others as the results of new chemical research appeared, or he moved on to other chemical, medical, and/or political issues. Mitchill's theoretical explanation of fever faded away, though he does not appear to have declared the theory "wrong." Although Mitchill stopped writing about his theories of septon, Barker still believed that alkaline therapy was efficacious and therefore continued its use in his practice.

CHEMISTRY, YELLOW FEVER, AND THE CONTAGIONIST/ ANTICONTAGIONIST BATTLE

The acceptance or rejection of Mitchill's new chemical explanation of disease was complicated by strong contemporary views on the yellow fever epidemics plaguing the Eastern United States port cities in the 1790s. Advocates of the contagionist (imported) explanation of yellow fever placed the blame on unhealthy refugees and their ships. Believers in the anti-contagionist (domestic/environmental) explanation claimed that the disease was caused by unhealthy locations, climatic conditions, and/or poor sanitation.[89] Of all the

---

and Philosophical: Chiefly Concerning Nitrous Oxide, or Diphlogisticated Nitrous Air, and Its Respiration (London: Printd for J. Johnson . . . by Biggs and Cottle, Bristol., 1800).

[87] "Medical and Philsophical News. Domestic. Progress of Pneumatic Medicine," vol. 4, 183–89.

[88] "Medical and Philsophical News. Domestic. Progress of Pneumatic Medicine."

[89] Historian Martin Pernick succinctly posed the debate: did "dirty streets or dirty foreigners" cause yellow fever? Martin S. Pernick, "Politics, Parties, and Pestilence: Epidemic Yellow Fever in Philadelphia and the Rise of the First Party System," in A Melancholy Scene of Devastation: The Public Response to the 1793 Philadelphia Yellow Fever Epidemic, ed. J. Worth Estes and Billy G. Smith (Canton, MA: Science History Publications/USA, 1997), 119–46. Though the terms "anti-contagionist" and "contagionist" have been used for at least 150 years according to the OED, most

febrile diseases troubling the United States at the time, it was yellow fever that caused the most discord in the American medical profession.[90]

In 1793 Mathew Carey wrote, "That it [yellow fever] is an imported disorder, is the opinion of almost all inhabitants of Philadelphia."[91] Various aspects of the new chemistry, of such interest to Barker, played a part in the battle for the hearts and minds of the public as well as physicians. In 1799, for example, the American Philosophical Society published a paper read by William Currie before the Society on October 2, 1795, in which he wrote that he was "next to certain" that the unwholesomeness of marshy low situations in the summer and autumn was due neither to putrefying vegetable and animal matter nor to "invisible Miasmata or noxious effluvia" but rather to "a deficiency of the oxygenous portion of the atmosphere."[92] He ridiculed the supporters of the domestic origin of yellow fever and their "imaginary change in the constitution of the atmosphere . . . in conjunction with putrid exhalations . . . [that] gives origin to the malignant and destructive yellow fever. . . . And till those gentlemen subject the atmosphere to eudiometrical experiments" their

modern historians emphasize a spectrum of disease theory between the two poles. Physicians spoke of predisposing and precipitating causes of disease complicating the anti-contagionist /contagionist dichotomy. The idea of "such a polarity is anachronistic and simplistic." W. F. Bynum, "Cullen and the Study of Fevers in Britain, 1760–1820," in *Theories of Fever from Antiquity to the Enlightenment*, ed. W. F. Bynum and V. Nutton (London: Wellcome Institute for the History of Medicine; Medical History, Supplement no. 1, 1981), 142. Hudson emphasizes that "among physicians there were few absolute anticontagionists" and that in the early nineteenth century most of the controversy involved yellow fever, cholera, and plague. See Robert Hudson, *Disease and Its Control* (Westport, CT: Greenwood Press, 1983), 146; Rosenberg, *Explaining Epidemics*, 283–85, 96–98; Apel, *Feverish Bodies, Enlightened Minds: Science and the Yellow Fever Controversy in the Early American Republic*, 7–8, 14, 145–48.

[90] Lloyd G. Stevensen, "Putting Disease on the Map: The Early Use of Spot Maps in the Study of Yellow Fever," *Journal of the History of Medicine and Allied Sciences* 20 (1965): 228.

[91] Mathew Carey, *A Short Account of the Malignant Fever, Lately Prevalent in Philadelphia: With a Statement of the Proceedings That Took Place on the Subject in Different Parts of the United States*, 2nd ed. (Philadelphia: Mathew Carey, 1793), 18; Apel, *Feverish Bodies, Enlightened Minds: Science and the Yellow Fever Controversy in the Early American Republic*, 11–32.

[92] William Currie, "An Enquiry into the Causes of the Insalubrity of Flat and Marshy Situations," *Transactions of the American Philosophical Society* 4 (1799): 135. Currie suggested the possibility of a chemical means of inhibiting putrefaction, but decided drainage, cultivation, and filling would be more appropriate, all old ideas. See also James C. Riley, *The Eighteenth-Century Campaign to Avoid Disease* (New York: St. Martin's Press, 1987), 93.

theories deserve "no more respect than the visionary opinions which prevailed in the dark ages of Gothic ignorance."[93]

Although the District of Maine did not suffer the yellow fever epidemics occurring further south, Barker did treat a few cases and must have been interested in the contagionist/anticontagionist debate. Medicine's inability to separate yellow fever from other febrile conditions causing jaundice, bloody stools, systemic symptoms, and a high mortality compelled him to add "Yellow-Fever" to his first published articles, beginning in 1798: "On the Febrifuge Virtue of Lime, Magnesia and Alkaline Salts in Dysentery, Yellow-Fever and Scarlatina Anginosa."[94]

BARKER THE "DANGEROUS INNOVATOR"

Was Jeremiah Barker taking a professional risk in the late 1790s by his use of limewater and alkaline salts for various diseases?[95] Why was this

[93] The eudiometer was originally used by Enlightenment reformers who were hoping to reduce disease by garnering the support of Royal patrons, who, after seeing the "scientific data," would help fund the clean-up of factory sites, marshlands, graveyards, etc. Lissa Roberts, "Eudiometer," in *Instruments of Science: An Historical Encyclopedia*, ed. Robert Bud and Deborah Jean Warner (New York: The Science Museum, London and the National Museum of American History, Smithsonian Institution in assoc. with Garland Publishing, Inc., 1998), 232–34. William Currie, *A Sketch of the Rise and Progress of the Yellow Fever, and the Proceedings of the Board of Health, in Philadelphia, in the Year 1799: To Which Is Added, a Collection of Facts and Observations Respecting the Origin of Yellow Fever in This Country; and a Review of the Different Modes of Treating It* (Philadelphia: Budd and Bartram, 1800), 67–68. A eudiometer is "an instrument for determining the purity of the air." Coxe, *The Philadelphia Medical Dictionary*. The word is derived from Greek, eudia: fine weather + -meter. The device measures changes in volume occurring when gases combine. During the 1770s, the pneumatic experiments of Joseph Priestley led to a new technology commonly known as eudiometry. Simon Schaffer, "Measuring Virtue: Eudiometry, Enlightenment and Pneumatic Medicine," in *The Medical Enlightenment of the Eighteenth Century*, ed. Andrew Cunningham and Roger French (New York: Cambridge University Press, 1990), 281–318, see 282. Though Priestley's test for the "goodness of air" measured dephlogisticated air, that is, oxygen, it was thought that the instruments could be used to determine healthy from unhealthy sites that should be quarantined. Experiments with the eudiometer led to Lavoisier's discovery that water was not an element, but rather a compound made up of oxygen and hydrogen. See Dovovan, *Antoine Lavoisier*, 1993, 141–42. Within a decade, however, eudiometer readings were found to vary little from site to site and were not correlated with mortality patterns. See Riley, *The Eighteenth-Century Campaign to Avoid Disease*, 50–51.

[94] *Medical (The) Repository* 2, no. 2 (1798): 147–52.

[95] Jeremiah Barker, "An Account of a Malignant Fever, Sporadically Formed, in Falmouth, County of Cumberland, District of Maine," *Medical Repository* New Series

regular physician, preceptor-trained by a well-educated physician and generally practicing in the accepted manner of his time, exposing himself to being called a "dangerous innovator" by using and encouraging the use of alkaline remedies?

At end of the eighteenth-century, professional identity was closely connected to therapeutic intervention.[96] Barker's use of alkaline therapy might have been considered a "disease specific therapy [that] was considered ethically suspect . . . and no scientific physician willingly admits the existence of specifics."[97] Fortunately for Barker, alkaline therapy was an adjunct to the standard care that soon had the authority of Mitchill's and his own published articles to bolster his claims of therapeutic efficacy.

Historian Charles E. Rosenberg, in a classic article, emphasizes the importance to the physician–patient relationship of "exhibiting" a drug, meaning that the drug should produce a "particular physiological end."[98] This means that the patient and doctor must see and/or feel the effects of the drug. The use of lime-water and alkaline salts, which decreased the peptic symptoms of heartburn and indigestion and made many people feel better promptly, thus may have been seen to be effective in treating fever.

Though it is important to remember that Barker was treating the "virulent acidity" causing fevers, he "exhibited" drugs that, rather than producing salivation, nausea, vomiting, diarrhea, or perspiration, instead quickly made the patient's belly or chest feel better. Patient and doctor sensed a physiological response to the medication and, if the patient recovered from the fever or whatever disease was being treated, both would assume that the medication "worked." For example, Barker noted that his use of one to two ounces (30–60 cc) every thirty to sixty minutes diminished the "thirst for water, so generally complained of" by patients with epidemic fever, abdominal pain, frequent

---

19, no. 3 (1818): 286–90. It is interesting to note that Barker, who had been publishing yearly until 1807, did not publish this article reporting an epidemic in 1809 until 1818, the year he retired from active practice.

[96] John Harley Warner points out that "the integrity of regular therapeutics could not be radically challenged without an implicit threat to regular professional identity." John Harley Warner, *The Therapeutic Perspective: Medical Practice, Knowledge, and Identity in America, 1820–85* (Cambridge, MA: Harvard University Press, 1986), 12.

[97] Warner, *The Therapeutic Perspective*, 62, but for the discussion of The Principle of Specificity, see 58–80.

[98] Charles E. Rosenberg, "The Therapeutic Revolution: Medicine, Meaning, and Social Change in Nineteenth-Century America," *Perspectives in Biology and Medicine* 20, no. 4 (1977): 485–506.

stools, or vomiting.[99] He recorded that the alkaline treatments were "grateful to her stomach . . . abated the sense of heat in the stomach . . . [alleviated] the distressing pain and anguish at the stomach, &c."[100] Thus Barker may have weathered the storm of criticism because his alkaline therapy actually worked to relieve symptoms associated with fever.

Barker reported on many patients who experienced various febrile conditions and were treated with alkali, as evidenced in his casebooks, manuscript, and in some of the articles he published in the *Medical Repository* from 1798–1818. For example, in 1800 he wrote, "The success that has attended the use of alkaline remedies in this fever [with jaundice, abdominal pain, nausea, vomiting, and deafness], not only in my hands, but in the hands of several of my brethren, has attracted the particular attention of many among us; so that, unless the patient is under a course of alkalies during the fever, we are accused of neglecting the most necessary means."[101] Barker was still reporting on the use of alkaline salts and lime to treat an epidemic caused by "tainted meat" in 1818 in the *Medical Repository*.

A weekly newspaper, the *Portland Gazette and Maine Advertiser* of September 15 and 22, 1806, included an article of nearly six full columns by Jeremiah Barker about the efficacy of alkalies in the treatment of fevers and the fumigation of rooms and ships. He wrote that his observations had been published in the *Medical Repository* and republished in the *London Reviews* as well as in Germany, and included the names of at least thirty-three philosophers, physicians, journal articles, and books to bolster his arguments. Barker expressed his desire to "aid the efforts of the Massachusetts Medical

---

[99] Barker, "On Febrifuge Virtues of Lime, Magnesia and Alkaline Salts in Dysentery, Yellow-Fever and Scarlatina Angiosa. In a Letter from Dr. Jeremiah Barker, of Portland, (Maine) Dated May 30 1798," 148–49. Perhaps limewater and alkaline salts should be added to Oliver Wendell Holmes's 1860 list of medicines *not* to be thrown into the sea. "Throw out opium . . . throw out a few specifics our art did not discover . . . throw out wine . . . and I firmly believe that if the whole material medica, as now used, could be sunk to the bottom of the sea, it would be all the better for mankind,—and all the worse for the fishes." Oliver Wendell Holmes, "Currents and Counter-Currents," in *Medical Essays: 1842–1882*, ed. Oliver Wendell Holmes (Boston: Houghton Mifflin Company, 1911), 202–203.

[100] Barker, "On Febrifuge Virtues of Lime, Magnesia and Alkaline Salts in Dysentery, Yellow-Fever and Scarlatina Angiosa. In a Letter from Dr. Jeremiah Barker, of Portland, (Maine) Dated May 30 1798," 148–49.

[101] Jeremiah Barker, "An Account of Febrile Diseases, as They Have Appeared in the County of Cumberland, District of Maine, from July, 1798, to March, 1800: Communicated in a Letter from Dr. Jeremiah Barker, of Portland, to Dr. Mitchill," *Medical Repository* 3, no. 4 (1800): 365.

Society in eradicating medical prejudices and disseminating useful knowledge and . . . exposing & suppressing empirical impositions, which rapidly increase; finally, in rendering the science of medicine more respectable and important in the view of mankind." He concluded by stating that alkalinization would benefit different parts of the United States "as long as filth, and putrefying substances continue to generate febrile poisons; and alkalines retain their correcting, cleansing, antidotal power."[102]

CONCLUSION

Extrapolating from Erwin H. Ackerknecht's "behaviorist approach," S. E. D. Shortt suggests "that if the medical elite were resistant to innovation, isolated general practitioners were doubtless even more so."[103] Barker would point out that the lack of reading by physicians was a major reason for the "hostility with which improvements in medicine have been pursued by empirics."[104] Fifty years ago Henry E. Sigerist asked us to study the work of ordinary physicians like Barker as well as the work of elites.[105]

One could argue whether Barker, who continued writing and editing *A History of Diseases in the District of Maine* for over thirty years and published over a dozen articles in the first and second US medical journals, quite fits into the category of "rank-and-file doctor." But with his background, education, and location he can hardly be called one of the elites. His apparent

[102] Barker, "On Febrifuge Virtues of Lime, Magnesia and Alkaline Salts in Dysentery, Yellow-Fever and Scarlatina Angiosa. In a Letter from Dr. Jeremiah Barker, of Portland, (Maine) Dated May 30, 1798"; Barker, "An Account of Febrile Diseases, as They Have Appeared in the County of Cumberland, District of Maine, from July, 1798, to March, 1800: Communicated in a Letter from Dr. Jeremiah Barker, of Portland, to Dr. Mitchill"; Jeremiah Barker, "Medical by Jeremiah Barker," *Portland Gazette and Maine Advertiser*, September 15 and 22, 1806, 1.

[103] S. E. D. Shortt, "Physicians, Science, and Status: Issues in the Professionalization of Anglo-American Medicine in the Nineteenth Century," *Medical History* 27, no. 1 (1983): 51–68; and Erwin H. Ackerknecht, "A Plea for a "Behaviorist Approach in Writing History of Medicine," *Journal of the History of Medicine and Allied Sciences* 22, no. 3 (1967): 211–14.

[104] Barker, "1806 Casebook," unpaginated.

[105] Henry E. Sigerist, *A History of Medicine*, vol. 1 (New York: Oxford University Press, 1967 [1951]), 14. Barker was already working on this manuscript by 1797. See Barker, "Dr. Barker of Portland, in the District of Maine, Is Preparing a Work for the Press, on Consumption and Fever. In This Work the Dr. Expects to Establish the Efficacy of Alkalies, in the Cure of Yellow Fever." There are numerous newspaper articles published in several Maine cities through 1820 discussing his work on the manuscript.

understanding of the new chemistry, or at least its rhetoric, may have helped him to secure patients, most likely of middle and upper classes, who might also be interested in and reading about chemistry. It's equally possible that his stance as an "innovator" turned patients away from his practice and drew criticism from his peers.

Jeremiah Barker is an example of a nonelite physician at the end of the eighteenth century who used the new acid/base, oxidation, and fermentation chemistry to provide an etiological rationale of disease and a treatment. The improvement his patients appear to have experienced probably had little to do with the "septic acid" and more to do with incidental symptomatic relief of peptic symptoms and dehydration and his own enthusiasm over the new chemical explanations. Acids would replace humors in Barker's understanding and treatment of many diseases.[106] But as John Harley Warner points out, an increase in the authority and status of physicians like Barker had less to do with "the content [than] the rhetoric of science."[107]

The new science had to be useful, whether it be the chemistry of manure and farming, manure on city streets, saltpeter for gunpowder, or nitrogen compounds in medicine. Historian Lester King writes that there are three aspects of a scientist: technology (not an issue in Barker's medicine), methodology (hypothesis and facts to confirm, refute, or modify the hypothesis), and knowledge (of the relevant literature) that provide "an insight denied to others."[108] Did Barker's scientific outlook give him an insight denied to others? Barker performed a few experiments and published over a dozen articles

---

[106] Barker discussed alkali treatment of skin lesions as well as fevers and intestinal aliments. See Jeremiah Barker, "Obstinate Eruption over the Whole Surface of the Body Cured by Chalk (Alkaline Earth, or Carbonate of Lime)," *Medical Repository* 3 (1800): 412–13. Others found that skin ulcers and cancers were acid when tested with litmus paper and seemed to improve with alkaline applications. H. C. Kunze, "Exteriments Proving the Acid Quality of the Pus, or Matter Formed on the Surface of Veneral and Cancerous Ulcers," *Medical Repository* 4, no. 3 (1800–1801): 297–98. and Samuel L. Mitchill, "Article IX. Arrangement of Facts Concerning Ulcers, Sores and Tetters; Showing How Agreeably These and Similar Affections of the Skin Are Healed, in Many Cases, by Alkaline Applications: In a Letter to Thomas Trotter, M.D. Physician to the British Fleet, Etc Dated New-York, September 20, 1800," *Medical Repository* 4, no. 2 (1801): 149–54.

[107] John Harley Warner, "Grand Narrative and Its Discontents: Medical History and the Social Transformation of American Medicine," *Journal of Health Politics, Policy and Law* 29, no. 4 (2004): 767–68.

[108] Lester S. King, *Medical Thinking: A Historical Preface* (Princeton, NJ: Princeton University Press, 1982), 294–309. Rather than a scientist, Barker probably would be considered a natural philosopher focusing on medicine, since the term "scientist" was just entering the lexicon circa 1834, as noted in the *Oxford English Dictionary*.

relating to chemistry and disease. Historians Shapin and Thackray might place him in the "third level" of scientific enterprise: a "cultivator of science, who patronized, applied, or disseminated scientific knowledge or principles."[109] There may have been many general physicians who worked at this level, but fortunately for us, Barker's work has survived and is available for study.

[109] Steven Shapin and Arnold Thackray, "Prosopography as a Research Tool in History of Science: The British Scientific Community 1700–1900," *History of Science* 12 (1974): 1–28.

CHAPTER 5

Thoughts to Consider While Reading Barker's Manuscript: Presentism, Whiggish History, and the *Post Hoc* Fallacy

To evaluate Barker's knowledge and treatments, the twenty-first-century reader must strive to avoid presentism, which is the tendency to use present-day ideas and perspectives to judge the past.[1] Barker, his patients, and his peers were just as intelligent as we are today, but they viewed the world differently, through the concepts available to them. Historian and physician Jacalyn Duffin notes that from a historical perspective, presentism and whiggish history[2] "could even be called sins or crimes," and clearly states

---

[1] J. Duffin, "A Hippocratic Triangle: History, Clinician-Historians, and Future Doctors," in *Locating Medical History: The Stories and Their Meanings*, ed. Frank Huisman and John Harley Warner (Baltimore: Johns Hopkins University Press, 2004), 432–49; L. Loison, "Forms of Presentism in the History of Science: Rethinking the Project of Historical Epistemology," *Studies in the History and Philosophy of Science* 60 (2016), 29–37; Oscar Moro-Abadía, "Thinking About 'Presentism' from a Historian's Perspective: Herbert Butterfield and Hélène Metzger," *History of Science* 47, no. 1 (2009), 55–77; Mary P. Winsor, "The Practitioner of Science: Everyone Her Own Historian," *Journal of the History of Biology* 34, no. 2 (2001), 229–45.

[2] Whiggish or whig history refers to a portrayal of the past as a series of events showing continual improvement until we reach the present. The name comes from the British Liberal Party's progressive philosophy, and its significance to historians from a book by a Professor of History at Cambridge University, Herbert Butterfield, *The Whig Interpretation of History* (London: G. Bell & Sons, 1931); Jacalyn Duffin, *History of Medicine: A Scandalously Short Introduction* (Toronto: University of Toronto Press,

that "It is unfair and anachronistic to blame predecessors for not saying, seeing, or knowing what could not yet be said, seen, or known."[3] Historian Lynn Hunt wrote "Presentism, at its worst, encourages a kind of moral complacency and self-congratulation . . . [and can lead to] attitudes of temporal superiority."[4] Instead, we should be attempting to understand what they were thinking and doing and not denigrate their thoughts and works.[5] Barker was following current theories and practice and was, in fact, attempting to go a step beyond by using the latest discoveries in chemistry to consider a new therapy.

The modern reader of Barker's manuscript will note the frequent post hoc fallacy,[6] referring to his assumption that a later event was caused by an earlier event, when in fact both events may be true but not be causally related. The cure may or may not be the result of the therapy—an observation that is just as true today as it was in the eighteenth century. This issue transcends the theory or philosophy being followed, whether it be correcting the humors, adjusting the tension of blood vessels or nerves, or using the genetic code to alter disease.

HOLISTIC AND BIOMEDICAL MODELS

The holistic approach[7] of Hippocrates and Galen endured for more than 1,500 years, emphasizing the correction of imbalances provoked by noxious air (miasma), inappropriate behavior, the environment, air, water, food, emotions, exercise, rest, and evacuations. All these factors helped to explain how diseases might be corrected by bloodletting and the use of emetics, cathartics, and enemas. Early modern investigations—on such subjects as

1999), 374; Adrian Wilson and T. G. Ashplant, "Whig History and Present-Centred History," *The Historical Journal* 31, no. 1 (1988): 1–16; A. R. Hall, "On Whiggism," *History of Science* 21, no. 51 Pt 1 (1983), 45–59.

[3] Duffin, *History of Medicine: A Scandalously Short Introduction*, 373–74.

[4] Hunt, Lynn, online comments: https://www.historians.org/publications-and-directories/perspectives-on-history/may-2002/against-presentism

[5] John C. Burnham, *What Is Medical History?* (Cambridge, UK: Malden, MA: Polity, 2005), 99–103.

[6] *Post hoc ergo propter hoc* translates to "after this, therefore because of this"—meaning that because an event occurred first, it must have caused a later event.

[7] The holistic approach refers to a form of medical treatment that attempts to deal with the whole person rather than merely the physical condition (OED).

anatomy by Andreas Vesalius in 1543, circulation by William Harvey in 1628, anatomical pathology by Giovanni Battista Morgagni in 1761, and tissue pathology by Marie François Xavier Bichat in 1800—provided a framework for future advances in medical science but did little to affect changes in medical therapeutics.

Barker practiced just at the close of this Hippocratic holistic tradition, which was winding down in the nineteenth century with the arrival of disease specificity. Medical science would soon incorporate Rudolf Virchow's cellular pathology (1858), Joseph Lister's surgical antisepsis (1865), Louis Pasteur's bacteriology (1860s), and Robert Koch's postulates and discovery of the tuberculosis germ (1880s).[8] With acceptance of the germ theory, concludes George Rosen, historian of public health, came an "incontrovertible demonstration toward the end of the nineteenth century that specific microscopic creatures rather than vague chemical miasmas produce infectious diseases."[9]

The biomedical model, reductionist medicine, positivistic scientific authority, and the numerical methods of Pierre Louis and others emerged in the second quarter of the nineteenth century. The trend toward reductionist medicine became even more powerful in the second half of the nineteenth century with the evidence that a particular bacterium caused a particular disease.[10] This perspective prompted the search for disease-specific treatments and advances in public health, but it tended to "marginalize or exclude the

[8] Joseph E. Davis, "Reductionist Medicine and Its Cultural Authority," in *To Fix or to Heal: Patient Care, Public Health, and the Limits of Biomedicine*, ed. Joseph E. Davis and Ana Marta Gonzalez (New York: New York University Press, 2016), 42–45. Koch's Postulates, 1880, then modified, established a causal relationship between a microorganism and a disease. Lester S. King, *Medical Thinking: A Historical Preface* (Princeton, NJ: Princeton University Press, 1982), 60–64. The Postulates: The microorganism or other pathogen must be present in all cases of the disease; the pathogen can be isolated from the diseased host and grown in pure culture; the pathogen from the pure culture must cause the disease when inoculated into a healthy, susceptible laboratory animal; the pathogen must be reisolated from the new host and shown to be the same as the originally inoculated pathogen.

[9] George Rosen, *A History of Public Health* (Baltimore: The Johns Hopkins University Press, 1958 [1993 ed.), 270. Chronic and noncommunicable diseases are generally thought to have multifactorial causation. The same is probably true of infectious diseases, though a particular organism must be present. For example, not everyone infected with the organism *Mycobacterium tuberculosis* suffers from tuberculosis. Some people have latent disease and will remain healthy; they carry live organisms but may never develop the disease. See J. Fuller, "Universal Etiology, Multifactorial Diseases and the Constitutive Model of Disease Classification," *Studies in History and Philosophy of Biological and Biomededical Sciences* 67 (2018): 8–15.

[10] "Reductionism" refers to the explanation of complex life science processes in terms of the laws of chemistry and physics alone.

crucial social and environmental determinants of disease."[11] Physicians were, and still are, unable to control all the variables in illness or disease and must regularly "pit the general against the particular," that is, offer explanations that apply to many people to make clinical sense. But the patient wants to be seen as unique and cares not that his or her clinical picture fails to match that of others; thus, the language and process of "patient-centered care" or holistic medicine was born (or rather reborn).[12] Neither approach—the holistic nor the biomedical/reductionist approach—is all right or all wrong. Some diseases or public health problems have a specific treatable or remedial cause that can be corrected by a biomedical/reductionist approach. Others, such as aging and chronic disease, require a holistic approach as well. They are not mutually exclusive, and in the best of worlds the two approaches can be combined.

Just after Barker's retirement in Maine 200 years ago, Dr. John G. Coffin in Boston delivered a series of lectures on preserving health. The 1819 prospectus stated, "the physician is chiefly occupied in the relieving and curing of diseases, while nature has ordained every man to be in a great measure the guardian and preserver of his own health, and for the very good reason, because he can better execute this trust than anyone else."[13] Like physicians today, Barker and his colleagues might have been able to prevent and cure certain conditions, but they could not correct all inappropriate behaviors, control all emotions, improve the environment, clean the air, purify the water supply, remove disease-causing organisms from food, or ensure adequate exercise and rest for their patients. Does Barker's *Diseases in the District of Maine*

[11] Joseph E. Davis and Ana Marta Gonzalez, eds., *To Fix or to Heal: Patient Care, Public Health, and the Limits of Biomedicine* (New York: New York University Press, 2016), 1–62. For more on specificity of diagnosis and holism see Charles E. Rosenberg, *No Other Gods: On Science and American Social Thought* (Baltimore: The Johns Hopkins University Press, 1997), 13–37 and 139–65.

[12] Kathryn Montgomery Hunter, *Doctors' Stories: The Narrative Structure of Medical Knowledge* (Princeton, NJ: Princeton University Press, 1991), 28–29; Rita Charon, *Narrative Medicine: Honoring the Stories of Illness* (Oxford; New York: Oxford University Press, 2006), 28. In 1996, the Institute of Medicine defined patient-centered care as "Providing care that is respectful of, and responsive to, individual patient preferences, needs and values, and ensuring that patient values guide all clinical decisions" though the term had been used earlier. Holistic medicine refers to medical treatment that attempts to deal with the whole person and not only with his or her physical condition. In general, the better physician always tried to accomplish holistic care before the term gained its current popularity.

[13] "Columbian Centinel," December 15, 1819, p. 2, col 4–5. John B. Blake, *Public Health in the Town of Boston 1630–1822* (Cambridge, MA: Harvard University Press, 1959), 240.

offer any perspectives on the problems we face today as patients, families, and physicians?

John Harley Warner maintains that in Barker's era "Therapeutic action . . . was . . . an essential element of professional identity." That is, a physician had to do something positive, generally to prescribe a medicine or some other action, and it was important that the physician had faith in that action.[14] Since antiquity, there had been a debate regarding the relative roles of nature and the healing arts in the sickroom. For example, Philadelphia's Benjamin Rush, one of Barker's mentors, believed that nature was an intruder in the sickroom and should be treated "as you would a noisy dog or cat [—] drive her out at the door & lock it upon her."[15] Increasing skepticism regarding medical therapy during the first decades of the nineteenth century revolved around the relative merits of nature healing versus the need for therapeutics such as bleeding, purging, and mercurials.

NUMERICAL METHODS AND RETROSPECTIVE DIAGNOSIS

Barker began his practice in the 1770s but the general use of numerical methods and statistical analysis, which might have altered some of his conclusions, did not reach American medicine until near the end of his life.[16] By the 1820s and 1830s physicians gradually embraced the use of numbers to guide their practice. For the United States, Pierre Louis in Paris influenced young American physicians training there. In his publications, using the numerical method first in 1825 and again in 1836, Louis wrote, "we infer that bloodletting has

---

[14] John Harley Warner, *The Therapeutic Perspective: Medical Practice, Knowledge, and Identity in America, 1820–85* (Cambridge, MA: Harvard University Press, 1986), 17–18.

[15] Warner, *The Therapeutic Perspective*, 18, and endnote #20 on p. 291. Warner is quoting from notes taken by John Austin at a lecture given by Rush in 1809.

[16] A few American reports used the numerical method during the first decades of the nineteenth century but "few if any of these doctors were at all systematic in gathering, organizing, or analyzing their data." James H. Cassedy, *American Medicine and Statistical Thinking, 1800–1860* (Cambridge, MA: Harvard University Press, 1984), 52–91, but particularly 57–58; P. C. A. Louis and Peter Martin, *An Essay on Clinical Instruction* (London: published by S. Highley, 32 Fleet Street, 1834); Jacob Bigelow, *A Discourse on Self-Limited Diseases: Delivered before the Massachusetts Medical Society, at Their Annual Meeting, May 27, 1835* (Boston: Nathan Hale, 1835).

had very little influence on the progress of pneumonitis, of erysipelas of the face, and of angina tonsillaris, in the cases under my observation."[17]

Another issue in reviewing a 200-year-old medical record is retrospective diagnosis, whether considering an epidemic or an individual patient. The clinical criteria used to name and analyze diseases change constantly as much by the alteration of medical theories as by the social and cultural milieu. Historians Risse and Warner observe, "One of the great temptations for scholars is to superimpose a modern disease classification on past nosology[18] and retrospectively build from patients records a false historical epidemiology that ignores the changing definition and construction of specific disease entities."[19] For example, what Barker and contemporaries termed yellow fever is not necessarily what we would call yellow fever today. The symptoms common to yellow fever—among them nausea, vomiting, jaundice, bloody stool, and fever—can be characteristics of a number of other diseases. Barker's yellow fever patients in Maine, especially, may very well have had another disease altogether. [20]

---

[17] P. C. A. Louis, *Recherches Anatomico-Pathologiques Sur La Phthisie* (Paris: Gabon, 1825); P. C. A. Louis, *Researches on the Effects of Bloodletting in Some Inflammatory Diseases, and on the Influence of Tartarized Antimony and Vesication in Pneumonitis with Preface and Appendix by James Jackson, Md*, trans. C. G. Putnam (Boston: Hilliard, Gray & Company, 1836), 22; Theodore M. Porter, *The Rise of Statistical Thinking 1820–1900* (Princeton: Princeton University Press, 1986), 157–58; Ulrich Tröhler, "The Introduction of Numerical Methods to Assess the Effects of Medical Interventions during the 18th Century: A Brief History," *Journal of the Royal Society of Medicine* 104, no. 11 (2011): 465–74.

[18] Nosology is a branch of medical science dealing with the classification of disease.

[19] G. B. Risse and J. H. Warner, "Reconstructing Clinical Activities: Patient Records in Medical History," *Social History of Medicine* 5, no. 2 (1992): 193. For an interesting look at retrospective diagnosis of a 1780 epidemic in Philadelphia called "bilious remitting fever" by Rush, later considered by some to be dengue, see R. M. Packard, "The Fielding H. Garrison Lecture: "Break-Bone" Fever in Philadelphia, 1780: Reflections on the History of Disease," *Bulletin of the History Medicine* 90, no. 2 (2016), 193–221. For Benjamin Rush's description, see Benjamin Rush, *Medical Inquiries and Observations*, 4th ed., 4 vols. (Philadelphia: Johnson & Warner, 1815), vol. 2, 229–39.

[20] Burnham, *What Is Medical History?*, 76–78; A. Karenberg, "Retrospective Diagnosis: Use and Abuse in Medical Historiography," *Prague Medical Report* 110, no. 2 (2009): 140–45. Margaret Humphreys, "Appendix II: Yellow Fever since 1793: History and Historiography," in *A Melancholy Scene of Devastation: The Public Response to the 1793 Philadelphia Yellow Fever Epidemic*, ed. J. Worth Estes and Billy G. Smith (Canton, MA: Science History Publications/USA, 1997), 183–98; Margaret Humphreys, *Yellow Fever and the South* (Baltimore: The Johns Hopkins University Press, 1992), 1–44; William Coleman, *Yellow Fever in the North: The Methods of Early Epidemiology* (Madison: University of Wisconsin Press, 1987), xiii–20; J. H. Powell, *Bring Out Your Dead: The Great Plague of Yellow Fever in Philadelphia in 1793*, (Studies in Health, Illness, and Caregiving) (Philadelphia: University of Pennsylvania Press, 1993), 29–44.

On the other hand, historians may find that modern technological advances, such as DNA recovery and sequencing, can validate a certain type of retrospective diagnosis. For example, the recovery of genomic data from bodies at plague gravesites has confirmed that *Yersinia pestis* is the bacterium that caused the mortality of the Black Death in London, England, 1348–1350. Rather than an increased virulence of the organism, a 2016 study suggests that factors other than microbial genetics, such as vector (black rat and flea) dynamics and host susceptibility, account for the epidemic and should be considered in analysis of past and future epidemics.[21] This is an example of reductionist medicine (in this case molecular genetics) recommending a more holistic approach to retrospective diagnosis.[22] Historian of science Laurent Loison described such critical presentism as "the elaboration of a reciprocal critical relation between scientific knowledge from different times. Its legitimacy comes from the acknowledgment of both the contingency and rationality of science."[23]

BARKER'S TREATMENTS, THERAPEUTIC EFFICACY, BACON, AND CONFIRMATION BIAS

Consider Barker's changing understanding of disease and therapy. Why did Barker, his medical peers, and many patients think that their treatments

---

[21] Kirsten I. Bos et al., "A Draft Genome of Yersinia Pestis from Victims of the Black Death," *Nature* 478 (2011): 506–10; Michal Feldman et al., "A High-Coverage Yersinia Pestis Genome from a Sixth-Century Justinianic Plague Victim," *Molecular Biology and Evolution* 33, no. 11 (2016): 2911–23. See also George Rice Carpenter, ed. *Daniel Defoe's Journal of the Plague Year*, Longmans' English Classics, vol. 4 (New York: Longmans, Green, and Co., 1895). And for a historical novel with modern genetic information added, see Geraldine Brooks, *Year of Wonders: A Novel of the Plague* (New York: Viking, 2001).

[22] "One can hardly imagine a rational argument supporting the claim that we should not take advantage of present-day technical and scientific advances to improve our understanding of the past world." Loison, "Forms of Presentism in the History of Science. Rethinking the Project of Historical Epistemology," 31.

[23] Loison, "Forms of Presentism in the History of Science. Rethinking the Project of Historical Epistemology," 36. And paraphrasing a comment on the same page: Awareness of the fleetingness of the present medical knowledge or medical "truth" is the best response to medical dogmatism. Again, replacing the word "scientific" with the word "medical," Loison concludes that critical presentism "acknowledges the contingent and rational dimensions of medical knowledge. Because medicine/science progresses, then it is legitimate for the present to serve as a yardstick for judging the past. But because the present is at the same time a contingent and fleeting norm, then the past becomes the privileged tool for criticizing the dogmatist temptation of present medicine."

worked? As previously discussed, historian Charles Rosenberg emphasized the importance to the physician–patient relationship of "exhibiting" a drug.[24] For example, if a patient took a drug with no obvious physical response, and then gradually recovered, both patient and doctor would assume that nature cured the illness, not the drug. If, on the other hand, the treatment resulted in twenty bowel movements, vomiting, and/or salivation (from mercurials such as calomel), and then the patient recovered, both patient and doctor would assume the drug "worked" to cure the disease. With few exceptions, unless the numerical method is used, one tends to confirm a theory by remembering results that fit one's theory and disregarding those that do not. Aware of this issue, philosopher and scientist Francis Bacon (1561–1626) wrote, "The human understanding when it has once adopted an opinion (either as being the received opinion or as being agreeable to itself) draws all things else to support and agree with it. And though there be a greater number and weight to be found on the other side, yet these it either neglects and despises, or else by some distinction sets aside and rejects."[25] Today, this source of error is referred to as confirmation bias.[26]

From the point of view of twenty-first century, Barker's use of fluid repletion (hydration) and alkaline therapy (antacids) might well have produced a physiological response obvious to both the patient and doctor, relieving dehydration by decreasing thirst and increasing strength, and relieving peptic symptoms such as indigestion, heartburn, and gastric distress, and this might happen in a patient with a disease that was actually much more serious than simple indigestion. But Barker believed that alkaline therapy was directed at the "septic acid of epidemic fever."[27] The rapid relief of peptic symptoms might convey to the patient and doctor that the medicine was having an effect on the

[24] Again, "exhibiting a drug" refers to the patient seeing and/or feeling the effects of the drug, that is, the drug should produce a "particular physiological end" that can be appreciated by the patient and doctor. Charles E. Rosenberg, "The Therapeutic Revolution: Medicine, Meaning, and Social Change in Nineteenth-Century America," *Perspectives in Biology and Medicine* 20, no. 4 (1977): 492.

[25] Francis Bacon, James Spedding, and Robert Leslie Ellis, *Novum Organum*, New Universal Library (London; New York: G. Routledge; E. P. Dutton, 1800), Aphorism XLVI, p. 73.

[26] "Confirmation bias" is the term used to describe errors produced when people selectively focus on evidence that supports their beliefs (or what they want to believe to be true) while ignoring evidence that would disprove their ideas. The modern scientific method requires one to seek to disprove one's theory.

[27] Jeremiah Barker, "On Febrifuge Virtues of Lime, Magnesia and Alkaline Salts in Dysentery, Yellow-Fever and Scarlatina Angiosa. In a Letter from Dr. Jeremiah Barker, of Portland, (Maine) Dated May 30, 1798," *Medical Repository* 2, no. 2 (1798), 147–52.

"septic acid" and, if the fever resolved, that it was likely the medicine had been effective in the cure.

Medical historians Wilson and Ashplant claimed, "What any human observer 'sees' is a function not simply of the object(s) [patient and illness] that observer is observing, but also of the observer's own categories, assumptions, values, expectations, hypotheses, preconceptions, purposes, interests, attitudes."[28] Barker's treatments may have relieved symptoms and saved lives, but perhaps not for the reasons he indicated in his manuscript. For example, Barker would probably use bloodletting in a patient with cough and shortness of breath, symptoms that today might be thought to be associated with congestive heart failure. The twenty-first century explanation of the effectiveness of bloodletting might be that the symptoms were alleviated by decreasing venous return to the heart, causing physiological and symptomatic improvement. Barker believed that he was treating symptoms provoked by excessive tension in the blood vessels or nerves (Cullen, Brown, Rush), symptoms that today are attributed to diminished myocardial (heart) function. His understanding or theory of the action of bloodletting differed from ours, but it seemed to work, and patients improved symptomatically.[29]

Historian Oscar Moro-Abadía wrote in 2009 that "the goal of historians should be to understand, as much as possible, past humans [physicians and patients] on their own terms. . . . Given that our scientific beliefs are continually reevaluated, there is no reason to consider modern science [and medicine] as a definitive achievement when examining past theories."[30] He continues, "historians have longtime suspected that the search for a "pure past" is utopic . . . understanding the past in its own terms as impossible to achieve, they [historians] should not renounce attempts to approximate it."[31]

Thus, we must try to see and understand medicine as Barker, his peers, and his patients experienced it in 1800. Today, for example, we know that mercurials act on the kidney as a diuretic. We also know that mercury is so highly toxic that we have even stopped using mercury thermometers, but as recently as the 1960s doctors were prescribing mercurial diuretics. In Barker's

---

[28] Wilson and Ashplant, "Whig History and Present-Centred History," 15.

[29] W. Bruce Fye, "Ernest Henry Starling," *Clinical Cardiology* 29, no. 4 (2006): 181–82. Louis J. Acierno, *The History of Cardiology* (New York: The Parthenon Publishing Group, 1994), 217–37.

[30] Moro-Abadía, "Thinking about 'Presentism' from a Historian's Perspective: Herbert Butterfield and Hélène Metzger," 57, 61.

[31] Moro-Abadía, "Thinking about 'Presentism' from a Historian's Perspective: Herbert Butterfield and Hélène Metzger," 71.

era, physicians watched for the production of catharsis, emesis, diuresis, and salivation (actually mercury toxicity), unaware that it was mercury's action on the kidney that relieved the shortness of breath associated with congestive heart failure, a condition not present in eighteenth-century conceptual understanding. Another example is Barker's use of digitalis (foxglove) to treat some of his patients suffering from dropsy (edema or swelling). His reasons were based on existing medical theories and the fact that both patient and doctor agreed that it worked, but he had no idea that he was treating heart disease.[32] Colchicine was and still is used to treat acute gouty arthritis, but in 1805 it was little used as it was considered "a very uncertain remedy."[33] Bloodletting, denigrated by many twenty-first-century observers, was used by Barker and his fellow physicians to treat patients with mania. It acted to quiet the patient, and if thoughtfully and carefully used, avoiding excessive loss of blood in the frail, the elderly, and the very young, it might prevent injury to the patient, family and friends. We could argue that today's therapies for mental illness are also not without risk. All medications and therapies have potential harm, both in Barker's time and today.

NATURE VERSUS ART IN MEDICINE—BEST AVAILABLE EVIDENCE AND THE BURDEN OF DISEASE

In 1835, the year of Barker's death, Jacob Bigelow wrote, "It is difficult to view the operations of nature, divested of the interferences of art [meaning medicine], so much do our habits and partialities incline us to neglect the former, and to exaggerate the importance of the latter . . . [the young student] will come at length to the conviction, that some diseases are controlled by nature alone."[34] Twenty-five years later, Dr. Oliver Wendell Holmes penned the

---

[32] ". . . there was absolutely no good reason for Hall Jackson or William Withering to think the drug's [digitalis] site of action could be the heart." J. Worth Estes, *Hall Jackson and the Purple Foxglove* (Hanover: University Press of New England, 1979), 149.

[33] The use of colchicum, the root of meadow saffron, was popularized in the 1760s to relieve the pain of gout, but the active ingredient, colchicine, was not isolated until 1833. J. Worth Estes, *Dictionary of Protopharmacology* (Canton, MA: Science History Publications, 1990), 51. *The Edinburgh New Dispensatory* of 1805, finds "it is at best a very uncertain remedy." The active ingredient, colchicine, had not yet been isolated. Andrew Duncan, *The Edinburgh New Dispensatory*, 1st Worcester ed. (Worcester: Press of Isaiah Thomas, 1805), 203.

[34] Bigelow, *A Discourse on Self-Limited Diseases: Delivered before the Massachusetts Medical Society, at Their Annual Meeting, May 27, 1835.*

following about medical therapeutics: "I firmly believe that if the whole materia medica, as now used, could be sunk to the bottom of the sea, it would be all the better for mankind,—and all the worse for the fishes."[35] We have to remind ourselves that in Barker's day there were very few remedies that pharmacologically helped the patient recover. Nature did the heavy lifting.

Different locations and time periods have changed the burden of disease, which means the impact of a health problem as measured by financial cost, mortality, morbidity, or other indicators. Urbanization brought added problems associated with the transportation of food, clean drinking water, and sewage removal. Rapid transport by land, sea, and air accelerated the spread of disease. In the late eighteenth century, perhaps less attention was given to gender issues, the social stigmata of sexually transmitted diseases, or the illnesses associated with urban or rural poverty and crowding. Some of the environmental and microbial causes of the infectious and vector-borne diseases that were of such concern to Barker would not be understood until the last quarter of the nineteenth century.

We might ask whether Barker was using the best available evidence in 1820. For the most part he cited the medical elites whose thought was most likely to reflect what was then considered medical "truth" or certainty. But medical certainty is elusive to say the least. In 1989, *New England Journal of Medicine* editor Jerome Kassirer, M.D., wrote "Absolute certainty in diagnosis is unattainable, no matter how much information we gather, how many observations we make, or how many tests we perform . . . our goal is to reduce the diagnostic uncertainty enough to make optimal therapeutic decisions."[36] The quest for certainty continues.[37]

The fact that a medication, procedure, or algorithm today is deemed "evidence based" does not mean it is an immutable certainty. Rules for evidence

---

[35] Oliver Wendell Holmes, "Currents and Counter-Currents," in *Medical Essays: 1842–1882*, ed. Oliver Wendell Holmes (Boston: Houghton Mifflin Company, 1911), 202–203. The essay was originally delivered to the Massachusetts Medical society in 1860. The full discussion is more nuanced. Holmes did exclude some medicines thought to be useful from his list to be thrown into the sea.

[36] J. P. Kassirer, "Our Stubborn Quest for Diagnostic Certainty. A Cause of Excessive Testing," *New England Journal of Medicine* 320, no. 22 (1989): 1489–91.

[37] "Roundtable on evidence-based medicine, charter and vision statement." Institute of Medicine, in *Leadership Commitments to Improve Value in Healthcare: Finding Common Ground: Workshop Summary*, The National Academies Collection: Reports Funded by National Institutes of Health, Washington, DC, 2009. In 2009 the Institute of Medicine Roundtable on Evidence-Based Medicine "set a goal that, by the year 2020, 90% of clinical decisions will be supported by accurate, timely, and up-to-date clinical information and will reflect the best available evidence."

have changed, but as new information from thousands of journals is added daily, we constantly face conflicting evidence and evolving "facts" regarding how patients or physicians should weigh the risks, benefits, and costs of any therapy. The seventeenth-century natural philosophy of Bacon and Descartes began "with skepticism—the setting aside of preconceived notions."[38] How did patients and physicians deal with that skepticism and inadequate or conflicting evidence 200 years ago and how do we deal with it today? Uncertainty continues to be an issue for patients, their families, physicians, governments, and the insurance and pharmaceutical industries.

Public health advances such as sanitary reforms led to cleaner food and water, better nutrition, and proper handling of sewage, which, combined with immunization, resulted in the rapid decline in infectious diseases and deaths in the twentieth century. These factors have had a much greater influence on health and longevity than touted "high tech" medical advances.[39] In 1850 Maine, according to the first US census collecting the causes of death, infectious diseases constituted four of the six leading causes of death. In 1900, the three leading causes of death in the United States were pneumonia, consumption (tuberculosis), and diarrhea/enteritis. By 1999, the leading causes of death were heart disease, cancer, and stroke.[40]

Medical historian Allan Brandt has commented, "The study of history is inevitably a dialogue with the present; the study of medical history is inevitably a dialogue with contemporary medicine."[41] Barker may give us a better sense of "when to act and when to subject received knowledge to skeptical

---

[38] Davis and Gonzalez, *To Fix or to Heal: Patient Care, Public Health, and the Limits of Biomedicine*, 36.

[39] Thomas McKeown, *The Modern Rise of Population* (New York: Academic Press, 1976). James Colgrove, "The Mckeown Thesis: A Historical Controversy and Its Enduring Influence," *American Journal of Public Health* 92, no. 5 (2002): 725–29; and Thomas R. Frieden, "A Framework for Public Health Action: The Health Impact Pyramid," *American Journal of Public Health* 100, no. 4 (2010): 590–95. There is some controversy regarding McKeown's analysis in the 1970s and 1980s that broad social and economic changes rather than public health or medical interventions were responsible for the rise in the world population from the 1770s. Most now agree that improved socioeconomic factors, rising living standards, better nutritional status, and cleaner water and food combined with sanitary reforms and immunizations to provide most of the increased longevity through the twentieth century.

[40] G. L. Armstrong, L. A. Conn, and R. W. Pinner, "Trends in Infectious Disease Mortality in the United States During the 20th Century," *JAMA* 281, no. 1 (1999): 61–66. "Achievements in Public Health, 1900–1999," *Morbidity and Mortality Weekly Report* 48, no. 29 (1999): 621–29.

[41] Allan M. Brandt, "Emerging Themes in the History of Medicine," *Millbank Quarterly* 69, no. 2 (1991): 201.

scrutiny."[42] An understanding of the medical past helps to decrease dogmatism and encourage appropriate skepticism from which the patient, the physician, and other health care professionals all benefit.[43] In 1929 philosopher George Santayana (1863–1952) wrote, "Skepticism is the chastity of the intellect, and it is shameful to surrender it too soon or to the first comer: there is nobility in preserving it coolly and proudly through long youth, until at last, in the ripeness of instinct and discretion, it can be safely exchanged for fidelity and happiness."[44] And in 1991 Kathryn Montgomery Hunter observed, "successes in medicine have obscured our understanding of medicine as an intellectual pursuit or as the exercise of practical wisdom in the face of uncertainty."[45] This is as true in 2020 as it was in 1820, and it is the essence of the art and science of medicine: the exercise of practical wisdom in the face of uncertainty.

CONCLUSION

Jeremiah Barker practiced physic from his homes in Stroudwater and Gorham and cared for patients from Bath to Biddeford, forty miles along the coast and ten to twenty miles inland, always with a copy of Rush on Fever and a notebook in hand. He recorded unusual cases and published at least twelve articles during the first decade of America's first medical journal. He studied medical epidemics, followed the science and chemistry of his day, and was willing to risk scorn when a new therapy seemed to be valuable. He corresponded with many of the leaders of medicine in the United States, including Lyman Spalding, Samuel Mitchill, Hall Jackson, John Gorham Coffin, and Benjamin

---

[42] Paraphrase of a comment in Hunter, *Doctors' Stories: The Narrative Structure of Medical Knowledge*, 40.

[43] D. S. Jones et al., "Making the Case for History in Medical Education," *Journal of the History of Medicine and Allied Sciences* (2014): 623–52.

[44] George Santayana, *Scepticism and Animal Faith; Introduction to a System of Philosophy* (New York: C. Scribner's sons, 1929), 69–70; Charles S. Bryan and Scott H. Podolsky, "Dr. Holmes at 200—the Spirit of Skepticism," *New England Journal of Medicine* 361, no. 9 (2009), 846–47.

[45] Hunter, *Doctors' Stories: The Narrative Structure of Medical Knowledge*, xix. Uncertainty was an issue in early modern thought as maintained an article focusing on Michel de Montaigne and Francis Bacon: Stephen Pender, "Examples and Experience: On the Uncertainty of Medicine," *British Journal for the History of Science* 39, no. 1 (2006): 1–28. And more recently, "Uncertainty is ubiquitous in medicine . . . [yet it] is often ignored as a subject in medicine . . . [and] results in overconfidence . . . in existing medical practices." S. Hatch, "Uncertainty in Medicine," *British Medical Journal* 357 (2017): 2180.

Rush.[46] He continued his medical education through the literature and the mail, and by visiting and making medical rounds with prominent physicians such as Dr. Lloyd, South End Boston, Dr. James Thacher, Plymouth, Dr. (later Gov.) John Brooks, Boston, Dr. Benjamin Waterhouse, Boston, Dr. Lyman Spalding, Portsmouth, and Dr. Richard Hazeltine, North Berwick.[47] He sought advice and support from history as much as science, practicing and writing during a period of enormous change in medicine.[48]

Barker's manuscript, together with his published articles, casebooks, and other material, constitutes a valuable resource on New England and American life, nutrition, public health, epidemics, and other aspects of health, disease, and healing. Not only does the manuscript describe particulars of his medical practice in rural Maine, but also it conveys his thoughts and changing philosophy related to the development and penetration of ideas advanced in the latest medical literature and his personal circle of communication. Optimistic and confident, Barker would probably have agreed with Dr. Josiah Bartlett's 1810 comment to the Massachusetts Medical Society that "more professional knowledge is at this time attainable in a single season, than was known to

[46] Lyman Spalding (1775–1821) had a distinguished career as a physician and educator, culminating in 1817 with his proposal for a national pharmacopoeia. Under Spalding's guidance, the first US Pharmacopoeia was published in December 1820 and represented a "nationwide professional consensus." Samuel Latham Mitchill (1764–1831) studied medicine in Edinburgh, helped found the College of Physicians and Surgeons at Columbia University, and became professor of chemistry, natural history, and agriculture at Columbia College. In 1797, with Elihu Hubbard Smith and Edward Miller, Mitchill founded, and for twenty-three years edited, the first medical journal in the United States, the *Medical Repository*. It was sometimes referred to as *Mitchill's Repository*. See R. J. Kahn and P. G. Kahn, "The Medical Repository—the First U. S. Medical Journal (1797–1824)," *New England Journal of Medicine* 337 (1997): 1926–30. Hall Jackson (1739–1797) was a prominent Portsmouth physician and surgeon who introduced digitalis to America. John Gorham Coffin (1769–1829) practiced in Boston, was an attending physician at the Boston Dispensary, and founded and edited the *Boston Medical Intelligencer*, a precursor to the *Boston Medical and Surgical Journal* and later the *New England Journal of Medicine*. He was also a founder and first secretary of what would become the Boston Medical Library, now part of the Countway Medical Library at Harvard Medical School. He also wrote on medical education in 1822. Joseph E. Garland, *The Centennial History of the Boston Medical Library, 1875–1975* (Boston: Boston Medical Library in the Francis A. Countway Library of Medicine, 1975).

[47] James Alfred Spalding, "After Consulting Hours: Jeremiah Barker, M.D., Gorham and Falmouth, Maine, 1752–1835," *Bulletin of the American Academy of Medicine* 10 (1909): 249.

[48] Frank Huisman and John Harley Warner, eds., *Locating Medical History: The Stories and Their Meanings* (Baltimore: Johns Hopkins University Press, 2004), 5. Huisman and Warner maintained that "Learned Western physicians before 1800 had long looked to history for much of the professional definition and authority that later physicians would derive from science."

Hippocrates, Galen, and their successors, till the beginning of the eighteenth century."[49]

In 1909 Maine medical historian James Spalding wrote that Barker "was the pioneer medical writer in Maine, at a time when even American Medical Literature was nothing but a reflection of the fashions of London and Paris. Barker's medical essays will stand comparison with many of today. . . . They tell us what he did and why. He was, I repeat, our first literary practitioner."[50]

[49] Josiah Bartlett, *An Historical Sketch of the Progress of Medical Science, in the Commonwealth of Massachusetts, Being the Substance of a Discourse Read at the Annual Meeting of the Medical Society, June 6, 1810, with Alterations and Additions to January 1, 1813* (Charlestown: s.n., 1813), 16. Josiah Bartlett (1759–1820) was a soldier of the Revolution, preceptorship trained, took various medical courses, was a ship's surgeon, took a full course at Cambridge (Harvard) and was given an honorary M.D. in 1791. Bartlett was active in the Massachusetts Medical Society and encouraging and contributing to the medical literature. Howard A. Kelly and Walter L. Burrage, *American Medical Biographies* (Baltimore: The Norman, Remington Company, 1920), 67–68.

[50] Spalding, "After Consulting Hours," 263.

VOLUME 1

The Jeremiah Barker Manuscript[1]

Chapter 1

THE MANUSCRIPT ALLUDED TO, contains a great variety of cases of insanity of both sexes, with practical observations. Some of these cases will be related in the following pages, after a few preliminary remarks. [2]

During my pupilage in Hingham from 1769 to 1772, I never saw a case of insanity, altho my Preceptor [Dr. Bela Lincoln][3] commanded an extensive practice in that town and some of its neighboring towns. I saw one Idiot, a girl of fifteen years old, whose face & gestures bore some resemblance to a monkey.[4] She never could be taught to speak, or do any work, tho she

---

[1] The Barker manuscript has been transcribed exactly as written, including crossed-out words, with original punctuation, grammar, and spelling. It is printed here in eighteenth-century fonts (Caslon and Garamond), as it might have been if published by Barker. Words that are not accepted spelling in 2020 are marked by the interpolation [*sic*] unless they represent archaic or obsolete spelling as found in medical dictionaries by Robert Hooper, *A Compendious Medical Dictionary: Containing an Explaination of the Terms in Anatomy, Physiology, Surgery, Materia Medica, Chemistry, and Practice of Physic: Collected from the Most Approved Authors* (London: Printed for Murray and Highley, 1799); John Redman Coxe, *The Philadelphia Medical Dictionary*, 2nd ed. (Philadelphia: Thomas Dobson, 1817); Robley Dunglison, *A Dictionary of Medical Science* (Philadelphia: Henry C. Lea, 1874); *The Compact Edition of the Oxford English Dictionary: Complete Text Reproduced Micrographically* (Oxford: Oxford University Press, 1971); *Oxford English Dictionary*, 2nd ed., online (Oxford: Oxford University Press). MS pagination is noted thus **2** at page changes. The Glossary provides explanation of unfamiliar medical and pharmaceutical terms.

[2] This paragraph is in response to a letter by George Parkman, M.D. Dr. Parkman wrote to Jeremiah Barker circa 1819, asking to read Barker's chapter on mental illness and promising to return it promptly. See the Jeremiah Barker Papers, Collection 13 at Maine Historical Society containing Barker's first chapter with Parkman offprints sewn with it.

[3] Barker studied medicine under Dr. Bela Lincoln (1733–1774) from 1769 to 1772. Lincoln, a graduate of Harvard College in 1754, apprenticed under Dr. Ezekiel Hersey, studied at London Hospital, and received an M.D. from the University of Aberdeen in 1765. Dr. Joshua Fisher, later to become president of the Massachusetts Medical Society (1815–1823), also had a preceptorship with Barker under Lincoln. Barker communicated with Fisher over the years. C. Helen Brock, "The Influence of Europe on Colonial Massachusetts Medicine," in *Medicine in Colonial Massachusetts 1620–1820*, ed. J. Worth Estes, Philip Cash, and Eric H. Christianson (Boston: The Colonial Society of Massachusetts distributed by the University of Virginia Press, 1980), 133; and Walter L. Burrage, *A History of the Massachusetts Medical Society* (Norwood, MA: Plimpton Press, 1923), 104.

[4] The term "idiot" did not always have the same insulting sense it has today. It is defined as "a fool; a natural; a changeling; one without the powers of reason." (Samuel Johnson's *A Dictionary of the English Language*, 1755 p. 1039) "Changeling" is often used to refer to a child who is considered undesirable, or who does not resemble his or her family. (OED) The current

attempted to imitate what she saw others do. Her mother saw a monkey, act its pranks, while pregnant with this child.[5]

The people in these towns were remarkably temperate in eating & drinking. D[r] Cheyne's dietetic rules were generally adopted by people, and most **2** of the physicians, of my acquaintance, pursued his mode of practice, particularly with respect to the liberal use of mercury, and recommended a diet, chiefly of milk & vegetables.[6] A glass of currant wine was the strongest spirit offered in our social meetings, and seldom used at the table, in dining hours. Malt beer & cyder were the common drinks. I never saw but one person intoxicated with spiritous liquors in that town, and the people were remarkably industrious.

From 1773 to 1780, I practiced physic in the County of Barnstable, Mass[tts].[7] The mode of living & habits of people, [were] very similar, excepting a few seamen, who used ardent spirits.

In the course of my practice, I never met with a single insane patient, nor heard of any. At times, I practiced among aboriginals, who lived in small villages. None of them pretended to possess any medical skill, or magic arts, but quickly called for a physician, when diseased.

They had the Gospel preached to them, by Missionaries, who received their stipend from England. These Indians were remarkable abstemious in eating and drinking. Fish with vegetables composed the chief of their food, and they were a sober & orderly people.

OED definition of idiot: "a person so profoundly disabled in mental function or intellect as to be incapable of ordinary acts of reasoning or rational conduct; *spec.* a person permanently so affected ... The older legal authorities in England defined an idiot as a person congenitally deficient in reasoning powers; this remained for a long time the common implication of the term."

[5] Since antiquity it was thought that a pregnant woman would produce a deformity in her child by being frightened by animals, witnessing disturbing events, or seeing a deformed individual. W. C. Shaw, "Folklore Surrounding Facial Deformity and the Origins of Facial Prejudice," *British Journal of Plastic Surgery* 34, no. 3 (1981): 240. "The sight of unusual creatures gave such stories of birth anomaly an exotic quality ... monsters had 'sometimes the look and figure of a Monkey,'" Turner, Daniel M. "Birth Anomalies and Childhood Disabilities." Chap. 9 In *The Secrets of Generation: Reproduction in the Long Eighteenth Century*, ed. R. Stephanson and D. N. Wagner, 217–37. (Toronto: University of Toronto Press, 2015), 223.

[6] Dr. George Cheyne (1671–1743) of Aberdeen, Edinburgh, and London. George Cheyne, *An Essay of Health and Long Life* (London: George Strahan etc., 1724), *Observations Concerning the Nature and Due Method of Treating the Gout* (London: G. Strahan, 1720), *The English Malady: Or a Treatise of Nervous Diseases of All Kinds* (London: G. Strahan, 1733), and *An Essay on Regimen, Together with Five Discourses, Medical, Moral, and Philosophical* (London: C. Rivington, 1740); Steven Shapin, "Trusting George Cheyne: Scientific Expertise, Common Sense, and Moral Authority in Early Eighteenth-Century Dietetic Medicine," *Bulletin of the History of Medicine* 77 (2003): 263–97.

[7] Barnstable County is a peninsula forming the southeast extremity of Massachusetts, now known as Cape Cod.

3

I never saw a case of insanity among them, neither did I ever hear of an insane Indian in other places, excepting when under the influence of spiritous liquors. Then they would sometimes commit murder, but not suicide. I never saw a case of insanity among those who had always been in indigent circumstances.

In 1780, I took up my residence in Gorham, District of Maine, and pursued the practice of physic in that, and several adjacent towns, 40 years. The mode of living and customs of people were very similar to those in Hingham & Barnstable, for several years, and mental diseases were of rare occurrence. In succeeding years, most of the people became less abstemious, and spiritous liquors were plentifully used, by young & old, male & female.

During my practice, in Maine, I met with many cases of insanity, and have been informed of numerous cases of this kind, in different parts of the District. I do not mean to suggest that spiritous liquors are the sole cause of this disease. ****4**** Too great indulgence in animal food, violent amorous passions, overstrained zeal, universalism, riches suddenly accumulated, avarice, a fear of starving tho affluent, disappointment, excessive anger, fright, Jealousy, and hereditary predisposition have also ~~given rise~~ been followed by insanity under my own observation.[8]

A number of cases, which have fallen under my particular care, together with those that have been communicated to me, will be related, in some order of time, according to their occurrence.

More cases of insanity, however, have come to my knowledge, where medical aid has not been requested, than those in which physicians have been consulted, for the disease has, unfortunately been considered by most people, beyond the reach of medical skill; so that they have been left to drag out their lives, often for a considerable length of time, when, they have not put an end to their existence, dangerous pests to society and grievous to beholders.

---

[8] Cotton Mather (c. 1662–1728), a Protestant clergyman who graduated from Harvard College and studied medicine, considered madness to be of divine origin. In *The Angel of Bethesda*, he wrote, "Denying the God that is above . . . render[s] me worthy to be smitten with madness." Cotton Mather and Society American Antiquarian, *The Angel of Bethesda* (Barre, MA: American Antiquarian Society and Barre Publishers, 1972), 130; Gerald N. Grob, *The Mad among Us: A History of the Care of America's Mentally Ill* (New York; Toronto: Free Press; Maxwell Macmillan Canada, 1994), 10–11; Martin Kaufman, Stuart Galishoff, and Todd Lee Savitt, *Dictionary of American Medical Biography*, 2 vols. (Westport, CT: Greenwood Press, 1984), vol. 2, 503. Barker listed the standard contemporary thoughts on predisposing causes of insanity. Norman Dain, *Concepts of Insanity in the United States, 1789–1865* (New Brunswick, NJ: Rutgers University Press, 1964), 3–27.

The following case is a remarkable instance.

5

Before the revolutionary war, a merchant in Falmouth[9] acquired a pretty large estate, in a few years, and his pride, as well as vanity were proportionately raised. He built an elegant house, and indulged freely every day in luxurious food, with wine & other spirits. Under these exercises of the mind & this mode of living, he became, at times, insane, in a peculiar manner, fancying himself to possess some spiritual intelligence and to be capable of rectifying what he thought was amis, in his own house, and in the houses of others. And this was to turn things upside down, piling one on another such as crockery ware, pictures & riding on the canter from house to house, dressed in fanciful garments, sometimes with a sword by his side, and bitterly offended at opposition.

But, strange to relate, he was for the most part, indulged in his whimsical notions without any control!

These paroxysms occurred once in two or three months, before they subsided. Then he became dull & dejected, for a time, saying nothing about what he had done, or making any apology, tho he sometimes injured peoples furniture & goods. On the contrary, he discovered a spirit of resentments, at the opposition, which he had sometimes met with, even in the recess of his disorder.

6

During this mental excitement he usually drank more spirit, than at other times, and indulged more greedily in animal food, sleeping but little. In this way, he was allowed to go on, and medical aid was not requested. His friends indulged him in his mad career, as he was opulent and full of self importance.

In his disordered state, he gave his money & goods lavishly, for small services, and thus wasted his estate considerably. At other times, he was remarkable avaricious, and gave very little to the poor & needy.

In 1775, his house was consumed by fire, with some of his goods. About the same time, he lost two children by sickness; all that he then had.

After these events, he continued rational, about two years, living on a farm in the country, in a more abstemious manner. After this, however, he received a quantity of goods from the West Indies, in payment of **7** a debt, which produced such an elevation of mind, that his disorder returned as usual and

---

9 Falmouth here may refer to Falmouth, Massachusetts, in Barnstable County (Cape Cod), where Barker practiced until moving to the District of Maine in 1780, although it is possible that the patient lived in Falmouth (name later changed to Portland) in the District of Maine.

continued to recur once in a few months for nearly forty years. During this long period means were used only twice. The first time was in Boston, where his disorder recurred, and meeting a physician, who did not bow to him, he knocked off his hat. The Doctor requested two strong men to hold him, while he drew a quart of blood from his arm, in the street. This moderated his phrenzy,[10] and he soon became rational.

After this he went to England, dressed in scarlet, pretending to be related to a certain Nobleman. There he became insane, and beginning to turn things upside down, was confined at Bedlam, in a straight jacket, debarred from spirits, and kept on a low diet. His reason was soon restored.

After his return, the disorder recurred, at times as heretofore, till he spent all his estate, and is now, vis 1820, a town pauper, at the age of 80 years clothed with humility, and **8** appearing to profess a Christian temper. See page 43 — Cases to be related in same order of time. [Clearly Barker intended to reorganize this entire chapter.]

Had this man been kept for some time in a well regulated Hospital, in the former part of his life under the care of a scientific physician, for the management of lunatics, he might probably have been cured.

About twenty years since he asked my advice, which was to live temperately in eating & drinking, also to be bled & purged freely, and to be salivated. To this he would not consent. Then I advised him to have a guardian appointed to take charge of his remaining estate. His pride, however, prevented this from being done.

Had the Mass^tts Lunatic Asylum been then established, it would have been the most proper place for this unhappy man, who has a poor, insane wife, and two daughters, in indigent circumstances![11] **9** His second wife, tho always affectionate and indulgent, met with repeated abuses from her husband, in his insane paroxysms. He accused her of spending his estate, and threatened her life, which greatly frighted her, so that she soon became insane, and incapable of paying any attention to domestic business.

I was once consulted by her friends. But as she was of a spare habit, evacuants were omitted. She complained of dizziness, with confusion of the mind; and she was very wakeful; pulse full and about 75. I directed the shower

---

[10] Probably "frenzy" or "phrensy," as there are numerous spellings of the word (OED).

[11] Through the efforts of Horace Mann, the Massachusetts legislature approved a bill to fund a state lunatic hospital in 1830 and, in 1833, the Worcester State Hospital opened. McLean Asylum, a private hospital founded by the trustees of the Massachusetts General Hospital, had admitted its first patients in 1818. See Grob, *The Mad among Us*, 23–53.

bath to be daily applied. This composed her mind, removed the dizziness and induced quiet sleep; so that she soon attended to domestic business with regularity. But the baths not being long continued, her mind again became confused, and filled with fearful apprehensions of being injured by her husband, in his insane turns; **10** so that she fled to her relatives for support, and is now, at the age of 75, preparing for a more happy state of existence.

In Jan. 1809, Miss L.H. of Scarboro,[12] aged 20, of a plethoric habit, and florid countenance, brought up in a farmers house, complained of universal heat; so that she could not comfortably remain in a room warmed by a common fire.

In July she became insane, and her friends confined her with cords, to prevent her from doing mischief.

The first of August I was consulted, when I drew a pint of blood tho her pulse did not indicate diseased action, neither did the blood appear unnatural. I then gave 15 grains of calomel and 20 of Jalap which operated freely, and directed calomel to be given; two grains night & morning. An ounce of mercurial ointments was also **11**
applied to her neck. I bled her five times in four weeks from the arm, taking a pint of blood each time; and twice from her feet, in like quantity; and gave a dose of Jalap and calomel after each bleeding.

Before bleeding she would rave and laugh, alternately; and made some attempts to hurt her attendants with a pair of scissors, which she had concealed. After bleeding she shed tears plentifully and complained of her head, which was ~~preternaturally~~ very hot to the touch. Cold water was repeatedly applied to her head, which replaced the heat, and was gratifying to her. After three bleedings a salivation took place profusely. Her reason gradually returned, and by the last of September, she was able to attend to domestic business as heretofore tho she was considerably emaciated, for she took very little **12** food in the course of her illness, and that consisted chiefly of vegetable matters. During her confinement she kept for the most part, quietly and was calm in the morning. In the afternoon her mind became much disordered with some increased action of the pulse.

In Jan. 1810, she had become plethoric and complained of heat of body, and pain in the head, together with fearful apprehensions that her friends wished to hite [sic] her. Bloodletting was mentioned by her relatives; but delayed.

---

[12] Scarboro is an alternative spelling of the more common Scarborough, Maine. It lies at the mouth of the Nonesuch River, 6.6 miles south of Barker's home in Stroudwater, part of Portland, Maine.

In Feb. she drank tea at a neighbours house, when she complained of heat & pain in her head. On her return, she leaped into a well of water, which extinguished heat and life!

13

On the 10th of April 1807, I was informed of a maniac, who was enchained. I repaired to his house, and was told by his wife, that about the middle of Feby he was seized with pain in his left eye, which soon passed into his right ear, that, in a few days, he became deranged in mind, and matter was discharged from his ear, that about the middle of March, a pint of blood was drawn which was covered with a white coat. A few hours after a neighbour gave him a small black powder which caused him to sleep six hours. When he awoke in wild distraction tore off his bandage and bled about another pint, which in some measure composed him. But he could not be reconciled to his wife and children, believing they were his enemies, and attempted to kill his oldest son.

The maniac begged me to take off his chain. I told him, if he would **14** let me anoint his neck, and give him some pills, he might be set at liberty. To this he consented. I then applied two ounces of mercurial ointment to his neck, and covered it with a flannel bandage, also gave a mercurial cathartic. In two days, a salivation took place in profusion, and an eruption appeared on his neck which swelled considerably. His reason then returned, and he became reconciled to his family, saying that he felt as tho he had been absent from home, among his enemies. He was then liberated, and attended to business, as heretofore. See page 10 [to reorder chronologically]

A few weeks after, he went to the raising of a building, where spiritous liquors were taken to excess, and he again became insane; so that his family were in danger. I furnished his wife with some more of the ointment & pills. But the patient would not consent to have them applied being told, by an empiric, that they contained poison mercury and advised that what had already been used, should be driven out **15**
of his blood & bones, by ardent spirit, some of which was given, but he grew so raving, that he was again enchained, and happy would it have been for society, if the empiric had been his copartner.

By their disuse, however his reason was restored, and he lived a sober life, many years till his death, by some other disease.

In 1819, I met with a scientific and experienced physician, in Maine, who informed me, that about five years since he was sent for to an insane person, who wished to put an end to his life, but not having sufficient courage desired him to his assistance him in the work. To this he agreed. The maniac then asked how he would proceed. By drawing blood from the veins, said the doctor. To this he agreed, believing that it would be an easy death. Two veins were then opened in each foot. After about two quarts were drawn, the patient became faint and asked if it was not time for him **16** to die. Not yet, replied the physician. After drawing another quart, the patient turned pale, and looked like a dying man. The ligatures were then taken off and a pleasant sleep ensued for a short time, when he awoke in the full exercise of his reason, astonished at his presumption in wishing for an untimely death full of gratitude to his Maker & physician. He continued in the enjoyments of health, both of body & mind, in the exercise of a Christian temper.

Many of late have committed suicide, which probably might have been prevented, by plentiful depletion.

In proof of this, several insane persons have cut their own throats and bled to a considerable degree, after which, their reason has been restored, and no further attempts have been made to put an end to their lives. —— Cases of this kind are recorded in my M.S. with many of a different description which are sent to Dr Parkman.[13]

17

Case of insanity communicated by Dr Pardon Bowen of Providence in 1820.[14] Some time since, a woman became so insane as to cut her own throat with a razor. She bled until no signs of life remained. I was then called and

[13] George Parkman (1790–1849), son of a wealthy Boston merchant, graduate of Harvard College and the University of Aberdeen Medical School, Parkman was very interested in mental illness. He visited Paris, studied under Philippe Pinel, in 1814 briefly ran a small private institution for the mentally ill, and in 1816 encouraged the trustees of Massachusetts General Hospital to add psychiatric facilities. E. T. Carlson, "The Unfortunate Dr. Parkman," *American Journal of Psychiatry* 123, no. 6 (1966), 724–28. Parkman's publications include George Parkman, *Proposals for Establishing a Retreat for the Insane* (Boston: Printed by J. Eliot, 1814), *Management of Lunatics: With Illustrations of Insanity* (Boston: John Eliot, 1817), and "Remarks on Insanity," *New England Journal of Medicine and Surgery* 7, no. 1 (1818), 117–30. On November 25, 1819, George Parkman wrote to Barker: "Sir, if your History of diseases is to present anything on the subject of Insanity, I should be gratified by the loan of that part of your M.S. which shall be returned without delay. Respectfully, George Parkman." Barker sent him volume 1, chapter 1, which was returned with copies of Parkman's own pamphlets and other materials about insanity, including a section of an 1823 book, pp. 43–69, on the subjects of delirium, mania, monomania, nymphomania, nostalgia, and epilepsy. These are roughly sewn together with chapter 1 and are included in Collection 13 at the Maine Historical Society, along with a handwritten note above the title of a twelve-page pamphlet: "A present from Samuel Parkman M.D. of Boston. Aug. 1820 for his Medical history." Apparently "Samuel Parkman M.D." is an error and should be George Parkman. Samuel Parkman (1751–1824), George Parkman's father, was not a physician, and the 1820 *Boston Directory* does not list a Samuel Parkman, physician.

[14] Pardon Bowen (1757–1826), the fifth son of Dr. Ephraim Bowen, practiced in Providence, Rhode Island. After graduating from Rhode Island College (now Brown University), he studied medicine under his brother William, and in 1783 studied medicine at the College of Philadelphia, called the University of Pennsylvania after 1791. In 1789 he signed on as a surgeon with a private-armed ship, only to be captured by the British several times. James Thacher,

viewing her as a dead person, thought it useless even to sew up the wound. Soon after, some signs of life appeared, and she revived tho in a confused state of mind. A large dose of laudanum was given and her reason was restored which she continued to enjoy.

A question then arose by some, which did the most good, the bleeding or the laudanum. It is well known that opium is not congenial to insane persons but she was prepared for its use by plentiful depletion when the opiate served to equalize the excitement and compose the mind.

18

"Parturition, says Dr Rush, is frequently followed by madness.[15]

My remedies for madness, in its first stage, or rather in all its stages of high excitement, are bleeding, purging and extremely low diet. In the use of the lancet, I am more influenced by the high temper & extravagant conduct of the patient; by the fierceness of the eyes, by the absence of sleep; and by cold feet with the above symptoms, than by the state of the pulse. In all diseases of the brain, Mr Hunter has well observed, the pulse now & then refuses to impart any knowledge of their force, seat or danger.[16] When the strength of the disease is concentrated to the brain, and other parts of the system are languid, I have substituted cups and leeches for venesection.

The liver, spleen & bowels all require the occasional use of calomel & Jalap, on account of the congestions **19** induced in them before and after madness.

If all the Blisters to the ankles I have found more useful than to the head and neck before the excitement of the brain is in part reduced. I learned this practice from Dr Willis soon after he cured the King of Great Britain.[17]

American Medical Biography: Or Memoirs of Eminent Physicians Who Have Flourished in America. To Which Is Prefixed a Succinct History of Medical Science in the United States, from the First Settlement of the Country (Boston: Richardson & Lord and Cottons & Barnard, 1828), 179–84.

[15] Benjamin Rush (1745–1813) studied medicine with John Redman, graduated from the College of New Jersey (Princeton), and studied in Liverpool, London, and Edinburgh. He practiced medicine and taught chemistry and clinical practice at the College of Philadelphia, later the University of Pennsylvania. He was interested in diseases of the mind and the humane treatment of patients suffering from mental disease and insanity. Benjamin Rush, *Medical Inquiries and Observations, Upon the Diseases of the Mind* (Philadelphia: Kimber & Richardson, no. 237, Market street. Merritt, printer, no. 9, Watkin's alley, 1812), 166–67, 251, 253. This book is considered the first American text on the subject of mental illness.

[16] John Hunter (1723–1793). John Hunter, *A Treatise on the Blood, Inflammation, and Gun-Shot Wounds*, 2 vols. (Philadelphia: Thomas Bradford, 1796), vol. 2, 50.

[17] Francis Willis (1718–1807), physician. Porter, Roy. "Willis, Francis (1718–1807), physician." *Oxford Dictionary of National Biography*. 23 Sep. 2004; Accessed 18 Apr. 2020. https://www.

If all the above remedies fail, recourse must be had to a salivation. There is no general disease in which its effects are more uniformly beneficial. I have known order to be established in the mind operations of the mind in a few hours after the patient complained of a sore mouth. But a much longer time is generally necessary for its cure.

The cold bath should follow the salivation, if any part of the disease should remain unsubdued after cordial diet & medicines. Great attention should be paid to the state of the mind. Every thing **20** associated with the cause of the disease, should be removed & objects calculated to revive pleasant & healthy associations of ideas should be sought after in company or in any place in which the person has been happy when sane.

When the temper or wrong associations ideas are highly extravagant, the mind should be soothed or diverted as if by accident, to other subjects.

When the aberrations of the mind become more feeble, they may be opposed by reason, amusements, by conversation, and even by ridicule. Gentle exercise, when practicable must not be neglected."

Medical Museum, Vol. 4. N'3.[18]

see page 39 bottom [where Currie will appear chronologically]

"D\u1d63 Currie has applied a very cold bath to more than one case of insanity, with brilliant success, but it was when the fit was at the highest."

Thacher's Dispensatory 3 Edition p. 613[19]

oxforddnb.com/view/10.1093/ref:odnb/9780198614128.001.0001/odnb-9780198614128-e-29578. Roy Porter, "Willis, Francis (1718–1807)," in *Oxford Dictionary of National Biography: In Association with the British Academy: From the Earliest Times to the Year 2000*, new ed., ed. H. C. G. Matthew and Brian Harrison (Oxford: Oxford University Press, 2004). Willis was a physician whose interest in the mentally ill led to his being called when George III showed symptoms of madness in 1788. His treatment included a straitjacket and blistering. The king's recovery in 1789 helped Willis's career.

[18] John Spence, "History of a Case of Mania, Successfully Treated, in a Series of Letters between Dr. John Spence and Dr. Benjamin Rush. Communicated to the Editor by Dr. Spence," *The Philadelphia Medical Museum* 4, no. 3 (1808): 129–48.

[19] James Thacher, *The American New Dispensatory Containing General Principles of Pharmaceutic Chemistry . . . With an Appendix, Containing an Account of Mineral Waters . . . And the Method of Preparing Opium. . . . The Whole Compiled from the Most Approved Authors, Both European and American*, 3rd ed. (Boston: Thomas B. Wait, 1817), 613. The first edition includes a forty-five-page abridged version of Dr. Currie's medical reports on the use of water. James Thacher, *The American New Dispensatory Containing General Principles of Pharmaceutic Chemistry. . . . The Whole Compiled from the Most Approved Authors, Both European and American* (Boston: T. B. Wait and Co., 1810), 408–53.

21

Some observations on Dr Rush's work, on "the disease of the mind."[20]
With remarks on the nature & treatment of insanity.

[The following long excerpt concludes on MS p. 39]

By George Hayward, M.D.[21]

"Among the improvements of modern medicine, we cannot boast the acquisition of any considerable ascendancy over the diseases of the mind.

Several causes have, no doubt, contributed to retard improvement in the medical treatment of the insane. As one of these may be mentioned, the fact is, that physicians have not, until within a few years, been agreed as to the seat of insanity.

Another cause may be, that though pathologists of the present day are pretty well satisfied that in all cases of insanity, the brain & its appendages, or both, are in some way disordered, they pretend not to say precisely how, yet from the extreme difficulty that has attended all investigations of the physiology of the mind, the subject seems to have been almost abandoned in despair by medical men. ****22**** But though we cannot examine by our senses, the faculties of the mind, as we do the organs of the body, nor understand the wonderful connection of matter and of mind, and their constant action & reaction on each other, yet much may be learnt, by an accurate analysis of our own intellectual faculties & operations. An intimate acquaintance with the philosophy of the human mind, is indispensable to him who would hope to treat its diseases with success. He may as well expect to understand the pathology of the body, without a knowledge of its structure and functions in health.

Another cause, probably, of the repeated failure of almost every attempt to relieve insanity, is, that mankind have too often considered the disease beyond the control of medicine, and the unfortunate patients have usually been abandoned to the care of ignorant or designing empirics; or when they have been placed under the direction of medical men, it is not in the early stages of their disease, it is, ****23**** in fact, usually permitted to continue so long,

---

[20] Rush, *Medical Inquiries and Observations*.

[21] George Hayward, "Some Observations on Dr. Rush's Work on 'the Diseases of the Mind.' With Remarks on the Nature and Treatment of Insanity," *New England Journal of Medicine and Surgery* 7, no. 1 (1818): 18–34. George Hayward (1791–1863) was a graduate of Harvard College and Yale College, and received an MD from the University of Pennsylvania in 1812. Though his major interest was surgery, he published on many nonsurgical topics. Haywood was a medical student during the year Rush published his *Medical Inquiries and Observations*.

that some organic changes are produced in the brain, before medical advice is obtained. Recent cases of insanity may be often cured, while those of long standing are almost always hopeless.

By a calculation that has lately been made in Great Britain, on a large scale, it appears, that of recent cases, seventy six patients of every hundred were relieved, while there were only nineteen out of the same number, whose disease had been of long standing. Perhaps, therefore, it should be adviseable to admit into public institutions, at a low rate, all patients whose disease was recent. This plan has been adopted, at one Asylum in Great Britain.[22]

Numerous treatises on mental derangement have appeared at different periods in Europe; but the work of D[r] Rush, published in 1812, is the only original one, ever printed in this country.[23]

24

From this circumstance, as well as from the fact of the alarming increase of insanity within a few years; and the uncommon attention which it has lately excited, in this vicinity, it was thought that an abstract of its contents might be interesting, if not instructive to some. In doing this, the writer has not confined himself exclusively to the views that the Author has taken of the subject; but has endeavoured to present, in as concise a manner as possible, the opinions of others, of equal eminence, on the nature & treatments of insanity.

The first chapter treats of the faculties & operations of the mind, and of the proximate cause of intellectual derangement. It also consists of remarks on the proximate cause of insanity. D[r] Rush endeavors to show, that it is not seated in the abdominal viscera, the nerves or the mind, except through the medium of the body; and his observations on these subjects are interesting and conclusive.

25

In attempting to establish his own theory, viz, that it is seated in the blood vessels of the brain, he seems not to have been so fortunate. In controverting this opinion of the Author, it is intended merely to say, that there seems not to be satisfactory evidence, that the proximate cause is in every instance, seated in the blood vessels, though there is no doubt that frequently an irregular & unhealthy action in them, may produce that state of the brain, which exists in insanity. What that precise state of the brain is, whether the whole, or a part

---

[22] Probably referring to the York Retreat founded by the English Quaker and merchant William Tuke in 1792. Grob, *The Mad among Us*, 27–29.

[23] Rush, *Medical Inquiries and Observations*.

only is affected, or what diseased action is going on in mental disease, it is impossible for any one to determine.

In the second chapter, the Author gives an account of the exciting ~~causes~~ and predisposing causes of insanity. The exciting causes are divided into such as act directly on the body, and such as act indirectly through the medium of the mind, according to Dr Arnold.[24]

26

The bodily causes are 1^t Those that are seated in the brain and its appendages, such as extravasated blood or water in the ventricles, &c. 2. There are external causes, that act mechanically on the brain, such as fractures, of the cranium, concussion of the brain, &c. 3^d There are causes which produce insanity, by their influence on the brain through the medium of the body in general such as fevers, inanition, excessive indulgence in venereal pleasures, and intemperance in living, &c.

The mental causes of insanity are intense study, close application of the mind to any subject that requires long watchfulness, and all the passions when they are not well regulated, especially excessive joy, grief, disappointed love, religious fanaticism, avarice, &c.

It appears from the best authorities that there are considerable more cases of insanity from mental than **27** corporeal causes. This fact which is noticed by Pinel & others, is confirmed by Dr Rush, who ascertained that of fifty maniacal patients, the disease of only sixteen was produced by corporeal causes.[25]

The predisposition to a disease, is that state of the body, which renders it peculiarly liable to be affected by its exciting causes. The predisposing causes of insanity are either hereditary or acquired. It has often been observed, that the children of persons who have been insane, are more liable to attacks of

---

[24] Thomas Arnold (c. 1742–1816) was considered one of the most prominent alienists in England at the end of the eighteenth century. His father set up a madhouse in Leicester in the 1740s. Arnold received an MD in 1762 from the University of Edinburgh, studying under William Cullen and Alexander Munro, and spent much of his life caring for the mentally ill. He was active in radical causes, particularly the "moral" treatment of the mentally ill. "Alienist" is a nineteenth-century term for one who specializes in mental illness, later called psychiatrists (OED). Alienists often acted as experts in trials when a determination of the defendant's sanity was needed. Peter K. Carpenter, "Thomas Arnold: A Provincial Psychiatrist in Georgian England," *Medical History* 33 (1989): 199–216. Arnold published a two-volume book on insanity in 1782 and 1786. Thomas Arnold, *Observations on the Nature, Kinds, Causes, and Prevention of Insanity, Lunancy, or Madness*, 2 vols. (Leicester, London: G. Robinson, T. Cadell, 1782).

[25] "Corporeal" means relating to a person's physical material body, as opposed to the spirit. Philippe Pinel (1745–1826) studied at Toulouse and Montpellier. In Paris he became a

delirium than others, and it cannot have escaped the notice of any that mania will oftentimes affect the ~~membranes~~ members of the same family of successive generations.

The disease does not, however, necessarily take place, though a predisposition may exist; for it may be prevented, if the exciting causes are avoided. A predisposition also may be acquired, by a frequent or long continued exposure to the action of some of the exciting causes. Some of these have been noticed. It **28** may be remarked, however, that <u>intemperance</u>, is probably the most frequent; as well as the most certain in its effects. [Underlining of the word <u>intemperance</u> is Barker's emphasis and is not found in the published journal article.]

The diseases of the mind assume such a variety of appearances, that it would be impossible to find an accurate account of all the symptoms, without exceeding the limits of this article.

The patients, in the beginning of the disease are usually wakeful, with a considerable elevation or depression of spirits, and ~~and~~ evident incoherence in their language, and excentricity, in their deportment & manners. The countenance is usually varying, at one time flushed, at another, pale & lifeless; the eye is sometimes unusually bright & penetrating, at others, dull, heavy, and stupid. The appetite for food is, for the most part, increased, the bowels are costive, the urine scanty & high coloured. The pulse is variable, sometimes hard & full, at others, preternaturally slow, then small & quick, or frequent & depressed. The senses of seeing & hearing are extremely **29** acute, while there is a morbid insensibility to cold. Sometimes the patients complain of pain, dizziness, and vertigo in the head, and are disturbed with uneasy sleep, and frightful dreams. Soon some extravagance will be discovered in their actions, and they take a strong dislike to their connections & friends. If nothing is done to allay these symptoms, the disease soon appears in its full force, and the patients become violent and impatient of restraint. The causes which have produced their insanity; as well as their former habits & dispositions, usually give a complexion to their disease. Insanity, in fact, appears under such aspects, that no two cases precisely resemble each other.

---

reformer, particularly with respect to the humane care of the insane. Philippe Pinel, *Traité Médico-Philosophique Sur L'aliénation Mentale: Ou La Manie* (Paris: Chez Richard, Caille et Ravier, 1801); and Philippe Pinel and David Daniel Davis, *A Treatise on Insanity, in Which Are Contained the Principles of a New and More Practical Nosology of Maniacal Disorders Than Has yet Been Offered to the Public: Exemplified by Numerous and Accurate Historical Relations of Cases from the Author's Public and Private Practice: With Plates Illustrative of the Craniology of Maniacs and Ideots* (Sheffield: printed by W. Todd, for Messrs. Cadell and Davies, Strand, London, 1806). John H. Talbott, *A Biographical History of Medicine* (New York: Grune & Stratton, 1970), 452–54.

The few symptoms that have been enumerated are only those of the most general kind. They are detailed, by Dr Rush, at some length, and with great accuracy.

Upon the prognosis of insanity, the Author has made a number of observations, and given several of the **30** signs of a favourable or unfavourable issue. The disease yields more readily in the young than the old, in women than in men, in those who have no children than in those who have. It gives way sooner when it is the consequence of corporeal, than of mental causes; and it is more difficult to cure, and more liable to return, when there is a hereditary predisposition, than under other other circumstances. Remissions, intermissions, and lucid intervals are favourable; so are abscesses, in various parts of the body, warm & moist hands, when the patients have previously had cold ones. Madness, which succeeds an organic injury of the brain, epilepsy, chronic headache, palsy, and fatuity, is generally incurable, while that arising from the common causes of fever, parturition, and intemperance in drinking, usually yields to the power of medicine. These are among the most prominent & important circumstances, connected with the prognosis of mania.

The only subject that remains to be noticed, and which is perhaps more important, than any that has spoken of, **31** is the moral & medical treatment of the insane. Within a few years, an entire revolution has been effected in the moral management of the insane.

Upon the first decisive symptoms of insanity, the patients should be removed from home, and placed under the care of strangers. This is necessary, in order to break up their old associations, and to obtain that control over them which their situation requires. At the first visit of the medical attendant, he should convince them, if possible, of the folly of resistance by showing them that it is in his power to restrain their greatest violence, and punish their excesses. The manners & language of the physician should always be gentle, dignified and affectionate. He should never condescend to trifle, or notice their [rude] & insolent remarks, except in the way of reproof. He should conscientiously fulfil every promise, and pay, in every instance, the strictest regard to veracity, in all statements he makes to them. If maniacs have been once deceived, they will never confide again in the same person. In those cases where they are violent, they may be prevented **32** from injuring themselves or others, by a strait waistcoat, or by hand cuffs, made of leather, to which cords may be attached. Their diet is to be regulated, in great measure, by the state of the system; it should, however, be mild, simple, and not very nutritious. Exercise, and even labour, in the open air, are useful to maniacs, adapted, as far as practicable, to their former mode of life. It may be observed also, that great advantage has been supposed to have been derived, from requiring a regular attendance on devotional exercises daily; as well as on the Sabbath, of all who are peaceable in their manners.

The subjects of an asylum should rarely be visited, except by the physician & attendants; the presence of strangers often increases their disease, or at least retards the cure. Relapses have taken place, from the exposure of patients to company, before their health was perfectly re-established.

The medical remedies should never be neglected. One of the most powerful & valuable of these is blood letting. The propriety of it is to be **33** determined by the state of the system; and it is particularly indicated in all recent cases, where there is frequency, strength, and fullness in the pulse. In cases of this sort Sydenham considers the use of the lancet highly important, and advises to draw blood, not only from the arm, but from the jugular vein.[26]

It is not unusual in mania, especially from corporeal causes, to meet with a depressed pulse, arising from what D[r] Rush terms suffocated excitement.[27] If bloodletting is performed, under these circumstances, the pulse rises, and frequently a cure is effected, if a large quantity of blood is drawn. There seems to be no remedy so well calculated as this, to diminish excessive arterial action in the brain; and the propriety of its use, in many cases of mania, is rendered evident, by the delicate structure of that organ, and the injury it would sustain, by a long continued plethora of its vessels; as well as from the benefit maniacal patients have frequently experienced, from spontaneous hemorrhages. **34**

In the recent affections of young subjects when bloodletting is employed, it should be copious, and its good effects are increased by compelling the patients to stand, while the operation is performed so as to produce fainting, and afterward confining them to diluting drinks, and a low spare diet. This, however, is proper only in those of plethoric habit.

There are cases also, where there is congestion upon the brain, and at the same time general debility. It is then that topical bleeding is indicated. This

---

[26] In a section titled "On the common madness"; Thomas Sydenham, Samuel Johnson, and John Swan, *The Entire Works of Dr. Thomas Sydenham, Newly Made English from the Originals: Wherein the History of Acute and Chronic Diseases, and the Safest and Most Effectual Methods of Treating Them, Are Faithfully, Clearly, and Accurately Delivered. To Which Are Added, Explanatory and Practical Notes, from the Best Medicinal Writers* (London: Printed for Edward Cave, at St. John's Gate, 1742), 609. Thomas Sydenham (1624–1689), with degrees from Oxford and Cambridge Universities, was a great clinician known by some as the father of modern medicine or "The English Hippocrates."

[27] Hayward, "Some Observations on Dr. Rush's Work," 30; Rush, *Medical Inquiries and Observations*, 23.

can be done by opening the temporal artery or external jugular vein, or by applying cups, or leeches; perhaps the last is most convenient, and equally efficacious with others.

There can be no doubt as to the propriety of treating insanity, as we do other diseases, according to the symptoms of each case; for surely no one will pretend that of all the remedies, which have **35** been tried, any one of them is entitled to the character of a specific.[28]

Cathartics have been long known to be useful, in the various forms of madness. In those cases where bloodletting is used, the saline purgatives are preferable, and Cullen recommends the tartrite of potash or soluble tartar, as more useful than any other.[29] When cathartic medicines are given to carry off the contents of the intestines, and at the same time, to promote the secretion of bile, and the other fluids that are poured into the intestinal canal, the submuriate of mercury is the most efficacious. This class of medicines, however, is used in various cases of mania, with a view of producing a determination[30] of blood to the abdominal viscera, and thereby relieving the brain from congestion, if that state of the organ should exist. On this account, aloes, which stimulates **36** the rectum, gamboge, scammony, and other drastic medicines have been employed. Many authors are of opinion that the hellebore, which is so repeatedly spoken of the ancients, as a remedy, and almost a specific for madness, owes its reputations, entirely to its cathartic properties.

Celsus directs the administration of cathartics of black hellebore, when the patients are sad & dejected, and emetics of the white [hellebore], when they are too much exhilerated.[31] This writer, in common with many others, speaks so highly of the good effects of hellebore, in maniacal cases, that it surely deserves trial. It is said that white hellebore oftentimes diminishes the

---

[28] "Specific" refers to a treatment that exerts "an invariable curative action on the disease . . . regardless of the particular patient or environment." Its mode of action was obscure as opposed to laxatives or cathartics. Until the 1860s "disease specific treatment . . . was considered illegitimate" (quackery). See John Harley Warner, *The Therapeutic Perspective: Medical Practice, Knowledge, and Identity in America, 1820–85* (Cambridge, MA: Harvard University Press, 1986), 58–80.

[29] William Cullen (1712–1790) was chair of medicine and chemistry at Glasgow and Edinburgh. William Cullen, *First Lines of the Practice of Physic with Supplementary Notes, Including More Recent Improvements in the Practice of Medicine by Peter Reid*, two volumes in one (Brookfield: E. Mirriam & Co. for Isaiah Thomas, 1807), 553–58.

[30] "A tendency or flow of the bodily fluids, now esp. of the blood, to a particular part" (OED).

[31] Aulus Cornelius Celsus (30 BC–AD 50) wrote eight surviving books devoted to medicine. He was not a physician, and the books "were written for a non-professional readership." He suggested that in medicine, "not just experience but reason" are required. Roy Porter, *The*

frequency of the pulse. This is evidently an argument in favour of its use, in some forms of mania.

D[r] Ferriar strongly recommends the use of tartrite of antimony, in small doses, in certain stages of **37** insanity, sufficient only to excite nausea, and thinks that by the use he has relieved several patients.[32]

Blisters to the head, are less used now, than in former years, though they are frequently applied to the back of the neck, arms, ankles and other parts of the body. It is probable that in cases where there is active inflammation, either on the brain or its membranes, they would have a tendency rather to increase than diminish it from their contiguity to the diseased parts. In recent cases, therefore, where the arterial action is great, cold applied to the head, in the form of water, snow or ice, is preferable to vesication. In chronic inflammation of the brain, however, the whole external surface of the head may be blistered with great advantage, and setons or issues in the neck, have been found beneficial.

The effects of mercury have been tried in some cases of insanity, until a slight salivation was produced; and, in a few instances the practice has been advantageous. It is probable that small doses of calomel, or the blue mercurial pill, might be given **38**
with benefit to melancholic patients, in whom the functions of the liver were deranged; and perhaps it would be justifiable to resort to some preparation of mercury, in cases of obstinate chronic mania with a view of exciting a new action in the system.

All authors are agreed, that baths, either of cold, temperate or warm water, are beneficial, in the various forms of madness. D[r] Ferriar recommends cold baths in melancholy, and warm in mania, while Pinel prefers the temperate in both cases.[33] The present opinion seems to be, that the warm bath, is one of the most powerful means that are used in the treatment of insanity.[x] [Here Barker refers the reader to his note [x] about Dr. Currie on the use of baths in mania at the bottom of MS p. 39]

Greatest Benefit to Mankind: A Medical History of Humanity (New York: W. W. Norton & Company, 1997), 70–71, 78. The writings of Celsus were rediscovered in 1443. Talbott, *A Biographical History of Medicine*, 7–8.

[32] John Ferriar (1761–1815) trained at Edinburgh University and was appointed physician at the Manchester Infirmary. A medical reformer, he was particularly interested in infectious diseases and hygiene, and he published four volumes of medical case histories beginning in 1792. John Ferriar, *Medical Histories and Reflections*, 1st American ed. (Philadelphia: Published by Thomas Dobson, at the Stone House, no. 41 William Fry, 1816).

[33] Pinel and Davis, *A Treatise on Insanity.*

The most important medical remedies of insanity, have thus been noticed; but it is only with a proper combination of these, with judicious moral management that any considerable degree of success can be anticipated.

"Of the uncertainties of our present state," says a celebrated moralist, "the most dreadful and alarming is the uncertain continuance of reason."[34] Is it not wonderful, **39** then, that so much zeal has lately been displayed in relation to the establishment of an asylum for the insane. It is a concern that equally interests all the members of the community, and everyone must have witnessed with delight, the pure zealous and signal benevolence, which our citizens have manifested. It is gratifying to think, that they can now lay claims to higher distinction, than they ever could have done before, by their earnestness in the cause of afflicted humanity. An institution founded for such laudable objects, and placed under the care of so many able & enlightened directors, will, with the blessing of Heaven, greatly contribute to ameliorate the condition of a distressed and suffering portion of our fellow beings."

New England Journal, No. 1. vol. 7
January 1818 [35]

x As Dr Currie has found the cold bath to be useful in mania, when the fit was at the highest. Of course the warm bath can only be beneficial in chronic mania, where the system needs to be invigorated.[36]

40

"A man, in the Philadelphia hospital, says Dr Rush, aged 68 years, and of a family subject to madness, was affected with mania in an uncommonly

---

[34] This quotation is found in Hayward, "Some Observations on Dr. Rush's Work," 34. William Perfect, M.D. (*Annals of Insanity*, 1787) opened his Preface with a quotation from *Rasselas*. John Haslam, M.D. (*Observations on Madness and Melancholy*, 1809) used the same quotation on his title page. The sentence that caught their imagination was Imlac's remark, "of the uncertainties of our present state, the most dreadful and alarming is the uncertain continuance of reason," a remark that evidently contributed to the increased interest in insanity at the time. Kathleen M. Grange, "Dr. Samuel Johnson's Account of a Schizophrenic Illness in Rasselas (1759)," *Medical History* 6, no. 2 (1962): 167.

[35] Hayward, "Some Observations on Dr. Rush's Work," 18–34. Also in the same issue is Parkman, "Remarks on Insanity."

[36] James Currie (1756–1805) of Scotland lived in Virginia from 1771 until 1776, when he returned to Scotland. He was interested in the use of water as a therapeutic modality. James Currie, *Medical Reports, on the Effects of Water, Cold and Warm, as a Remedy in Fever, and Febrile Diseases; Whether Applied to the Surface of the Body, or Used as a Drink: With Observations on the Nature of Fever; and on the Effects of Opium, Alcohol, and Inanition* (Liverpool: Printed by

violent degree. But it yielded to 17 bleedings, 10 or 12 ounces at time, purging every second or third day, and a low diet, in six weeks. He is now with his family, in New Jersey, in good health."

1807
[Philadelphia] Medical Museum.v.4 n.3.[37]

In Autumn 1819, a young man, in Maine was seized with typhous fever, and treated with common evacuants, followed with stimulants. The fever terminated in about 4 weeks and left him insane. At times he attempted to commit murder. At other times he would take of[f] his cloaths and aim at the water. In the spring he ceased to speak and became considerably emaciated.

In May, by the advice of a physician, he was bled freely, and stramonium was given which produced a cutaneous eruption. His reason was soon restored. D[r] Barton, in his Materia Medica, speaks of a case of Mania, where stramonium produced biles, on various parts of the body and reason was restored.[38]

41

In Nov. 1818, a young woman in Maine of an irascible temper, became insane. She wandered into a field in the evening and cut her throat with a razor, so that she bled till she was unable to walk. In the morning, she was found, and her reason was restored, tho "almost frozen to death," as she expressed herself. By suitable nutriment, her blood was soon regenerated, with health of body and a sound mind.

About this time, a butcher in Maine under perplexed circumstances, became insane, & cut his throat, ~~which~~ so that he bled till he was restored to reason, which continued a year when he again became insane and cut his throat to such a degree, that he bled even unto death!

J. M'Creery, for Cadell and Davies, London, 1797). Currie's book was reprinted in an abridged form in Maine: James Currie and Benjamin Vaughan, *An Abridgment of the Second Edition of a Work, Written by Dr. Currie, of Liverpool in England: On the Use of Water, in Diseases of the Human Frame; and on Fever, Opium, Strong Drink, Abstinence from Food, and the Passages through the Human Skin: With Occasional Remarks* ([Augusta, ME] and by the Booksellers of Boston, New-York, and Philadelphia: Printed by Peter Edes; sold by Mr. Edes of Augusta, and Mr. Bass of Hallowell, 1799).

[37] Spence, "History of a Case of Mania," 129–148; This "Extract of a letter from Dr. Rush" is found on p. 148.

[38] Barker is probably referring to Benjamin Smith Barton, *Collections for an Essay Towards a Materia Medica of the United-States*, 2nd ed. (Philadelphia: Printed for the author by Robert Carr, 1801). His nephew later published a botany; see William P. C. Barton, *Vegetable Materia Medica of the United States, or, Medical Botany: Containing a Botanical, General, and Medical History, of Medicinal Plants Indigenous to the United States: Illustrated by Coloured Engravings, Made after Original Drawings from Nature, Done by the Author*, 2 vols. (Philadelphia: Printed and published by M. Carey & Son, 1817). "Biles" is an early spelling of "boils" (OED).

In 18— A wealthy farmer, who was deprived of several lucrative offices, became insane, imagining that he was surrounded with enemies. Soon after he cut his throat, so as to bleed considerably. His mind then became calm, and he lamented his rash conduct in attempting to destroy his own life. Still he believed that his farm would not be productive enough to support his family, and he should become **42** a pauper. In this state of mind, he lived so abstemiously that he became greatly emaciated, tho his bodily strength was such that he would do considerable labour, without complaining of fatigue. Under this course, his reason was perfectly restored, and he returned to his usual mode of living, tho with great regularity & temperance. His flesh was soon regained, and health enjoyed.

Some years since, an aged woman imagined that she should become poor, tho in comfortable circumstances. She took but very little food, and became much enfeebled. At length, while attempting to swallow a hard crust of bread, it struck in her throat and produced great distress of body & mind. I was then called, and gave her but little encouragement that it could be removed. She then said, with much grief, that for some time past she had thought that she should starve to death; but now she must be choaked to death with bread and considered herself a vile sinner ——I directed her to hold water in her throat to soften the crust which soon passed down and she became a rational woman no longer distrusting Providence.

43

[Top of page: Barker notes that p. 43 is "to follow p. 8"—the case that begins with "Before the revolutionary war, a merchant in Falmouth . . ." MS p. 5–8]

While in my pupilage with Dr Lincoln of Hingham, he was sometimes consulted in cases of insanity, which occurred in distant towns. The mode of treatment consisted chiefly in bleeding, purging and a low diet (so that he was accused by some physicians, of <u>starving</u> his patients.) But good success, generally attended his practice in such cases.

The cathartic which he used, was composed according to the following Receipts, which he obtained from Dr Brattle of Cambridge, Mass. in 1769, an experienced physician, who considered it highly efficacious in cases of insanity.[39]

---

[39] William Brattle was born in Cambridge in 1702, graduated from Harvard in 1722, and served as a lawyer, preacher, physician, soldier, and legislator. He was a captain of an artillery company in 1733, a major general in the militia, and at times a member of the General Court and the Council. A Loyalist, he moved to Halifax, Nova Scotia, in 1776 and died there in October of that year. D. Hamilton Hurd, *History of Middlesex County, Massachusetts, with Biographical Sketches of Many of Its Pioneers and Prominent Men*, 3 vols. (Philadelphia: J. W. Lewis & Co., 1890), vol. 1, p. xxxviii.

R$_x$ Pul. Helleb. Nig. — — — — —Ʒii [symbol for scruple, 20 grains]

Agaric   — — — — — Ʒii [symbol for ounce]
Cologunit.   — — — — — Ʒi
Scammon.   — — — — — Ʒss
Asa Fat.   — — — — — Ʒiss
Calomel   — — — — — Ʒis
Syr. e spin. cen. L.S. pro. mol.
S. t. — Sumend. Ʒi ad Ʒii
pro cathartic.
Deob. vel allerat. 10. $^{grs.}$
repeated according to the urgency of the symptoms.

44
In succeeding years, I have frequently used this cathartic in Mania, and found it to be considerably drastic, producing irritation in alimentary canal, sometimes tenesmus, and, in this way, it appeared to alleviate mental derangement keeping the patient on a low vegetable diet, bloodletting, particularly in recent cases, being prenzised,[40] and occasionally wetting the head with cold water; but not so as to produce reaction. Also warm water to the feet & legs, and draw blood from the feet when indicated.

This mode of practice has been attended with success; but since 1800, I have found that mercury, given so as to excite salivation, has much more expeditiously removed maniacal complaints; for the knowledge of which, I acknowledge myself indebted to D^r [Elihu Hubbard] Smith of New York. Med. Repos[itory] Vol 1.[41] where a violent maniacal affection was readily removed, by salivation, produced by mercurial unction.[42]

45
This case of "Mania," recorded by Dr Smith, I think, might with propriety, be termed, "Delirium Vigilans," for the patient, a delicate young girl, did not

---

[40] Probably "frenzy" or "phrensy" (OED).

[41] E. H. Smith, "Article VI Case of Mania Successfully Treated by Mercury," *Medical Repository* 1, no. 2 (1797): 181–84. Several subsequent editions of the early volumes of the *Medical Repository* appeared. For example, the 3rd edition of volume 1 is dated 1804. See R. J. Kahn and P. G. Kahn, "The Medical Repository—The First U.S. Medical Journal (1797–1824)," *New England Journal of Medicine* 337 (1997): 1926–30.

[42] In 1812 Rush wrote, "mercury acts by abstracting morbid excitement from the brain to the mouth; by removing visceral obstructions, and by changing the cause of our patient's complaints, and fixing them wholly upon his sore mouth." Rush, *Medical Inquiries and Observations*, 105.

sleep for 14 days, and strong cords would not confine her, ~~and she went naked, taking but~~ tho she took very little food. But as soon as a phalysm [*sic*] [43] was produced, she became tractible [*sic*], and sleep took place without opium.

I have met with many cases of this in the course of my practice of late years, and always found that after salivation, sleep succeeded without opiates, and if the brain in its disease is affected in the manner described, by Dr Hayward in his dissections, I cannot conceive that opium is eligible, at least, until congestion & inflammation are removed, by some other means.

see Dr Haywards diss[ertation] N.Engl Journal[44]

[Barker notes] Turn back to page 13 [the case that begins "On the 10th of April 1807, I was informed of a maniac, who was enchained . . ." MS p. 13] In 1807. Case of Mrs Noyse [of] Falmouth who ceased to converse or take food cured by OS [oral] – Salivation & cath^s – then select from Notes, other cases in succeeding years.

46

In Autumn 1819, a middle aged man, in Maine, who had been for some time previous in the habit of taking ardent spirits to excess according to the fashionable mode of drinking, was attacked with a convulsion fit, of the epileptic kind, to which succeeded a diarrhœa attended with flatulency and distention; tho his appetite for food & spirits continued, and he indulged in both to excess. Under these circumstances he became insane, not only when under the influence of spirit which always produced temporary insanity; but at other times; so that he was very illnatured, beating & abusing friends breaking furniture, particularly glass & crockery ware; and using very profane language. The diarrhœa became habitual and continued to molest him night & day, sometimes 8 or ten times in 24 hours in abundant profusion for the most part free from any bilious tinge or pain and it continued much the same

---

43 From context, I believe that Barker means "ptyalism" or the excessive secretion of saliva frequently associated with the therapeutic use of mercury.

44 George Hayward, "Some Remarks on Delerium Vigilans; Commonly Called 'Delerium Tremens,' 'Mania a Potu,' 'Mania a Temulentia,'" *New England Journal of Medicine and Surgery* 11 (1822): 235–43. George Hayward (1791–1863) of Boston was a surgeon with an A.B. from Harvard in 1809, and an M.D. from the University of Pennsylvania in 1812. He studied abroad under Astley Cooper and others and became the Harvard's first professor of the principles of surgery. He must have had some interest in mental illness, as he published this article and another in 1818; see footnote 21. For more biographical information see Howard A. Kelly and Walter L. Burrage, *American Medical Biographies* (Baltimore: The Norman, Remington Company, 1920), 508–509.

for more than a year, tho various means were taken to restrain the discharges, viz emetics, cathartics, opiates, alkalies &c.

At the expiration of this term he repaired to my house and put himself under my care, that is in ~~Dec^r~~ Nov. 1820.

47

During the month of Decr. his diarrhœa was more profuse than hereto-fore, and his appetite was impaired; pulse 120 in a minute; and considerable thirst for acid drinks so that he was confined to the house the chief of the time with very little expectation of a recovery, and impaired in mind. His flesh wasted and he appeared to labour under a consuming hectic [fever] from inflammatory irritation in the intestinal canal, tho he was free from any pulmonary complaints which had in former years molested him.

In this month he abstained from spirits and made use of milk with its preparations, and salt fish with sea bread [hardtack] together with bitters after decoction, ~~with~~ and occasional doses of opium & calomel.

At the close of the month, his health was in great measure restored, and his diarrhœa had almost wholly ceased. At the first of Jany he returned home and passed a pretty comfortable winter able to endure fatigue and exercise. In the Spring however he made free use of spirits, and again became insane as heretofore, with a return of his diarrhœa and borborigmi, appetite voracious particularly for ~~animal food~~ fresh meat which always made him worse.

48

In May he returned to my house greatly disordered in body & mind, and he had a great thirst for spirits which he took to excess at times as well as animal food; so that his mind was greatly deranged; yet his strength often was such that he could walk to Portland & back again with little fatigue. He was at times, particularly when under the influence of spirits, disposed to do mischief and sometimes threatened to injure his friends.

I again debarred him from spirits and means to procure any; put him on a low diet without much animal food, save salted fish. In June & July he was able to labour in the field and could do ~~could do~~ considerable work altho his diarrhœa continued to molest him several times in the day as well as by night so that he was deprived of much sleep unless procured by opium, but this increased his insanity, and was laid aside. In October his bowels became regular, and his reason was restored. He then returned home.

49

Some years since, a woman, in Maine, became so insane that she thought it sinful to eat any kind of food; of course she took very little. But she soon became irascible, and attempted to hurt her friends, by blows, &c, so that she was enchained. After remaining several months thus confined, without any mitigation of her disorder, few means being used, she was liberated and conveyed in a chaise, into another town, among strangers, distant thirty miles. Her reason was then restored, and continued.

A zealous religious exhorter, in process of time, ceased to speak a single word on any occasion, for about a year; tho apparently in health, eating drinking & sleeping as usual. At length he was conducted to a river, distant a quarter of a mile, and preparation made to throw him into the water. He then opened his mouth and begged to be released, which was granted. After this he conversed as usual; and blamed his friends for not employing medical aid. The reason assigned for not speaking was "a fear of uttering something which should be sinful." ——What better means could have been used? devised?

50

Some years since, a young man in Maine, became insane, and was so turbulent mischievius that it was thought proper to confine him. But he was so noisy, that a cave was dug in the ground near the house, for his accommodation. The weather however, becoming cold his feet were frozen to such a degree that a great discharge took place. His reason was then restored, and he was liberated. In process of time when his feet were restored to soundness, he complained of a strange feeling in his head, and fearing that he should again become insane, and so as suffer confinement as heretofore he put an end to his life with a halter! This case serves to show the power of counter stimulants & evacuations, in insanity. ——When the discharge ceased and his mind became disordered, should not some other stimulint [*sic*] have been applied and evacuations have been made to relieve the mind brain?

D[r] Barton[45] says that in case of mania he at length gave the stramonium datura to the extent of Cc grains at a dose. When the patient had continued on this dose for some time she broke out into boils on various parts of her body, and was thus cured.

51

[Missing; torn out. Only a torn stub of paper remains.]

52

---

[45] Probably Benjamin Smith Barton (1766–1815), who had studied with William Shippen in Philadelphia and subsequently at the University of Edinburgh and elsewhere. He returned to teach at the medical school at the College of Philadelphia (the University of Pennsylvania after 1791).

See last page, bottom. [Note at the top of this page—may refer to Dr Barton or to something on the missing page 51.]

Under the indirect operation of these effects is included that deterioration from the original perfection of the constitution of species and that susceptibility to disease, of which I have just spoken.

The powers exercised in the processes of disease are the same as those which maintain the system in a state of health diverted from their natural course & operation. Every phenomena may be clearly attributed to the ordinary vital laws, and there is in fact, considerable resemblance between the processes of disease & those of health, as to the general plan on which they proceed.

The powers of life have an instinctive tendency to resist the operation, & remove the effects of the operation of those external agents which are disposed to injure the organs, or derange the functions. This is a genuine principle of action, and all disease, except that which is produced by mechanical injury, is directly or indirectly the result of this principle. Indigestible food excites vomiting & diarrhœa for its expulsion. Poisons excite the same action in a more violent degree.

53

On Suppuration

"Suppuration, says Dr Ware,[46] is so important a part of the process of inflammation, and so intimately connected with its other stages, that one cannot enter upon the consideration of the former, without embracing a view of some of the general principle of the latter. These do not refer to any particular stage of the process, but to inflammation as a whole, as consisting of a series of connected functions existing for some definite purpose; which is accomplished by different degrees, and a different exercise of the same powers, according to the nature of the purpose and the opinions of the system and of the past.

If we would attain to a right understanding of suppuration, we ought to understand the object originally proposed by nature; in the

---

[46] John Ware, *Medical Dissertations on Hemoptysis or the Spitting of Blood, and on Suppuration, Which Obtained the Boylston Premiums for the Years 1818 & 1820* (Boston: Cummings and Hilliard, 1820), 54–95. John Ware (1795–1864) was born in Hingham, Massachusetts, and received a Harvard B.A. in 1813 and an M.D. in 1816. He practiced in Boston, became coeditor of the *New England Journal of Medicine and Surgery*, and later edited the *Boston Medical and Surgical Journal*. Ware would become the Hersey Professor of Medicine at Harvard and president of the Massachusetts Medical Society. See Kaufman, Galishoff, and Savitt, *Dictionary of American Medical Biography*, vol. 2, 773–74; Kelly and Burrage, *American Medical Biographies*, 1190–91.

establishment of such a function; to what degree it is simply as a general principle that it should take place in those cases where there is an obvious tendency to produce it; what is the state of the parts which preceeds it; and what the actions by which it is accomplished. These principles embrace the fundamental principles of inflammation; and those laws which regulate its progress from its mildness & simplest, to its most severe & complicated forms.

Supposing a human body in the most perfect health of which it is capable there seems to be only two means by which disease should ever be produced. **54** First, by a spontaneous imperfection in the actions of some of its organs, which deranges the natural relations its functions maintain with each other and the reciprocal influences they exert. Second, by the operation of external causes with different parts of the body; which operation is of two kinds, and will produce disease in two different ways. 1st By an immediate primary derangement, as is the case with all injuries, poisons, indigestible food &c or 2^d by exciting trains of action in the system not essentially morbid which yet result, at a greater or less distance of time, in the establishment of disease.

Disease is probably never established in the first of these ways, since this necessarily implies an original tendency in the system to its existence. The gradual decay of the powers & organs, in old age, is the natural provision for the cessation of life, and seems to be the only one had in view in the construction of the system. But this is something very different from an original tendency to disease; this would amount to a direct provision for the extreme of evil, of which I believe there is no example in the creation. Considered abstractly, it is believed that everything in the human body is established in the best possible manner for its own well being, so for as its organs & powers are concerned.

55

That if every natural appetite was universally [indulged], the functions might be performed in the same degree of perfection as at first, till exhausted by old age, were they not not subject to the influence of external causes. It is to this influence, combined with the unnatural indulgence of our appetites, that we are to attribute our liabilities to disease; and not merely to ~~attribute our liability~~ these circumstances operating on individual, but to the influence they have exerted for ages, upon generation after generation, till the constitution of the species has deteriorated from its original perfection; so that we are now born with a predisposition to disease. It is in consequence of this that we daily see individuals who come into the world with such imperfections of constitution or of particular parts, that even when in health, it is obvious that the regular series of their functions will finally end in the establishment of some fatal malady.

Considered merely in relation to our physical constitutions, [our habits of life in society are artificial and pernicious.]"[47]

---

[47] Ware, *Medical Dissertations on Hemoptysis*, 56. Barker's handwritten chapter 1 of volume 1 ends here, but Ware's paper on suppuration continues for another forty pages.

PROPOSALS FOR PUBLISHING
A HISTORY
OF

DISEASES IN THE DISTRICT OF MAINE,

Commencing in 1772, and continued to the present time.

CONTAINING ALSO,
Some Account of Diseases in New-Hampshire,
and other parts of New-England,

WITH

BIOGRAPHICAL SKETCHES,

Of learned and useful Physicians, both in Europe and America,
as well as other Promoters of Medical Science.

TO THIS IS ANNEXED
An inquiry in to the Causes, Nature, increasing Prevalency,
and Treatment of

CONSUMPTION

WHICH IS MAINTAINED TO BE CURABLE,
If proper means are seasonably and duly employed,

8 vo [handwritten]
CONTAINING ABOUT 400 PAGES —
PRICE TWO DOLLARS IN BOARDS,

Written so as to be intelligible to those who are destitute of Medical Science :

BY JEREMIAH BARKER, Esq. F.M.M.S.[1]

NAMES   RESIDENCE   No. Copies

---

[1] Jeremiah Barker was elected Fellow of the Massachusetts Medical Society (M.M.S.) in 1803. He accepted the honor in a letter of July 12, 1803, to Dr. Joseph Whipple (1756–1804), who was corresponding secretary of the M.M.S. from 1800–1805. The letter is in the Center for the History of Medicine at the Countway Library of Medicine, B MS c 75.2. See also Walter L. Burrage, *A History of the Massachusetts Medical Society* (Norwood, MA: Plimpton Press, 1923), 23. On

About 100 subscribers have been procured in Maine [and]
other states in New England.
Subscribers in Gorham: Dudley Folsome, Elisha Bax[ter],
Jacob S. Smith, Reuben Nason, Joseph Adams,
Asa Rand, now of Boston. — George Parkman of [Boston]
who requested a subscription paper to procure subs[cribers.]
Subscribers in Portsmouth
Ammi R. Cutter, and 10 other physicians, all in that town.
Joshua Fisher of Beverly, who took a paper.
Thomas Manning of Ipswich procured four on a paper.
Daniel Cony of Augusta took a paper for subscription.
In Boston, Dr Parkman & Dr Coffin took papers.
In Providence Drs Bowen & Wheaton took papers.
In New York President Spalding and Professor Mitchill took papers in
order to procure subscriptions —— &c

June 30, 1804, Barker, along with Nathaniel Coffin, Shirley Erving, Dudley Folsom, Stephen Thomas, and Aaron Kinsman, petitioned the Council of the M.M.S. to appoint a District of Maine Medical Society that would include York, Cumberland, and Lincoln counties and would meet in Portland. "Nothing came of their attempts to form a society." Burrage, *A History of the Massachusetts Medical Society*, 331. This application for District of Maine Medical Society is in the collection at the Center for the History of Medicine at the Countway Library of Medicine, Nathaniel Coffin, B MS c 75.2. When Maine became a state in 1820, the Maine Medical Society held its first meeting and was incorporated the following year. A possible contradiction is found in Spalding's writings: "district medical societies were formed at Augusta in 1797, in Knox and Lincoln in 1804, and York and Cumberland about 1811." James Alfred Spalding, *Maine Physicians of 1820; a Record of the Members of the Massachusetts Medical Society Practicing in the District of Maine at the Date of Separation* (Lewiston: Lewiston Print Shop, 1928), 6. Please note that an image of this page appears in the Introduction as Fig. 1.8 on page 16.

Chap. 2.ᵈ

IN 1780, FINDING the air on Cape Cod injurious to my constitution and physicians being numerous, I removed to Gorham, in the County of Cumberland, District of Maine, adjoining Falmouth,² eight miles north of Portland, where the air was salubrious, the land fertile, and under good improvement. Gorham was first settled by Capᵗ John Phinney, of Barnstable, in 1736;³ and he was soon followed by many families from that town & county; as well as from other parts of New England, people of steady habits.

In 1780, the town contained about 200 families. It now contains more than three times that number. The Rev. Josiah Thacher, aged about 40, was then Pastor.⁴ He was sound in doctrine, but unsound in health. He had been troubled from some years with a catarrhal cough, which terminated in a fatal pulmonic affection in 18__.⁵ His whole family, eight in number, died in succeeding years, of pulmonary affections, concerning which, some account will hereafter be given.

The following adjacent towns, exclusive of Portland, were destitute of physicians, although they contained from 80 to 200 families, viz Falmouth, Cape Elizabeth, Windham, Raimond, [*sic*] Otisfield, Standish, Buxton & Limington.

My practice soon extended into all these towns, so that opportunities were afforded of noticing the mode of living habits and diseases. The people in general were enterprising, industrious and temperate. Indian corn & grain of

---

² Falmouth here refers to Falmouth in the District of Maine, named in 1658. Part of the town of Falmouth "commonly called the Neck" was renamed Portland in 1786. William Willis, *Journals of the Rev. Thomas Smith and the Rev. Samuel Deane . . . With Notes and Biographical Notices and a Summary History of Portland* (Portland: Joseph S. Bailey, 1849), 429, 580. Falmouth on Cape Cod, in what is now Massachusetts, was settled in 1660 and was named Falmouth in 1690. William Willis, *The History of Portland*, facsimile ed. (Somersworth, New Hampshire Publishing Company and Maine Historical Society, 1972; Portland: Bailely & Noyes, 1865), 95.

³ Hugh D. Mc Lellan, *History of Gorham, Maine* (Portland: Smith and Sale, 1903), 74.

⁴ Josiah Thacher [Thatcher]. Born in Lebanon, Connecticut, he graduated from Princeton College in 1760 and settled in Gorham in 1767. "He was dismissed from the pastoral office in Gorham in 1779 . . . [and was] thence a Judge of the Court of Common Pleas from 1784 to 1799." Willis, *Journals of the Rev. Thomas Smith and the Rev. Samuel Deane*, 211.

⁵ Thacher died in Gorham on December 25, 1799. Mc Lellan, *History of Gorham, Maine*, 187–89.

different kinds were raised in abundance on burnt land in the **3** interior towns, and the arable lands were very productive; so that bread & meat, particularly pork, were raised in great plenty; as well as vegetables. Many cows were kept by the farmer and large quantities of butter were made, with considerable cheese, which were exchanged in Portland, for such articles as were needed. Among those very little distilled spirit was purchased. Neither was there a single retailor in any of these towns, save one; and there was no distillery in the District of Maine; so that spiritous liquors were very sparingly used. But this state of things, respecting the use of spirits, did not continue for long to be our happy portion; for the Elements of Brown[6] were, in a few years, introduced among us, when distilleries were erected, and retailors placed in many towns, dealing out this liquid fire, in abundant profusion.

Physicians in the County of Cumberland in 1780. D[r] Nathaniel Coffin, whose medical education was compleated in London, who commanded an extensive practice in physic, Surgery and obstetrics, with good success.[7] D[rs] Watts[x] & Louther[x] all of Falmouth, now Portland.[8] D[r] Robert

---

[6] The "Elements of Brown" refers to *The Elements of Medicine; or, a Translation of the Elementa Medicinae Brunonis* by John Brown (1735–1788). At least ten editions were published in the United States between 1790 and 1814, though Barker may well have read a British edition in the late 1780s. Robert B. Austin, *Early American Medical Imprints: 1668–1820* (Arlington, MA: The Printers' Devil, 1961; reprint, 1977). Brown, a student of William Cullen (1712–1790) of Edinburgh, developed a very popular system of medicine called "Brunonism," which maintained that continuous stimuli, with the normal "excitability" of organs, would constitute a state of health. Deviations from the norm were referred to as sthenic if excitation was too strong and asthenic if too weak; sedatives were used in cases of "too much" and stimulants if "too little" excitation. Because alcohol was a major stimulant therapy in Brown's system, Barker's refers to it at this point in the manuscript. Brown influenced Rush, who helped guide Barker's practice, but Rush later rejected treatments using alcohol. Lester S. King, *Transformations in American Medicine: From Benjamin Rush to William Osler* (Baltimore: Johns Hopkins University Press, 1991), 49–52; Lester S. King, *Medical Thinking: A Historical Preface* (Princeton, NJ: Princeton University Press, 1982), 232–33; John H. Talbott, *A Biographical History of Medicine* (New York: Grune & Stratton, 1970), 472–74; and Fielding H. Garrison, *An Introduction to the History of Medicine*, 4th, reprint ed. (Philadelphia: W. B. Saunders, 1929), 314–15.

[7] Dr. Nathaniel Coffin (1744–1826) studied medicine under his father, and at age eighteen traveled to London, where he studied from 1763–1765 at Guy's and St. Thomas's Hospitals under Hunter and others. He began practice at age twenty-one and went on to receive an honorary degree of Doctor of Medicine in 1821 from the College of Brunswick (Bowdoin College). Coffin was the first president of the Medical Society of Maine. James Thacher, *American Medical Biography: Or Memoirs of Eminent Physicians Who Have Flourished in America. To Which Is Prefixed a Succinct History of Medical Science in the United States, from the First Settlement of the Country* (Boston: Richardson & Lord and Cottons & Barnard, 1828), 229–34; Willis, *The History of Portland*, 796–97; Howard A. Kelly and Walter L. Burrage, *American Medical Biographies* (Baltimore: The Norman, Remington Company, 1920), 234–35.

[8] Dr. Edward Watts moved to Falmouth, later Portland, about 1765; his father, Judge Samuel Watts, lived in Boston. Dr. Watts opened an apothecary shop and practiced medicine. He died suddenly in Wells, Maine, on June 9, 1799, while returning from Boston. Willis, *Journals of the*

Southgate of Scarborough,[9] who devoted the former part of his life, to the practice of physic. In the latter part, he was appointed a Judge of the Court. D[rs] Russel[x] and [x]Jones of North Yarmouth.[10] Bridgum of New Gloucester,[11] Goss[x] of Brundswick [*sic*] and Swett[x] of Gorham.[12] In the County of York, D[rs] Porter and Fairfield[x] of Saco, Chaise[x] of Fryburgh.[13] In the County of Lincoln, D[rs] Cony of Augusta, Theobauld[x] of Pownalborough, [blank in manuscript] of Newcastle and Shepherd[x] of Waldoborough [*sic*].[14]

Rev. Thomas Smith and the Rev. Samuel Deane, 351, and Willis, *The History of Portland*, 856. Dr. John Louther or Lowther came to Falmouth Neck (Portland) from Tuxford, county of Nottingham, England, in 1765. He had served seven years in a hospital in England before moving to Portland, where he practiced and "was connected with" an apothecary shop. He died in 1794. Willis, *The History of Portland*, footnote #4, 377–78. [Barker's small superscript [x] may indicate an intention to add a footnote about certain names, as he did in chapter 1 and elsewhere.]

[9] Dr. Robert Southgate, born in Scituate, Massachusetts, in 1741, settled in Scarboro, Maine, in 1771 and practiced there until his retirement in 1796. He then became Judge of Common Pleas for York County until his death in 1833. Spalding, *Maine Physicians of 1820*, 28.

[10] Dr. Edward Russell of Cambridge, Massachusetts, a graduate of Harvard, class of 1759, arrived in North Yarmouth about 1765. Though he had been ordained as a minister, he never accepted a parish and practiced medicine until his death in 1785. William Hutchinson Rowe, *Ancient North Yarmouth and Yarmouth, Maine, 1636–1936* (Yarmouth, ME, Southworth-Anthoensen Press, 1937), 335. Dr. David Jones moved from Abington, Massachusetts, to North Yarmouth (later called Yarmouth) shortly after the Revolutionary War, during which he had served as a naval surgeon. He bought a farm and practiced there until his death in 1822. His widow served as the community dentist for many years. Rowe, *Ancient North Yarmouth and Yarmouth, Maine, 1636–1936*, 335; Spalding, *Maine Physicians of 1820*, 102–103.

[11] Dr. William Bridgham, fourth son of John and Joanna (Comer) Bridgham, was born 1756. The 1790 census shows him living in New Gloucester, Maine, where he resided until his death in 1837. Little, George Thomas, *Genealogical and Family History of the State of Maine* (New York: Lewis Historical Publishing Co., 1909), 1591.

[12] Dr. Ebenezer H. Goss came to Brunswick, Maine, after the Revolution and practiced there until he moved to Paris, Maine, in 1804. George Augustus Wheeler and Henry Warren Wheeler, "History of Brunswick, Topsham, and Harpswell, Maine Including the Ancient Territory Known as Pejepscot," Curtis Memorial Library, see Part II, Chapter 9: "Diseases & Accidents, Freshets," p. 312. Dr. Stephen Swett arrived to practice medicine in Gorham, Maine, in 1770, briefly served in the Revolutionary War, and died in 1807. Mc Lellan, *History of Gorham, Maine*, 281.

[13] Dr. Aaron Porter was born in Boxford, Massachusetts, in 1752, studied medicine under Dr. Thomas Kittredge of Andover, and practiced in Saco, Maine, for almost forty years. He retired to Portland in 1810 and died there in 1837. Spalding, *Maine Physicians of 1820*, 139–40. Dr. Josiah Fairfield came to Pepperrellboro (now Saco) about 1770, practiced for a short time, and relinquished medicine for mercantile business. He died of consumption in 1794, and his epitaph reads, "as a man, a physician, and a magistrate." George Folsom, *History of Saco and Biddeford* (Somersworth Portland: New Hampshire Pub. Co. Maine Historical Society, 1975), 272. Dr. Josiah Chaise (Chase) was born in West Newbury, Massachusetts, in 1741, read medicine with Dr. Enoch Sawyer of Newburyport, and served with General Paleg Wadsworth on the Penobscot Expedition. He moved to Fryeburg, Maine, in 1780 and practiced until his death by drowning in the Saco River in 1796 (personal communication; Fryeburg Historical Society, May 20, 2017).

[14] For Dr. Cony, see Footnote 106 on page 77 of the Introduction. Dr. Ernst Friedrich Philip Theobald, born in Doeringheim, Hesse Cassel, Germany, in 1750, became a physician after

All these physicians have been faithful labourers in the medical field and useful **4** practitioners. But it is to be lamented that many of them have made so few records of extraordinary cases, which occurred in their intensive practice.

Physicians, at this time, in Maine, are numerous, perhaps 200, who are, in general, regularly educated and labouring to promote the cause of medical science. It is sincerely hoped that they will not be negligent in recording cases, which occur in their practice, for their own benefit, as well as that of their successors.

In 1818, a scientific physician in Boston observed to me, that if every physician would record a case, only once a month, for publication, they would make a valuable acquisition to our medical libraries, and tend much to promote the cause of medical science.

The Rev. Thomas Smith was the first settled Minister in Falmouth, now Portland.[15] He was ordained in 1727, over about 40 families. Besides Divinity, he devoted a part of his time to the study of medicine, particularly the works of Dr Cheyne.[16] Being an Invalid from his youth, he paid particular attention to his dietetic rules, which benefited his constitution, and he lived to the age of 94 years, able to preach, till within a few years of his death, which took place in 1795.

---

graduating from the University of Göttingen in 1774. A soldier in the Hessian army, he was captured and after the war moved to Pownalborough, later called Dresden, where he died in 1809. Spalding, *Maine Physicians of 1820*, 167–68. Dr. Shephard is surely Dr Johannes Martin Schaeffer, as that name translates from German, meaning Shephard. He came to Broad Bay (Waldoboro, Maine) circa 1762. Dr. Schaeffer was apparently neither a doctor of theology nor of medicine. There are many stories about him, both as a religious leader and physician. He moved to Warren, Maine, in 1790 and died there in 1794. Jasper Jacob Stahl, *History of Old Broad Bay and Waldoboro*, 2 vols. (Portland, ME: Bond Wheelwright Co., 1956), vol. 1, 334–39.

[15] Rev. Thomas Smith was born in Boston on March 10, 1702, and graduated from Harvard College in 1720. He first visited and preached in Falmouth in 1725, was invited to minister the settlement in 1726, and accepted the offer January 23, 1727. Dr. Barker knew Rev. Smith and, in 1782, "obtained much information, relative to his [Smith's] successful practice." See MSS pp. **4**, **5**, and **18** of this chapter. Smith's diary (1720–88) provided Barker with early Maine medical history otherwise unavailable. Rev. Smith died May 25, 1795. Willis, *Journals of the Rev. Thomas Smith and the Rev. Samuel Deane*, 30.

[16] Dr. George Cheyne (1671–1743) of Aberdeen, Edinburgh, and London struggled with his own obesity, gout, and hypochondriasis. Cheyne's works that may have been studied by Rev. Smith include: George Cheyne, *The English Malady: Or a Treatise of Nervous Diseases of All Kinds* (London: G. Strahan, 1733); George Cheyne, *Observations Concerning the Nature and Due Method of Treating the Gout* (London: G. Strahan, 1720); George Cheyne, *An Essay on Regimen. Together with Five Discourses, Medical, Moral, and Philosophical* (London: C. Rivington, 1740); Talbott, *A Biographical History of Medicine*, 177–79; Steven Shapin, "Trusting George Cheyne: Scientific Expertise, Common Sense, and Moral Authority in Early Eighteenth-Century Dietetic Medicine," *Bulletin of the History Medicine* 77 (2003): 263–97.

His most troublesome complaint in the former part of his life was indigestion, to remedy which he made a liberal use of testaceous powders, and used
friction **5** with a flesh brush. At times he used the cold bath. His breakfast, as he informed me, consisted of chocolate with milk, for more than fifty
years of his life. He generally dined at a late hour on animal food, but ate no
supper. He was a great friend to mercury, ~~which he often prescribed~~ particularly turpeth mineral, which he often prescribed, as an emetic, and sometimes
as a salivating means, with good effects. One case will briefly be related. M^rs^
Johnson, one of his paritioners, lost her three first children by abortion. Her
minister was consulted, as she informed me, who prescribed a mercurial salivation, which she went through. After this, she had four sons and a daughter,
who grew up with vigorous constitutions; and are now, save one who lately
died, useful members of society. Mrs Johnson died in 1815, aged 96 years,
having enjoyed a sound constitution, since her salivation. [See Figure vol.1.2.1]

The diseases which I found most prevalent were Pneumonia, Rheumatism,
slow fevers[17] and consumption.

For more information about Rev. Smith, see Patricia A. Watson, *The Angelical Conjunction: The
Preacher-Physicians of Colonial New England* (Knoxville: The University of Tennessee Press,
1991), 4–5, 149–50. Watson points out that the "intimate relationship between religion and
healing in New England created an environment ideally suited to encourage the minister to
combine prayer with practical medical techniques not unlike those used by the lay practitioners."
She notes that the religious and political instability as well as economic forces encouraged such
practice. Rev. Smith is one of the twenty-nine ministers she studied who entered practice between 1711 and 1730. On November 7, 1748, Smith wrote the following in his diary: "I am
hurried perpetually with the sick; the whole practice rests on me, and God gives me reputation
with satisfaction of mind, as being a successful instrument in his hands." Willis, *Journals of
the Rev. Thomas Smith and the Rev. Samuel Deane*, 134. Whether compassion, socioeconomic
factors, or both led Smith to practice medicine and ministry can only be surmised.

[17] Fever at the end of the eighteenth century generally meant "shivering, a quick pulse, and
heat," and of the three, rapid pulse was the most important characteristic. Lester S. King, *The
Medical World of the Eighteenth Century* (Huntington, NY: Robert E. Krieger Publishing
Co. Inc., 1958; reprint 1971), 125–28. Fever is the topic of Cullen's first 106 pages. William
Cullen, *First Lines of the Practice of Physic with Supplementary Notes, Including More Recent
Improvements in the Practice of Medicine by Peter Reid*, two volumes in one (Brookfield: E.
Mirriam & Co. for Isaiah Thomas, 1807). Slow fever appears in Coxe's 1817 medical dic-
tionary as "febris lenta" without further definition. John Redman Coxe, *The Philadelphia
Medical Dictionary*, 2nd ed. (Philadelphia: Thomas Dobson, 1817), 211. Slow fever may refer
to what, in the twentieth century, "seems to be what we call typhoid fever," but Huxham
mentions only that the pulse "is quick, weak and unequal, sometimes for a few minutes slow,
nay intermitting." John Huxham, *An Essay on Fevers with Introduction by Saul Jarcho* (Canton,
MA: Science History Publications [reprint 1988], 1757), xiv, 40–49; H. F. Harris, "Slow Fever,"
Journal of the American Medical Association 49 (1907), 406–411; John Duffy, *Epidemics in
Colonial America* (Baton Rouge: Louisiana State University Press, 1953), 222–23. An excellent discussion of the complicated language of fevers is found in Christopher Hamlin, *More

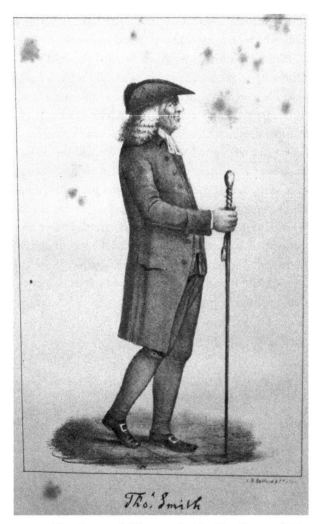

FIGURE VOL.I.2.I. The Reverend Thomas Smith. The Reverend Thomas Smith, Minister of the First Parish Church of Portland, Maine. Image from Willis, William. *Journals of the Rev. Thomas Smith and the Rev. Samuel Deane, . . . With Notes and Biographical Notices and a Summary History of Portland.* Portland: Joseph S. Bailey, 1849.

In succeeding years, inebriation, Insanity, palsy, apoplexy, dropsy, Jaundice, erisepilas and cancers, enlarged the list. The Quinsy & rickets were of frequent occurrence among children, and epidemical distempers, at times, invaded all classes of people.

In the treatment of these diseases, such practical observations as have been made, and obtained from others, will be detailed, **6** in the hope that some light may be thrown on their causes and nature.

They will be related, in some order of time according to their occurrence, excepting consumptive cases, which will be reserved for the concluding part.

We cannot learn from the records of physicians or others, that any epidemical disease had occurred in the District of Maine, since its first settlement, which was only about the beginning of the eighteenth century, until 1735, when, according to the records of the Rev. Thomas Smith of Falmouth, the throat distemper appeared in the western part of the County of York, and progressed eastward.[18]

October 31ᵗ a fast was held, on account of the sickness, which broke out at Kingston N. Hampshire, and had got as far as Cape Porpoise, carrying off a great many children; as well as young persons, and alarming the whole country.

This epidemical distemper appeared in May, in Kingston, and spread gradually through that township, during the summer. Of the first 40 who had the disease, none recovered. In August, it began to make its appearance at Exeter [New Hampshire], and in September in Boston. It continued its ravages through the succeeding winter & spring; and did not disappear until the end of the next summer.

In the Province of New Hampshire, not less than one thousand persons of whom nine hundred were **7** under twenty years of age, fell victims to this malignant distemper. In Boston 4000 persons had the same disease; and one hundred & fourteen died. In Haverhill, Massᵗᵗˢ there died of the same disease, from Nov. 17ᵗʰ 1735, to October 6ᵗʰ 1737, 199 persons. This disease gradually spread westward, and was two years in reaching the river Hudson, about 200 miles, in a straight line from Kingston. It continued its progress, with some interruption, until it spread over all the colonies.[19]

In the summer of 1736, the measles was prevalent in Falmouth.

Than Hot: A Short History of Fever, Johns Hopkins Biographies of Disease (Baltimore: Johns Hopkins University Press, 2014), 23–53.

[18] For details of this epidemic, see Ernest Caulfield, *A True History of the Terrible Epidemic Vulgarly Called the Throat Distemper, Which Occurred in His Majesty's New England Colonies between the Years 1735 and 1740* (New Haven: Yale Journal of Biology & Medicine for the Beaumont Medical Club, 1939), 25–27, for comments on Maine; Duffy, *Epidemics in Colonial America*, 113–22 and, for consideration of diphtheria and scarlet fever, 13–37. On page 114, Duffy points out that the eighteenth-century physician, when confronted with a serious sore throat and associated symptoms including diphtheria and scarlet fever, had numerous names for it: "throat disease, throat distemper, throat ail, canker ail, malignant quinsies, putrid, malignant, or pestilential sore throat, cynache trachealis, angina suffocative, and malignant angina."

[19] Extracts from the Journals of the Rev. Thomas Smith, in Willis, *Journals of the Rev. Thomas Smith and the Rev. Samuel Deane*, 82–83. Entries from the Smith Diary are accurately paraphrased in Barker's manuscript.

In Autumn, the slow fever & throat distemper were of frequent occurrence; but not mortal.

In Jan. 1737 the throat distemper broke out a fresh, and proved mortal in York & Wells. The disease also appeared in several places in Falmouth. Three children died.

In March, the distemper, which seemed to be gone, broke out again in several houses.

In May, the distemper was mortal in North Yarmouth. Seventy five died in that town. Forty nine in Falmouth, and twenty six in Cape Elizabeth.

In September the distemper appeared in Scarborough. 2 or 3 children died.

In October the distemper continued bad in Scarborough. Not one has lived, that has had it of late!

Nov. three children died in Falmouth, and the Pleurisy fever, which prevails, has proved mortal in North Yarmouth. All that have had this fever died, save one.

Decr. the throat distemper is mortal in Cape Elizabeth. One Mourton buried 3 out of 4.

1738 April, the Canker distemper is at N. Yarmouth. **8** The disease also appeared in Milton, Woburn and Cape Ann.

August the throat distemper prevails in Falmouth, at the falls, and proves universally mortal.

Nov. The disease is still exceeding bad at Saco.

From 1722 to 1734 nothing extraordinary is recorded relative to the weather. The winter months were generally very cold, and the snow was about 3 or 4 feet deep on a level, seldom disappearing till April. In Jan. Feb. & March 1734, the weather was generally pleasant. April the 4, as hot a day as the generality of summer. June, vegetation very rapid. July; we hear that people die, at Boston, of the excessive heat.

1735, Jan. Though cold at times, there has been much pleasant & moderate weather this month.

Feb. 28. This has been a summer month, only 2 or 3 cold days. April 17. Quite hot. 21. same.

August 11. There has been an abundance of rain.

1736. Feb. a close cold winter. April 10, a hot day. July, grashoppers plenty. Sept. very dry.

1737. Jan. The ground frozen 4 feet deep. April 25. no grass at all. May 2. many cattle have died. July. grashoppers plenty. October It was never known to be so dry. Decr 18. no northwesters as yet.

1738. Jan. The month comes in warm, like the beginning of April. 23^d Two things are remarkable, relative to the wind, for several months past. One is, that the wind always comes about with the sun. The other, that after foul weather, the wind comes as far as S. W. and except once or twice no further. April 14, unusually hot weather. May 24. Abundance of rain. July grashoppers. The drought came on very severely and prevailed in such a manner, as the like was never known.

9

1739. April 30. No rain for about a month past, except a small shower. August 31. We have had more hot weather there four days past than all the summer together. Sept. 17 a severe white frost, which killed the tops of potatoes. Oct. 3. The cold weather prevails as far as Boston. A very healthy year.

1740. Jan. 25th we have had a close week with our children, all having the quinsy; as well as others of us. It seems to be going through the country. The weather in Jan. generally fair & pleasant. Feb. 18. A summer winter. We had only two snows, and sledding but three weeks. 27. Warm southerly weather. March 3. A summer day. 10. the same 18. warm. April 23. Exceeding hot. August 10. An uncommon season of hot weather this summer.

1741. 1742. 1743. & 1744. No diseases recorded, except in Dec^r, 1744, mention is made of its being a sickly dying time, at North Yarmouth with the slow fever.

1745. October. It is generally a very sickly and dying time through the country, with the usual nervous or slow fever.

Dec. 19. Several children have died of the quinsy and throat distemper.

In these five years, the snow is said to be 4 feet deep in March, save the two last.

1746. 1747. No diseases mentioned.

1748. August. I don't know whither I was ever so hurried in the ministry, so constantly praying with the sick and at funerals. There is an asthmatic quincy[20] prevailing among the children, that proves dreadfully mortal. Nine

---

[20] Quinsy, quincy, and other spellings: see Glossary entry. Here it refers to inflammatory sore throat, tonsillitis. (In the twentieth century, quinsy commonly means peritonsillar abscess.) See Calvin Jones, *A Treatise on the Scarlatina Anginosa: Or What Is Vulgarly Called the Scarlet Fever, or Canker-Rash. Replete with Every Thing Necessary to the Pathology and Practice, Deduced from Actual Experience and Observation* (Catskill, NY: M. Crosswell & Co, 1794); James Thacher, *American Modern Practice* (Boston: Ezra Read, 1817), 397–99. The term "asthmatic" refers here to difficulty breathing, generally with wheezing.

10 children have died lately at N. Yarmouth with the canker ail.[21] I am hurried perpetually with the sick. The whole practice rests on me, and God gives me reputation and satisfaction of mind, as being a successful instrument in his hands.

In March there was five feet of snow on the ground.

May. 15th unusually hot & dry. 31st All the talk is about the heat & drought, never the like. June. Exceeding rain & cold. 14th An epidemic cold prevails. July, the grass is all burnt up. 19th rain. August, very dry & hot. Oct. no moisture in the ground.

1749. No diseases recorded.

1750. October, an epidemical fever in Gorham as also in Falmouth, spreading over the parish.

1751, April. A melancholly time, on account of the epidemic fever. July, a time of health.

1752. Jan. remarkably cold; snow very deep. A pleuritic fever prevails at Biddeford, and proves very mortal. Also in Wells.

1753. April, an epidemic rash prevails, not mortal.

1754. Jan. The throat distemper in Falmouth; several died.

1755. Nov. Eight children and one adult died of the throat distemper in New Casco. 17th, at a quarter past 4 in the night, there was a most amazing shock of an earthquake. Several shocks followed, in the course of a week.[22]

1756, September. It is a sickly time generally through the country. At Saco, the throat distemper has killed 14 children. At Dunston[23] they have the fever & ague; and at Scarborough, N. Yarmouth & Falmouth, the slow fever and dysentery.

---

[21] "Ail" is a general term for sickness or disease, from the Saxon. Dunglison, *A Dictionary of Medical Science* (Philadelphia: Henry C. Lea, 1874); Canker ail probably refers to scarlatina anginosa or scarlet fever. Thacher, *American Modern Practice*, 400–408.

[22] Webster records the following: "On the 18th of November [1755], America sustained a violent and extensive shock; but its effects were not very calamitous. The fish in the ocean did not escape without injury. Two or three whales, and multitudes of cod were seen, a few days after, floating on the surface of the water." Noah Webster, *A Brief History of Epidemic and Pestilential Diseases with the Principal Phenomena of the Physical World Which Precede and Accompany Them and Observations Deduced from Facts Stated*, 2 vols. (Hartford: Hudson and Goodwin, 1799), vol I, 245.

[23] Dunston or Dunstan once referred to a tract between the Scarboro and Nonsuch Rivers near Portland named for Dunster, England, the former home of some of the early settlers. Phillip R. Rutherford, *The Dictionary of Maine Place-Names* (Freeport, ME: Bond, Wheelwright Co, 1971), 38.

July; We are visited with worms, which have destroyed whole fields of English & Indian corn in divers places. A wet summer, and very hot. **11**

1757. General health till Dec[r] when an epidemic cough prevailed. A cold, wet ~~summer~~ spring. Dec[r] very cold.

1758. Sept[r]. The epidemic cough we had all the last winter, now again prevails in every house, particularly among children. Oct[r] hundreds of children are sick with the cough & fever in the parish. A cold wet summer.

1759. Jan. The measles is spreading through the towns, in this part of the country. March, several died.

1760. Sept. It is as sickly a time in Boston, as has been known. Sickly here also.

1761. March 12th. An astonishing earthquake in all the New England Colonies. 31st A sickly dying time.[24]

From 1762 to 1773. No mention is made of any diseases save a cancer in the lip which proved fatal, after going through a mercurial salivation.

1773. Jan. The measles is now spreading here. Sept. There is an epidemical vomiting & purging with fever, among the children & others, attended with a considerable degree of mortality.

From 1773 to 1776. No diseases are recorded.

1776. March. The peripneumony is prevalent Falmouth and very mortal.

April. The epidemic sickness is everywhere through the country, a proper pestilence.

From 1776 to 1780. No diseases are mentioned, except that the dysentery was prevalent at the westward, and very mortal, not leaving a child three years old in Mystic!

See Extracts from the Journals kept by the Rev. Thomas Smith. By Samuel Freeman Esq.[25]

---

[24] Noah Webster writes, in "1761, in America; an earthquake during its [influenza's] prevalence." See Webster, *A Brief History of Epidemic and Pestilential Diseases (Hartford, 1799)*, vol. 2, 32. Influenza: see Glossary entry. In the eighteenth century it referred to contagious epidemic catarrh, but the term itself refers to the influence of the stars and naturally occurring phenomena such as earthquakes.

[25] Samuel Freeman, *Extracts from the Journals Kept by the Reverend Thos Smith from the Year 1720 to the Year 1788, with an Appendix Containing a Variety of Other Matter Selected by Samuel Freeman* (Portland: T. Todd & Co., 1821). See MHS Collection 684. William Willis later published these journals: see Willis, *Journals of the Rev. Thomas Smith and the Rev. Samuel Deane.*

12

"The cyanche maligna, putrid sore throat, or throat distemper,[26] as it has been called, says Dr Warren, made its appearance at Boston, in September, 1735, after a very cold and wet summer. It commenced in the May preceeding at Kingston, New Hampshire, an inland town, situated on a low sandy plain.

The first person seized with it was a child, who died in three days. About a week after, three children, in one family, at the distance of four miles from the first, were successively attacked, and died on the third day. It continued spreading in that town, and gradually made its way, in the course of the summer & following winter to Boston, and many of the neighboring towns, and did not cease till the end of the next summer. The whole of its extent was from Maine to Carolina. The subjects were usually children.

The attending symptoms were a pain in the head & back, soreness of the throat, and swelling in the glands of the neck; pulse frequent, but small & soft; the tonsils somewhat inflamed at first, the velum pendulum palati & uvula in the same condition, with whitish or ash coloured spots on their surfaces. Dr Holyoke [Salem, Massachusetts] informs me, that, when it did not prove fatal, on the second or third day, which it frequently did, it was almost universally attended with great erosion & excoriation about the fauces, inside of the mouth, lips & chin, and wherever the saliva was lodged; and that these parts became covered with a white apthous [*sic*] slough, painful & corrosive. Even the extremities of the fingers, when they were besmeared with the saliva, were corroded. A sister of the Doctor, twelve months old, as he well remembers, lost the nails of the fingers from the acid quality of the matter.

---

[26] This represents a long excerpt, "Section III, Throat Distemper," from John Warren, *View of the Mercurial Practice in Febrile Diseases* (Boston: T. D. Wait & Co., 1813). Warren begins with the 1735 epidemic of throat distemper, as earlier described in Rev. Smith's diary. Warren (1753–1815), after receiving an A.B. from Harvard College in 1771, studied under his brother, Dr. Joseph Warren. John Warren was influential in founding Harvard Medical School and became its first professor of anatomy and surgery in 1782. See Kelly and Burrage, *American Medical Biographies*, 1193–96; Talbott, *A Biographical History of Medicine*, 381–83. Dr. Jeremiah Barker and Dr. John Warren had similar medical training, an American preceptorship, though Warren also had a college degree. Dr. Bela Lincoln, Barker's teacher, was a student of the same Dr. Ezekiel Hersey who endowed the Hersey Professorship of Anatomy and Surgery at Harvard in 1791; John Warren was the first person to hold that chair. Cynache maligna or gangrenosa is defined in 1817 as "the malignant quincy" and in 1874 to include diphtheritic and gangrenous pharyngitis. "Cynache" comes from the Greek, "I choke," and "quincy" is an abbreviation of the French "squinancie" which is derived from the Greek for "dog throttling," all meaning bad sore throat. See Coxe, *The Philadelphia Medical Dictionary*; Robley Dunglison, *A Dictionary of Medical Science* (Philadelphia: Henry C. Lea, 1874); and Henry Alan Skinner, *The Origin of Medical Terms*, 2nd ed. (Baltimore: The Williams & Wilkins Company, 1961), 347.

13

In these cases, calomel,[27] given frequently & liberally, and young children, he observed, for the most part, bear it remarkably well, was the only medicine which could be depended upon to stop the progress of the erosion.

A remark, offered by the Doctor, that the cynanche has of late years, ~~has~~ appeared in a form somewhat different, in which the debility is too great to admit of a free use of mercury, is exactly correspondent with my own observation on the disease, as it appeared here a few years past.

But it is further observed, when the angina is extreme, unless the prostration of strength is very great, an emetic of turpeth mineral, given at, or soon after the attack, is frequently attended with the happiest effect, the stomach, fauces, & breast, being greatly relieved by the dislodgement of vast quantities of viscid phlegm. All copious evacuations were generally hurtful, especially bleeding.

That the disease in 1735, was not contagious, was the opinion of the physicians of that day. It had been supposed, on its first appearance in Boston, to be nothing more than a cold; but when its mortality in New Hampshire was known, it spread the utmost degree of terror through the town and vicinity.

The house, in which the first person was seized, was shut up; but it was soon discovered, that the persons particularly exposed, escaped infection, whilst others at a distance, in every quarter, who had no communication with the sick, did not take it; and in no instance was it conveyed by the clothes, to the families of those who had visited them; but was supposed to proceed from an impure atmosphere.

The number of those, who had the distemper in Boston, was four thousand, of whom, one hundred & fourteen died, which is one in thirty five. The whole number of inhabitants was, at that time, estimated at sixteen thousand. In the whole state, about one thousand persons fell victims to this disease.

14

In 1754 & 55, it again made its appearance in some parts of Massachusetts & New Hampshire.

In 1784, this disease also spread through most of the towns in New England. Since which, it has never been generally prevalent, in any considerable part of this State. Sporadic cases have indeed frequently been seen in

---

[27] Calomel: see Glossary entry. For the use of mercury in fevers in general, see Thacher, *American Modern Practice*, 284–88.

Boston; but, though sometimes extremely malignant, they have never become general.

In January 1802, some instances of extreme virulence occurred, and began to produce an alarm in the town; but, a more specific epidemic, the measles, having made their appearance, the latter end of January, the inhabitants were happily relieved from their anxiety, and the throat distemper was overpowered & subdued by this welcome substitute.

The first appearance of this disease was about the latter end of December 1801. The symptoms at first, were remarkable paleness, extreme weakness, pain in the limbs, slight soreness of the throat, a white tongue. On examining the fauces, in this stage, the tonsils were not remarkably inflamed or tumefied; not so much as in a common sore throat from cold. On the second day, an efflorescence usually commenced on the arms, neck & breast, which gradually extended over the whole surface without affording any relief. In some cases, the respiration was laborious. One case assumed the form of a common cynanche tonsillaris, the breathing having been, from the beginning, of that hoarse stridulous kind, which often attends the most threatening species of this disease. The glands of the neck were much swollen. On the third or fourth day, the efflorescence, in the more violent cases, assumed a deeper shade of red, bordering on purple; and in proportion to the cutaneous eruption, was the danger of the disease.

At this period, an aphthous coating[28] was discovered **15** on the velum of the palate, and on the tonsils. Gangrenous sloughs were cast off from these parts; so that the action of swallowing was much interrupted. A regurgitation through the nose ensued, on attempting to swallow. On the fifth day, the patient usually either died, or shows marks of amendment. In one case, however, the disease was protracted to the third week, and proved fatal at last.

In one instance, the first stage had passed over, before any apprehension of danger had been exited; and within twenty-four hours from the seizure, the extremities became cold, the pulse sunk, and was intermittent; and petechial spots made their appearance over the whole body; and without much complaint in the throat. The patient died within sixty hours of the attack. Another case assumed nearly the same form; tho in a less violent degree, and terminated in the same manner, on the fifth day.

The prostration of strength was so remarkable, from the beginning, the pulse so extremely frequent and small, and the tendency to putrefaction so

---

[28] See Glossary entry for "aphthae"; ulcerations in the throat.

obvious, that it was judged necessary to commence immediately with tonic & antisceptic [*sic*] medicines. Sometimes, however, cleansing the stomach & fauces with an emetic of ipecac. Bark & wine were then prescribed in as large quantities as could be taken, with elixir vitriol diluted with water; and in case of aphthae or erosions of the tonsils & uvula, great advantage was derived from diluted muriatic acid, applied with a small mop or sponge, to the parts afflicted.

For the swellings of the parotid glands, nothing was so efficacious as the application of cold water, or vinegar and water, by cloths kept constantly wet with these fluids. The drinking of cold water was in some instances, attended with the happiest effect. One patient, recovered from the most desperate state of the disease, by drinking in the course of two or three days, several pails full, discharging most of it immediately from the stomach.

16

Blisters were sometimes used to the neck, and behind the ears; but never, so far as I could discover, with any advantage; on the contrary, by preventing or rendering inconvenient the application of cold water, they were decidedly injurious.[29] The subjects were chiefly children, and adult females of weak & slender constitutions. It was remarkable that the most malignant instances, were those of two young ladies, who died at an early period of the disease.

Mercury was not used in this disease for the purpose of affecting the glands, or of acting on the system at large; but only in doses of three or four grains, combined with some auxiliary article, as a mild cathartic.

---

[29] As Barker was writing his manuscript and John Warren, his journal article, there were major changes in theory and practice of medicine. A number of "systems" of medicine were based on theoretical concepts that had developed over the centuries, some employing the same treatments but with differing rationales. One system for example, considered disease an excess of excitement that could be drained off by cathartics such as calomel, emetics, counterirritants (blisters), or bleeding. Blisters could be raised by applying cantharides or Spanish fly to the skin, producing painful vesicles. Physicians "exhibited a drug"; that is, the drug had to have a physiological effect on the patient, or physician and patient would assume the medicine didn't work. If, after cantharides was applied and a blister formed, or calomel (mercury) given and salivation occurred, and the patient improved, the drug had worked. If the patient got better without such a physical manifestation, however, the patient and doctor would assume that the drug was not responsible for the improvement. See Charles E. Rosenberg, *Explaining Epidemics and Other Studies in the History of Medicine* (New York: Cambridge University Press, 1992), 9–31; John Harley Warner, *The Therapeutic Perspective: Medical Practice, Knowledge, and Identity in America, 1820–85* (Cambridge, MA: Harvard University Press, 1986), 83–161. This therapeutic behavior was beginning to change in the period from 1800 to 1830. But at the Massachusetts General Hospital in the 1820s, 46.3 percent of patients were still being blistered and 57.1 percent were given calomel. See Warner, *The Therapeutic Perspective*, Table 1 on p. 117.

The prevalence of what was called a putrid diathesis, and the marks of debility so predominant in the progress of the disease, prevented practitioners from using this medicine, notwithstanding the advantages that had attended it in most of the former periods of its prevalence in the New England States.

In 1773, mercury had been generally supposed serviceable; but the character of the disease, at that time, appeared to be different. The use of mercury in putrid diathesis was at least hypothetical; and indeed, strong prepossessions were entertained against it. At that time, an emetic or a cathartic, if it operated briskly, was sure to be followed by prostration of strength, and aggravation of symptoms.[30]

D^r. W. Bailies observes that in the ulcerated sore throat, which prevailed at Dighton in 1785 & 6, mercurials were not found to be attended with **17** the same advantage as when it appeared there fourteen years before.

Communication to M. M. S.[31]

D^r. Rush used calomel in small doses, in all stages of scarlatina anginosa, which appeared at Philadelphia, in 1783 & 4. Sometimes he added a few grains of calomel to his gargles.[32]

This disease had some appearance of being contagious. Whenever it attacked an individual of a family, most of the children, and some of the adults were, within about six or seven days, seized with the same distemper, unless immediately removed from the atmosphere of the sick. In every instance,

---

[30] Here Warren seems to be questioning the use of mercurials or at least expresses less enthusiasm than others from earlier times. Mercurials were still being used quite extensively by many experienced, well-educated regular physicians, though questioned by some.

[31] William Baylies (Bailies) (1743–1826) graduated from Harvard College in 1760 and then studied medicine under Dr. Elisha Toby of New Bedford. Practicing in Dighton, Massachusetts, Baylies was one of the original members of the M.M.S. He published "An Account of the Ulcerated Sore Throat as It Appeared in the Town of Dighton in the Years 1785 and 1786." *Massachusetts Medical Society Papers* 1 (1790), 41–48, and reprinted in the M.M.S. "Medical Communications" 1 (1808). See Kelly and Burrage, *American Medical Biographies*, 77–78, and Clifford Shipton, *Biographical Sketches of Those Who Attended Harvard College; Sibley's Harvard Graduates, Vol. 14: 1756–1760* (Boston: Massachusetts Historical Society, 1968), 552–55.

[32] Scarlatina anginosa: see Glossary entry. Rush's "An Account of the Scarlatina anginosa as it appeared in Philadelphia in the years 1783–4" is found in Benjamin Rush, *Medical Inquiries and Observations*, 2nd ed., 4 vols. (Philadelphia: J. Conrad & Co., 1805), vol. 1, 137–65. On pages 144–45 Rush states, "[in] every case that I was called to, I began the cure by giving a vomit joined with calomel. . . . I gave the calomel in every stage of the disease." His treatment of scarlatina anginosa, which yielded to "copious blood-letting, and other depleting remedies," did not change between 1793 and 1800. See "Additional Observations upon the Scarlatina anginosa" in Benjamin Rush, *Medical Inquiries and Observations*, 4th ed., 4 vols. (Philadelphia: Johnson & Warner, 1815), vol. 2, 249–51 (the page numbers in this edition are actually printed as 245–47 but should be 249–51 to be consistent with the chapter preceding and following "Additional Observations."

where this was complied with, the infection was evaded. In my own family, the distemper was discovered in one of my children; and having been a witness to the horrors attendant on its footsteps in the family of a friend, and apprized of the apparent activity of the contagion, I immediately separated the rest of the family, by a removal into the country, and they avoided the disease.

The marks of this distemper, by which it was distinguished from inflammatory sore throat, were the following.

The subjects of the first were generally infirm persons, especially females; of the latter, the healthy and athletic.

The former disease, I believe, originated from contagion; the latter is known to arise from cold and is sporadic.

18

The former was a constitutional distemper, attended with vomiting or purging, acute pain in the back of the head, erysipelatous redness of the fauces, and a scarlet eruption on the skin, with quick and weak pulse; the latter was chiefly local or confined to the throat with full and hard pulse, and symptomatic fever.

The former became ulcerous, with sloughs of a cineritious colour; the latter frequently terminated in suppuration."

View of the mercurial practice. 1813.[33]

"I remember to have heard a little anecdote, says D[r]. Holyoke of Salem, Mass[tts] which may be worth relating — A practitioner, in a neighboring town, of great repute & extensive practice, being called to attend a young woman dangerously ill of the throat distemper, in 1735, having ordered her, among other things, four or five grains of calomel, was astonished the next day, to find her relieved, greatly beyond his expectations. On enquiring of his pupil, to whom he had given his directions, whether his prescription had been followed, he found that his patient had taken thirty grains of calomel; to which mistake he attributed the cure. From this time forward, in every dangerous case, he used this medicine in much larger doses than before."

Med. Repos. vol. 1.[34]

---

33 Warren, *View of the Mercurial Practice in Febrile Diseases*, 137–45.

34 Edward Augustus Holyoke, "'A Letter to Dr. —; in Answer to His Quiries Respecting the Introduction of the Mercurial Practice in the Vicinity of Boston, Mass.' Salem, Mass, Dec. 1797.," *Medical Repository* 1, no. 4 (1798): 500–503. Dr. Holyoke (1728–1829), whose father, also Edward Holyoke, had been President of Harvard College from 1737 to 1769, graduated from Harvard College in 1746. He began his medical practice in Salem in 1749, and was the first president of the M.M.S. from 1782–1784. Burrage, *A History of the Massachusetts Medical Society*, 15, 37–40; Kelly and Burrage, *American Medical Biographies*, 547–48.

In January 1740, when the quinsy, was prevalent in Maine, all the Rev. Thomas Smith's children, six in number, ages from nearly nine to one year, and some adults, were attacked with this disease. They all recovered; and turpeth mineral was the chief means employed; as an emetic & alterative.

In 1748, when "an asthmatic quinsy, and canker ail, were prevalent, and dreadfully mortal, among children," he speaks, in his Journal, of being "a successful instrument, in the hands of God, in curing these diseases." Turpeth mineral was liberally used and found to be highly efficacious.

In 1782, I was consulted by him, in case of sickness, and obtained much information, relative to his successful practice, in these and other inflammatory diseases, by the use of turpeth mineral.

Chap 3.ᵈ

FROM 1780, TO 1784, no extraordinary diseases appeared in the District of Maine, as far as my observations extended, neither was there any thing uncommon in the weather or seasons.[1]

In Feb. 1784, the Measles was prevalent in Maine.

In the spring of 1784, some unusual appearances took place in the wounds & bruises, even trivial ones, which baffled the skill of the Surgeon, and issued in the death of the patient.

In April, I was called to Capt. Graffam of Windham,[2] aged 60, of a good habit, who broke the skin of his leg over the tibia. The wound readily inflamed and was attended with great pain. Febrile disturbance took place, with a swelling of the leg, and, in about one week, it put on a gangrenous hue. The wound turned black, and red streaks extended up the thigh to the body. He died in 14 days.

Several other very similar cases occurred in my practice, where slight wounds soon became gangrenous, and terminated fatally, under the common mode of treatments, viz. discutient poultices, spiritous fomentations & astringent lotions of a decoction of the bark, with preparation of lead, and covering the wounds with Turner's cerate.[3]

---

[1] Barker moved from Barnstable, Massachusetts, to the District of Maine in 1780.

[2] Capt. Caleb Graffam, born in Scarborough, Maine, in 1711 or 1713, cleared nine acres and built a garrison house on lot No. 61 in New Marblehead, now Windham, Maine, in 1749 and was a garrison soldier there in 1757. When the town was incorporated in 1762, Caleb was elected first selectman and later town moderator. His gravestone in the Smith Cemetery in South Windham indicates that he died in November 1784. There are numerous sources with conflicting dates. Thomas Laurens Smith, *History of the Town of Windham* (Portland ME: Hoyt & Fogg, 1873).

[3] Turner's Cerate: see Glossary entry. Daniel Turner (1667–1741) was a British surgeon and physician who wrote many books, including *De morbis cutaneus: A Treatise of Diseases Incident to the Skin*, 1714, possibly the first book in English devoted to diseases of the skin. H. C. G. Matthew and Brian Harrison, *Oxford Dictionary of National Biography: In Association with the British Academy: From the Earliest Times to the Year 2000*, new ed. (Oxford: Oxford University Press, 2004); Andrew Duncan, *The Edinburgh New Dispensatory*, 1st Worcester ed. (Worcester: Press of Isaiah Thomas, 1805), 648–49.

Besides, gentle emetics and cathartics were given, on account of the attending fever; and these were generally followed with a decoction of the bark, and wine, as soon as the febrile disturbance began to subside, when the fever was supposed to assume a putrid form. Very few recovered.

20

Soon after, I was called in consultation to a patient of Dr Watts who had suffered a simple fracture of the leg, with a bruise on the skin. Altho treated according to rule, in a few days inflammation and gangrene took place. The leg swelled and was beset with watery blisters which discharged an ichorous matter. The swelling soon extended to the body and life was extinguished.

Local inflammation chiefly from injuries were more frequent and intractable during the year than I ever knew them to be before or since. The subjects of these complaints were chiefly males and apparently of good constitutions.[4]

How extensive these morbid affections were I could not learn, but was informed that they occurred in different parts of the country.

In the spring of 1784, several women were attacked with fever in the puerperal state, even after favourable travails; and, in most all, the disease proved fatal, at least in my own practice.[5]

---

[4] After two pages describing men dying in 1784 with fever and inflammation resulting from trivial wounds or bruises, Barker continued with twenty pages on an epidemic, beginning in the spring of 1784, of "women attended with fever in the puerperal state." He had never seen an epidemic of fever and death in the puerperal state before or after 1784. He read books and articles on the subject and then wrote, "The ill success which attended my practice induced me to write to several aged & experienced physicians in different portions of Mass. for advice as puerperal fever had never appeared among us, excepting in a few sporadic cases." See mss **21** Exacerbations of virulent Group A Streptococcal puerperal sepsis have occurred through the years, and one can hypothesize that in 1784, a virulent Streptococcus affecting men and women visited Maine. See L. Nathan and K. J. Leveno, "Group A Streptococcal Puerperal Sepsis: Historical Review and 1990s Resurgence," *Infectious Diseases in Obstetetrics and Gynecology* 1, no. 5 (1994), 252–55. This article also makes reference to books by Leake and Gordon cited by Barker.

[5] Drs. Jeremiah Barker of Gorham and Nathaniel Coffin of Portland carried on a public argument over the prevention and cure of puerperal fever. Their letters, beginning with Barker's, were published in alternate issues of the *Falmouth Gazette*, February 12, 19, and 26, and March 5 and 12, 1785. The *Falmouth Gazette*, the first newspaper printed in the District of Maine, began publication January 1, 1785. See Ronald Banks, *Maine Becomes a State* (Middletown, CT: Wesleyan University Press, 1970), 13. For further discussion of this controversy, see the Introduction, chapter 2. See also Laurel Thatcher Ulrich, "'The Living Mother of a Living Child': Midwifery and Mortality in Post-Revolutionary New England," *The William and Mary Quarterly* 46, no. 1 (1989): 27–49, with the Barker/Coffin controversy discussed 40–45. Though there was some animosity in 1784 and 1785, Coffin and Barker together signed a request to the Massachusetts Medical Society dated June 30, 1804 requesting the formation of

Soon after, I was called in consultation to a patient
of Dr Watts' who had suffered a simple fracture
of the leg, with a bruise on the skin. Altho treated
according to rule, in a few days, inflammation and
gangrene took place. The leg swelled and was beset
with watery blisters which discharged an ichorous
matter. The swelling soon extended to the body and
life was extinguished.

Local inflammations chiefly from injuries were
more frequent and untractable during the year
than I ever knew them to be before or since. The
subjects of these complaints were chiefly males and
apparently of good constitutions.

How extensive these morbid affections were I could
not learn; but was informed that they occurred in
different parts of the country.

In the spring of 1784, several women were attacked
with fever in the puerperal state, even after favourable travails; and, in most all, the disease proved
fatal, at least in my own practice.

The fever commenced with rigor, on the 2' or 3' day
after delivery, followed by heat, pain, tension and
soreness of the abdomen on pressure, together with
thirst, pain in the head, a flushing in the face and
sometimes delirium, with a hot & dry skin and
great anxiety of the precordia. pulse frequent,
small and sometimes tense, with a shortness of breathing, high coloured urine, a change of the quality of
the lochia, and, sometimes suppression with tenesmus.
In some the fever was ushered in with a vomiting
of matter resembling what is ejected in cholera.
When the fever had continued about one week,
the inflammatory symptoms subsided, and the disease put on what was called a putrid form, and

FIGURE VOL.I.3.I. **Page of Barker manuscript beginning discussion of childbed fever.** An example of a page of the Barker manuscript, Volume One, Chapter 3, p. 20, in which he begins a discussion of the 1784–1785 epidemic infections that included childbed fever and various other severe infections.

The fever commenced with rigor, on the 2^d or 3^d day after delivery, followed by heat, pain, tension and soreness of the abdomen on pressure, together with thirst, pain in the head, a flushing in the face, and sometimes deliriums, with a hot & dry skin and great anxiety of the precordia; pulse frequent, small and sometimes tense, with a shortness of breathing, high coloured urine, a change of the quality of the lochia, and, sometimes, suppression with tenesmus. In some the fever was ushered in with a vomiting of matter resembling what is ejected in cholera.[6] When the fever had continued about one week, the inflammatory symptoms subsided, and the disease put on what was called a putrid form; and **21** a bilious diarrhœa supervened, with great exhaustion. At length the stools became involuntary, often black, and death soon closed the scene.

In the summer the disease became more malignant, and was truly alarming, for few women escaped a greater or lesser degree of the distemper, and it might with propriety be called an epidemic fever, which continued to prevail in many parts of the country throughout the year, with a considerable degree of mortality.[7]

My practice extended into several towns northerly to the distance of thirty miles; so that I had many opportunities of making observations.

District of Maine Medical Society to be part of the Massachusetts Medical Society. Nathaniel Coffin, Jeremiah Barker, Shirley Ervin, Dudley Folsom, Stephen Thomas, Aaron Kinsman, "Letter to the the Massachusetts Medical-Society Requesting Permission to Allow a District of Maine Medical Society," in *Coffin, Nathaniel*, Countway Library Harvard (Portland, Maine, 1804), B MS c75.2.

[6] In 1785 "cholera" was defined as "an excessive vomiting and purging." John Redman Coxe, *The Philadelphia Medical Dictionary*, 2nd ed. (Philadelphia: Thomas Dobson, 1817), 129. Charles E. Rosenberg maintains that before 1817 there had "never been a cholera [Asiatic] epidemic outside the Far East." It first appeared in the United States in 1832. Charles E. Rosenberg, *The Cholera Years: The United States in 1832, 1849, and 1866*, reprint, 1987 (Chicago: The University of Chicago Press, 1962), 1.

[7] In epidemic form the "case fatality rate was high—70 to 80 percent, compared with 25 to 30 percent in the sporadic form." Christine Hallett, "The Attempt to Understand Puerperal Fever in the Eighteenth and Early Nineteenth Centuries: The Influence of the Inflammation Theory," *Medical History* 49 (2005): 1–28. The author also points out that the disease may be "complex and difficult to interpret" so doctors may disagree on early postpartum diagnosis of headache, shaking chills (rigors), extreme heat, perspiration, and thirst as well as increasing abdominal pain and distension. The pulse may be elevated, and blood may be sizy and buffy, discussed elsewhere, as signs of inflammation. One of the main issues is deciding whether the disease is inflammatory with abnormalities of circulation and blood, in which case the appropriate therapy would be copious bloodletting. If childbed fever is considered putrid, caused by "acrid or morbific matter, then bloodletting would be contraindicated. Hallett discusses the problems and that "uncertainty and conflict" prevailed until the acceptance of germ theory and bacteriology during the last third of the nineteenth century.

The means which I used were emetics, cathartics and saline draughts; as also blisters. When the fever subsided the bark was freely given with tonic bitters. Very few recovered. All where the fever was high, and the abdomen tense, died. Those who did recover were spare enfeebled habits, where the fever was very moderate.

The ill success which attended my practice induced me to write to several aged & experienced physicians in different portions of Mass. for advice, as puerperal fever had never appeared among us, excepting in a few sporadic cases, which yielded to common means.

I could not find that any of my correspondents had known this fever to prevail in America, as an epidemic. They referred me to Dr Denman,[8] and other British Authors, who had written on puerperal fever. These books I procured. These writers supposed that acrid bile, unwholesome food and bad air, chiefly fomented this disease, and began with emetics & cathartics **22** followed with the bark & columbo root.

Dr Denman considered bleeding as hazardous, and when we consider the situation of child bed women, we should be apt to conclude that this operation would be unnecessary or injurious.[9]

Dr Leake[10] observed that in the puerperal fever which prevailed in and about London in 1770, the depression of strength was so sudden & great, that few of the patients could turn in bed, even so early as the 2^d or 3^d day from the attack; that the lochia was not obstructed nor deficient in quantity or quality; and that a considerable pressure above the pubes did not occasion pain; while the same degree of pressure between the stomach and umbilical region, produced a pain almost intolerable; and in those who died, the omentum was found in a state of suppuration. Dr Leake's description of puerperal fever, says Dr Terriere of Canada, comes the nearest to what I have observed, of any of the British Authors. I have found good effects from emetics and gentle

---

[8] Thomas Denman (1733–1815) wrote many books on midwifery. Barker may have used Thomas Denman, *Essays on Puerperal Fever, and on Puerperal Convulsions* (London: J. Walter, 1768), or a more "contemporary" text, Thomas Denman, *An Introduction to the Practice of Midwifery* (London, J. Johnson, 1782).

[9] Denman, *Essays on Puerperal Fever*, 20–23.

[10] John Leake, *Practical Observations on the Child-Bed Fever* (London: J. Walter, 1772). "Leake (1729–1792) insisted on the contagious nature of puerperal fever." See Leslie T. Morton, *A Medical Bibliography (Garrison and Morton)*, 4th ed. (Aldershot, NH: Gower Publishing Company, 1983), # 6269.

cathartics, but in most cases, I am deterred from bleeding, tho in many, I have taken two ounces to advantage.[11]

Being informed that this fever was equally prevalent in New Hampshire, particularly in Portsmouth, I wrote to Dr Cutter[12] in Autumn, an experienced physician in that town for advice. He referred me to the same writers who were his guides; so that he pursued a very similar **23** mode of practice, with the addition of fermenting cataplasms to the abdomen, composed of flower & yeast. Still he observed that the disease was attended with a great degree of mortality; and that he had made no examination by dissection.

Soon after I was permitted to open two of my patients who died of this fever, and had an oppertunity of seeing another inspected.

I put a middle aged woman to bed in Windham after a laborious travail, in which no depleting means were used. The placenta adhered, so that it was extracted with difficulty. She died in two weeks, with puerperal fever. On dissection the uterus was found inflamed & gangrenous. Other marks of inflammation appeared in the viscera of the abdomen.

I put another woman to bed, aged 30, in Buxton, after a favorable travail, in every respect. Puerperal fever, however, invaded in the usual manner. The stomach was evacuated on the 2^d day from the attack with Ipecacuan, and the bowels with Glaubers salts, pulse small, frequent and tense. Neutral salts were occasionally given, and she was fed chiefly with water gruel. The abdomen soon became tense, painful & sore to the touch. The fever continued nine days, with great thirst, when a diarrhœa took place ~~and~~ which continued five days, and she died greatly exhausted.

On dissection, twelve hours after death, the inside of the stomach was found red & inflamed; the texture of the villous membrane destroyed, grumous blood appearing in its stead; a black **24** liquor was also contained in the stomach. The intestines contained a yellow fluid, and were distended with air. The omentum was considerably wasted and of a red colour.

---

[11] Born in France, Dr. (La) Terriere, or Pierre le Sales Laterriere (1747–1815), was apprenticed and then studied in Paris and London hospitals. In 1766 he moved to Canada and later attended Harvard for an M.B.; in 1810 he received an honorary M.D. from the same institution. Helen Brock, "North America, a Western Outpost of European Medicine," in *The Medical Enlightenment of the Eighteenth Century*, ed. Andrew Cunningham and Roger French (New York: Cambridge University Press, 1990), Appendix pp. 132–33.

[12] Dr. Ammi Ruhamah Cutter Jr. (1735–1820) graduated from Harvard College in 1752. He apprenticed to Dr. C. Jackson and began practice in Portsmouth, circa 1758–1759. J. Worth Estes, *The Changing Humors of Portsmouth: The Medical Biography of an American Town, 1623–1983* (Boston: The Francis A. Countway Library of Medicine, 1986), 15.

After this I saw a woman inspected who died of this fever, in about ten days, after an abortion of seven months gestation. She had been of a costive habit, and when the fever invaded she was attended with great pain in the bowels, ~~with~~ which soon became ~~tenseion~~ & ~~soreness~~ to the touch. In this case, the rectum was found gangrenous and partly destroyed; so that glysters, &c passed through the aperture.

These appearances convinced me that the disease was highly inflammatory in the onset, and that ~~bleeding~~ the lancet was eligible, <u>before,</u> if not after delivery. I was further induced to believe that bleeding was expedient, in this fever, on account of the salutary effects of hemorrhage which sometimes took place from the uterus, before and after delivery, to a considerable extent, so that the patient was greatly exhausted. In these cases no fever insued, and the patients soon recovered.

It then appeared to me, that a mode of prevention ought to be attempted. I therefore, drew a pint of blood, which was sometimes repeated, in plethoric habits, in time of travail; also gave one emetic & cathartic; and debarred my patients entirely from spirits, which were always used at such times; and sometimes freely, **25** keeping them on a low diet, without any animal food, in a well ventilated apartment, without any curtains, on mattrass or straw beds.

Many, indeed all who conformed to these rules, either escaped the fever, or were but slightly affected. After parturition, indian gruel & rice were ~~were~~ the chief articles of food allowed, the first week, with milk & water for common drink; keeping the bowels soluble with castor oil or Glaubers salts.

"I am of opinion, says Dʳ Terriere, that this fever assumes its form principally from circumstances, preexisting in the system, the circumstance of parturition, I would consider, only as an exciting cause; that it is inflammatory in its onset; and putrid in its progress."

"The complication of inflammatory and putrid symptoms, often puzzles the practitioner, who hesitates in doubt, whether he shall adopt the antiphlogistic or tonic plan."

Dissertation on puerperal fever. 1789.[13]

"I once dissected a woman, says Dʳ Brickell of Savannah, who died of a most violent puerperal fever. The whole surface of the peritoneum, strictly so called, as well as the parts of it which gave the exterior coats to the intestines, uterus, bladder &c, had with other marks of high inflammation, **26** a coat

---

[13] Pierre de Sales La Terriere, *A Dissertation on the Puerperal Fever* (Boston: Samuel Hall, 1789).

of pus, like that observed in the corner of an inflamed eye; and as thick as broadcloath."

"Should enteritis, peritonitis, epiploitis, or any other inflammation ensue, I apply the antiphlogistic means; but with reserve, on account of the natural discharges. I sometimes draw blood from the arm; and in cases of extreme violence, I have repeated this operation three times in one day, with the happiest effects." Med. Repos. v.2. 1798.[14]

In the London Medical Repository, for May 1815, five severe cases of puerperal fever, are reported, by Wm Galskill [*sic*], Surgeon.[15] The plan consisted in bleeding, which was repeated six times, in one case, in four days, till the frequency of the pulse was diminished; and a sensible alteration was made for the better; and in purging till the alvine discharges exhibited a more favourable appearance. They all recovered.

Drs Gordon, Armstrong and Hey, British physicians, have carried bleeding to a great extent in this fever, and found it successful. See New England Journal. vol.4&5.[16]

In the course of my practice, two instances of convulsions occurred, in time of travail. Opiates, nervines & glysters, were the chief means used; but they terminated fatally; one without being delivered; the other soon

[14] John Brickell, "Theory of Puerperal Fever. Communicated in a Letter to the Editors of the Medical Repository, by Dr. John Brickell, of Savannah," *Medical Repository* 2, no. 1 (1799): 15–23. John Brickell was born in Ireland in 1749 and attended King's College (now Columbia University in New York) until the activities of the institution were suspended in 1776. After the Revolution he practiced in Savannah, Georgia, where he died in 1809. Howard A. Kelly and Walter L. Burrage, *American Medical Biographies* (Baltimore: The Norman, Remington Company, 1920), 142.

[15] William Gaitskell (1773–1833) was a member of the Royal College of Surgeons and Society of Apothecaries. He wrote that for four years there had been many cases of puerperal fever and reported five cases successfully treated by venesection. He stated that "I have taken the precaution to wash myself and change my clothes before visiting the uninfected" and illustrated the contagious nature of puerperal fever thus: "A midwife lost a patient in puerperal fever; the next she attended at another part of the town died of it; and then another, at a different part. She was greatly alarmed, and consulted Dr. Ramsbotham what she should do. He properly advised her to quit practice and London for a fortnight. She did so; and the mischief ceased." William Gaitskell, "Five Cases of Puerperal Fever Successfully Treated, with Remarks," *The London Medical Repository* 3, no. 17 (1815): 365–71. According to local lore, a tunnel led from Gaitskill's London (Rotherhithe) house on Paradise Street to the Thames, where children were paid to provide corpses from the river for him to dissect for study and teaching.

[16] " 'A Treatise on the Puerperal Fever Illustrated by Cases, Which Occurred in Leeds and Its Vicinity in the Years 1809–1812' by William Hey, Jr., London 1815," *New England Journal of Medicine and Surgery* 5 (1816): 85–98. This paper cites the works of Gordon and Armstrong, "Puerperal Fever," *The New England Journal of Medicine, Surgery and Collateral Branches of Science* 4, no. 4 (1815): 397–98.

after. — I was informed of another case, treated in like manner, where the patient was delivered in a convulsion fit, after a very laborious travail, and survived; but she became incurably insane!

27

Remarks on puerperal fever, By Dʳ Channing, Lecturer on Midwifry, in Harvard University:

"The puerperal state, in some seasons, seems unusually liable to disease, and in such seasons, puerperal fever is occasionally to be met with. It does not occur, however, with the frequency and other circumstances, which would constitute in a genuine epidemic."

"During a puerperal epidemic, physicians have observed that all puerperal patients are liable to its attacks. The ease with which labour is accomplished affords no promise of exemption from the disease. This has frequently been adverted to, by the best writers on this subject.

The means of prevention may be reduced to two. The first consists in adopting during labour that treatment which experience has sanctioned as the best for puerperal fever, occurring after delivery. The second is facilitating or rather hastening, by artificial means, the termination of labour. In the first, prompt bleeding is expedient. That prompt bleeding and purging also, which are among the best means of treating puerperal fever may be used, with a view principally to remove threatening ~~symptoms~~ disease, during labour, and without danger, may be argued from the most successful treatment of puerperal convulsions. This consists in suddenly taking from the system a large quantity of blood. It might be further proved, by recurring to cases of severe arterial ~~action~~ hemorrhage, in which recovery after delivery seems scarcely retarded; and from the fact that where fever has happened, after such hemorrhage, the indication for bleeding has been **28** as great, as in other cases, and has been attended with success.

See Armstrong on puerperal fever. [cited above]

Dʳ Gordon of Aberdeen, assures us, that in a very fatal puerperal epidemic of that city, of those who were freely purged the day after delivery, only one died of the fever."[17]

---

[17] Alexander Gordon, *A Treatise on the Epidemic Fever of Aberdeen* (London: G. G. and J. Robinson, 1795). Gordon (1752–1799) studied medicine in Aberdeen and Edinburgh. After five years in the Royal Navy he left and developed an interest in midwifery, studying under Thomas Denman and William Osborne in London. He returned to Aberdeen, and several years later became involved in a severe epidemic of puerperal fever from 1789 to 1792. As in Portland and Gorham, Maine, epidemic puerperal fever had apparently not previously been

"The management of the puerperal state, viz. that which immediately follows delivery, with a view of preventing puerperal fever, may form a subject of a future communication."   New England Journal. vol.6.1817.[18]

"With respect to the quantity of blood drawn in convulsions, occurring in labour or during pregnancy, says Dr Dewees, Lecturer on Midwifry in Philadelphia,[19] I have but one rule, bleed as long as the convulsions continue frequent & powerful, and the determination to the head evident, by the swelling and lividity of the face, projection of the eyes &c. I have often taken, with the happiest effect an hundred ounces in a few hours. The first bleeding especially should always be large. If the orifice be small and the blood only trickle down, it will do harm, by allowing the blood vessels gradually to contract on their contents, once this fail in diminishing their vigour. Blood should be drawn from a large orifice, and a large vein. I have sometimes set two streams going, one from each arm; at other times opened the Jugular.

This remedy must be used promptly, before effusion has taken place in the brain. I examined the head of a woman who died from this kind of convulsion. The longitudinal sinus of the dura mater contained about three ounces of blood; the left ventricle was filled with bloody serum."

29

"I am convinced that this milk fever[20] is in great measure if not altogether of artificial origin. It never occurs to patients who strictly follow my directions after delivery. It is the product of improper regimen. When women who are not predisposed to fever, are kept quiet, from all stimulating drinks,

---

known to exist in Aberdeen. Gordon observed that the "disease tended to be confined to the practice of a small minority of midwives . . . [and he therefore suspected] could be carried from patient to patient by doctors and midwives." His early observations, epidemiology, and treatise, like those of Ignatz Semmelweis and Oliver Wendell Holmes some fifty years later, damaged his reputation. "Gordon, Alexander (1752–1799), Physician," in *Oxford Dictionary of National Biography* (Oxford: Oxford University Press, 2018). For further reading on Gordon and the early history of childbed fever, see Loudon, Irvine. *The Tragedy of Childbed Fever*. Oxford ; New York: Oxford University Press, 2000, 1–57.

[18] Walter Channing, "Practical Remarks on Some of the Predisposing Causes, and Prevention, of Puerperal Fever, with Cases," *New England Journal of Medicine and Surgery* 6, no. 2 (1817): 157–69.

[19] William Potts Dewees (1768–1841), a graduate of University of Pennsylvania, lectured in midwifery, became adjunct professor in 1825, and full professor in 1834. He published several books on midwifery and diseases of children. Kelly and Burrage, *American Medical Biographies*, 309.

[20] "The secretion of milk on the second or third day is commonly attended with a slight fever, and the breasts become turgid and painful." James Thacher, *The American New Dispensatory Containing General Principles of Pharmaceutic Chemistry . . . The Whole Compiled from the Most Approved Authors, Both European and American* (Boston: T. B. Wait and Co., 1810), 634–35.

from animal food and broaths, who have cool & diluting drinks, or water, toast water, balm tea, &c. who have fresh air freely admitted into their rooms, who have frequent changes of clothes, who have their bowels freely opened, on the 2^d or 3^d day, never have the milk fever, as it is termed."

"There are few cases of disease occurring during pregnancy or labour so alarming and serious in its consequences, as Hemorrhagy. The most effectual remedy is the <u>acetite of lead</u>, called sugar of lead. I have uniformly, however, made it a rule, where the pulse was tense, to diminish its vigor by bloodletting from the arm before its exhibition. The blood should be taken pretty suddenly away, so as to induce <u>syncope</u>, without a great loss of blood, and an enama [*sic*] may be ~~given~~ used. The acetite of lead may then be given from three grains to ten every half hour until its object is obtained. It should always be combined with a small quantity of opium. An aqueous solution of the lead, viz a drachm to a pint of water, has been thrown up the vagina, in the early months of pregnancy to advantage, in considerable discharges of blood. In addition to this I have seen a very alarming hemorrhagy suppressed by a stream of cold water, from a considerable height on the belly of the patients; keeping the feet & legs warm, by flannels, bottles of warm water, &c."

Med. Repos. vol.ii.[21]

---

[21] William P. DeWees, "Art. 4. An Abridgment of Mr. Heath's Translation of Baudelocque's Midwifery with Notes by William P. Dewees, Md. Lecturer on Midwifery in Philadelphia. 8vo. Pp. 685. Philadelphia. Bertram and Reynolds. 1807," *Medical Repository* 5 (1808): 291–96. This article is found in vol. 11 (of the whole) or 2nd hexade no. 5 (1808). Barker is making an excerpt of the DeWees excerpt found on p. 293 of the journal article. *Mr. Heath's Translation of Beaudelocque's Midwifery* was published in 1790.

Chap. 3ᵈ4.ᵗʰ

DURING THE WINTER of 1784 & 5, the puerperal fever continued to prevail in Maine, tho with decreasing malignancy and mortality. Since which it has not appeared among us, excepting in a few sporadic cases, which seldom proved fatal.

In Dec.ʳ 1784, the throat distemper appeared in the County of Cumberland; and in Jan. 1785 it was considerably prevalent, moreso, in the interior towns than on the sea coast.

The distemper first appeared in the County of York, in the Autumn of 1784, and progressed eastward into the County of Lincoln. It was attended with a considerable degree of mortality, particularly among children; and some adults succumbed under the disease.

We had Huxham, Brooks and Fothergill for our guides.[1] But the direful malady seemed to bid defiance to the means, which were generally used, at least in my own practice, and continued to rage till the Autumn of 1786, when it subsided.

The degeneracy of the humours, into "a sort of aqua fortis," as described by Tournefort, in his voyage to the Levant, vol.1. p.133, where this malady prevailed, was truly alarming, and much greater than I had ever seen before.[2]

---

[1] John Huxham (1692–1768), John Huxham, *A Dissertation on the Malignant, Ulcerous Sore-Throat* (London: J. Hinton, 1757). Richard Brookes (fl.1721–1763), R. Brookes, *A History of the Most Remarkable Pestilential Distempers That Have Appeared in Europe for Three Hundred Years Last Past: With What Proved Successful or Hurtful in Their Cure. Together with the Method of Prevention and Cure of the Plague. Founded Upon the Experience of Those Who Were Practitioners When It Raged. Laid Down in Such a Manner That the Generality of People May Be Able to Manage Themselves. By R. Brookes M.D.* (London, Printed for A. Corbett, at the Old Hand and Pen, over against the Chapel in Russel-Court, near Covent-Garden; and J. Roberts, near the Oxford-Arms in Warwick-Lane,1721). John Fothergill (1712–1780), John Fothergill, *An Account of the Sore Throat Attended with Ulcers* (London: C. Davis, 1748). See Leslie T. Morton, *A Medical Bibliography (Garrison and Morton)*, 4th ed. (Aldershot, NH: Gower Publishing Company, 1983), #5049, #5050.

[2] Joseph Pitton de Tournefort (1656–1708), professor of botany and medicine at Montpellier. Joseph Pitton De Tournefort, *Relation D'un Voyage Du Levant, Fait Par Ordre Du Roy, Contenant L'histoire Ancienne & Moderne De Plusieurs Isles De L'archipel, De Constantinople, Des Côtes De La Mer Noire, De L'arménie, De La Georgie, Des Frontières De Perse & De L'asie Mineure* (Paris: De L'Imprimerie Royale, 1717).

In two or three days from the attack, a thin corrosive sanies flowed from the nose of children, so acid as to excoriate the lips & cheeks, where it came in contact. The same sort of matter, generated by ulcers in the throat, passed into the stomach & bowels, produced pain & anguish, vomiting & purging, till death closed the scene. Gentle emetics & cathartics, with opiates were used; but they only afforded temporary relief; so that few, thus affected, recovered.

31

In others an efflorescence of an ersipelatous colour appeared on the 2^d or 3^d day, over the whole body, with considerable fever, and sometimes delirium.

A sudden retrocession of this eruption sometimes proved fatal in a short time, when medical aid was not at hand. My own wife suffered this retrocession on the 5th day, and sunk into a cold sweat with great faintness; pulse scarcely to be felt. Volatile alkali in wine was freely given, with snakeroot tea, and a warming pan was moved round her body & limbs, applying bottles of hot water to the feet. The efflorescence soon returned, with a full pulse, and desquamation took place. She recovered. When this eruption took place, the throat was much less affected; and the contrary.

In some cases among adults the fauces were so highly inflamed, and the tonsils so tumefied that swallowing was greatly impeded and they were beset with small ulcers, which discharged a corrosive matter; so as to excoriate the throat and produce great anguish, with a quick tense pulse. Bleeding, however, was not practiced, on account on account of the supposed putrid tendency of the disease. — A gangrenous affection soon took place which destroyed life.

Gargles of various kinds, were prescribed, according to Dr Fothergills directions, such as sage tea and rose leaves in vinegar with honey. Also contrayerva & liquorice, tincture of myrrh, &c. But such gargles always increased the anguish. Bland oils & mucilages were congenial, and seemed to afford the most relief, for a time. But the fever and inflammation increased inspite of these means or any others that were used.

32

Mercury was recommended by some, particularly turpeth mineral as an emetic & alterative; as also mercurial cathartics, on account of the inflammatory symptoms and corrosiveness of the humours; as also likewise antiphlogistics. But mercurials were reprobated by others, as being dangerous medicines tending to dissolve the blood, debilitate the system, and increase putrefaction; so that peoples minds were greatly perplexed; and these means were sparingly used or entirely neglected; for we had no authority from our Authors, to use such medicines. Tonics & stimulants, therefore, were the chief means employed, with a view of preventing putrefaction, by keeping up the tone of the vessels.

Whatever success attended others, in this way, I confess that ill success attended my practice in most cases.

In every case where there was a frequent tense pulse, great heat and difficulty of breathing, and where warm pungent stimulants were used, a gangrenous affection took place, with great corrosion of the throat; and the disease proved fatal. In such cases there was no eruption nor cutaneous efflorescence. But in spare habits and delicate constitutions, where the symptoms were moderate, an eruption often took place, without much inflammation or ulceration of the throat. In such cases the disease generally terminated favourably and desquamation took place without the use of any tonic or stimulating means.[3]

Among children, the distemper was so mild, in some cases, that few means were required or used and they soon recovered.

33

"Observations and Remarks on the Putrid Malignant
Sore-throat, from 1784 to 1786.
By a Gentleman of the Faculty."
Said to be Dr Hall Jackson
"Portsmouth, New Hampshire
printed by John Melcher, 1786."[4]

Introduction.

"At a time when a most pestilential & contagious disease is making its progress through a country, marking its way with the most calamitous

---

[3] This probably represents what we would today call diphtheria, though severe "strep throat" can have a similar presentation. "The clinical diagnosis of diphtheria is based on the constellation of sore throat; adherent tonsillar, pharyngeal, or nasal pseudomembranous lesions; and low-grade fever. The systemic manifestations of diphtheria stem from the effects of diphtheria toxin and include weakness as a result of neurotoxicity and cardiac arrhythmias or congestive heart failure due to myocarditis. Most commonly, the pseudomembranous lesion is located in the tonsillopharyngeal region. Less commonly, the lesions are located in the larynx, nares, and trachea or bronchial passages. Large pseudomembranes are associated with severe disease and a poor prognosis." William R. Bishai and John R. Murphy "Diphtheria and Other Corynebacterial Infections," in *Harrison's Principles of Internal Medicine*, 19th ed., ed. Dennis Kasper et al. (New York, NY: McGraw-Hill, 2014).

[4] "Observations and Remarks on the Putrid Malignant Sore-throat, from 1784–86 by a Gentleman of the Faculty" has been established to have been written by Hall Jackson. "Jackson's authorship is verified by the inscription in the copy in the American Antiquarian Society, Worcester, Mass." See J. Worth Estes, *Hall Jackson and the Purple Foxglove* (Hanover: University Press of New England, 1979), 242–43, note #35.

circumstances, any attempt to investigate the real nature of the disorder, to mitigate its violence, and if possible, to prevent its destructive effects, is not only in itself laudable; but a duty highly incumbent on those who have the lives of their nearest connections, friends & neighbors committed to their care. This consideration alone, has produced the following observations & remarks. They were thrown together at a late hour, after the fatigues of a busy day, as well for the authors own satisfaction, as the purpose of adopting some concise and regular method of treating a disease, which is so rapidly spreading, and in all probability will become general amongst us. They were shown to some medical friends, at whose pressing solicitations, they are now, with the utmost diffidence, submitted to the public inspection.

The author is not unaware that he has laid himself open to criticism & censure. But he will as patiently bear the one as be regardless of the other, should he stimulate those of superior abilities & more **34** extensive medical knowledge to improve on these imperfect hints, and favour the public with their opinions, that from the united endeavours of all, some effectual method may be obtained to mitigate the violence of so distressing a disease."

Observations & Remarks
on the Putrid Malignant Sore-throat.[5]

The present putrid malignant sore throat, as far as we can learn, first made its appearance in Sanford, Coxhall,[6] and several other new settled towns, in

---

[5] Putrid sore throat probably refers to what twentieth- and twenty-first-century clinicians call diphtheria; the presence of pseudo membranes favors diphtheria as the etiology. The first accurate account of this disease was by Pierre Bretoneau in 1821 and was so named in 1826 from the Greek diphtheria, "leather," as a description of the pseudo membrane seen in the back of the throat. The disease was described in Hippocrates *Epidemics III* and by Fothergill; see Fothergill, *An Account of the Sore Throat Attended with Ulcers*. The 1735 epidemic in New England is mentioned earlier in Barker's manuscript, volume 1, chapter 2, MS pp. 6–8, 12–13, 18. Various epidemics from ancient times may at times have been caused by Streptococcal or Parainfluenza infections and were given names such as putrid sore throat, croup, and others emphasizing certain aspects of the disease. It was not until 1883 that Edwin Klebs described the bacterium causing diphtheria; a year later Friedrich Loeffler first cultured it. See Kenneth F. Kiple, *The Cambridge World History of Human Disease* (Cambridge; New York: Cambridge University Press, 1993), 682–83. See also Henry Alan Skinner, *The Origin of Medical Terms*, 2nd ed. (Baltimore: The Williams & Wilkins Company, 1961), 142.

[6] These are two towns in southern Maine. Sanford was incorporated in 1768. Coxhall was settled in 1767, incorporated in 1778, and renamed Lyman in 1803. William Williamson, *The History of the State of Maine: From Its First Discovery, A.D. 1602 to the Separation, A.D. 1820, Inclusive* (Hallowell, ME: Glazier, Masters & Co., 1832), vol. 2, 465.

the upper part of the county of York, District of Maine, in the fall of the year 1784. Since which it has been slowly spreading, though more rapidly in the back towns than towards the sea coast.

The three last years have not been marked with any remarkable circumstances as to the weather, or state of the air. The two last winters were not uncommonly severe, and the summers have been remarkably temperate, nor has any great degree of dry or moist weather prevailed. A foggy day or night has scarcely been known in any part of the seasons, and more generally health never prevailed through the country, excepting in the summer of 1784, when puerperal fevers were remarkably common through the country in general, and proved fatal to a great number of women.

Whatever may be the remote or predisposing cause of the present disease, must remain one of those **35** mysteries that baffle human researches. Blindly to puzelle [*sic*] for peccant causes, is oftentimes as futile & absurd, as prescriptions founded on prejudice & conjecture are unjustifiable.

The author has had an oppertunity of seeing a considerable number under the present disease, and has most attentively marked the symptoms, compared them with the disorders that he thought similar, as described by a number of authors. He has taken the opinion of some aged and formerly eminent practitioners; and on the whole, he is persuaded that the present contagious disorder is a disease <u>sui generis</u>. It differs from that destructive disease that formerly prevailed in this country, known by the name of the <u>Throat Distemper</u>. This was a dreadful disease indeed! much more mortal than the present one; often destroying in a few hours after the attack, while the innocent victim was diverting with its toys, and its fond parents unsuspicious of danger. Many were suddenly carried off when no marks of the disease appeared, more than a superficial pustle [*sic*] or small inflamed ulcer on a finger or a toe. He has not seen nor heard of any like effects in the present disease. It may not, however, be improbable, that the former malignant disease may associate with the present one; as they are both disorders of a highly putrid nature, the disposing cause in the air, and constitutional disposition in the habit, may produce them both in the same season. Yet out of a considerable number, he has not seen more than one or two, who have appeared to have had the real <u>Throat distemper</u>. Nor is the present **36** disorder that which often prevails, and is commonly called the Scarlet fever. This is most evident, from numbers that are now under the present disease, who heretofore have had the Scarlet fever, a disease that has not been known to attack the same persons a second time.

Besides, an efflorescence always appears in the Scarlet fever, indeed it is a characteristic of the disease.[7] But in the present disorder, one third, at least, are free from every appearance of eruption.

The ulcerous sore throat of D[r] Huxham, the cynanche maligna of D[r] Cullen, are in many cases a good description of the present disease; the putrid sore throat of D[r] Brooks more accurate; the scarlatina anginosa of D[r] Withering he has not seen.[8] The present putrid sore throat is contagious, more so with children, frequently with those ~~of more advanced life~~ from twenty to thirty years of age; and those of more advanced life, do not always escape. It is a disease of a highly putrid nature; this is most evident from the appearance of the sloughs & ulcers in the throat; the offensive putrid smell of the breath, so soon after the patient begins to complain; and the petechial spots which in many cases are dispersed over different parts of the body. The attack is often sudden, and the symptoms increase very rapidly. Persons have been perfectly well at noon, in the evening in the most disagreeable circumstances; a most violent fever, pain & stiffness in the neck; the uvula and tonsils so swelled as almost to close up the throat. In others the symptoms advance more slowly, beginning with slight rigors & sickness. **37** But in all, sooner or later, there is great increased heat, restlessness, difficulty of breathing, with an exceeding full & quick pulse; and very soon the uvula, and tonsils, and in some the whole inside of the throat will be covered with white, or ash coloured spots, which enlarge & become thick sloughs; the tongue exceeding foul at the basis and in young subjects, a remarkable drowsiness. All these symptoms increase, and are greatly aggravated towards the evening. On the second or third day, an efflorescence of a deep erysipelatous colour appears, more especially on the face, neck, breast and hands, all which appear to be a little swelled; the fingers more evidently so, and in many, tinged in a remarkable manner. If these parts

7 Simple scarlet fever was thought to be "a variety of Scarlatina Angiosa." James Thacher, *American Modern Practice* (Boston: Ezra Read, 1817), 367–68.

8 Drs. Huxham, Cullen, and Brook[e]s have been mentioned. Dr. William Withering (1741–1799) was an Edinburgh trained physician and botanist best known for his work on digitalis (foxglove). William Withering, *An Account of the Foxglove, and Some of Its Medical Uses: With Practical Remarks on Dropsy, and Other Diseases* (Birmingham: M. Swinney for G, GJ, and J Robinson, London, 1785). Withering is mentioned here for William Withering, *An Account of the Scarlet Fever and Sore Throat, or Scarlatina Anginosa; Particularly as It Appeared at Birmingham in the Year 1778* (London: T. Cadell &c., 1779).

be accurately viewed, an infinite number of small pimples, of an intense scarlet colour, will be perceived. But here, different from other eruptive disorders, the patient gains no relief, nor are the symptoms the least extenuated by this large despumation on the skin. On the contrary, the pain, heat, and anxiety increase. At night a delirium frequently comes on, which generally goes off in the morning, with an abatement of the other symptoms; but returns again with equal violence towards the evening.

The tongue & mouth become more foul; the sloughs in the throat increase, so as almost to prevent breathing; these are frequently thrown off in large flakes, and leave deep, painful, and sometimes bleeding ulcers behind them; from the inside of the nostrils, especially in ~~young~~ children is discharged large quantities of a thin putrid matter, of a most corrosive nature, excoriating whatever it touches. In infants, this virulent matter often passes down the <u>œsophagus</u> into the stomach and **38** intestines, bringing on sickness, vomiting and violent purgings; the fine membrane that lines the larynx is corroded off; the <u>epiglottis</u> looses its action, by which every thing the child endeavours to swallow, passes the wrong way, as the common phrase is, strangles, and it flies back through the nose; a hoarseness ~~and~~ with hooping, which is generally a fatal symptom, however mild and favourable other appearances may be, comes on; suffocation and death suddenly take place. About the 5th day, sometimes sooner, and sometimes a day later, all the symptoms become more & more aggravated; the heat, restlessness, difficulty of breathing, and delirium constant; the pulse small, but excessive quick; the sloughs in the throat thicker, and change to a livid colour; the fœtor from the breath intolerable; the efflorescence on the skin disappears, or becomes of a dark crimson colour, with petechial spots dispersed about on the legs, thighs, and sometimes other parts of the body; the difficulty of breathing increases; the patient falls into a stupor, and death suddenly closes the scene.

Those that have the disease more favourably, generally have an abatement of all the symptoms on the 4th day; the efflorescence on those that have it; for as was observed before, one third of the patients have no appearance of eruption, disappears; the sloughs in the throat seperate and come off; and leave ulcers that readily heal. In some, a hardness & tumefaction of the parotid glands remain, in others a dry hoarse cough; these, however, soon give way to proper remedies.

From a consideration of the foregoing symptoms we are led to conclude, that the present disorder is a disease of a highly putrid nature; and that the indications of cure are to be sought for only, in such remedies as may obviate the tendency to putrefaction, quiet the septic ferment in the habit, and support the system. **39** The tonic, as well as antiseptic powers of the Bark must render it a medicine not only proper; but highly necessary, in this disorder.

The virtues of the Bark, when taken in substance, in full doses, in putrid disorders, stands unrivalled by all other remedies. But there are many cases where it appears highly necessary; but it cannot be got down, or the stomach will not retain it; and the disease now under consideration, affords many instances of this kind. To obviate this difficulty, we have now a method of conveying into the habit, a sufficient quantity of this noble medicine, by the means of a pediluvium, recommended by Dʳ Alexander. The salutary effects of this medicine, when used in this way, have been abundantly experienced by practitioners in this town, in low fevers, and other disorders of a putrid kind.

Dʳ Percival informs us, that it has been found, that the hand, after being well chafed, will imbibe in an hour, near an ounce and a half of warm water; and allowing that the surface of the hand is to that of the whole body, as one to sixty, the absorption of the whole, in the same space of time, would amount to upwards of seven pounds.[9]

The fact related sometime since, in the newspapers, of a British sea officer, who was wrecked on a desolate island in the West Indies, where no fresh water was to be obtained, that his thirst was sufficiently prevented, or allayed, in that intensely hot climate, by frequently wetting his shirt in the sea, and putting it on, under his other clothes, that he continued in that situation for a long time before relieved, and that the only inconvenience he found was a fret on the skin, from the incrustation of the salt, when the aqueous particles were absorbed. And the curious fact related by Dʳ Chalmers, of a negro man, gibbetted in Charleston, South Carolina, in March 1759, who had eat nor drank but little **40** for some time before he was put up; yet he regularly voided, every morning, a large quantity of urine, imbibed by the body, from the dews of the evening, and besides this, a sufficient quantity to support perspiration by day; and he adds, had these fluids been of a nutritious quality, he might have been kept alive for a considerable length of time.[10]

---

9 Thomas Percival, *Experiments on the Peruvian Bark* (London: L. Davis & C. Reymers, 1768). Thomas Percival (1740–1804) of Manchester, England, is known today for his influence and writings on medical ethics.

10 Lionel Chalmers, *An Account of the Weather and Diseases of South-Carolina*, 2 vols. (London: Edward and Charles Dilly, 1776), vol. 1, 51. Lionel Chalmers (c. 1715–1777) was born in Scotland and trained at Edinburgh. He lived and practiced in Charleston, South Carolina, for over forty years and recorded local weather observations between 1750 and 1760.

From these facts, it cannot be doubted, that warm water, fully impregnated with the Bark, and other antiseptics, may be conveyed into the body, in very considerable quantities, by the absorbing vessels; and that too with a very good purpose, in all cases where the bark is required. In disorders where great putridity prevails, Virginia snakeroot, and camomile flowers, may be added to the pediluvium with a very good intention.

Out of a considerable number that have been visited with this disease, in Portsmouth; and the neighbouring towns, it has proved fatal in a few instances; excepting a boy nine years old, at Kittery, all were infants that have died; they suffered from a defluxion of the putrid matter on the lungs.

On the 17th of August last, the author had an oppertunity of seeing W. J. H. of Somersworth,[11] a man naturally of a good constitution, and about 23 years of age; the disease had been sometime in the family; it was the eighth day of his sickness; and he then appeared to be just expiring; the circulation had so far ceased that no pulse could be perceived; his countenance was sunk, a cold clammy sweat pervaded the whole body, and he was universally putrid. Early in his sickness a blister had been drawn, on one of his arms, the whole limb **41** was tumefied to a surprising degree, and that part where the blister had been laid, had become a dead sphacelus; yet he continued 24 hours after those alarming appearances. What expectations could be had, in any remedies equal to the sovereign specific virtues of the bark, early pushed to the utmost extent?

This instance is mentioned to show the very great tendency to putrefaction in this disease.

The author conceives that he cannot do better, in this place, than transcribe a passage from the late celebrated D[r] Fothergill;[12] whose name & works will be revered as long as gratitude and the love of merit shall continue in the world.

"The use of the bark, in the cure of this disease, putrid sore throat, was unknown to the early practitioners. It is but of late that this celebrated medicine has been used with freedom, in this, as well as in other putrid diseases, and with great advantage."

---

[11] Somersworth, New Hampshire, on the Salmon River that forms the border between Maine and New Hampshire near Berwick, Maine.

[12] John Fothergill (1712–1780) See Fothergill, *An Account of the Sore Throat Attended with Ulcers*.

"The difficulty of prevailing on children, afflicted with this distemper, to take any kind of medicine, put me early on trying the bark in clysters, and sometimes where these seemed very little chance of relieving them by any means. To very young children two or three drachms of the bark, in fine powder, have been given every six hours, in four ounces of broth, as a clyster, adding a small quantity of the <u>Elect. Scordio</u>, to the second or third; if the first was discharged too speedily; and this has been the means of saving many, when not a drop of any medicine, and scarcely any kind of nourishment could be swallowed."

Adults may take half a drachm of the powder, in an ounce and a half of the decoction, warmed with any grateful compound water, every two or three hours, taking particular care to prevent any considerable tendency to diarrhœa, from the use of the medicine. Free, but not **42** cold air, plenty of liquid nutriment & generous, with constant attention to keep the patients clean, their mouths and throats often washed, and their lined [*sic*] often changed, contribute greatly to the cure of this disease. While their skin is covered with that deep efflorescence, if they are at all sensible, they often complain of the least admission of cold air, and very frequently of much sickness and oppression, "if the efflorescence disappears."

"To favour the eruption, it will always be proper to put those who are seized with this distemper to bed, as early after the seizure as possible, and to give the mild and cordial diaphoretics. As a preservative, I have often recommended the bark to be given both in decoction & substance, with the addition of such a quantity of the volatile tincture of <u>Guaicum</u>, as may render it gently purgative."

The author will now take the liberty of communicating the method that has been generally pursued by the practitioners in this place, and which at present, he believes they find no occasion essentially to alter.

In many cases the disorder is so mild as to require little more than keeping warm; at bed time, taking a draught of cyder or wine whey, a little sage being previously boiled in the milk. The mouth & throat may be washed with barley water, rose leaves & sage tea, with a little vinegar, and as much honey as will leave it agreeably acid.

In cases where the attack is severe, beginning with sickness and vomiting, it has been thought adviseable to encourage it by a few grains of Ipecac, or camomile flower tea. If after the operation of the medicine, the symptoms do not abate, the following Julep will, for the most part, effectually restrain the stomach.

43

R. Sal. Absinth. vel Tartar. gr. 20. Succ. Limon. oz. ss. Ol. Menth. pip. gut. 3. vel. Essent. Menth. pip. gut. 20. Tinct. Thebaic. gut. 40. Aq. Font. oz. 2. M. F. Julep.[13]

If the oil of peppermint is used instead of the essence, it should be previously rubbed with a little sugar, and the water added by degrees. A spoonful of this Julep, more or less according to the age & circumstances of the patient, is directed to be taken every hour, until the stomach is quieted. In cases where there is no sickness or disposition to puking, an emetic has seldom been prescribed; but rather have directed them to take a spoonful of Mindererus spirit, every four or six hours, as occasion may require, through the disease.

But where the symptoms are more urgent, the tendency to putrefaction great, the sloughs large & thick, and the breath offensive, recourse must be had to more efficacious remedies. Six ounces of bark, four ounces of camomile flowers, and two ounces of Virginia snake root, are directed to be boiled or rather infused for four hours in ten quarts of water, in a close vessel, and the patient to soak his feet and legs in this infusion, made a little more than lukewarm, one hour at least, morning & evening, and oftener, if the symptoms are alarming. A decoction of bark, snake root & camomile flowers is also to be taken once in four or six hours, and the bark freely in substance, if it can be got down. Here it may be observed, that not an instance has been seen, even where a most phlogistic diathesis appeared to prevail, that the symptoms were the least exaggerated from this treatment of the disorder; but, on the contrary, the heat and restlessness have abated, a gentle diaphoresis taken place, which is far from being natural in this disease; ****44**** the skin, in general, being remarkably dry.

In cases where a delirium comes on in the evening, and the patient has been any time costive, a milk clyster is directed, taking care, if more than one or two stools are procured, which will sometimes be the case, to restrain the bowels with a proper dose of Paragoric Elixir.

In the evening, when the accession has been very great, and the patient uncommonly restless, it has been found necessary to give some gentle sedative draught.

---

[13] Roughly interpreted: R$_x$. Salt of Absinthe OR Tartar (Lixivia) 20 grains, Juice of lemon ½ oz, Peppermint Oil 3 grains OR Essence of Peppermint 20 grains, Tincture of Opium 40 grains, Spring Water 2 oz.—Combine to make a Julep. Terms for these and other preparations may be found in the Glossary.

With regard to the throat, they are directed to receive the steam of boiling vinegar, honey and myrrh into the mouth through an inverted funnel, or the nose of a coffee pot; and where a gargarism can be used, the following one has been found very efficacious in bringing off the sloughs, and deterging the ulcers.

R. Aq. Fontan. oz. 6. Mel oz. 1. Tinc Myrrh. oz. ss. Spt. Salis. Marini. q. s. M. F. Garg.[14]

Here the quantity of spirit of salt is not mentioned, as this must be regulated by the throat; for if the sloughs have seperated and come off, very little can be endured; otherwise, from ten to twenty drops may be sufficient. The patient need not be fearful of swallowing any of this gargarism; the myrrh, as well as spirit of salt are antiseptics.

It is with great difficulty that children can be brought to manage either the steam or gargarisms properly, and with infants impossible. Great attention, however, should be paid to the cleansing the nose, mouth & throat, by washings, injections, and every method that can be devised.

It frequently happens that the parotid glands are much swelled; painful, and hard. In such cases the following liniment has been used with advantage. **45** R. Camphor. drachm. 2. Ol. Amygd. vel. Olivar. oz. 2. Spt. sal. ammoniae drachm 2. misce.[15]

A small quantity of this may be rubbed into the part; afterwards a fermenting cataplasm of milk, beergrounds[16] or yeast, with oatmeal may be applied.

As to blisters, a promiscuous use of them is far from being thought adviseable. In some languid cases they may be useful, yet the inflammation, painful sloughs, deep ulcerations, and even mortifications, that have taken place, seem to be more than a counter balance for all their good effects. But it is impossible to overcome the prejudices of some; and we often find blisters applied without consulting the physician. In such cases, and when any of the above disagreeable appearances take place, the before mentioned cataplasm, with the addition of some onions, sliced small and previously boiled in the milk, will be found one of the easiest & best applications.

---

[14] Roughly interpreted: R$_x$. Spring Water 6 oz., Honey 1 oz, Tincture of Myrrh ½ oz, Spirits of Sea Salt as much as suffices—Combine to make a Gargle.

[15] Roughly interpreted: R$_x$. Camphor 2 drachm, Oil of Almonds OR Olive Oil 2 oz, Spirits of Ammonium 2 drachm—Combine.

[16] The grounds, or thick sediment of beer; a mucilage.

The author, in September 1785, attended the wife of Mr B. R. of York. She had the disorder severely indeed; the whole of the tonsils were mortified. A blister had been drawn on one arm and leg; these limbs were swelled to an astonishing degree. No description can give an idea of the pain she suffered in them. The parts where the blister had been laid, were also mortified. Yet with a constant use of the pediluvium with bark, camomile flowers & snake root, the red bark taken freely in substance; and the frequent use of the gargarism before mentioned, she recovered. There was so great a loss of substance in the throat, that she could scarcely utter a word intelligibly, and for many months, whatever she attempted to swallow returned as freely by the nose. The mortified **46** blisters separated and came out, leaving the bones nearly bare; and it was some months before they were fully incarned and healed; and nature has in a surprising and unexpected manner overcome the difficulty in her throat.

In cases where blisters are thought necessary, it has been found much better to apply them to the neck over the tonsils, than on the limbs.

In some cases the putrid fœtor from the breath is not only intolerably offensive to the attendants; but to the patients themselves. The fixed air emitted from the effervescence of chalk and sharp vinegar, mixed ~~with~~ in pretty large quantities, in a bowl, and placed near the patients mouth, will be found very advantageous.

Faintness is frequently a symptom in this disease; genuine Madeira wine, will be found the best antiseptic cordial that can be taken.

If after the disorder is gone off, a swelling & hardness of the parotid glands remain; keeping the part warm, friction with soft flannel, and in obstinate cases, a small quantity of mercurial ointment, rubbed into the part, and a dose or two of calomel with rhubarb will remove the complaint.

It has happened with some patients, especially those more advanced in life, that on the decline of this disorder, they have been attacked with violent pains in the limbs, not unlike those of the rheumatism; and in some few instances, they have so far lost the use of them, as to be unable to stand on their feet or make use of their hands. In these cases, the volatile tincture **47** of Guaicum, or the saw dust of the Lignum vitæ, has speedily put an end to those complaints.

The cough & œdemetous swelling of the limbs, that some times remain after the disease, are best removed by a continuance of the bark.

It may be objected, by some, that few remedies are proposed. It was not the authors intention to prescribe for every symptom that might arise in this disorder; his endeavour was to point out the real nature and tendency of a disease that has become so general, under so many names & titles; as also to adopt some rational method of cure instead of the numberless remedies constantly recommended; indeed, in all cases, more especially in one where so little can be swallowed, a few well chosen powerful remedies are to be preferred to a farrago of insignificant stuff that can serve only to tease the patient and obstinately determine him against every remedy, however important and necessary.　　　　　　　　　　　　　Portsmouth November, 1786.

These "observations & remarks" were not received till after the throat distemper had subsided; so that an oppertunity of trying the Bark externally was not afforded. Neither can I learn that any of my medical brethren, in Maine, made use of it in this way.

In the spring of 1786, I met with a gentleman from Quebec, who informed me that the throat distemper had been prevalent in that City, the year past, and that spirit of sal. ammoniae mixed with olive oil was liberally used, by physicians ~~both~~ externally over the tonsils, and, internally, to great advantage. ****48****

This disease also appeared in the southern parts of New England, about the same time, called by Dr William Baylies of Dighton, the ulcerated sore throat, ~~and~~ who speaks highly of Marsh Rosemary in the disease, as an emetic & expectorant, in a medical communication to the M. M. Society. as it appeared in that town, in 1785 & 1786.[17] ****49**** Some account of the throat distemper, or Scarlatina Anginosa, as it appeared in Beverly, Mass^tts. communicated to me by Joshua Fisher, M. D. ~~and~~ member of the Mass. Medical and Philosophical Society.

Dated ~~July 1.^t 1796~~ Beverly, July 1.^t 1796.

"You wish to have some information respecting the ulcerous sore throat. We have had it here, and I assure you, I hope never to see it again.

It assumes a great variety of forms, hence the variety of names. The Spaniards call it <u>garrotillo</u>, from the ratling in the throat. I have heard this noise formerly; but only in one case, in this town. It has been called ulcerated sore throat; but I have seen no ulcerations; putrid sore throat; but it was not more putrid than the small pox by inoculation. Scarlatina Anginosa best expresses the disease as it appeared here. Yet there was often no eruption;

---

[17] Dr. William Bailies (Baylies) published "An Account of the Ulcerated Sore Throat as It Appeared in the Town of Dighton in the Years 1785 and 1786." *Massachusetts Medical Society Papers* 1 (1790): 41–48, and reprinted in the M.M.S. "Medical Communications" 1 (1808). Clifford Shipton, *Biographical Sketches of Those Who Attended Harvard College; Sibley's Harvard Graduates, Vol. 14: 1756–1760* (Boston: Massachusetts Historical Society, 1968), vol. 14, 552–55.

sometimes it was crimson instead of scarlet; and sometimes there was no sore throat. The disease was sometimes local; but generally universal & highly inflammatory, with quick, hurried, irregular pulse, very much resembling, in some cases, the Yellow fever, as described by Dʳ Rush.

The <u>virus</u> of the disease did not incline to pass off by the skin; but kept continually pouring in on the primæ viæ. The matter thrown off by evacuations was either a green liquid, or gelatinous substance. The crisis of the eruptive fever generally took place on the 5ᵗʰ day; but the crisis of the fever was by no means, the crisis of the disease, for it continued sometimes, without any abatement, as long as 14 days.

50

The intentions of cure, with me, were to evacuate the morbid matter as fast as possible; and, in the mean time to counteract the symptoms. As an emetic I generally gave 5. or 6. grains of turpeth mineral with 8. or 10. ᵍʳˢ of pan. antim. or 15 or 20 grains of calomel; and if this did not give the patient considerable relief, I repeated the dose till it did, sometimes four doses in 24 hours, and afterwards as the stomach required, or the sick could bear. As a cathartic I generally gave calomel at first sometimes from $\mathbf{3}$i to $\mathbf{3}$ii[18] were required to affect the intestines. When the canal became sore and irritated I mixed castor oil with the calomel, sometimes a decoction of Jalap was convenient.

With a view of counteracting the symptoms I depended chiefly on blisters applied to the throat, breast or stomach; and mercurials were freely exhibited. But I generally found it difficult to affect the salivary glands; when I could the disease yielded.

The sick could bear no kind of astringent till the primæ viæ were properly cleansed and the violence of the fever was subdued. In the progress of the disease opiates were often useful, especially at night.

Tumors & suppurations about the throat, discharges from the ears, eyes &c appeared to me, to arise from a want of evacuations.

It would be highly agreeable to be able to get a clear idea of the fermentation which produces the violent acrimony ~~which~~ prevalent in this disease; and to be able to counteract it without powerful evacuants; but of this I see little prospect. In some places the distemper had been more inclined to putridity; so that fewer evacuants & more astringents have been required."

---

[18] 1–2 scruples; see Glossary.

51

Chap 5.

DURING THE MONTHS of Nov. & Dec. 1797, and January Feb. & March 1798, the Scarlatina Anginosa was prevalent in almost every town in the county of Cumberland, Maine. It likewise prevailed in other parts of the District.

The disease was ushered in with nausea & sometimes vomiting, to which succeeded chilly fits, followed by increased heat, pain & soreness of the throat, which soon became inflamed, and sooner or later, according to the violence of the fever, put on a gangrenous hue with a fœtid breath. In some cases the throat was swelled to such a degree, both externally & internally, that deglutition & speach were almost prevented, and the patient was very thirsty, pulse small & tense.

Not being authorised to bleed, and mercury being disapproved of by most of my medical brethren, in this disease, on account of its supposed putrid tendency, and never having seen any good effects from pungent stimulating medicines, in the primary stages of this distemper, my views were directed to the use of <u>alkalines</u>,[1] from their known tendency to check and even remove apparent putrescency in inanimate substances; as well as from their salutary effects in other kinds of fever in preceeding years.[2]

---

[1] Jeremiah Barker, "On Febrifuge Virtues of Lime, Magnesia and Alkaline Salts in Dysentery, Yellow-Fever and Scarlatina Angiosa. In a Letter from Dr. Jeremiah Barker, of Portland, (Maine) Dated May 30, 1798," *Medical Repository* 2, no. 2 (1798): 147–52.

[2] Though alkaline salts and limewater continued to be used for years as antacids and absorbents as well as lithonotriptic (drugs that dissolve uric acid stones), their use in putrid fevers was at issue. See William Cullen, *First Lines of the Practice of Physic with Supplementary Notes, Including More Recent Improvements in the Practice of Medicine by Peter Reid*, two volumes in one (Brookfield: E. Mirriam & Co. for Isaiah Thomas, 1807), 426. J. Worth Estes, "Therapeutic Practice in Colonial New England," in *Medicine in Colonial Massachusetts, 1620–1820: A Conference Held 25 & 26 May 1978*, ed. Frederick S. Allis (Boston: The Colonial Society of Massachusetts, 1980), table XI. Guenter B. Risse, *Hospital Life in Enlightenment Scotland: Care and Teaching at the Royal Infirmary of Edinburgh* (Cambridge: Cambridge University Press, 1986), 200. Andrew Duncan, *The Edinburgh New Dispensatory*, 1st Worcester ed. (Worcester: Press of Isaiah Thomas, 1805), 414. For help with terminology, see J. Worth

Accordingly, after evacuating the stomach & bowels, my efforts were particularly directed to counteract the virus, or noxious cause; as well as to reduce inflammation. To effectuate these important purposes, alkaline remedies were liberally employed, particularly an aqueous solution of the carbonate of potash, which evidently appeared to reduce the fever, and to remove that peculiar fœtor, which constantly attended. This alkaline solution was used externally as well as internally, generally combined mixed with aqua calcis for internal use; and the sick rooms were carefully ventilated. **52** Cold water impregnated with cream of tartar, was freely drank, and Glauber's salts were used as a cathartic, which was repeated according to the degree of febrile action. A scarlet efflorescence took place in most cases, when the fever abated, and desquamation followed.

In some cases, there was no sore throat nor eruption; yet the attending fever was highly inflammatory. In three cases, which I saw, the virus was turned on the renal glands, producing bloody urine, mixed with skinny filaments, attended with great pain, heat & anguish.[3] In others there was distressing pain in the bowels and great thirst for water.

Besides these means, oils & mucilages were used to great advantage, viz olive oil, fresh butter & Gum arabic. The mouth & throat, when particularly affected were gargled with lime water. This was evidently beneficial. It was as congenial to the sores & ulcers, as it is to ulcerations & sores on the external surface. Epispastics were applied to the neck & breast. They produced a great

---

Estes, *Dictionary of Protopharmacology* (Canton, MA: Science History Publications, 1990). See also chapter 4 of the Introduction.

[3] Barker describes an associated rash in most of the more than fifty cases but that the "virus was turned upon the renal glands, producing bloody urine" in three cases. Barker, "On Febrifuge Virtues of Lime, Magnesia and Alkaline Salts in Dysentery, Yellow-Fever and Scarlatina Angiosa. In a Letter from Dr. Jeremiah Barker, of Portland, (Maine) Dated May 30, 1798." From the twenty-first-century perspective, this condition most likely represents group A beta-hemolytic streptococcus (*S. pyogenes*) infection causing glomerulonephritis, an inflammatory disease of the kidneys that may follow a beta-hemolytic streptococcus infection. As Barker describes it, the rash may be followed by desquamation, first described in the seventeenth century. Sydenham used the term "scarlatina" and differentiated it from measles. There were epidemics in the seventeenth and eighteenth centuries in Europe and North America, some with a high mortality. The organism was named and isolated in the late nineteenth and early twentieth centuries. Childbed (puerperal) fever and erysipelas can be caused by the same organisms. J. Ferretti and W. Kohler, "History of Streptococcal Research," in *Streptococcus Pyogenes: Basic Biology to Clinical Manifestations*, ed. J. J. Ferretti, D. L. Stevens, and V. A. Fischetti (Oklahoma City, OK: University of Oklahoma Health Sciences Center, 2016). Ferretti J, Köhler W. History of Streptococcal Research. 2016 Feb 10. In: Ferretti JJ, Stevens DL, Fischetti VA, editors. Streptococcus pyogenes : Basic Biology to Clinical Manifestations [Internet]. Oklahoma City (OK): University of Oklahoma Health Sciences Center; 2016–. Available from: https://www.ncbi.nlm.nih.gov/books/NBK333430/

discharge, and were very sore, attended in many instances with intollerable itching. A lotion of lime water readily allayed this itching, and disposed the sores to heal, which, in some cases, where the fever had been high, appeared gangrenous. Lime water was freely drank by many in this disease, and was found very grateful to the stomach.[4] In the latter part of the distemper, it was mixed with milk, which was thereby rendered congenial to the stomach, and afforded additional nutriment. Rice & indian gruel were also used, to advantage; and every thing of a heating, ~~pungent~~ stimulating nature was studiously avoided; from the beginning to the end.

53

I was called to two cases, which terminated fatally. These were all that I lost, out of more than fifty in this distemper, who were treated in this manner, with particular attention, being seasonably called.

In one of the fatal cases, a girl 12 years old, to whom I was called on the sixth day, the throat was gangrenous. The arm also became gangrenous where an epispastic had been applied. The breath was extremely fœtid, and her speech; as well as swallowing were in a great measure prevented. No physician had been called. She had taken a gentle emetic & cathartic, which were followed with warm, ~~pungent~~ stimulating teas, and cordial spiritous drinks! She died on the 12th day, and livid spots appeared on the skin, particularly about the neck & breast.

The other, a child of four years old, complained of a distressing pain in the bowels, and was very thirsty. The efflorescence, which had been small, readily disappeared; and the throat was not affected. Warm stimulating teas, gentle evacuants, opiates & tonics had been given; but no ease could be afforded. I was called on the 8th day, and was informed that she had laboured under a high fever, which had now abated. She died the next day. ——On dissection, by permission, twelve hours after death, the inside of the stomach was found red & inflamed; the texture of the villous membrane destroyed, grumous blood appearing in its stead. A black liquor was also contained in the stomach, which was in a contracted state. The intestines contained a yellow fluid,

---

[4] In his case books of 1806, Jeremiah Barker recorded an interest in the use of lime and alkaline salts, as discussed in chapter 4 of the Introduction. He concluded that "the exciting cause of fever was a virulent acid often generated in the stomach from substances undergoing putrid fermentation" and that alkaline therapy was useful. Jeremiah Barker's 1806 Casebook, Maine Historical Society, Collection 13, Box 1/5, unpaged. He subsequently published his work in: Barker, "On Febrifuge Virtues of Lime, Magnesia and Alkaline Salts in Dysentery, Yellow-Fever and Scarlatina Angiosa. In a Letter from Dr. Jeremiah Barker, of Portland, (Maine) Dated May 30, 1798."

and were distended with air. The omentum was considerably wasted and of a red colour. No other morbid affection could be discovered.

Another child in the family, a girl, six years old was soon after, attacked in a similar manner. I was called the fourth day, when the efflorescence which was **54** partial & light, had just vanished, when pain & anguish seized her bowels in a distressing manner, with great thirst; pulse quick & small. After gently cleansing the stomach and intestines with ipecac, and castor oil, an aqueous solution of pearl ash was freely given in flaxseed tea, which soon alleviated her distress, and anguish. A blister was also drawn over the stomach, and contrary to our expectations, she recovered.

I dissected a woman, in 1784, who died of a puerperal fever, and found the stomach in a very similar condition with the child inspected. I saw another puerperal case dissected, about that time, where the rectum was corroded and partly destroyed. I then accused the bile of being the mischievous cause; but I now believe that the ravages made in the stomach, intestines, throat, or other parts, must be imputed to the septic acid, which excites a fever of a different kind, from other febrile diseases, where no such virulency and degeneracy of the humours take place. Under these circumstances, Alkalines and oils are especially indicated; though not to the exclusion of the lancet nor mercury, as we have been taught by later experience of scientific physicians in the republic of medicine.

Although my patients generally recovered, under the antiphlogistic and alkaline plan, with copious evacuations from the stomach & bowels, yet I am persuaded that many, where the fever was highly inflammatory, suffered for the want of bleeding, and perhaps they would have been benefitted by mercury, as a cooperative mean.

55

In the months of November & December 1799, and in January & February 1800, an inflammatory fever, attended with a sore throat, prevailed in several towns, among adults; as well as children.[5]

The disease was ushered in with a pain & soreness of the throat, which soon swelled both externally & internally; redness of the fauces, and difficulty of swallowing; often with increased salival discharge; nausea and vomiting, increased heat over the whole body; redness of the face, with heavy & watery eyes; pulse quick and full, with considerable tension.

[5] Jeremiah Barker, "An Account of Febrile Diseases, as They Have Appeared in the County of Cumberland, District of Maine, from July, 1798, to March, 1800: Communicated in a Letter from Dr. Jeremiah Barker, of Portland, to Dr. Mitchill," *Medical Repository* 3, no. 4 (1800): 364–68.

In four or five days, the inflammatory action of the vessels abated, and a livid appearance was discoverable in the fauces, which became excoriated, and discharged a corrosive offensive sanies. A febrile disturbance continued until the ninth or tenth day from the attack, when a recovery or fatal termination of the disease took place.

The distemper generally proved fatal, where seasonable assistance was not employed.

Bloodletting on the first or second day to a considerable amount, according to the age of the patient & state of the fever, was evidently beneficial; and vomiting as well as purging always afforded relief. Calomel, if it produced a salivation, appeared to be productive of good effects, by unloading the glands and abating the swelling, but it did not appear to correct the virulence of the humors, or reduce the fever. Indeed it appeared to be productive of no effect, till the fever was reduced by bleeding, and this in many cases was repeated, before the mercury affected the mouth, and then, if the discharge was copious, the throat was relieved.

56

Blisters on the neck & arms produced a great discharge. The parts were very sore, and often highly inflamed. On this account, they were not attended with such good effects, when applied to the throat. Roasted onions, impregnated with oil, applied to the throat seemed to assist in abating the swelling and relieving the swallowing, when blisters to this part, often aggravated the complaints, and in some instances were followed by a gangrenous affection, which was checked by a lotion of the ley of wood ashes and covered with a plaister of hard soap. In some cases ashes was applied to advantage covered with lint.

With a view to subdue the febrile disturbance, after depletion, which I supposed was kept up by the virulence of the poisonous cause, I made a liberal use of lime water; as also a powder of sal absynth, and calcined oyster shells, together with linseed oil and flaxseed tea; often repeated.

These articles were certainly attended with salutary consequences; for where they were seasonally & duly employed, the virulence of the humors seemed evidently to be corrected; and the fever subsided. A decoction of the bark with mild bitters, ~~with~~ and nourishing food were then directed, and health was soon regained. In nearly one half of the highly inflammatory cases, the disease proved fatal; and, I believe, generally for want of seasonable assistance; for if depleting remedies were not employed on the first or second day, there was but little hopes of a favourable termination; but when they were, and the other remedies were duly administred [*sic*], the patient generally recovered.

57

In January & February 1803, the measles, which had been very prevalent in Maine, in 1802, appeared in several families in some towns, though mild; but no case occurred afterwards.[6]

During the spring, summer and autumn, of 1803, the sea port towns in Maine, were very healthy excepting a few sporadic cases of dysentery, which occurred in autumn. The scarlatina anginosa, however, prevailed in many of our inland towns, chiefly among children under puberty. This distemper made its first appearance in the western part of the district, early in the spring, at a considerable distance from the sea coast, and traversed all the counties of Maine, as far as the river St Croix[7] continuing its ravages till the close of the year; but with no great degree of mortality.[8]

I attended only a few cases in this disease, which occurred in scattered instances near the coast. I have taken pains, however, to obtain accounts of its character & treatment, from some physicians, who resided & practiced in sickly towns.

In those cases which I attended; as well as in those which were related or communicated to me, the first symptoms were loss of appetite and stomach sickness; chilliness, followed with more or less heat and pain in the head. Soon after, generally on the second day, a soreness of the throat and difficulty of swallowing took place, with a redness of the fauces, and swelling of the tonsils. A hoarse cough sometimes occurred. On the third day, white sloughs appeared in the throat; an eruption on the skin supervened, attended with a frequent & full pulse, and thirst for water. The inflammatory action of the vessels generally abated on the fifth or sixth day; but a febrile disturbance, with exacerbations & remissions, often molested the patient till the 12th or 14th day. On the 5th or 6th day, the sloughs were generally **58** thrown off, leaving ulcerations, which discharged a corrosive ichor.

---

[6] Jeremiah Barker, "An Account of the Measles, and Some Other Distempers, as They Appeared in Several Towns in the District of Maine, from January, 1802, to January, 1803. Communicated by Dr. Jeremiah Barker, of Portland," *Medical Repository* 2nd hexade, vol. 1 (1804): 125–34. Barker reported caring for 140 patients with measles in 1802 and 1803.

[7] The St. Croix River became part of the border between Maine and New Brunswick, Canada with the signing of the Treaty of Paris on September 3, 1783. Due to "an imperfect map" and involvement of several rivers, the present border was not agreed upon until the Webster-Ashburton Treaty of 1842. James S. Leamon, "Maine in the American Revolution, 1763–1787," in *Maine: The Pine Tree State from Prehistory to the Present*, ed. Richard William Judd, Edwin A. Churchill, and Joel W. Eastman (Orono: University of Maine Press, 1995), 161–62, 346–47.

[8] Jeremiah Barker, "An Account of Diseases as They Appeared in Several Parts of the District of Maine, from January, 1803, to January, 1804: Communicated in a Letter from Dr. Jeremiah Barker to Dr. Mitchill," *Medical Repository* 2nd hexade, vol. 3 (1805), 132–40.

Under these circumstances, the disease generally terminated favourably, by the seasonable use of emetics, cathartics, alkalines, oils and epispastics. But when the fever was ardent, in the first stage, with a tense pulse, the throat much inflamed, and the breathing difficult, which was generally the case, bloodletting was called into aid, and found to be very beneficial. Calomel too was employed in such cases, with a view of producing a salivation; and when this took place the inflammation in the throat evidently abated. But a second bleeding was often required before the inflammatory action of the vessels was so far reduced as to allow the mercury to operate. Vesicating the external surface with cantharides or mustard was also attended with good effects, if seasonably done.

In cases of this description, when medical aid was not called in season, the fauces soon became gangrenous, the stomach oppressed, and the abdomen tense, with labourious breathing, and a cold sweat, presaging a speedy dissolution, which generally took place.

A physician, who attended many patients in this disease, informed me, that in some cases, the fever was highly inflammatory, yet the throat was not affected; that the stomach was greatly oppressed; and that the matter thrown off by emetics & cathartics was of a green hue, and that great thirst attended.

I was also informed by another physician, that in two of his patients, in this distemper, a violent <u>tenesmus</u> took place, on the 4th day, with an eruption around the <u>anus</u>, the verge of which was beset with sloughs and eroding ulcers. These were children; one of which died.

59

A few cases which fell under my notice will be related.

Case 1.

In the autumn, I was called to a child, 18 months old, in this disease. It had sores behind the ears when invaded. These sores readily became inflamed, and discharged a corrosive ichor for several days. The throat, in this case was but slightly affected; and the febrile disturbance subsided on the 5th day, but the use of an emetic, an aqueous solution of pearl ash and occasional doses of castor oil, with a diet of water gruel. It soon recovered.

Case 2.

A girl, aged seven years, complained on the 3^d day when I was called, of sickness at the stomach, pain in the throat and head, difficulty of swallowing & thirst; pulse frequent and rather full; the tonsils were much swelled, the fauces very red and interspersed with sloughs.

The stomach and intestines were then freely evacuated, with tartar emetic & Jalap & calomel. Olive oil and an aqueous solution of alkaline salts were liberally given. An epispastic was applied to the back of the neck, extending over the tonsils, and an oily poultice to the throat. Olive oil was used externally, as well as internally, and preferred on account of its known good effects in other cases of poison. The cantharides produced great inflammation on the skin; the discharge was very copious, and in the progress of the disease attended with a very troublesome itching. On the 4th day, the inflammation in the throat abated, which together with the fever, subsided on the eighth day.

Case 3.

A girl, aged four years, complained on the 5th day, when I first saw her, of great thirst, a hoarse cough, and the breathing was laborious. The eruption had disappeared, and the abdomen was tense. The fauces appeared gangrenous; the tongue dry & livid; pulse quick & weak. She died on the 8th day.

Case 4.

A woman of a slender habit, aged 30, was seized with this disease; tho her throat was but slightly afflicted, and the **60** fever was moderate. An emetic & cathartic were given, and an eruption took place on the 3d day; but it disappeared on the 5th, when she became faint and greatly oppressed at the stomach, pulse low & feet cold. Bottles of hot water were put to the feet; a large sinapism was applied to the region of the stomach, and snakeroot tea was given with wine whey. The efflorescence returned in half an hour, with a full pulse, and desquamation soon took place. She recovered.

Case 5.

A boy, fourteen years old, of a full habit, was seized with the usual symptoms of this disease. On the 2d day he took an ounce of salts; but on the 3d day at 10 o'clock A.M. when I was called, his fauces were highly inflamed, and of a livid hue; his breathing was very difficult, and he had a dry hoarse cough; pulse full & tense. I then drew a pint of blood, which alleviated his breathing, and the fauces assumed a florid red colour. Another dose of salts with two grains of tartar emetic was given, which operated as a powerful cathartic. An epispastic was applied to the back of his neck, and two grains of calomel were given, once an hour. At six o'clock P.M. the difficulty of breathing increased, and the fauces again acquired a livid hue. Another pint of blood was then drawn, with similar good effects. Immediately after, an emetic was given, which produced six ejections & four dejections. A large sinapism was applied to the breast, which highly inflamed the skin. His complaints gradually subsided, and he recovered.

I believe, with Dr Darwin,[9] that the <u>deleterious material</u>, which produces Scarlatina, becomes mixed with the saliva, and is carried into the stomach; and I presume that all **61** the phenomena of this disease depend on the primary action of that poison, on this organ, excepting the inflammation of the tonsils, which may have arrested a part of the virus, because this disease has existed, and even proved fatal, without any morbid affection of the throat. In a fatal case of scarlatina, which I dissected in Nov. 1797, the throat was not affected; but the stomach was inflamed & disorganized.

Soon after, I attended another patient, in this disease, where the virus appeared, by the complaints to be ravaging the stomach, while the throat escaped. These complaints, however, were removed by an emetic of ipecac, and a cathartic of castor oil, followed with an aqueous solution of alkaline salts, tho not given till the 4th day. Hence I infer, that if the stomach could be duly evacuated, and alkalized, on the first day of the invasion of fever, before any considerable morbid associations should be formed, the febrile poison might generally be subdued, and the disease prevented. But this "<u>golden oppertunity</u>" is seldom afforded to physicians!

In November & December 1804, the scarlatina anginosa prevailed in several towns on the sea coast. It commenced its ravages in the western part of Maine, and progressed eastward, while most of our inland towns escaped. I attended a considerable number of patients in this disease, which, in most instances, assumed a great degree of malignancy.[10]

During the winter and spring of 1805, the distemper continued to prevail, on the sea coast, with increasing malignancy, among adults, as well as children.

62

The disease appeared under two forms or states; the one was highly inflammatory, unattended with exanthemata or any apparent virulency of

---

[9] Dr. Erasmus Darwin (1731–1802) of Litchfield, England, was Charles Darwin's grandfather. See Erasmus Darwin, *Zoonomia, or the Laws of Organic Life*, Vol. 1 (New York: T. and J. Swords, 1796), Genus 3 number 11 on scarlatina.

[10] Jeremiah Barker, "An Account of the Weather and Diseases in the County of Cumberland, District of Maine, from January, 1804, to January, 1805: Communicated in a Letter from Jeremiah Barker, M. D. Of Portland, to Dr. Mitchill," *Medical Repository* 2nd hexade, vol. 4 (1807): 137–40.

the humours. In some of those cases the swelling of the throat was so great that deglutition and speech were almost entirely prevented, at times; in a few instances wholly suspended; pulse frequent, small & hard. Cases of this description made up about one third of my patients, which were generally adults.

Under these circumstances bloodletting, emetics, cathartics, blisters, and a mercurial salivation were attended with salutary effects, when seasonably employed, otherwise the disease generally proved fatal.

When depleting means were sparingly used, as was some times the case, indeed too often, in my own practice, glandular swellings on the neck frequently took place, which terminated in suppuration. I opened several of these tumours of about a weeks duration. The matter discharged was of a bottle green hue, and very fœtid. In others, the body & limbs swelled, as in anasarca. This complaint generally yielded to mercurial purges, digitalis and friction with olive oil. Blisters on the legs were also useful. But when the lancet was seasonably & duly used, with other depleting means, these morbid affections, to my knowledge, did not occur.

In Jan. 1805, Susan Bond of Falmouth, where ~~the disease~~ many sickened, aged 17 years, was attacked with this disease.[11] I was called on the 2^d day, at night, when she complained of pain in the head with universal heat, pulse frequent and hard. Her throat was highly inflamed, and the tonsils much swelled. She could not be prevailed on to be bled. An emetic & cathartic, however, were given, and two grains of calomel every hour till the 4th day. A **63** blister was also applied to the back of the neck, and an oily poultice to the throat. At this time, she was speechless, and could not swallow. She then consented to be bled. A pint of blood was drawn from a large orifice, which was sizy & buffy. This afforded great relief, and she could soon swallow. In a few hours, a copious salivation took place, and her speech returned. The salivation continued about one week, when her complaints were in a great measure removed, and she soon recovered. Many adults were invaded in a very similar manner, and when seasonably bled & salivated, they recovered.

The other form of the disease exhibited all the symptoms described by Drs Huxham & Fothergill. It was confined chiefly to children under 14 years old.

---

[11] Susan Bond, possibly a daughter of merchant William Bond of Portland, and thus one of the four "free white females" in the home listed in United States. Bureau of the Census, *Heads of Families at the First Census of the United States Taken in the Year 1790: Maine* (Spartansburg, SC: The Reprint Company, originally printed by the Government Printing Office, Washington, 1908, 1978), 24.

In most cases a corrosive ichor was discharged from the nose, and sometimes from the ears, which inflamed & excoriated the parts adjacent. Epispastics produced unusual inflammation & exulcerations; so that they were commonly applied to the extremities; and roasted onions with oil to the throat.

In the treatment of this form of the disease, I dispensed with bleeding in the three first cases, suddenly attacked in one family, from six to ten years of age, by the advice of a consulting physician, on account of the supposed putrid nature of the disease; accordingly, tonics or antisceptics, [*sic*] as they were called, were used externally & internally after evacuating the stomach & bowels. But they all died, gangreniously [*sic*] affected. After this I let blood to the amount of half a pint, in children 8 or 10 years old; sometimes it was repeated, tho the pulse was small, yet frequent. The blood in some was sizy & buffy; in others, it was of a loose texture and dissolved. This last appearance, was considered, by some, as a symptom of putridity, not indicating the use of the lancet, or even mercury, lest they should further dissolve the blood, and increase ~~putridity~~ putrescency.

Modern physicians,[x] however, have corrected these views, and maintain, from indubitable experiments, that putrefaction never takes place in the blood of living animals; also that gangrene is an effect of inflammation.

"Dissolved blood, says D[r]. Rush, in the first stage of fever, indicates a repetition of the lancet. Of this I have had frequent experience since the year 1793."

Med. observations.[12]

[x]Seybert, Moore, Lind, &c.[13]

64

After bleeding, according to the urgency of the symptoms, I evacuated and alkalized the stomach & intestines. An aqueous solution of alkaline salts

---

[12] Benjamin Rush, *Medical Inquiries and Observations*, 2nd ed., 4 vols. (Philadelphia: J. Conrad & Co., 1805), vol. 4, 325–27.

[13] Adam Seybert (1773–1825), born in Philadelphia, studied under Casper Wistar and graduated from the medical department of the University of Pennsylvania in 1793. He was a physician, chemist, and statesman who served in the US Congress from 1809 to 1815 and 1817 to 1819. Howard A. Kelly and Walter L. Burrage, *American Medical Biographies* (Baltimore: The Norman, Remington Company, 1920), 1037–38; Adam Seybert, *An Inaugural Dissertation: Being an Attempt to Disprove the Doctrine of the Putrefaction of the Blood of Living Animals* (Philadelphia: T. Dobson, 1793). Probably John Moore (1729–1802), John Moore, *Medical Sketches: In Two Parts* (London: A. Strahan and T. Cadell, 1786). James Lind (1736–1812), James Lind, *A Treatise on the Putrid and Remitting Marsh Fever, Which Raged at Bengal* (Edinburgh, C. Elliot, 1776); James Lind, *Essay on Diseases Incidental to Europeans in Hot Climates with the Method of Preventing Their Fatal Consequences*, 5th ed. (London: J. Murray, 1792).

was liberally given and often repeated with a view of correcting the virulency of the humors, and of preventing, or stopping the progress of putrefaction in the alimentary canal, and removing the fœtor, which always attended this disease. Calomel was given in small doses, with a view of producing a salivation, which was easily effected, when bloodletting was premised, and this always relieved the throat, in proportion to the soreness excited in the mouth. An epispastic on the neck was productive of similar effects, by inflaming the skin. Soap dissolved in lime water was used to advantage as a lotion for excoriations of the virus, and epispastics.

This appeared evidently to correct the virulency of the humors. A mixture of olive oil with lime water was used internally to advantage in excoriations of the throat and morbid affection of the stomach produced by swallowing the matter generated from ulcers in the fauces; and it appeared evidently to be productive of as good effects as it is known to produce in burns and scalds.

A diarrhœa sometimes took place about the 5. or 6th day which caused a sudden retrocession of the exanthemata. I lost one patient thus circumstanced. On this account I omitted cathartics in the eruptive state, and occasionally used oily glysters. I frequently rubbed calomel with pearl ash in water, which being decanted, left the calomel possessed of a salivating, but not of a cathartic power. This was suggested to me, by Dr Shirley Erving of Portland,[14] who was in the habit of using it, in this way. He also used lime water and alkaline salts, particularly sal sodæ in this distemper, and had a high opinion of their efficacy, as correctors and febrifuges.

65

When the above mode of practice was regularly pursued, the fever subsided without any alarming gangrenous affection, and the patients generally recovered.

It was remarked that several who had passed through the highly inflammatory form of this disease; were some weeks after, invaded with the exanthematous form; and the contrary. It was also observed that bleeding, in the eruptive state, did not tend to produce a retrocession of the virulent

---

[14] Dr. Shirley Erving (1758–1813) was born in Boston, attended Boston Latin, and entered Harvard College in 1773, but left when the war began. He studied medicine with Dr. James Lloyd of Boston, continued his training in Europe, and in 1789 moved to Portland, where he practiced and was connected with "an apothecary establishment." He returned to Boston in 1811. William Willis, *The History of Portland*, facsimile ed. (Somersworth, New Hampshire Publishing Company and Maine Historical Society, 1972; Portland: Bailely & Noyes, 1865), 803–804.

efflorescence; but rather facilitated its expulsion, and the desquamation. Since this eventful time, diseases of this kind, have not, to my knowledge, appeared in the District or State of Maine.[15]

From 1795, to 1806, while epidemic fevers prevailed in Maine, the hooping cough was of frequent occurrence, chiefly among children, and generally more obstinate than in preceeding years. The distemper has seldom appeared in this State, to my knowledge, since 1805.

In 1801, when this disease was very prevalent and attended with febrile disturbance, a number of children died, and others recovered with great difficulty. Physicians were rarely consulted for the means commonly used offered but little relief. They consisted chiefly of emetics, cathartics, demulcents & opiates.

The nature of the disease was not understood; and it was considered, by many, beyond the reach of medical skill; so that it proved fatal in many instances, under convulsive tortures.

"The hooping cough, says D[r] Gamage,[16] seems to have been less understood, than any other disease of so common occurrence. It is but **66** recently, that any attempt has been made to ascertain the true character & seat of this distemper."

"D[r] Watt of Glasgow,[17] has lately obliged the profession and society with a very able work on this subject, and this appears to be the first attempt of a philosophical investigation of the disease. He lost two of his own children, by this disease, which were examined after death; and the disorder was found to be of the class of inflammatory complaints. He was, therefore, led to adopt a mode of practice different from that in common estimation. This consisted in a more liberal use of the lancet, from which he experienced the happiest of consequences."

---

[15] This paragraph was written sometime around March 15, 1820, the official date when Maine separated from Massachusetts and the District of Maine became the State of Maine.

[16] William Gamage, "On the Hooping Cough," *New England Journal of Medicine and Surgery* 6, no. 3 (1817): 213–28.

[17] Robert E. Watt (1774–1819), physician to the Royal Infirmary of Glasgow, published Robert E. Watt, *Treatise on the History, Nature, and Treatment of Chincough: Including a Variety of Cases and Dissections. To Which Is Subjoined and Inquiry into the Relative Mortality of the Principal Diseases of Children, and the Numbers Who Have Died under Ten Years of Age, in Glasgow, during the Last Thirty Years* (Glasgow: John Smith & Son, 1813). The etymology of the word "chincough," or whooping cough, is discussed in Watt's book; other names include "kinkcough (term used in Scotland) and the Latin "pertussus" used by Sydenham, Huxham, and Cullen. See Watt, *Treatise On . . . Chincough*, 17–21. See also John H. Talbott, *A Biographical History of Medicine* (New York: Grune & Stratton, 1970), 475–77.

"Dissections have shown that the seat of this disease, is in the mucous membrane of the trachea & bronchia. As to its essence, we shall remain, probably, in the dark. All that we are able to discover, are the effects of inflammation; and to this cause, we must attribute all that is either distressing or dangerous in the disease. Inflammation is uniformly present, and makes an essential part of the disease; and, like other inflammatory diseases, the hazard is in proportion to the degree of inflammation and its extensiveness. Such means, therefore, should be used as are most effectual in reducing inflammation. Among these, bloodletting holds the first **67** place, and it should be used without delay. It often happens that a first bleeding effects no apparent benefit, when a second or a third accomplishes the object."

"I have, on record, ten cases of hooping cough, whose symptoms, tho violent, were rendered mild by a simple bleeding, where emetics &c afforded no relief. The subjects were from four to ten years of age, and the quantity taken from each, was from four to eight ounces of blood. In some cases, bloodletting was repeated. A lad six years old, had a pain in the side, and was bled three times; six ounces at first and four twice after. He recovered. Next to bloodletting, antimonial emetics and cathartics of calomel afford the most efficient means."

See New England Journal.[18]

In the course of my practice, in the County of Barnstable, from 1774, to 1780, I met with a considerable number of cases of Quinsy or Croup, a kindred disease. But I never made use of the lancet, neither did I even hear of its being used, by any of my brethren, in this disease. The means generally employed, were emetics of tart antim. and cathartics of Jalap & calomel, squills and blisters. The disease generally proved fatal, sometimes in 24 hours from the attack. The tonsils were often swelled to such a degree, that swallowing was greatly impeded, and they appeared to be much inflamed.

In 1780, when I removed into the District of Maine, and in succeeding years, I have found that the Croup was more frequent among children than on **68** Cape Cod, tho seldom with much swelling of the tonsils. In Maine, I found that bleeding was practiced, by some physicians, followed by emetics, particularly of turpeth mineral. Blisters were applied to the throat; and mercurial cathartics were given; also oximel of squills was freely used. When these means were seasonably and duly employed many recovered. But medical aid

[18] Gamage, "On the Hooping Cough," 213–28.

was often neglected till the disease was so far advanced, that the means were ineffectual. Indeed the nature of the disease was not well understood, as no examinations were made after death.

Professor Hosack, of N. York, divides croup into three stages, viz. the first or forming stage, where the disease is merely local; the second, or inflammatory stage, where the constitution sympathises with the local affection; the third, or post febrile, in which effusion has taken place, forming a false membrane.[19]

"If we see the child, says Dr Sweetser, before the last stage, except perhaps very early in the first, we should always commence the treatment with general bloodletting; and the Jugular vein is the most eligible. In the first stage, it will not always be requisite to employ bleeding to the same extent, as when general inflammation is present. But if the child is roburst [*sic*] & plethoric, and the difficulty of breathing considerable, we should let blood, pretty freely. When general inflammation supervenes, with great difficulty of breathing, we ought to bleed till fainting is induced, which is the principal means to be depended upon, taken from a large vein and large orifice. In a child from two to six years old, from five to eight ounces at once, or more, according to existing circumstances. When an emetic is given in the very onset of the disease, within a few hours, it is generally sufficient to restore to the diseased parts their healthy action, and effect a cure or lay a foundation for the cure.

69

In the last stage, when effusion has taken place, expectorants are indicated by emetics of blue vitriol at short intervals; supporting the powers of life by suitable nutriment. I have found a decoction of seneka the most powerful medicine, says D^r. Archer, in croup, but it should only be used in the last stage.

---

[19] David Hosack (1769–1835), physician, surgeon, and teacher in New York City, taught at Columbia College of Physicians and Surgeons and helped to found the Rutgers Medical School and Bellevue Hospital in 1820. Hosack was the physician who attended Alexander Hamilton at his duel with Aaron Burr at Weehawken, New Jersey, in 1804. He wrote a number of papers and started and edited (with John W. Francis) the *Medical and Philosophical Register* in 1810. See Kelly and Burrage, *American Medical Biographies*, 561–62. For his stages of croup, see David Hosack, *The Modern Practice of Physic, Exhibiting the Characters, Causes, Symptoms, Prognostics, Morbid Appearances, and Improved Method of Treating the Diseases of All Climates*, the 4th American from the 5th London ed. (New York: Collins & Company, 1817), 887. Though he was writing about "croup, he was likely dealing with diphtheria when describing the "false membrane." See previous notes on diphtheria. Reference to Hosack's stages is found in James Thacher, *American Modern Practice* (Boston: Ezra Read, 1817), 242.

Bronchotomy has succeeded, in some cases when the common remedies fail, or when called at a late period.

Prize dissertation: 1820.[20]

"In some fatal cases of croup, says Professor Jackson, which I have examined, the mucous membrane of the larynx has been found highly inflamed; but without any false membrane or lining of coagulable lymph."

In a late case of croup, a child fifteen month old was bled to the amount of six ounces from the external Jugular vein, 24 hours from the attack. A very long continued faintness ensued. In a few hours the respiration altered, and was nearly natural in twelve hours after bleeding. The child recovered.

N. E. Journal. [1813].[21]

"Bleeding, says Dr Gamage, is now recommended by most authors as a remedy for croup. But most direct it in quantities so small, as to do no good. In every case which I have seen, violent inflammation was present."

"On examining the body of a child four years, old, who died of this disease, the mucous membrane of the larynx & epiglottis shew marks of being highly inflamed. At the beginning of the trachea, a factitious membrane began and lined the whole trachea and bronchial branches. The redness was evident through the trachea."

Boston March 1816.[22]

"The application of Leeches, says Dr Hamilton of Edinburgh, is followed by a considerable flow of blood; but this discharge is so tardy, that it does not

---

[20] William Sweetser (1797–1875) was born in Boston and practiced in Boston; Burlington, Vermont; and New York City. He was professor of medicine at the University of Vermont from 1825 to 1832 and held the same chair at Bowdoin College from 1845 to 1861; he also taught at other schools. Sweetser was awarded the Boylston prize in 1820. William Sweetser, *Dissertations on Cynache Trachealis or Croup and on the Functions of the Extreme Capillary Vessels in Health and Disease; to Which Were Awarded the Boylston Premiums for the Years 1820 and 1823* (Boston: Cummins, Hilliard & Co., 1823), 3–62.

[21] J Jackson, "On Croup," *New England Journal of Medicine and Surgery* 1 (1812): 383–84.

[22] William Gamage (1780–1818). William Gamage, "Cases of Croup," *The New England Journal of Medicine, Surgery and Collateral Branches of Science* 6, no. 1 (1817): 24–29; W. J. Gamage, *Some Account of the Fever Which Existed in Boston during the Autumn and Winter of 1817–18. With a Few Remarks on Typhus* (Boston: Wells & Lilly, 1818). A copy with his comments and cases is with the Barker Collection 13, Box 2/4 at Maine Historical Society. This was originally "intended and prepared for the New-England journal of medicine and surgery."—See Robert B. Austin, *Early American Medical Imprints: 1668–1820* (Arlington, MA: The Printers' Devil, 1961), no. 810. See also Gamage, "On the Hooping Cough."

often check the progress of the disease. The lancet, therefore ought always to be first used; and the external Jugular is the proper vein to be opened. Leeches may be employed as auxiliaries." Obser. On Croup. 1821. [23]

70

We find no account of a false membrane, in this, nor the preceeding favorable case; for, as it is an effect of violent inflammation, its formation was prevented by sufficient bleeding. When this has not been practiced, a false membrane is often formed, which renders the case much more hazardous. Various means have been successfully used to dislodge and eject this substance from the trachea. Turpeth mineral, in small doses, with oxymel of squills, and a decoction of Seneka have often proved effectual.

D[r] Reddelin of Wismar, relates a case of a child 19 months old, who, on the third day of this disease, could not swallow, and rattled in the throat, when he insinuated a mixture of Spanish snuff and marocco[24] into the nostrils, by means of a quill, which excited sneezing & vomiting. This occasioned the discharge of two long membraneous cylinders from the trachea, and the child recovered.

"Professor Recamier of Paris has recently succeeded in curing three cases of croup which threatened suffocation, by means of the injection of milk & water, by the mouth & nose, at the same time, so as to excite violent convulsions of the throat and muscles of the larynx. In all these cases, portions of false membrane were expelled." This must be in the 3[d] stage.[25]

With regard to the choice of emetics in croup, turpeth mineral has been considered by experienced physicians, the most efficacious, for more than half

---

[23] Alexander Hamilton, *A Treatise on the Management of Female Complaints, and of Children in Early Infancy, 8th ed., revised and enlarged; with hints for the treatment of the principal diseases of infants and children. By Dr. James Hamilton, Junior . . . ed.* (Edinburgh: Edinburgh, Printed for Peter Hill & Company; and sold by Longman, Hurst, Rees, Orme, and Brown, and T. & G. Underwood, London, 1821). Edinburgh's Alexander Hamilton (1739–1802) wrote this treatise that went through at least five editions and was printed in Edinburgh and the United States. See also Gamage, "On the Hooping Cough," 213–28.

[24] Spanish snuff consists of *Nicotiana tabacum*, tobacco leaves that were introduced from the New World to Europe by Spanish explorers soon after 1492; see glossary. Arnold James Cooley, *A Cyclopaedia of Practical Receipts, and Collateral Information in the Arts, Manufactures, and Trades, Including Medicine, Pharmacy, and Domestic Economy* (London: J. Churchill, 1845), 712. Morocco was a source of snuff from the seventeenth century onward. Richard Reece, "Croup . . . Dr. R. Reddelin of Wismar," *The Monthly Gazette of Health* 7 (4th ed.) (1822): 274.

[25] Professor Recamier, "New Treatment of Croup," *New England Journal of Medicine and Surgery* 13 (1824): 103. Joseph-Claude-Anthelme Recamier, "New Treatment of Croup," *London Medical and Physical Journal* 1 (July to December 1823): 258. He was chief physician at the Hotel-Dieu in Paris since 1806.

a century. I well remember that between 1760, & 70. Drs Otis & Stockbridge of Scituate Mass^{tts}. successfully used this mean in croup.[26] It has also been preferred to any other, by Dr Fisher of Beverly, who informed me, a few years since, that he never lost a patient in croup, and always used turpeth mineral as an emetic & alterative. About two grains was the usual dose as an emetic for a child two years old, and from half a grain to a grain, as an alterative, once an hour or oftener, according to existing circumstances.

71

In the course of my practice, in Maine, I have often been called to children in the first stage of croup, and found that an emetic of turpeth mineral would readily remove the disease. But much oftener in the second stage, when the inflammation was so violent, that no means were effectual. Bleeding, however, followed with an emetic of turpeth mineral and alterative doses, were sometimes successfully used, together with cathartics of Jalap & calomel, blisters and squills.

In the third stage, small & often repeated doses of the turpeth, with a decoction of Seneka, have, in some instances, proved effectual, by ejecting a factitious membrane.

This preparation of mercury produces its salutary effects in small doses, and acts readily on the parts affected, with the greatest safety; whereas calomel is slow in its operation; and such large, as well as repeated doses are required to produce the desired effect, as sometimes prove injurious, as has been noticed by Dr Ives[27] and others.

---

[26] Charles Stockbridge was one of the charter members of the Massachusetts Medical Society when it was incorporated in 1781. Walter L. Burrage, *A History of the Massachusetts Medical Society* (Norwood, MA: Plimpton Press, 1923), 16. "Dr. Otis" may refer to James Otis (1734–1807), who began practice in Scituate, Massachusetts, in 1760, but more likely his father, Dr. Isaac Otis, whose practice began in 1719, since Barker was talking about a half a century of efficacy of turpeth mineral in croup. Samuel Deane, *History of Scituate, Massachusetts, from Its First Settlement to 1831* (Boston: J. Loring, 1831), 114, 318.

[27] Ansell W. Ives (1787–1838) was born in Woodbury, Connecticut, studied under physicians such as Elisha North and Valentine Mott, and then graduated from the College of Physicians and Surgeons of Columbia University in 1814. Ives republished with notes and additions, James Hamilton and Ansel W. Ives, *Observations on the Use and Abuse of Mercurial Medicines in Various Diseases and an Appendix by Ansel W. Ives* (New York: Bliss & White, 1821). Kelly and Burrage, *American Medical Biographies*, 594–95, and Stephen W. Williams, *American Medical Biography; or, Memoirs of Eminent Physicians, Embracing Principally Those Who Have Died since the Publication of Dr. Thacher's Work on the Same Subject* (Greenfield, MA, 1845: [Millford House, Inc. Reprint, 1967], 1845), 304–307.

In many other diseases, calomel is considered more eligible, especially if a salivation is desirable; and in some cases, corrosive sublimate and mercurial ointment are allowed to be preferable to either.

72

"There is no disease, says Dr Ives, the nature & treatment of which is more settled, in the United States, than Croup. It is known to be of a highly inflammatory character and very rapid in its progress & termination. When encountered in the attack it is almost certainly subject to medical control, but as certainly fatal if left to itself or improperly treated. The customary mode of treatment is in perfect conformity to this view of the disease, viz. by emetics, copious bloodletting, active cathartics, blisters, warm bath, &c. Emetics are first mentioned because they are generally prescribed on the invasion of the disease; for at that period it generally appears to be entirely local, and, whether, at this time it depends on spasm or inflammation, it is commonly arrested by an emetic before symptomatic fever ensues.

With regard to the use of calomel in croup, it is now, so far as my information extends, only employed as an auxiliary. Indeed I know not that it has ever been regarded, in this country, in any other light. Mercury was used, combined with other medicines, in this disease, in New England, as early as the middle of the last century, and Dr Rush, in an essay on Cynanche Trachealis, written more than twenty years ago, advised the use of calomel after bloodletting, vomits & purging. At the present time calomel is also in general use, when the disease is protracted and dangerous."[28]

"My own child, aged twenty months, was attacked with this disease, the last winter, in the afternoon, having slept some hours in a room where the floor was wet. At ten o'clock he awoke with a dry shrill cough, wheezing & difficult respiration. Gave him instantly half an ounce of ol. oliv. without any relief. In ten minutes gave a dose of antim. tart. solution which operated in fifteen minutes, and continued to puke, at short intervals, till 12 o'clock, when he was much exhausted, but not perfectly relieved. At two o'clock gave ten grains of calomel, which operated freely as a cathartic, after quiet sleep, when the cough & difficulty of breathing returned, the **73** surface became heated with a frequent hard pulse. He was constantly nauseated with antimony. At twelve o'clock he took twelve ounces of blood from a large orifice in the Jugular vein, a large blister was applied to his throat. He was partially relieved for two or three hours, when all its symptoms began to increase. He

---

[28] Benjamin Rush, *Medical Inquiries and Observations*, 4th ed., 4 vols. (Philadelphia: Johnson & Warner, 1815), vol. 2, 225–28.

was then put into the warm bath, and the antimonial solution continued till he vomited. At five o'clock he lost two or three ounces of blood from the same orifice, and his bowels were opened by an injection. Eight o'clock, same evening, the cough still sonorous, breathing difficult and the pulse wiry. Eight ounces of blood were then taken from the temporal artery, which induced complete syncope. From this time, from three to five grains of calomel, were given every three hours; symptoms much abated during the night. The next morning the difficulty of breathing and symptomatic fever increased notwithstanding the continued use of nauseating medicines, and the evacuations produced by the calomel from the bowels. At 11 o'clock A.M. pulse hard and one hundred & thirty in a minute, and the skin still flushed. From six to eight ounces of blood were then taken from the temporal artery, which again induced fainting. At twelve o'clock began to give three doses of Tinc. Digitalis every two hours, and at four o'clock P. M. the bath was repeated. The circulation became less rapid, and heat more natural; has frequent evacuations of green matter from the bowels; the calomel is continued, and, during the night gave alternately the antimony & digitalis. The next morning, the third day of the disease, gave a strong decoction of Polygalia Senega so as to cause vomiting, continuing the calomel. He is rapidly convalescing. In one week from the attack he was walking about the room after having lost in less than twenty four hours, about thirty ounces of blood, and taken in three days from ninety to one hundred grains of calomel. Perfect health was soon restored."

74

[Crossed out page]: ~~Some years since, a child of Mr Samual Sands of Buxton, was attacked with croup, aged three years. I was called on the second day, when the breathing was very distressing, with a hoarse cough; pulse quick & small. I drew half a pint of blood from his arm which produced paleness, and the breathing was relieved, but the hoarse cough continued. Twelve grains of calomel were then given, which operated several times, as an emetic and cathartic. The next day, it was almost free from cough & hoarseness, tho no expectoration took place, neither did it appear that a factitious membrane had formed; for the child soon recovered. Hence I conceive that if the inflammation is removed by a membrane has formed, bloodletting being premised, Turpeth mineral, squills & seneka are considered as the most eligible expectorants.~~

~~Dr John Archer of Maryland used mercury in the advanced stage of croup, freely & frequently, in order to assist the operation of seneka in separating the membrane.~~

Dr James Anderson of Edinburgh has given eighteen grains of calomel in 24 hours, to children of three years old, in doses of two or three grains every hour, and in one urgent case, of a child four years old, forty five grains in 50 hours. In seven cases thus treated, not one died.

It is remarkable that a liberal use of mercury in young children, very seldom produces a salivation, and never infuses the stomach or bowels, unless these organs are inflamed.

"I have never known an infant to be salivated, says Dr John Warren of Boston, notwithstanding I have given, in some instances, large quantities with this view.

Perhaps the means, with which the primæ viæ is apt to be lived at this age, may prevent the medicine from entering the lacteals. And I have reason to think that its action of the intestines is also weakened by this cause, so that some more active cathartic is generally combined, in order to insure its operation." View of Mercurial Practice.

From this view of things, we may easily account for the beneficial effects of emetics & cathartics, in diseases of children; as well as of alkaline salts and earths, in order to remove accumulated mucus, and correct acidity which so often abound, instead of ardent spirits, which are so commonly used in infantile diseases, to the destruction of health and often of life.

75

Chap. 6.

IN MARCH 1781, I was called to the Rev. Ephraim Clark[1] of Cape Elizabeth, aged 55, labouring under pneumonia, which required two bleedings, &c. He was a powerful Evangelical preacher, and had so infused his lungs by loud speaking that, for several years past, he had been troubled with a catarrhal cough, and suffered frequent attacks of pulmonic inflammation, which always yielded to bleeding. He continued, however, to preach till the age of 75, when he died of a pulmonic fever.

He was well acquainted with the use of the lancet, and always carried it with him; so that in his parochial visits, he often found it useful, as his people were in the habit of being bled, not only in sickness; but in health, as a preventive of disease, particularly in the spring months. By this means excessive action in the bloodvessels was prevented and as the summer approached, they performed their labour with ease & activity, more free from inflammatory affections.

As I had the chief of the practice in that town from 1786, to 1812, opperotunities were afforded of observing their mode of living, diseases &c. Farming & fishing were their chief employment. They were in general temperate in eating & drinking; so that inflammatory fevers were of rare occurrence. Indeed the inhabitants were so healthy that no physician could find sufficient encouragement to tarry long among them, altho the town contained in 1810, 1415 souls. In the course of my practice in Maine, I noticed more aged people in that town, than in any other, where people were much more numerous. Many lived to the age of 90 and upwards. Among these females made up the greater part, who had lived very abstemiously; and many of the

---

[1] The Rev. Ephraim Clark (1722–1797) was minister of the Second Parish Church in Cape Elizabeth, Maine, from 1756 until his death on December 11, 1797. A protracted religious controversy marked the early years of his service. He served as an army chaplain during the Revolutionary War in Cambridge, Massachusetts, in 1776 and was on the Bagaduce Expedition at Castine in the summer of 1779. William B. Jordan, *A History of Cape Elizabeth, Maine* (Portland, ME: House of Falmouth, Inc., 1955), 290–95.

most aged had always been poor & needy, tho blessed with health and length of days.

76

I met with a healthy middle aged woman, on the cape, who informed me that she had been bled more than twenty times, in the course of her life, chiefly as a preventive of disease. She lived to a great age, and was by no means singular in this depleting mode of conduct.

It was said by some, who had been among the Aboriginals, that bleeding was frequently practiced by them, not only in disease, but in the healthy state. This has been verified by Alexander Henry Esq. of New York, in his "Travels in Canada and the Indian territories, between the years of 1760 and 1776."[2]

"The Indians, he says, are in general free from diseases, and an instance of their being subject to dropsy, gout or stone, never came within my knowledge. Inflammations of the lungs are among their most ordinary complaints, and rheumatism still more so; especially with the aged. Their mode of life, in which they are so much exposed to the wet & cold, sleeping on the ground, and inhaling to night air, sufficiently accounts from their liability to these diseases. The remedies on which they most rely, are emetics, cathartics and the lancet; but especially the last. Bleeding is so favourable an operation among the women, that they never loose an oppertunity of enjoying it, whether sick or well. I have sometimes bled a dozen women, in a morning, as they sat in a row along a fallen tree.

In most villages, particularly in those of the Chippeway's, this service was required of me, and no persuasion of mine could ever induce a woman to dispense with it." Henry's Travels.[3]

Pulmonary consumption rarely occurred in Cape Elizabeth. Perhaps their mode of living and frequent depletion tended to prevent pulmonary affections.

77

Slow fevers sometimes occurred in that town in autumn, tho with little or no nervous affection.[4] Bleeding was very seldom neglected in the onset

---

[2] Alexander Henry, *Travels and Adventures in Canada and the Indian Territories between the Years 1760–1776* (New York: I. Riley, 1809). Alexander Henry (1739–1824) was a fur trader and merchant who spent a great deal of time with the Indians and traveling back and forth between Michigan and Montreal. John A. Garraty and Mark C. Carnes, *American National Biography* (New York: Oxford University Press, 1999), vol. 10, 604–605.

[3] Henry, *Travels and Adventures in Canada and the Indian Territories between the Years 1760–1776.*

[4] As mentioned earlier, slow fever may have been what we would today call typhoid fever. The word "typhoid," meaning "typhus-like," was used from the seventeenth century, but it was not

of the fever, which commonly terminated in 14 days, and the patient readily recovered. I attended a woman, in this fever, aged 90 years, whose pulse was intermitting. Twelve ounces of blood were drawn, and the intermission ceased. The fever subsided in 14 days, by the conjoint aid of other depleting means, without nervous affection; and she enjoyed comfortable health, nine years longer, on a diet chiefly of milk and farinaceous substances.

In other towns where the mode of living, fashions, customs and employments of people were different, inflammatory diseases of various kinds, were of more frequent occurrence.

In April 1782, Robert Higgins[5] of Standish, aged 16 years, who was employed in tending a saw mill by night, as well as by day, where spiritous liquors are freely used, was seized with <u>hemiplegia</u>. He remained in this condition, unable to move his arm & leg of the palsied side, about three weeks before I was called. Having no other idea of the nature of the disease, than a stagnation of fluids in the small vessels of the affected parts, I drew a pint of blood from the ~~affected~~ paralytic arm and evacuated his bowels with aloes.[6] Three days after, on a second visit, finding his affected limbs equally motionless, I drew another pint of blood, and being much engaged in practice, directed Capt More, a neighbour, who could use a lancet, to draw half a pint of blood from the arm or foot, once in three days, and to give a dose of aloes as often till some change should be produced. **78** After fifteen bleedings and as many cathartics of aloes, the palsy was removed and his limbs were readily restored to their usual activity.[7]

---

until the mid-nineteenth century that the disease typhus was clinically separated from the disease typhoid. This was years before the organism, Salmonella, was isolated. John Huxham, *An Essay on Fevers with Introduction by Saul Jarcho* (Canton, MA: Science History Publications [reprint 1988], 1757), xiv, 40–49; C. S. Bryan, S. W. Moss, and R. J. Kahn, "Yellow Fever in the Americas," *Infectious Disease Clinics of North America* 18, no. 2 (2004): 275–92.

[5] Robert Higgins (1769–1844) was born in Standish, Maine, married Sarah Whitney of Gorham January 21, 1790, and died April 21, 1844 at seventy-five years of age. See Hugh D. Mc Lellan, *History of Gorham, Maine* (Portland: Smith and Sale, 1903), 831.

[6] Physicians were aware that brain trauma and bleeding can cause palsy or hemiplegia, especially when associated with mental status changes and generally in older individuals. This teenager apparently did not have changes in mental function or Barker would have written so; thus the case was more difficult to explain and treat. James Thacher, *American Modern Practice* (Boston: Ezra Read, 1817), 542–45; William Cullen, *First Lines of the Practice of Physic with Supplementary Notes, Including More Recent Improvements in the Practice of Medicine by Peter Reid*, two volumes in one (Brookfield: E. Mirriam & Co. for Isaiah Thomas, 1807), 404–13.

[7] A brief look at the state of neurology in 1780 might be helpful to put Barker's treatment in perspective. Emanuel Swedenborg (1688–1772) noted different functions for different cerebral loci, thus suggesting that damage to one part of the brain might cause paralysis; however, his work remained unnoticed until the 1880s. Stanley Finger, "Chapter 10: The Birth of Localization

Here I would observe that in my hurry of business, I never enquired nor was informed of the termination of this case, till July 1807, when Mr Higgins came to my house in Falmouth, and informed me that a few days previously, while mowing grass in the heat of the day, he was seized with a paralytic affection of his left arm, and that Dr How[8] had drawn off a pint of blood, which afforded some relief. He wished, however, that I would furnish him with such means as he took when I was called to him in 1782. —I then enquired how his case terminated at that time, and he gave me the information of his being bled and evacuated, as above related, when he was restored to health, which had continued till the present attack. I furnished him with some aloes, and directed another bleeding. His complaint was removed, and he is now in the enjoyment of health, a laborious farmer.

A knowledge of the termination of this case brought a number of disagreeable reflections to my mind; for, a few years after this occurrence, I met with Dr John Browns "Elements of Medicine,"[9] in which I found that palsy

---

Theory," in *Handbook of Clinical Neurology*, ed. Michael J. Aminoff, François Boller, and Dick F. Swaab (Amsterdam, Elsevier, 2009), 117–18; Fielding H. Garrison and Lawrence C. McHenry, *History of Neurology. Rev. and Enl. With a Bibliography of Classical, Original and Standard Works in Neurology, by Lawrence C. McHenry, Jr* (Springfield, IL: Thomas, 1969); John H. Talbott, *A Biographical History of Medicine* (New York: Grune & Stratton, 1970), 202–204. Boerhaave in Leyden, who taught William Cullen, so important in the education and philosophy of Benjamin Rush and of Barker, "was instrumental in getting Swammerdam's" work published. Christopher U. M. Smith, "Chapter 9: Understanding the Nervous System in the 18th Century," in *Handbook of Clinical Neurology*, ed. Michael J. Aminoff, François Boller, and Dick F. Swaab (Amsterdam, Elsevier, 2009), 107–108. Galenic doctrine of neurology involved the inhalation of external air, which becomes a vital spirit in the heart and is transferred to the brain, where the cerebral ventricles transfer the animal spirits to the nerves, which were considered hollow tubes until the work of Antony van Leeuwenhoek (1632–1723) and others. The contributions of people like Leonardo da Vinci (1452–1519), Andreas Vesalius (1514–1664), Thomas Willis (1621–1675), Marcello Malpighi (1628–1694), John Hunter (1728–1793), Paul Broca (1824–1880), and many others, were important in the evolution of our understanding of the neurological system in health and disease. For further details of the eighteenth-century understanding of neurology, see Smith, "Chapter 9: Understanding the Nervous System in the 18th Century," 107–14; Finger, "Chapter 10: The Birth of Localization Theory," 117–28; and Marina Bentivoglio and Paolo Mazzarello, "Chapter 12: The Anatomical Foundations of Clinical Neurology," in *Handbook of Clinical Neurology*, ed. Michael J. Aminoff, François Boller, and Dick F. Swaab (Amsterdam, Elsevier, 2009), 149–68; Garrison and McHenry, *History of Neurology. Rev. and Enl.*, 91–136.

[8] Dr. Ebenezer Howe (April 21, 1773–June 4, 1841) was born in Sturbridge, Massachusetts, and moved to and practiced in Standish, Maine. He was the second doctor to practice there, having arrived after the death of Dr. Isaac Thompson in June 1799. Personal communication with the Standish Historical Society, Charles Ruby, curator, 2018.

[9] John Brown, *The Elements of Medicine; or a Translation of the Elementa Medicinae Brunonis* (London: J. Johnson, 1788).

was considered by him, as a disease of debility, requiring internal stimulants; and recollected several cases of hemiplegia, which had since occurred in my practice, and were treated according to his plan, without succeeding in a single instance.

Thus, we see some of the unhappy consequences of the fascinating Brunonian doctrine,[10] which ought studiously to be avoided.

79

Since this account from Mr Higgins, I have met with several cases of palsy; some of which have been cured, others alleviated by bleeding and cathartics. A few of these cases will be related together with observations of others, relative to the nature & treatment of this disease; as well as apoplexy, a kindred malady, which afford much instruction, and evidence great practical improvement.

In Autumn 1807, Mrs Thoms of Falmouth, aged 60, of a gross habit, was attacked with hemiplegia, which deprived her of speech, and motion of her limbs on the left side, pulse full & slow. I drew a pint of blood from the affected arm, and evacuated her bowels with Jalap & calomel, of each 15 grains, which afforded considerable relief, tho her limbs remained in some degree, benumbed, with languor & inactivity. By repeated cathartics, chiefly of aloes, she gradually recovered, to a tolerable state of health, excepting a numbness of the arm.

In April 1808, she was again attacked in a very similar manner, when one of my pupils was called, in my absence, and drew a pint of blood; but no relief was afforded. She then wished him to draw another pint, which being done, faintness ensued. Her paralytic complaints were readily removed, and her limbs restored to their usual activity. Since which she has enjoyed good health, losing a pint of blood every returning spring, as a preventive, and occasionally taking an aleotic cathartic, living abstemiously.

In Autumn, 1808, Mr John Watson of Salem,[11] aged 62, who lived in a genteel stile, indulging freely in the best of meats & drinks, suffered an

---

[10] Brunonian Doctrine refers to the concepts of John Brown (1735–1788), a Scottish physician who proposed that most diseases were the result of excess or deficiency of excitability. Most diseases were treated by stimulants such as wine, spirits, and opium. W. F. Bynum, "Cullen and the Study of Fevers in Britain, 1760–1820," in *Theories of Fever from Antiquity to the Enlightenment*, ed. W. F. Bynum and V. Nutton (London: Wellcome Institute for the History of Medicine; Medical History, Supplement No. 1, 1981), 143. Lester S. King, *Medical Thinking: A Historical Preface* (Princeton, NJ: Princeton University Press, 1982), 232–33, and Talbott, *A Biographical History of Medicine*, 472–74.

[11] Salem, Massachusetts, rather than Salem, Maine, which was first settled in 1815. There were a number of Watsons in Salem, Massachusetts, in the eighteenth century.

attack of the remitting fever, attended with difficulty of speaking. After the fever subsided his hands became very numb, and the difficulty of speaking continued.

In the spring of 1809, he became much enfeebled and his spirits were so depressed that he had **80** no inclination to exercise. After dinner he generally slept a while, and often complained of distress at the pit of the stomach. His countenance was fresh, tho his flesh wasted, particularly in his limbs. The restorative & stimulant plan was pursued, but to no advantage. As the summer approached, he became still more enfeebled, and the numbness increased, so that he dispaired of obtaining any relief.

The last of June, my advice was requested, by Mr John Watson Jn^r his son, secretary of the insurance office in Portland, who related his case to me. I sent him a copy of Mrs Thom's case, to be submitted to the consideration of his physician, who drew 110 ounces of blood, in the course of ten days, as Mr Watson informed me. His limbs became more active after each bleeding, and his other complaints were greatly alleviated. His strength increased by thus lessening the superabundant load of blood; and he lived several years, enjoying a pretty comfortable state of health. ——So sensible was Mr Watson of the benefit received from bloodletting, that I was remunerated with ten dollars, for thus suggesting its utility.[12]

Soon after, a gentleman in Maine, aged about 70, who lived luxuriously, and at times, took a glass or two of madaira, [*sic*] was attacked with hemiplegia, and difficulty of speaking. He was bled twice freely, by a scientific physician, and his bowels were evacuated with Jalap & calomel. Aleotic cathartics were occasionally given. He soon recovered and lived abstemiously, with respect to meats & drinks, finding that wine was offensive and impeded digestion.

A few years after, while feasting at a luxurious supper, he was seized with apoplexy, so as to be entirely deprived of speech and motion. Enemas were given, but without effect. He expired in two days. Would not an emetic have been more eligible?

Another gentleman, aged about 65, who indulged freely in animal food, and used very little exercise, **81** while heartily eating at a late supper, amidst great hilarity, was suddenly attacked with palsy, for which stimulants were used, and at times the cold bath; but to no advantage. He lived a diseased inactive life several years before his death.

---

[12] The amount of $10 in 1809 is roughly equivalent to $204 in 2020.

A middle aged man in ~~Boston~~ Mass^tts of a corpulent habit, a noted "<u>wine bibber</u>," and voracious eater, attended a ball; and in the midst of his giddy whirls, dancing the "<u>black Joke</u>,"[13] was seized with apoplexy; and sunk into the shades of darkness, without the use of any depleting or evacuating means!

Were it necessary, I could relate many cases of palsy, and even apoplexy, where the patients have died under the use of stimulating means without any depleting remedies; but shall proceed to a description of the ~~improvements~~ discoveries which have been made relative to the nature of palsy and the improved mode of treatment, in this disease; as well as apoplexy.

In the 53 number of the New York Medical Repository, we are furnished with "An account of the efficacy of bloodletting & cathartics, in the cure of palsy, with observations on that disease, communicated by Dr Hunting Sherrill, of Clinton, formerly resident in the New York Alms-House, to Edward Miller, M.D. Professor of the Practice of Physic in the University of New York, dated June 30th 1810."[14]

"Those who have made examinations of the brain, after death, in persons who have been affected with palsy, have ascertained that there is generally a compression of the origin of the affected nerves, owing to an extravasation of blood, or an effusion of fluid, in some part of the brain. This observation is supported by a number of writers, among whom may be mentioned John ~~John~~ Hunter, Townsend and John Bell. And this appears **82** to be the immediate cause of the nerves & muscles, dependant on them, having lost their powers of action. Conformably with these principles, I made use of some remedies, which it appeared, were directed to the true pathology of this disease, in several cases which came under my care, in 1808, the principle of which were bloodletting & cathartics. I was warranted in using bloodletting

---

[13] "'The Black' [or Black Joak] was a widely popular street song in England in the early 1700s. That it was extremely vulgar and bawdy probably in no small way contributed to its continued popularity into the nineteenth century in that country and its colonies (including America). Irregular in form in many versions, its opening phrase has six measures, while the second has ten." Andrew Kuntz, "The Fiddler's Companion: A Descriptive Index of North American and British Isles Music for the Folk Violin and Other Instruments," http://www.ibiblio.org/fiddlers/BLACK.htm#BLACK_JOKE_[1].

[14] Hunting Sherrill, "An Account of the Efficacy of Blood-Letting and Cathartics in the Cure of Palsey, with Observations on That Disease; Communicated by Dr. Hunting Sherill, of Clinton, Duchess County, (N.Y.) Formerly a Resident in the New-York Almshouse, to Edward Miller, Professor of the Practice of Physic in the University of New-York. Dated June 30th, 1810," *Medical Repository Comprehending Original Essays and Intelligence* 3rd hexade, vol. 2, no. 1 (1810): 35–42.

from the following observations in Hunter on the blood, part 2. chap. 1. In palsy, he says, "we ought to bleed at once very largely, till the patient begins to show signs of recovery; and to continue it till the patient becomes faintish."[15] By accomodating this remedy to the morbid actions of the arterial system, there appears to be no impropriety in continuing it, as long as the state of the pulse, and continuance of the symptoms indicate it. Cathartics are used to promote absorption from other parts of the body in a variety of cases. D[r] Rush informs us, that he has long observed their good effects in palsies, and other cases of congestion in the brain; with this intention they were used to relieve the oppressed nerves."

Several cases are recorded which serve to show the efficacy of bloodletting & cathartics in palsy. One will be related.

D. McLain, aged 28, was brought to the Alms house on a cart, on the 8 of July, 1808, completely helpless, from a paralytic affection of the left side. The left arm & leg hung motionless; he had considerable stupor, and a numbness of the whole left side, and of the tongue. He was entirely deprived of speech. **83** By signs, it appeared that he had pain in his head, and some distress in the region of the stomach. He was suddenly attacked on the 4th of July, previous to which he had enjoyed good health. His pulse was small, slow & tense. An emetic was given on the 9th which discharged much foul mucous matter. The emetic was repeated on the 10th & 12th by which his tongue and stomach were somewhat relieved. He was now put on a course of cathartics of calomel gum. gamb.[16] & aloes of each 10 grains, which operated pretty briskly; there were repeated once in four or five days. Rubefacients and friction were occasionally used.

August 1st. He had recovered the use of his speech in some measure also the use of his leg; pulse small & tense; appetite rather improved. As his complaints had remained stationary for ten days past, he was now bled to 16^oz which produced some faintness. After bleeding the pulse was better. Bleeding was repeated whenever the pulse became tense, which was about once a week. The quantity of blood taken at each bleeding was from 12 to 24 ounces. He has been gradually recovering since pursuing this depleting plan. The cathartics were repeated once a week; and the bleeding once in two weeks.

---

[15] The actual quotation reads: "we ought to bleed at once very largely, especially from the temporal artery, till the patient begins to show signs of recovery; and to continue it till the patient becomes faintish." John Hunter, *A Treatise on the Blood, Inflammation, and Gun-Shot Wounds*, 2 vols. (Philadelphia: Thomas Bradford, 1796), vol. 1, 203.

[16] Gum resin of Gambogia; see "Gamboge" in Glossary.

Octr 1. He has perfectly recovered the use of his leg, and walks out, without a staff. He converses well, enjoys very good general health, and has acquired considerable flesh."

Other cases were successfully treated by bleeding and cathartics, without emetics.

84

Some observations on Paraplegia in Adults. By Matthew Baillie, M.D. &c. Fellow of the Royal College of Physicians, &c.[17]

Hemiplegia is the most common form of paralysis in Adults; paraplegia, however, is said to have increased considerably within the last 15 or 20 years. Paraplegia is usually supposed to arise from some affection of the spinal cord; but it has occurred to Dr B. to find, with other medical men, that where no accident has affected the spine, by outward violence, this gradual loss of power, in the lower parts of the body, has arisen from a disease affecting the brain itself.

It is the object of D^r B's paper to elucidate the fact; and it is said that symptoms of increased action within the head will generally be discovered, even in the early stages of such cases. The upper extremities are also some times affected with numbness, without a corresponding derangement being found in the cervical vertebræ. The dissection of one case is given, in which morbid congestions were found in the brain, with serous effusion within the cavities, and in the theca of the spinal marrow. Recovery sometimes occurs, in cases of paraplegia, tho, he says, no plan of treatment is very successful in such cases. Bleeding, alterative medicines, electricity, friction & blisters, with setons to the neck comprise what he recommends.

Much obscurity still hangs over these complaints. In the first place, dissections of the spinal cord are seldom made; and hence diseases may be attributed to ~~diseases~~ affections of the brain, which have commenced in the vertebral canal. In the second place, the readiness which exists in the brain to be affected, in spine cases, has not, perhaps, been sufficiently attended to. Symptoms of cerebral disorder are often found in pure affections of the spinal cord. In one case, where inflammation of the spinal cord, at the top of the lumbar vertebræ took place, some weeks after a wrench in skaiting, pressure on the tender part of the spine, produced the most alarming affections of the head & heart, confusion, dimness of sight, syncope, convulsions, **85** and

---

[17] Matthew Baillie (1761–1823) was a physician and anatomist in London. Matthew Baillie, "Some Observations upon Paraplegia in Adults," *Medical. Transactions of the. Royal College of Physicians of London* 6 (1820): 16–26.

an almost total cessation of the heart's action, were amongst these symptoms; the breathing at the same time being very laborious. In one instance, these symptoms followed the slight pressure which was made by changing the position of the body in bed. We have heard also, one of our friends quote another fact, which points at the same consentaneous action between the head and the spinal marrow; the observation that women who have distorted spines, are often affected by intractable headaches.

On the other hand, we witnessed the dissection of a case of paraplegia, a few weeks ago, which materially tended to prove D^r. Baillie's observations. A girl was seen to squint; paraplegia gradually supervened. The symptoms of head disease, however, kept pace with the paraplegic affection, so that a few days before she died, which was about three months after the attack. She was much emaciated & paraplegic; her head lolled from side to side; her arms were equally affected; her mouth was open, and her appearance nearly idiotic. But she had no pain in the head, and there was an evident falling in of the fourth & fifth cervical vertebræ.

After death, congestion was found in the vertebral canal; but no derangement of structure; whilst, in the head, the brain & membranes were much loaded with blood; much water was found in the cavities; and a large broken down, or ulcerated mass was discovered in the substance of the left half of the pons varolii."

New England Journal. vol. 10. N° 1.[18]

86

"Nature, says Boerhaave, has cured palsy, with a great and continued looseness." He also observes that palsy may be occasioned by every cause creating apoplexy, which when gentle goes off with large bleeding from the piles; as well as other hemorrhages."   Aphorism. 1030.[19]

"A sudden attack of palsy, in an inebriate, says Dr Mann, immediately after a fit of intoxication, the patient having lost his reason, was succeeded

[18] Mathew Baillie, "Some Observations on Paraplegia in Adults," *New England Journal of Medicine and Surgery* 10, no. 1 (1821): 84–85. Barker read Baillie's article in the journal's "Selections"; the article original article is found in the *Medical Transactions published by the College of Physicians of London* 6 (1820): 16–26.

[19] Aphorism 1030 discusses apoplexy, but Aphorism 1017 states, "A gentle Apoplexy . . . [may be relieved] with large Bleeding from the Piles for a long while." Gehard Van Swieten, *An Abridgement of Baron Van Swieten's Commentaries Upon the Aphorisms Of . . . Herman Boerhaave . . . : Concerning the Knowledge and Cure of Diseases / by Colin Hossack. . . . In Five Volumes; Vol. III* (London: Printed for Robert Horsfield and Thomas Longman 1774), 167.

by vomiting & purging of blood, which continued 24 hours, when by the use of calomel & ipecac, the person, in a few days, was restored to reason & health."   Prize dissertation. 1803.[20]

Again, An inebriate, after large potations of ardent spirits, was found apoplectic in his bed. An intestinal hemorrhage soon succeeded, and removed the effects of the spiritous excitement from the brain."

Medical Sketches, 1816.[21]

Notwithstanding the successful treatment of palsy, by bloodletting & cathartics; as well as the beneficial effects of hemorrhages, in this disease, most all to whom I have been called labouring under palsy, have been un-willing to loose blood, on account of their weakness of body and imbecility of mind, chosing rather to take stimulating articles, even spiritous liquors, as remedies, tho the disease was induced, in many instances, by the fashionable & habitual use of ardent spirits; so that some, whose lives have been spared, remain helpless, speechless paralytics, disparing of a recovery; and the longer the disease remains uncontrolled, the more unyielding it becomes!

In the course of my practice I have met with many cases of Apoplexy, as well as palsy; and found that they were generally induced, by overeating and hard drinking; and that aged people, who are apt to indulge too freely, are most liable to these diseases. The state & condition of the stomach, **87** should, therefore, be taken into consideration, on their approach; as well as the brain. The first question should be respecting the quantity & quality of the food last taken. If it should appear that the stomach has been overcharged, an emetic should be given, without hesitation, after drawing a suitable quantity of blood, in order to relieve the brain & oppressed nerves. Indeed, if blood cannot conveniently be drawn, an emetic should by no means be dispensed with. I have known many deaths to take place in apoplexy, from too great in-dulgence in food, where no attention was paid to the stomach.

---

[20] James Mann (1759–1832); "Prize Dissertation" refers to the Boylstonian Prize won by Mann in 1803. Barker is referring to James Mann, *A Dissertation Upon the Cholera Infantum; to Which Are Added, Rules and Regulations, as Preventive Means of the Autumnal Diseases of Children; Which Gained the Boylstonian Prize for the Year 1803* (Boston: Young & Minns, 1804). See Robert B. Austin, *Early American Medical Imprints: 1668–1820* (Arlington, MA: The Printers' Devil, 1961), no. 1189. Mann won the same prize in 1806 on the topic of "dysentery" as noted in Josiah Bartlett, *A Dissertation on the Progress of Medical Science in the Commonwealth of Massachusetts* (Boston: T. B. Wait and Co., 1810).

[21] James Mann, *Medical Sketches of the Campaigns of 1812, 13, 14. To Which Are Added, Surgical Cases; Observations on Medical Hospitals; and Flying Hospitals Attached to a Moving Army. Also, an Appendix, Compromising a Dissertation on Dysentery* (Dedham [MA]: H. Mann and Co., 1816), 35. See Austin, *Early American Medical Imprints: 1668–1820*, no. 1190.

A short time since, an aged man, in Maine, was seized with apoplexy, in the night, after a late plentiful supper of salted mackerel & potatoes. He was bled, by his physician, and cathartics were given; but they did not operate. He expired in 48 hours. An emetic might probably have afforded relief, by disgorging the contents of his stomach.

Case of Apoplexy related to me by Joshua Fisher, M.D. &c of Beverly.

"In 1774. I was sent for to a poor man, who was attacked with a fit of apoplexy, but not being at home, another physician was called, who, in vain attempted to bleed him, and pronounced his case desperate. Three days after, hearing that the patient was alive, I made him a visit, and found that he was incapable of voluntary motion, with a slow, stertorous breathing; which had been his situation since the attack; and that, in the mean time, nothing had passed into his stomach. ——I found, on inquiry, that, on the day of his attack, he ate voraciously of a beef steak, and drank freely of ardent spirit. I then gave 10 or 12 grains of tart emet.[22] which operated in less than an hour, and threw up large pieces of beef, which did not appear to have undergone any change, **88** except enlargement. By the help of a finger they were disengaged from his throat. He could then speak, and move himself. — By the aid of cathartics, he soon recovered."

See New England Journal vol.1. for a particular account of this case, with instructive remarks, and dissections.[23]

"It is not rare, says Professor Tourtelle, to see aged men die with apoplexy, indigestion, &c from partaking too freely in the pleasures of the table. The repast of the evening should be light; for when the stomach is surcharged with aliments, the energies are too much concentrated in the epigastrium, and digestion is laboriously performed; the brain, excited by the action which it partakes with the epigastrium suffers too much tension, and its unhappy consequences."

"The grand rule of temperance, consists in taking only a sufficiency of food, to satisfy natural hunger, and that of the most simple kind. All animals, except man, follow this rule, which is directed by instinct. But man, endowed with reason, gives himself up to excesses; and is as much an enemy to himself, as he

---

[22] Tartar emetic. See "Tartrite of Antimony" in Glossary.

[23] John C. Warren, "Cases of Apoplexy, with Dissections," *New England Journal of Medicine and Surgery* 1 (1812): 34–41, 154–59. The "Case of Apoplexy related to me [Barker] by Joshua Fisher" is found on page 154–55 as "A letter from Joshua Fisher, M.D., vice-president of the Mass. Med. Soc. Beverly, March 6, 1812."

is to society. He has served on his table, at a great expense, the productions of both hemispheres, surcharged with nourishment. He only quits the repast to kindle new flames in his entrails. Strong liquor taken in profusion, make a volcano of his stomach, which burns the whole system, and rapidly consumes life! — Intemperance is as injurious to the moral, as it is to the physical part of man, and depraves the faculties of the soul."   Principles of health.[24]

89

Cases of Apoplexy, with Dissections.

By John C. Warren, M. D. [25]

Abridged.

"Every fact, in pathological anatomy, is worthy of preservation. Every morbid appearance, which has not been noticed, or at least not generally known, should be recorded and given to the world, especially if it serve to illustrate obscure doctrines and points of practice. The treatment of apoplexy, in its first stage, is a fair subject for the application of these remarks; as it has been a source of division & discussion among physicians ever since the days of Van Helmont.[26] We have not been able to discover that the appearance of the stomach, in patients, who have died of apoplexy has been carefully observed, by any of the writers on this disease. On the contrary, it is found that most of them have neglected even to name this organ, in their descriptions.

Case 1.

Major L. enjoyed good health till 60, when he had some slight attacks of indigestion, and two or three fits of faintness. At last, while apparently in good health, he was seized with a fit of apoplexy. He had dined about half an hour before, on what are usually called pancakes, with a large quantity of cider without other solid or liquid food. He afterwards walked to the place of his daily occupations, where he sat down to repose himself, a few minutes; then rising to go to his desk, he suddenly fell, and expired. In a few minutes, when I saw him, there was not any pulse, not the least appearance of life remaining.

---

[24] Etienne Tourtelle, *The Principles of Health (Elements of Hygiene . . . From the Second French Ed.; Translated by G. Williamson* (Baltimore: John D. Toy, 1819). Editions had been available in French since 1796.

[25] Warren, "Cases of Apoplexy, with Dissections."

[26] Jean Baptiste van Helmont (1577–1644) was born in Brussels and took an M.D. degree at Louvain. He practiced and assembled his concepts of medicine in *Ortus Medicinae* (Origins of Medicine) published in Amsterdam in 1648. Talbott, *A Biographical History of Medicine*, 90–92.

Dissection

In about 24 hours, the body was examined, in the presence of a number of physicians. The face, neck & upper part of the trunk, were of a purple colour. When the scalp was cut, a great quantity of venous blood streamed from the wound. The cranium being opened, the dura mater was seen of a darker colour than usual. Not only were the large vessels of the brain filled; but the most minute branches were injected with blood in a fluid state. The lungs were of a healthy aspect. The cavities of the heart, and first portion of the aorta, were full of black fluid blood.

90

On opening the stomach we were astonished at seeing the quantity of food it contained. The mass had a slightly acid odour, and no perceptable change had been effected on this mass by the action of the gastric powers. This being removed, we examined the internal or mucous coat. — The greater part of this coat was of as deep a red colour, as would accompany a high degree of inflammation. The redness was greatest in the pyloric portion of the stomach, where it was very deep and uniform.

Case 2.

The Rev. President W.[27] enjoyed good health till 40. He was then affected with slight attacks of indigestion. His habits of living were those of studious and sedentary men, except during the two last years of his life.

It seems that he had dined profusely on the parts of a certain kind of meat pie, nearly resembling the species of food in Case 1. He remained in his house, conversing pleasantly till six o'clock; three hours after dinner, when he suddenly complained of want of air. The window being opened he attempted to reach it; but fell into snoring apoplexy. Medicines were given, and attempts made to bleed him, without success; and he expired in an hour.

---

[27] This is almost certainly the Rev. President Samuel Webber (1759–1810), president of Harvard College 1806–1810, Hollis Professor of Mathematics and Natural History. John Collins Warren performed an autopsy and dissection on him in July 1810, the original report of which can be found in Warren's manuscript *Surgical Notes, 1808–1826* [1.K.62]. Though the account in the *New England Journal* has greater detail, many of the elements, including the meat pie and the coagulum of black blood, are common to both accounts. Personal communication with Jack Eckert at the Harvard Center for the History of Medicine.

Dissection.

At eleven o'clock, the next morning, we examined the body. The veins on the surface of the brain, were moderately distended with blood; but nothing very remarkable was seen in this organ till we cut deep into the left hemisphere. Below, and on the left side of the ventricle was discovered the immediate cause of death; a large coagulum of black blood discharged, probably from a considerable branch of the arteria callosal [probably the anterior communicating artery]; for we distinctly saw the branches of **91** this artery running towards the coagulum and could almost fix on one at the fatal source of the effused fluid.

The substance of the heart was tender & livid; all its cavities contained black fluid blood. The lungs were found; and the abdominal organs, in a healthy condition. The stomach was very full. Its contents consisted of a brownish mass, destitute of any peculiar appearance or smell. The veins were peculiarly distinct as seen through the outer coat. The internal or mucous coat had an <u>extremely deep red colour</u>, especially near the pyloric orifice and was tender.

A sufficient number of pathological facts might be adduced to show the influence of the stomach on the brain. The sick headach is an evident example. In this disorder the brain is severely affected, as is shewn by the intense pain &c. During this affection the stomach labors under severe oppression. An emetic is oppertunely given, perhaps by nature unassisted, and this organ relieved of its offensive contents. The pain then ceases, and the brain clears, like the sky, after a sudden storm. Persons laboring under indigestion often experience strange sensations in the head. — A lady dreadfully affected with this disorder, while growing worse, began to complain of strange feelings in her head, like insanity. The symptoms of dyspepsia increasing, she was at last attacked with terrible fits of epilepsy, which continued to occur for some weeks. — When she began to recover from ~~the~~ indigestion the fits went off, and have never reappeared.

Is not the stomach the seat & throne of Enoch[28] as well as convulsion fits, with children & adults? Some observations will be ~~made~~ noted relative to these disorders, in the sequel.

---

[28] This is probably a reference to the *Book of Enoch* and Enoch as a knower of secrets. It is an ancient Hebrew apocryphal religious text ascribed to Enoch, great grandfather of Noah. There is an extensive body of literature on this book, translations, and meanings by various religions.

92

Chap. 7.

Chap. Hydrophobia.

THE ANCIENTS, SAYS Dr Mead,[1] have at large described the symptoms of this disease, as Galen, Dioscorides, Cælius Aurelianus &c.[2] That this disease is accompanied with a delirium is almost the common opinion both of the Ancients & Moderns. This delirium is supposed to proceed entirely from an indisposition of the body, owing to the alteration made in the blood, by the saliva of the mad dog.

That we may rightly understand this, we may take notice that the Rabies, or madness in a dog, is the effect of a violent fever. Neither is it amis to add that Joannes Faber, in the dissection of one who died at Rome of the bite of a mad dog, and a hydrophobia succeeding, found the blood coagulated in the right ventricle of the heart; the lungs wonderfully red & tumefied; but especially the throat, stomach & bowels, bearing the marks of the inflammatory venom.[3]

---

[1] Richard Mead (1673–1754) was a British physician who trained at Leyden and obtained an M.D. from Padua in 1695. He was elected physician to St. Thomas's in London, but it was not until 1707 that Oxford accepted his medical degree from Padua, allowing him admission to the College of Physicians. He became one of the leading physicians in Britain, attending such people as Charles II and Sir Isaac Newton. John H. Talbott, *A Biographical History of Medicine* (New York: Grune & Stratton, 1970), 186–88.

[2] Galen (AD 129–c. 210) is discussed in the introduction. Pedanius Dioscorides (AD c. 40–90) was a Greek physician, writer, botanist, and pharmacologist. Cælius Aurelianus was a fifth-century Roman physician and writer from North Africa. Arturo Castiglioni, *A History of Medicine*, 2nd ed. (New York: Alfred A. Knopf, 1947), 215–17, 49.

[3] Johannes Faber (1574–1629) was born a German Protestant in Bamberg, orphaned by the plague as a one-year-old, raised as a Catholic, and served as a papal physician in Rome. He was professor of medicine at the University of Rome and Keeper of the Vatican Garden, a friend of Galileo Galilei, and apparently coined the word "microscope." Sabina Brevaglieri, "Science, Books and Censorship in the Academy of the Lincei. Johannes Faber as Cultural Mediator," in

The same observation has been made by others, in bodies dead of this disease. In one case, a part of the liver was inflamed, the lungs parched & dry, and the inner coat of the stomach so mortified, that it might be abraded with ones fingers. In another the stomach discovered the marks of an erosion with something like a gangrene, and suffusion of blood, here & there.

Galen wisely advises to enlarge the wound, by making a round incision about it; to cauterise it with a hot iron, and apply drawing medicines, so as to keep up a discharge forty days. But when these means are omitted various antidotes are prescribed and vulgar trifles. But the greatest & surest cure of all, is frequent submerging or ducking the patient in water, mentioned by Celsus. But after the dread of water it is considered incurable.

Essay on Poisons. N. 2.[4]

93

"There is scarce any poison known, says Boerhaave, whose malignancy is so terrible, and occasions such prodigious changes in men, as dog madness. Some people are immediately affected with the symptoms of this disease, some not till twenty years, after they are bit, and some are more or less disordered all the while, between its first occasion, and its last scenes.

The anatomy of bodies has shewn that the organs of swallowing are most times inflamed, and there is a bilious glue of several colours in the stomach; the gall bladder is full of black choler; the pericardium is quite dried up; the lungs are surprisingly full of blood; the heart is full of almost all dried up blood; the arteries full, the veins empty; the brain and medulla spinalis are drier than usual, &c. The method to preserve one that is bit requires that the whole affected place be scarified very deep, and blood be drawn to a great quantity, by means of large glasses[5], burning the same deep with a red hot iron, so as to produce suppuration for a long time.

Conflicting Duties: Science, Medicine and Religion in Rome, 1550–1750, ed. Maria Pia Donato, Jill Kraye, and Institute Warburg (London: Warburg Institute, 2009), 133–57.

[4] Richard Mead, *A Mechanical Account of Poisons* (Dublin: S. Powell, 1736), 55, "Essay II Of the Tarantula and the Mad Dog," with marginalia by Jeremiah Barker, is found in the Jeremiah Barker Papers, Coll. 13, Maine Historical Society, Box 2/5.

[5] Scarified . . . glasses: "The apparatus for local bloodletting by cupping consists of a scarificator and a glass, shaped somewhat like a bell. The scarificator is an instrument containing from sixteen to twenty lancets which are so contrived, that when the instrument is applied to any part of the body, the whole number of lancets are by means of a spring pushed suddenly into the skin to a depth at which the instrument has previously been regulated. As only the small vessels can be punctured, very little blood would be discharged from them were not some method taken to promote the evacuation. This is commonly done with a cupping-glass; the air within the cavity of which being so rarefied by heat as to produce a very considerable degree of suction." James Thacher, *American Modern Practice* (Boston: Ezra Read, 1817), 668.

Immediately after the first signs of this evils invading, it ought to be treated like a disease of the fiercest inflammatory kind, letting blood out of a large orifice, of a large vessel, to a large quantity and even to swooning; then giving glisters. These must be repeated boldly, and even more than prudence would allow of in most diseases. In the intervals, he must be blinded and thrown into a cold pond, or be made wet with the continual throwing of water upon him, till he doth not seem any more to be afraid of water, then force him to drink a large quantity of water, and procure him sleep in this way; with a thin diet. **94** Nor ought we to dispair of finding out, one time or other, a peculiar antidote for this poison." Aphorisms.[6]

"The dread of water, says D^r. Rush, Med. Obser. vol.2,[7] is said to give a specific character to hydrophobia; but this symptom often occurs in diseases from other causes. As soon as the disease discovers itself, whether by pain in the wounded part, or any other symptoms, the first ~~thing~~ remedy indicated is bloodletting; and to be effectual, it should be used in the most liberal manner. The loss of 100 to 200 ounces of blood will probably be necessary in most cases.

In the 40th volume of the transactions of the Royal Society of London, there is an account of a man being cured of hydrophobia, by Dr Hartley, by the loss of 120 ounces of blood.[8]

In the Medical Essays of Edinburgh, vol. 1. p. 212, there is an account of a dreadful hydrophobia being cured by an accidental & profuse hemorrhage, from the temporal artery.[9]

---

[6] Herman Boerhaave, *Boerhaave's Aphorisms: Concerning the Knowledge and Cure of Diseases Translated from the Last Edition Printed in Latin at Leyden, 1715*, Classics of Medicine Library (London: R. Cowse and W. Innys in St. Paul's Church-Yard, 1715). Gerard Swieten and Herman Boerhaave, *Commentaries Upon Boerhaave's Aphorisms Concerning the Knowledge and Cure of Diseases. By Baron Van Swieten, Counsellor and First Physician to Their Majesties the Emperor and Empress of Germany; Perpetual President of the College of Physicians in Vienna; Member of the Royal Academy of Sciences and Surgery at Paris; H. Fellow of the Royal College of Physicians at Edinburgh; &C. &C. &C. Translated from the Latin*. Vol. 11 (Edinburgh: printed for Charles Elliot, Parliament Square. Sold by J. Murray, Fleet Street, London, 1776), Monograph, 139–234.

[7] Benjamin Rush, *Medical Inquiries and Observations*, 4th ed., 4 vols. (Philadelphia: Johnson & Warner, 1815), 193–211.

[8] David Hartley and Fr Sandys, "VI. Another Case of a Person Bit by a Mad-Dog, Drawn up by David Hartley, M. A. And Mr. Fr. Sandys, Communicated to the Royal Society by Francis Wollaston, Esq; F. R. S," *Philosophical Transactions* 40, no. 448 (1738): 174–76.

[9] John Innes, "An Inflammation of the Stomach, with Hydrophobia, and Other Uncommon Symptoms; by Dr. John Innes, Fellow of the College of Physicians, and Professor of Medicine in the University of Edinburgh," *Medical Essays and Observations* 1 (1752): 227–32.

Bleeding, however, has been used, in some cases of hydrophobia without success. But in all such cases, it was probably used out of time, or in too sparing a manner. The credit of the lancet has suffered in many other diseases, from the same causes."[10]

95

An account of a case of Hydrophobia successfully treated by copious bleeding and mercury. In two letters, from Dr Robert Burton, of Bent [Creek)], in the State of Virginia, to Dr Benjamin Rush, of Philadelphia.[11]

Bent Creek, August 21, 1803.

Sir. Believing that you are always disposed to encourage any thing, which may throw light on the treatment of diseases, I take the liberty of addressing to you the following case of hydrophobia, requesting a line or two, if you think it deserving your attention.

On the 4th of July, 1803, at nine o'clock in the evening, I was desired to visit Thomas Brothers, aged twenty eight years. I was informed by the person who came for me, that he had been bitten by a dog, which his friends suspected to be mad. I found him in the hands of four young men, who were endeavouring to confine him; and merely prevent him from injuring himself or friends. He recognized me, and requested me to give him my hand, which he made a violent effort to draw within his mouth. Concious of his inclination to bite, he advised his friends to keep at a distance, mentioning that a mad dog had bitten him. His symptoms were as follows, viz. a dull pain in his head, watery eyes, dull aspect, stricture & heaviness of the breast, and a high fever.

Believing as you do that there is but one fever, I determined to treat this case as an inflammatory fever. I, therefore, drew 20 ounces of blood, and as he refused to take anything aqueous, I had him drenched with a large dose of calomel & Jalap.

Jul 5th. 4. A.M. finding his symptoms worse, I drew 16 ounces of blood, and applied two large epispastic plaisters to his legs, hoping thereby to relieve the oppression of the precordia and other symptoms.

---

[10] Rush, *Medical Inquiries and Observations*, vol. 2, 193–211; see p. 202.

[11] Robert Burton, "An Account of a Case of Hydrophobia Successfully Treated by Copious Bleeding and Mercury. In Two Letters, from Dr Robert Burton, of Bent(Creek), in the State of Virginia, to Dr Benjamin Rush, of Philadelphia. Dated Bent-Creek (Virginia) August 21, 1803, and Sept. 18, 1803," *Medical Repository* 8, 2nd hexade, vol. 2 (1805): 15–18.

96

Twelve M.[12] was informed, that one of his friends had permitted him to take a stick in his mouth, which he bit so as to loosen several of his teeth. As he craved something to bite, I desired his friend to give him a piece of lead, which he bit until he almost exhausted himself.

One P.M. finding but little alteration, I drew 18 ounces of blood; and had him drenched with the antimonial powders.

Two P.M. He slept until half past three, when he awoke, with the disposition to bite; oppression, &c, but not so violent.

July 6th 8 A.M. found him biting the bed clothes; his countenance maniacal, his pulse synocha, with a stricture of the breast, difficult swallowing, laborious breathing, and a discharge of saliva. I took away 24 ounces of blood, gave him a dose of calomel & Jalap, and continued the powders.

Twelve M. drew 16 ounces of blood and gave him laudanum.

Five P.M. found him in a slumber, his skin moist, and his fever and other symptoms much abated.

July 7th 8 A.M. was informed that he had only two paroxysms during my absence; and that he had lost 16 ounces of blood, agreeably to directions. Notwithstanding the favourable aspect the disease wore, I resolved to bleed him twice more, and then to induce an artificial fever by mercury, which would predominate over the hydrophobic. I, therefore, drew 10 ounces of blood, and requested his friend to take 18 ounces at night; to rub in a small quantity of mercurial ointment; and to give a mercurial pill every four hours.

July 8th. 9 A.M. found him convalescent, but continued the mercurial unction & pills.

July 9. 10 A.M. found his gums sore, and discontinued the mercury.

July 15th, 1 P.M. found him well; but with a considerable degree of debility.

97   Philadelphia, August 29, 1803.

Dear Sir,

Accept my congratulations on your rare triumph over a case of hydrophobia. I give you great credit for your boldness in practice. You have deserved well of the profession of medicine.

In order to render your communication more satisfactory, permit me to request your answer to the following questions,

---

[12] "M." is mid-day. Noah Webster, *An American Dictionary of the English Language. With an Introd. By Mario Pei*, reprint of 1828 ed. published by S. Converse, 2 vols. (New York and London: Johnson Reprint Corporation, 1970).

1. On what part of the body was the wound inflicted? And how long was the interval between the time of his being bitten, and the attack of the fever?
2. Did he discover any avertion from the sight of water; and did he refuse to swallow liquids of any kind?
3. What were the appearances of blood drawn? Did it differ in different stages of the disease?

Your answer to the above questions will much oblige your sincere friend,

Benjamin Rush

Dr Burton.

Bent Creek, Virg. Sept. 18, 1803.

Sir. I regret that business of an indispensable nature prevented me from being more particular.

The part bitten was a little above the union of the solæus & gastrocnemius muscles, which form the tendoachillis.[13] The interval between the time of his being bitten and the attack of the fever was 24 days.

He was, I was told, dull & solitary a few days previous to the attack. A few minutes before it, his friends found him 200 yards from the house, apparently in a deep study. He has informed me, since his recovery, that he had a slight pain in the wound, attended with itching, and an uneasiness in the inguinal gland, several days before the fever. He refused to swallow liquids; and the sight of water drew him into a convulsive agitation. The blood was not examined.

I am, Sir, yours, &c

Robert Burton.[14]

Dʳ. Rush.

98

"When a wound is made by the bite of a rabid animal, says Dʳ Mann, it should be immediately washed with warm water. The use of this is to wash away the poison, which may be lodged within the wounded flesh; and lest this washing might not, in every case, cleanse the wound of the poison, the part wounded should be removed by a knife. Still apprehending that the knife

---

[13] Soleus and gastrocnemius are the calf muscles, which unite to become the Achilles tendon.

[14] Worldwide, approximately 53,000 people die of rabies each year; recovery from rabies is rare. A. C. Jackson, "Recovery from Rabies," *New England Journal of Medicine* 352, no. 24 (2005): 2549–50; R. E. Willoughby Jr. et al., "Survival after Treatment of Rabies with Induction of Coma," *New England Journal of Medicine* 352, no. 24 (2005): 2508–14.

might not have reached beyond the poison, it is adviseable to apply some caustic upon the wound. The muriate of mercury, the nitrate of silver, and arsenic have severally been employed in these cases. These caustics will destroy the parts or neutralize the virus, so as to prevent its hydrophobous effects on the system. Nine persons have been treated after this method, within a few years. It is presumed on evidence conclusive, that the fatal hydrophobous symptoms were, in the above cases, obviated by these means; for in every instance, animals bitten by the same dog, and on the same day, became rabid and died of that disease.

Of the preventive means, every regular physician is well informed. It is solely for the benefit of the uninformed citizens that they are now communicated to the public. The same method of prevention may be employed on the cattle and other domestic animals, as on the human species; and no doubt is entertained, but they will be accompanied with equal success.

The poison of rabid animals appears to be slow in producing its specific effects on the system. It may possibly be lodged on the wounded part, and remain some days, in a dormant state, before it is absorbed and generally diffused. This is, however, a mere conjecture, and therefore should not induce so much security as to delay the **99** employment of the knife and caustic one minute. The above means become a certain preventive, when immediately applied; uncertain when delayed many hours.

James Mann"[15]

Wrentham 1810.   Boston Patriot.[16]

Use of a volatile alkali as a counter poison.

M[r] Dubarnard, [sic] of France, has given an account of the successful treatment of three persons bitten by mad dogs. He describes his method in the following terms. "The wounds were dilated and well washed with a strong solution of sea salt, and afterwards seared with a red hot iron. Immediately after, a blistering plaister was applied to each of the wounds. The suppuration

---

[15] James Mann (1759–1832) of Wrentham, Massachusetts, graduated from Harvard College and then studied under Dr. Samuel Danforth. He was a physician in the American Revolution and the War of 1812. Howard A. Kelly and Walter L. Burrage, *American Medical Biographies* (Baltimore: The Norman, Remington Company, 1920), 758–59.

[16] A Boston newspaper, the *Boston Patriot* (1809–1816) later became the *Boston Patriot and Daily Chronicle*, and then the *Boston Patriot & Daily Mercantile and Advertiser*. Though the manuscript reads "1810," Barker is actually citing the following article from 1816 in which Dr. Mann presents ten cases from Massachusetts; two from Medway, one from Franklin, five from Foxborough, one from Mansfield, and one from Stoughton. "Medical. For the Boston Patriot; Hydrophobia, or Canine Madness," *Boston Patriot* 16 (December 14, 1816): 1.

was copious, and kept up for a month, by gentle epispastics. After the first dressing, the patient was put upon the use of the volatile alkali. This he took three times a day, for a fortnight, to the amount of fifteen drops in two ounces of water. After this the dose was altered to twenty drops twice a day, and continued until the thirty fourth day from the accident. It was then discontinued, having never been omitted but twice during the whole time, and then in the morning for the sake of taking mercurial pills. On the 44 day from the bite, the patient went about his usual business. Another person, bitten by the same dog, and not treated according to this plan, died on the 26th day, with all the symptoms of confirmed rabies.

The Medical Society of the department of Gers [in southern France], where M[r] D. practices, has expressed an opinion on the treatment in the following words. "The treatment employed by M[r] Dubernard is predicated on correct principles. According to the theory & experience of the best practices, it is a matter of primary consequence to destroy the hydrophobic **100** virus by the actual cautery. With the same intention he has subjected to a long suppuration, the flesh tainted with the venom, that it may be freed from every vestige of poison. But he has not stopped there. His prudence taught him to prescribe internally the remedies proper to subdue the poison, which might have slipped into the channels of the circulation, and by these means he had enjoyed the satisfaction of seeing the individuals whom he had under his care entirely preserved from the canine madness."

Paris Journal de Commerce, Aug[r] 7th 1805. [17]

Treatment of persons who have been bitten by mad dogs. D[r] Joseph A. Gallup[18] of Woodstock in Vermont, in July 1806, made to D[r] Mitchill

---

[17] Published in Mr. Dubernard, "Use of Volatile Alkali as a Counter-Poison (from the Paris Journal De Commerce, Aug. 7, 1805)," *The Medical Repository (and Review of American Publications on Medicine)* 2nd hexade, vol. 3 (1806): 423–24.

[18] Joseph Adam Gallup (1769–1849) was born in Connecticut and lived in New Hampshire before moving to Vermont, where he spent most of his life. In 1798 he was one of the first two students to be granted a Bachelor of Medicine at the new Dartmouth Medical School under Nathan Smith. He taught medical students at the Castleton Medical Academy (Vermont Academy of Medicine after 1822), and then in 1823 joined the new medical department of the University of Vermont. In 1815 Gallup published a book on Vermont medical history similar to what Barker was attempting for Maine: Joseph A. Gallup, *Sketches of Epidemic Diseases in the State of Vermont* (Boston: T. B. Wait & Sons, 1815). See Frederick Clayton Waite, *The Story of a Country Medical College: A History of the Clinical School of Medicine and Vermont Medical College, Woodstock, Vermont 1827–56* (Montpelier: Vermont Historical Society, 1945), 29–47; Oliver S. Hayward and Constance A. Putnam, eds., *Improve, Perfect, and Perpetuate: Nathan Smith and Early American Medical Education* (Hanover: University Press of New England, 1998), 27, 50, 105–107; and John A. Garraty and Mark C. Carnes, *American National Biography* (New York: Oxford University Press, 1999), vol. 8, 660–62.

the following communication. "I communicate to you the following, not as containing anythink [*sic*] new or interesting, except as it goes to show at what period attempts may be made to eradicate the canine virus after it is communicated to the system. Perhaps many facts of this kind, brought together, might establish some points of much importance in the pathology of the disease."

"Gilbert Wait, about 28 years of age, was bitten by a dog known to be mad, on the outer side of the left arm, about three inches from the Joint of the wrist, on the 23ᵈ of March, 1805. On the 17ᵗʰ of April, being 25 days, he called on me for advice, he having omitted it, until the principal part of the animals had died, that had been bitten, the same and preceding day by the same dog. There died within 21 days, a dog, two hogs and a sheep, with all the symptoms of canine madness. Two other dogs on being taken sick were killed, and in an adjacent town, several other animals, bitten by the same dog next day, died about this time.

101

The wound made by the teeth was healed over with a smooth cicatrix, without inflammation. All the unusual feelings were a slight numbness, and pain by turns in the affected part. I made a circular incision, so as to inclose both punctures of the teeth, and took out all the part bitten. At the bottom, about half an inch deep, was a black spot, being the very lowest part of that the tooth pierced, which was about the bigness of a peppercorn. I then applied some some alkaline caustic, dressed the wound with empl. vesicat.[19] and, by the help of poultices, directly brought on a plentiful discharge. This discharge was kept up until the next October, by occasionally applying the caustic. I could not tell whether the poison had entered the lymphatics, and if it had, many doubts lay on my mind whether it could be dislodged by any internal remedies. With a view of doing all I could, and, if erring, to err on the safe side. He was bled to the amount of 20 ounces, took calomel twice a week as a cathartic, a solution of corrosive sublimate in brandy, so as to nauseate twice a day; as also from 6 to 8 grains of camph. twice a day. These measures were continued about two months. He had no hydrophobic symptoms; but seemed to manifest more inquietude and restlessness, than is common for patients, not labouring under actual pain. It being now fifteen months and upwards since the bite, I feel but little apprehension of his being afflicted with the malady."

Med. Repos. vol. 10.[20]

[19] See "Vesication" in the Glossary.
[20] Joseph A. Gallup, "Treatment of Persons Who Have Been Bitten by Mad Dogs," *Medical Repository* 2nd hexade, vol. 4 (1807): 199–200.

102

An account of the strange <u>effects of a bite, by a mad dog</u>. "On or about the 18th of May, 1793, Asa Felton of Danvers, Mass^{tts} a person of a plethoric habit and sanguine complexion, as he was walking with his old dog, trotting by his side, attempted, by holding out his hand, as usual, to play with him; on which the dog snapped, and made with his tooth, in an old scar, on the back of his hand, a slight wound, which caused him to suspect that the dog was mad, which soon proved to be the fact, by the same dog, on the next day, biting a heifer, and attempting to bite a yoke of oxen; but was prevented. The dog was then killed, and about fifteen days after, the heifer run mad & died. The wound on Mr Feltons hand, which yielded but little blood, ~~was~~ soon healed without any surgical application; and for above five years after, he continued in general good health, labouring hard, eat & drank heartily, made no application to any physician for medicine nor advice; tho, during the above term, he frequently desired his wife, if he should be seized with illness, to have him immediately confined. By this it appears that he was apprehensive of suffering sad consequences of the bite, in some future time; as he was invariably unwell every year after the bite, at the time he was bitten; and in the course of the five years aforesaid, he at times would appear very froward, peevish & passionate, more than he used to be. For about a year past, he had suffered greatly with inquietude of mind, by night & day; he slept but little and was troubled with frightful dreams as tho he was falling into deep water, in his well, &c. In the night he often complained of **103** great thirst, and of burning pain in the back of his hand. At times he has suffered grievous mental derangement, would often tell that he had seen the Devil, and that he should come to want, and made several attempts of suicide, once by throwing himself out of the scuttle of his house, and falling nearly thirty feet, on hard ground, by which fall his collar bone was broken, and he for a little time stunned, tho he never after would own that he had any knowledge of his going out at the scuttle, or falling from it. Sometimes he has been found lying on the ground by the side of his horse; at such times he would complain of giddiness in his head, which caused him to dismount and lie down. This some people would attribute to intoxication; but it has been often observed, that after his lying & resting for a short time, he would rise, mount his horse, and steadily proceed on his business. At other times, when riding out to a neighbours house, and had come within six or eight rods of the door, an impression would suddenly seize on his mind, tho to all appearance perfectly sensible, that he could not ride one step further; but must dismount from his horse and travel into the house upon all fours, which he would do; and after setting & conversing about the business which he went upon, he would mount his horse again, and ride home. At other times, when setting in company, tranquil in mind to appearance, at home or abroad, he would suddenly cry out with a terrible loud and irregular voice, as if he was seized with pain. On asking him the reason, he would say, I can't help it. — Are you in pain? No but I can't help it.

For some months past, he has been troubled with weakness, and great pain in his hips, and lower extremities, which rendered him unable to walk.

104

The foregoing are some of the strange & uncommon symptoms which attended Mr Felton, for almost two years past, and on the 11th day of July last, he became delirious, fancying himself possessor of great riches, and owner of the whole earth; that the angels in Heaven, and all creatures were subject to him. On the 12th day, he continued much on the same subject, proclaiming it with a loud voice, and with little or no cessation. On the 13th day, at times, he was attacked with spasms, and extreme trembling, which would cause the bed to shake under him. The 14th, 15th & 16th days, he continued howling, snapping his teeth at the corners of the pillow, and biting the bed clothes, gaping & curling up his tongue, and making many other canine gestures. During all the six days, he slept not one minute; nor could 15 grains of crude opium, with ~~other~~ liquid preparations, as laudanum, in large quantities, given each day, cause the least appearance of drousiness upon his eyes, till the latter part of the 16th day of July last, when his voice & strength began to fail, and about seven o'clock in the evening, he began to drouse a little, and before eight he died, in the 42^d year of his age. He left a wife & six children."

Printed in the Salem Gazette of July 28th 1798, and transmitted to me by a medical friend.[21]

105

Dear Sir, Letter from Dr Rush to Dr Miller.

"In the first number of the 5th volume of the Medical Repository, Dr Physick has supposed death from Hydrophobia to be the effect of a sudden & spasmodic constriction of the glottis, inducing suffocation, and that it might be prevented by creating an artificial passage for air into the lungs, whereby life might be continued long enough to admit of the disease being

---

[21] Asa Felton died on July 16, 1800. The date of the article "Account of the Strange Effects of a Bite by a Mad Dog" is incorrect in Barker's manuscript; it was published in the *Salem Gazette*, July 29, 1800, p. 3. The identical article was published in the *Massachusetts Mercury* (Boston), August 1, 1800, p. 2; *Independent Gazetteer* (Worcester, MA), August 5, 1800, p. 4; *Federal Spy* (Springfield, MA) 11 August 1800, p. 1; *Greenfield Gazette* (Greenfield, MA) 16 August 1800 p.4; *Hampshire Gazette* (Northampton, MA), August 20, 1800, p. 1.

cured by other remedies.[22] The following account of a dissection is intended to show the probability of the Doctor's proposal being attended with success.

On the 13th of September, 1802, I was called with D[r] Physick,[23] to visit, in consultation with D[r]. Griffiths,[24] the son of William Todd Esq. aged five years, who was ill with the disease called Hydrophobia, brought on by the bite of a mad dog on the 6th of the preceding month. The wound was small and on his cheek near his mouth; two circumstances which are said to increase the danger of wounds from rabid animals. From the time he was bitten he used the cold bath daily, and took the infusion of anagallis, until the 9th of September, when he was seized with a fever, which at first resembled the remittent of the season. Bleeding, purging, blisters and the warm bath were prescribed; but without success. The last remedy appeared to afford some relief, which he manifested by paddling in the water. At the time I saw him, he was much agitated, had frequent twitchings, laughed often; but with this uncommon excitement in his muscles & nerves, his mind was unusually correct in all its operations. He discovered no dread of water except in one instance, when he turned from it with horror. He swallowed occasionally, about a spoonful of it at a time, holding the cup in his own hand. The quick manner of his swallowing, and the intervals between each time, were **106** such as we sometimes observe in persons, in the act of dying of acute diseases. Immediately after swallowing water, he looked pale, and panted for breath. He spoke rapidly and with much difficulty, particularly when he attempted to pronounce the words carriage, water & river. He coughed and breathed as patients do in the moderate grade of the Cynanche trachealis. The dog made a similar noise, in attempting to bark, the day before he was killed. We proposed making an opening into his windpipe; but while we were preparing for the operation, such a change for the worse took place, that it was not performed.

---

[22] Philip Syng Physick, "Case of Hydrophobia: Communicated by Dr. Philip Syng Physick of Philadellphia to Dr. Miller," *Medical Repository and Review of American Publications* 5, no. 1 (1802): 1–5.

[23] Dr. Philip Syng Physick (1768–1837) was a surgeon who graduated from the University of Pennsylvania, studied under John Hunter in London, and was house surgeon at St. George's hospital for one year. He then spent a year in Edinburgh, after which he returned to Philadelphia to practice surgery, was active at the Pennsylvania Hospital, and taught surgery at the medical school. Talbott, *A Biographical History of Medicine*, 370–71.

[24] Probably Dr. Samuel Powell Griffiths (1759–1826), founder of the Philadelphia Dispensory, who had trained in Philadelphia, France, London, and Edinburgh. He became Professor of Materia Medica at the University of Pennsylvania in 1792. Talbott, *A Biographical History of Medicine*, 468–69.

A cold sweat, with a feeble & quick pulse came on, and he died suddenly, at 12 o'clock at night.

On dissection, I discovered the following appearances. All the muscles of the neck had a livid colour, such as we sometimes observe, after death, in persons who have died of the sore throat. The muscles employed in deglutition & speech were suffused with blood. The epiglottis was inflamed, and the glottis so thickened and contracted as barely to admit a probe of the common size. The trachea below it was likewise inflamed & thickened, and contained a quantity of mucus, such as we observe, now & then, after death, from Cynanche trachealis. The œsophagus shew no marks of disease; but the stomach had several inflamed spots on it, and contained a matter of a brown appearance, and which emitted an offensive odour.

From the history of this dissection, and of many others in which much fewer marks appeared of violent disease in parts whose actions are essential to life, it is highly **107** probable death is not induced in the ordinary manner, in which malignant fevers produce it; but by a sudden or gradual suffocation. It is the temporary closure of this aperture, which produces the dread of swallowing liquids; hence the reason why they are swallowed suddenly, and with intervals, in the manner that has been described; for should the glottis be closed during the time of two swallows, in the highly inflamed state of the system, which takes place in this disease, suffocation would be the immediate & certain consequence. Solids are swallowed more easily than fluids, only because they descend by intervals, and because a less closure of the glottis is sufficient to favour their passage into the stomach.

An aversion from swallowing liquids is not peculiar to this disease. It occurs occasionally in the Yellow fever. It occurs also in the disease, which has prevailed among the cats, both in Europe & America, and probably in both instances, from a dread of suffocation in consequence of the closure of the glottis, and sudden abstraction of fresh air.

The seat of the disease, and the cause of death, being I hope, thus ascertained, the means of preventing death come next under consideration. An artificial aperture into the windpipe alone bids fair to arrest its tendency to death, by removing the symptom, which generally induces it, and thereby giving time for other remedies to produce their usual salutary effects in similar diseases. In the middle & northern States of America the disease is commonly attended with so much activity and excitement of the blood vessels, as to require copious blood letting & other depleting remedies.

108

Should this new mode of attacking this furious disease be adopted and become generally successful, the discovery will place the ingenious gentleman who suggested it, in the first rank of the medical benefactors of mankind.

Before I conclude my letter, I have only to add a fact which may tend to increase confidence in a mode of preventing the disease, which has been recommended by Dr Haygarth, and used with success in several instances. The same dog which bit W. Todd's son, bit, at the same time, a cow, a pig, a dog, and a black servant of W. Todd; The cow & pig died; the dog became mad, and was killed. The black man, who was bitten on one of his fingers, exposed the wound for some time, immediately after he received it, to a stream of pump water; and washed it likewise with soap & water. He escaped the disease. I am not, however, so much encouraged by its happy issue, in this case, as to advise it in preference to cutting out the wounded part. It should be resorted to where the fears of the patient, or his distance from a surgeon, render it impossible to use the knife."   Med. Repos. vol. 7.[25]

Philadelphia July 27, 1803.

109

"A case of Hydrophobia, successfully treated by Mercury; communicated to the Medical Society of the State of New York, by Dr Westell Willoughby, of Hermiker [sic—should be Herkimer] county; and transmitted to the Editors, by Nicholas Romayne, M.D. &c President of that Society.[26]

A son of M^r. Abraham Vankyning, of Newport, in the county of Hermiker [sic], aged 12 years, was bitten by a rabid dog on the 28th of April 1807. On the 30th of the same month, about 48 hours after the bite, he became

---

[25] Benjamin Rush, "An Account of the Examination of the Body of a Little Boy Who Died of Hydrophobia; Intented to Show the Probable Success of Dr. Physic's Proposal for Preventing Death by Making an Artificial Opening into the Windpipe," *Medical Repository* 2nd hexade, vol. 1, no. 2 (1804): 105–09.

[26] Westel Willoughby Jr. (1769–1844) was born in Goshen, New York, and practiced in Newport in Herkimer County. He was one of the founders of the College of Physicians and Surgeons in Fairfield, was active in county and state medical societies, became a judge, and held several state and national political offices. Nicholas Romayne (1756–1817) of New York began his medical education at King's College (Columbia College after the Revolutionary War) and continued at Edinburgh, London, Paris, and Leyden. He taught medicine at Columbia College and later at Rutgers College. In 1806 Romayne was elected president of the New York County Medical Society and, in 1810, the New York State Medical Society. Richard P. McCormick, *Rutgers: A Bicentennial History* (New Brunswick: Rutgers University Press, 1966), 32; Garraty and Carnes, *American National Biography*, vol. 18, 796–97.

indisposed with suspicious symptoms of madness; such as dejection of spirits, difficult deglutition, which at that time was considered, by the parents, as originating from worms in the throat, a peculiar avertion to light expressed by endeavouring to avoid it, and by covering himself so closely with the bed clothes as to shut out every ray. On the first day of May, I visited the patient, and at that time, learned the above statement from his parents. I found him labouring under the whole catalogue of symptoms, as described by different writers, in cases of hydrophobia, viz. impatience of light, a peculiar aversion to his friends, great thirst, violent febrile excitement, and whenever water was presented to him, an attempt to drink invariably produced a constriction of the throat, which was immediately followed by violent spasms of the whole system; with an attempt to bite every thing which came in his way; and in spite of the utmost precaution, he did actually bite out pieces of his own flesh. Finding him in this situation, and being fully persuaded of its being a case of canine madness, I had no expectation of giving him relief; having never before seen a case of this kind, **110** except among the animal tribe. Being fully satisfied from the general failure of remedies in healing the complaint, that there was scarcely any chance of relief, I concluded not to [be] influenced by any thing which I had read on the subject. Finding the patient labouring under violent vascular action, in consequence of excessive excitement, as soon as the paroxysm was off, I had recourse to blood-letting, and took away such a quantity as to remove the tension, and lessen arterial action. Having seen that the presence of his friends, the admission of light, and an attempt to swallow any liquids, seemed as the immediate causes of spasms, I endeavoured to re-move all these evidently hurtful powers. At the commencement of every par-oxysm, the spasms began in the throat; the pharynx first undergoing morbid derangement; from thence they extended to the hand, which had been bitten, and afterwards universal spasms ensued with a constant attempt to bite. These paroxysms generally continued from 10 to 20 minutes. After reducing the in-flammatory action, with the lancet, I thought best, on the ground of various authorities, together with my own knowledge of the medical properties of mercury, to give it a fair trial in this case. As the throat appeared to suffer pri-marily in this disease, I determined to give calomel in the following way.

I mixed about two drachms of calomel, with twice its quantity of dry sugar, and after blending them well together, I gave a teaspoonful of the mix-ture once in 20 minutes, until it proved violently emetic & cathartic. After which I gave it in smaller quantity and more frequently; taking particular care to keep the fauces & throat constantly overspread with it. **111** In this way, it was taken up quickly by the absorbants, and speedily affected the glands of the mouth. Within 12 hours from the first exhibition of the calomel, a gentle ptyalism was produced; upon which the violence of the symptoms abated; the paroxysms growing lighter and lighter, until they disappeared entirely. The salivation was kept up a few days. After this, to my astonishment and the disappointment of every one who saw him, he was happily restored to his disconsolate friends.

What is peculiar in this case, is, that the child was bitten by a puppy of six months old; which had never been bitten, to the knowledge of any one. The bitch, which brought the pup, while in the state of gestation, was known to have been bitten by a dog actually mad. After her whelps were weaned, the bitch was killed; she having never shown any symptoms of Hydrophobia.

After this time another of the puppies sickened, had every appearance of canine madness, and was killed. Two others, of the same litter have not sickened.

The patient becoming diseased, so soon after the bite is as novel, as the other circumstances are remarkable; yet I do not hesitate, in believing the case to have been strictly hydrophobia; and the cure to have taken place in consequence of the quantity of calomel given, and the particular manner mode in which it was given, aided by the lancet.

In the first stage of this case it was violently inflammatory. Had I pursued the stimulant & antispasmodic plan, recommended by many, instead of the depleting plan, it requires very little discernment to pronounce what would have become of my patient.

Med. Repos. vol. 12.[27]

---

[27] Westell Willoughby, "A Case of Hydrophobia, Successfully Treated by Mercury; Communicated to the Medical Society of the State of New York, by Dr Westell Willoughby, of Hermiker County; and Transmitted to the Editors, by Nicholas Romayne, M.D. &C President of That Society," *Medical Repository* 2nd hexade, vol. 6, no. 2 (1809): 135–37.

Chap. 8. [marked Chap. 7 in MS.]

FROM 1786, TO 1789, there was no appearance of any epidemical diseases in the District of Maine, as far as my observations extended, and fevers, wearing a malignant aspect, were of rare occurrence.

In 1787, the interior towns being supplied with a number of physicians, I removed to Stroudwater in Falmouth, near Portland, where my practice became more extensive on the sea coast; sometimes sixty miles eastward;[1] so that I had further oppertunities of making medical observations.

In the course of my practice, ~~during this period~~ I was consulted in many cancerous cases, besides some in preceeding years.[2] Various ~~means~~ medicines were used, and the knife was sometimes employed. But I was not so fortunate as to be instrumental in making a single cure, till 1795. I shall, hereafter describe these cancerous affections with my ill success; as also the success which

---

[1] By "eastward," Barker meant he was traveling northeast along the coast. Sixty miles in that direction would take him approximately to the town of Waldoboro traveling overland and St. George by sea. From Portland, one would speak of going "down" to Waldoboro, because the "eastward" coastal towns of Maine are downwind for sailboats; hence the term "Down East."

[2] This chapter is primarily about anasarca and dropsy, but Barker launched it with a discussion of cancer because fluid retention is seen with many cancers. Thus he referred to Cullen's nosology and the Class Cachexia under which the Orders of Emaciations (diminished bulk) and Swellings are listed. W. F. Bynum, "Cullen and the Study of Fevers in Britain, 1760–1820," in *Theories of Fever from Antiquity to the Enlightenment*, ed. W. F. Bynum and V. Nutton (London: Wellcome Institute for the History of Medicine; Medical History, Supplement No. 1, 1981), 137. Cullen concluded that one of the causes of watery swelling or dropsy is obstruction of the free return of venous blood including obstruction of the vessels of the lungs, valve ossifications, obstruction of the liver, and "scirrhosities of the spleen and other viscera. . . . But the cause most frequently interrupting the motion of the blood through the veins, is the compression of tumors existing near them; such as . . . scirrhous or steatomatous tumors in the adjoining parts." William Cullen, *First Lines of the Practice of Physic with Supplementary Notes, Including More Recent Improvements in the Practice of Medicine by Peter Reid*, two volumes in one (Brookfield: E. Mirriam & Co. for Isaiah Thomas, 1807), 592–602, particularly 593–95. "Scirrhous," or "scirrhus," refers to a tumor, hard, sometimes knotty and painful, most frequently affecting glands, terminating in cancer. John Redman Coxe, *The Philadelphia Medical Dictionary*, 2nd ed. (Philadelphia: Thomas Dobson, 1817), 380, and see OED.

has attended the means used for cancers, since 1795, not only in my own hands; but much more abundantly in the hands of others.[3]

In March 1788, I was called to a man in Cape Elizabeth, aged 50, of a gross habit who had lived in the fashionable way of drinking ardent spirits. He had been troubled with general anasarca[4] several months. At this time he

---

[3] In 1817 cancer was defined as a "painful, scirrhous tumor of the glands, generally becomes ulcerated." Coxe, *The Philadelphia Medical Dictionary*, 104. Hippocratic writings suggest that cancer results from an excess of black bile (one of the four humors). Galen believed that the deposition of the black bile in places such as breasts, tongue, and lips led to tumors, some of which were crab-shaped; hence the word "cancer" is derived from the Latin word for crab. The circulation of blood (Harvey) and the lymphatic system (Aselli) were described in the early seventeenth century, leading Descartes to suggest the "lymph theory" of the etiology of cancer, that is, the lymph fluid may leak out of lymph ducts, causing a benign tumor that with fermentation or degeneration may become malignant. Boerhaave (1688–1738), teaching in Leiden, considered cancer a result of inflammation. By the beginning of the eighteenth century the lymph theory had gained acceptability, though the humoral theory was still playing a role in the thoughts of those teaching and writing about cancer. Damianus Johannes Theodorus Wagener, *The History of Oncology* (Houten: Springer, 2009), 8, 12, 17, 19, 22–27. Cancer in its "full-blown state, has been recognized since antiquity. The properties of a hard swelling, destructive invasion, ulceration, pain, and fatal outcome were characteristic. By the eighteenth century advanced cancer was quite readily defined, but the early stages were not readily identified." Lester S. King, *Medical Thinking: A Historical Preface* (Princeton, NJ: Princeton University Press, 1982), 100–103. For a brief review of thoughts on cancer from Hippocratic times to the mid-nineteenth century, see Siddhartha Mukherjee, *The Emperor of All Maladies: A Biography of Cancer*, 1st Scribner hardcover ed. (New York: Scribner, 2010), 46–56. Life-expectancy charts are very numerous and complicated, and several factors may explain why cancer appears to have been a less common cause of death circa 1800. At that time, life-expectancy at birth was between thirty and forty years, but if one avoided death due to numerous childhood diseases and reached the age of twenty, one had a reasonable chance of reaching fifty to sixty years of age. J. David Hacker, "Decennial Life Tables for the White Population of the United States, 1790–1900," *Historical Methods* 43, no. 2 (2010): 45–79. And for five New Hampshire towns and Boston, see J. Worth Estes, "Therapeutic Practice in Colonial New England," in *Medicine in Colonial Massachusetts, 1620–1820: A Conference Held 25 & 26 May 1978*, ed. Frederick S. Allis (Boston: The Colonial Society of Massachusetts, 1980), table IX, 313. Life-threating infections for which there were no efficacious therapies available were a much more common cause of death; some of these infections may have occurred in people who had a cancer, but an infection would be regarded as the cause of death. Hall Jackson's well-studied Portsmouth, New Hampshire, practice revealed that only one of ninety-one deaths between 1775 and 1794 was attributed to cancer. J. Worth Estes, *Hall Jackson and the Purple Foxglove* (Hanover: University Press of New England, 1979), 124. The "Statement of Deaths" in Philadelphia, from January 1807 to January 1809, lists cancer as a cause of death in 18 out of 4,316 deaths. Health Board of, "Statement of Deaths, with the Diseases and Ages, in the City and Liberties of Philadelphia, from the 2d of January 1807, to the 1st of January 1809. Communicated by the Board of Health," *Transactions of the American Philosophical Society* 6 (1809): 403–407.

[4] Anasarca (dropsy, fluid retention), see Glossary entry. For more information on diagnosis and treatment of dropsy and anasarca in America in the early nineteenth century, see James Thacher, *American Modern Practice* (Boston: Ezra Read, 1817), 554–60. In the twenty-first century we know that anasarca can be caused by a number of conditions including liver disease, renal failure, congestive heart failure, severe malnutrition, malignancy, and others.

was swelled to a great degree, with difficulty of breathing & cough. Various means had been used; but to no advantage. I prescribed such medicines as had been directed by Dr Monro[5], but the swelling continued to increase with his other complaints. D^r. Hall Jackson[6] of Portsmouth was then consulted by letter, who sent me some of the **113** Digitalis or Fox-glove, with some account of the success which had attended his practice, of late, by this mean in Anasarca. Two drachms of the dried leaves were directed to be infused in half a pint of boiling water four hours, a tablespoonful of which was to be given, night & morning. This acted as a very powerful diuretic; and by pursuing this course, one week, the swelling was in great measure removed, with his other complaints. Friction was then used with tonic bitters, together with occasional doses of the digitalis, and his health was soon restored.

~~Two~~ In succeeding years, many cases of anasarca occurred in my practice, which in most instances yielded to an infusion of the digitalis. In some cases bleeding and cathartics were premised to advantage. But the digitalis did not succeed in any other species of dropsy.[7] A similar observation was made to me by Dr Jackson.

Ascites was of frequent occurrence, but it seldom yielded to the remedies commonly used. Tapping was sometimes practiced; but the water generally

---

[5] Donald Monro (1727–1802) of Edinburgh. Donald Monro, *An Essay on the Dropsy* (London: E. Wilson & T. Durham, 1755). Monro also mentioned cancer as a cause of dropsy; see pp. 11–13. He postulated the cause of dropsy to be "a weakness or laxity of the fibers." See Estes, *Hall Jackson and the Purple Foxglove*, 156.

[6] Hall Jackson (1739–1797) was a prominent Portsmouth physician and surgeon who had a special interest in dropsy throughout his career. See Estes, *Hall Jackson and the Purple Foxglove*, 141. He introduced digitalis (foxglove) to America within six months of the publication of William Withering, *An Account of the Foxglove, and Some of Its Medical Uses: With Practical Remarks on Dropsy, and Other Diseases* (Birmingham: M. Swinney for G, GJ, and J Robinson, London, 1785). See Estes, *Hall Jackson and the Purple Foxglove*, 141–63. We know that within two years, Barker wrote to Jackson and obtained some digitalis. Estes notes a letter "from Doctor Barker, a gentleman of eminence in his profession in Portland [illegible], with an account of the foxglove in the case of Capt. Frickey of that place" (p. 217). Withering was aware that digitalis was not effective for all cases of dropsy, for example with ovarian tumors: "but I wish it not to be tried in ascites of female patients, believing that many of these cases are dropsies of the ovaria." Estes argues "that there was absolutely no good reason for Hall Jackson or William Withering to think that the drug's site of action could be the heart" (p. 149).

[7] We know today that the effects of digitalis are primarily on the heart, a fact not known in Barker's and Hall Jackson's day. Digitalis is not efficacious in all anasarca, ascites, or edema, or in all cases due to heart disease, but it is certainly much less likely to benefit those with liver and renal failure, malignancy, or malnutrition. For a review of dropsy, ascites, and anasarca, see Steven J. Peitzman, "Swollen with Dropsy," in *Dropsy, Dialysis, Transplant: A Short History of Failing Kidneys*, Johns Hopkins Biographies of Disease (Baltimore: Johns Hopkins University Press, 2007), 1–23.

collected again in a longer or shorter time, and the disease terminated fatally. In a few instances tapping was successfully employed, and there was no further collection of water.

In 1786, Miss Watson of Gorham[8] aged about 40, was tapped by D^r. Coffin of Portland, in case of Ascites of 20 years standing, till then unsuspected altho she was very large. In other respects she enjoyed good health, able to walk several miles, and attend domestic business. Few means had been used excepting occasional doses of Jalap, when costive. Forty two quarts of water were drawn off at once, which was clear **114** and free from any ill smell. No faintness ensued. I attended her after the operation with Dr Rea of Windham[9] who first suggested that she was dropsical. The chief means used was an daily embrocation of a strong decoction of white oak bark for several weeks, with a suitable bandage. The water never collected again, and she enjoyed good health many years, when she died of pneumonia.

In the spring of 1800, Mark Wilson of Falmouth, aged 50, a sea man, who had been in the habit of drinking ardent spirits rather freely, was seized with the usual symptoms of ascites. He also complained of pain about the region of the liver, and his skin was yellow. Cathartics & diuretics of various kinds were employed, among which were Jalap, calomel & digitalis; but to no apparent advantage. In September following, after violent exercise in handling of bricks, he was attacked with vomiting & purging of blood without pain. I was then called when the patient informed me that he several quarts of blood had been evacuated which afforded some relief. Mercurial cathartics and the Digitalis were occasionally given, with other means; but the abdomen continued to enlarge, and there was a paucity of urine. Soon after I was called again in consultation with D^r. Jones of North Yarmouth[10], when we drew off six quarts of sizy yellowish water by tapping. Tonic embrocations as in the former case,

---

[8] Miss Watson may be Martha Watson, who was born December 4, 1743; no record of marriage or death is found. Or it may be her sister Susanna, born February 1, 1746, who married Isaac Skillings, January 8, 1766. Both women were daughters of Eliphet (deacon of the Congregational Church of Gorham after 1750) and Elizabeth Watson. See Hugh D. Mc Lellan, *History of Gorham, Maine* (Portland: Smith and Sale, 1903), 809.

[9] Dr. Caleb Rea Jr. (1758–1796) studied under Dr. Holyoke of Salem and was a naval ship's surgeon during the Revolution, finally settling in Windham in about 1788. James Alfred Spalding, *Maine Physicians of 1820; a Record of the Members of the Massachusetts Medical Society Practicing in the District of Maine at the Date of Separation* (Lewiston: Lewiston Print Shop, 1928), 142–43.

[10] Dr. David Jones had been a naval surgeon, became a member of the Massachusetts Medical Society, and was one of the signers of the 1804 petition to establish a District Society in Maine in 1804. Spalding, *Maine Physicians of 1820*, 102–103.

together with friction were daily used, as also aleotic cathartics occasionally. His health was soon restored. He died in 1806, of apoplexy, without any return of his dropsical complaints.

115

Case of Anasarca, communicated by Dr D. G. Barker of Sedgwick, Maine.[11]

"In Autumn, 1816, Mrs Morse of Bluehil, [*sic*][12] aged about 40, was invaded with Anasarca. The swelling increased to a great degree and extended to her face; so that she was almost blind, and a general torpor took place. She was attended by an experienced physician, but the usual remedies failed of producing the desired effect. In Jan. 1817, she was considered incurable. In Feb. I was requested to visit her, and found the disorder as above described. Twenty ounces of blood were then drawn, which produced great faintness and prostration of strength. The next day a dose of Jalap & calomel was given, which operated freely. The swelling then abated to a considerable degree. A few days after, an abortion took place; being six months advanced in pregnancy. The swelling in a short time wholly subsided; but her eye sight remained much impaired. A Seton was put into her neck, and tonic means were used. Her health was restored in about three months."[13]

"A very strong man, says Dr Monro, on the authority of Hildanus,[14] aged 30, was seized with an Anasarca; his optic nerves were obstructed, and he gradually became blind; but having discharged from the nose about four pounds of blood, he was soon restored to health, in every respect but that of his blindness, from which he was never wholly free."

---

[11] Dr. David Gorham Barker (1784–1830) was Dr. Jeremiah Barker's son, the third of five children.

[12] Probably Elizabeth Roundy Morse, born September 16, 1775. Rufus George Frederick Candage and Bluehill Historical Society, *Historical Sketch of Bluehill, Maine* (Ellsworth, ME: Hancock County Publishing Company, 1905), 14.

[13] This is almost a textbook description of preeclampsia, which occurs most commonly in pregnant women over forty years of age and after the twentieth week of gestation. Dropsy (edema), anasarca, and loss of vision are common, and it may lead to seizures (eclampsia) and death. The likelihood of fetal death is increased five times. Preterm delivery or, in this case spontaneous abortion, may cure the condition, although blindness, by several mechanisms, may persist.

[14] Guilelmus Fabricius Hildanus, also called Wilhelm Fabry and Fabricius von Hilden (1560–1634) studied in Italy and France, was called the father of German surgery, and practiced in Bern. Arturo Castiglioni, *A History of Medicine*, 2nd ed. (New York: Alfred A. Knopf, 1947), 480. The work of Hildanus, including a large chapter on ophthalmology, was edited posthumously in 1646 and published as "*Opera observationum et curationum medico-chirurgicarum.*" Wolfgang Straub, "The Ophthalmology of Fabricius Hildanus in the 17th Century," *Documenta Ophthalmologica* 74 (1990), 21–29.

"A man who laboured under a dropsy & fever was much relieved by an hemorrhage from the nose, which happened twice or thrice every day, for the space of three weeks. The swelling decreased, and the distemper was **116** totally dispelled, by the use of diaphoretics & diuretics."

"In Dec. 1758, a lad, aged 16 years, had a universal anasarca, with difficulty of breathing; a small quick pulse, and paucity of urine of a high colour. The complaint was of four weeks standing, brought on by sitting up three nights successively with a sick companion. Cathartics & diuretics were given; but to no advantage. He died. On opening his body, the lungs were found inflamed; as also most of his intestines, though he had never complained of any acute pain in these parts."

"Sponius[15] affirms that a man in a dropsy, which had increased rather than diminished by the use of hydragogues & diuretics, was cured by 20 bleedings."

Essay on Dropsy. p. 45.[16]

D[r] Rush relates a number of cases, in his own practice, as well as others, where bloodletting & spontaneous hemorrhages were productive of salutary effects in <u>tonic</u> dropsy, arising from too much action in the arterial system.

In <u>atonic</u> dropsy,[17] he recomments [sic] such stimulating substances as increase the action of the arterial system. viz aromatics, metalic tonics, &c also diuretics, generous diet, pressure, friction exercise &c.

Med. Obser. vol. 2[d].[18]

An account of two cases of Dropsy, cured by the loss of blood, communicated to D[r] Rush, by D[r] Wallace, in Virginia.

"In 1802, Kemble, aged 55, after much exposure to cold and wet during the winter, was early in March attacked with the usual symptoms of dysentery, but not in violence sufficient to confine him to bed. Bloody mucous stools, tormina & tenesmus continued about five weeks, when they gradually subsided; but a colliquative **117** diarrhœa followed, occasioning great emaciation & debility. About the middle of May, he complained of an abdominal increase, which, about the middle of June had arisen to as complete

---

[15] Charles Spon (1609–1684), Charles Spon and Hipprocates, *C. Sponii . . . Sibylla Medica: Hippocratis Libellum Prognosticon Heroico Carmine Latine Exprimens* (Lugduni, 1661).

[16] Monro, *An Essay on the Dropsy*, 45.

[17] Atonic dropsy, or dropsy of debility with a quick and weak pulse, little of no fever or thirst is discussed in Thacher, *American Modern Practice*, 559–60.

[18] Benjamin Rush, *Medical Inquiries and Observations*, 2nd ed., 4 vols. (Philadelphia: J. Conrad & Co., 1805), vol. 2, 153–89, particularly 175–82.

an abdominal dropsy as I ever saw. At this time, I was called to him, and explained the nature of ascites. But he refused the use of any internal remedies; adding, he never had, nor would take any physic. After some persuasion, he consented to the loss of blood. His pulse strongly indicated bleeding. I drew 20 ounces, which was buffy. He was sensibly relieved in his feelings, and that night discharged more urine, than was usual for him to discharge in forty eight hours.

The next morning I repeated the bleeding and found the blood buffy. When I left him I directed the loss of 16 ounces of blood every third day, until he should lose three pounds more. My directions were complied with.

The third week after I left him, he visited me on horse back, 30 miles distant; not a symptom of dropsy remaining. In a few weeks he recovered his flesh.

M^rs —— aged 45; was in April last, attacked with symptoms of universal dropsy. She was swelled from head to foot. In this state, her catamenia flowed immoderately for ten days. She took no remedies. The dropsy entirely disappeared. Her urine was discharged in full quantity on the approach of the hemorrhage.

M^rs —— as is usual at her age, previous to the entire cessation of the catamenia, has menstruated irregularly for the last twelve months. In July, the hydropic symptoms returned & increased until the middle of the last month, when I was called to her, and found her head, abdomen, superior & inferior extremities **118** very much swelled. She could not walk across the room, without losing her breath; pulse tense & hard, urine scarce, very costive; and an immoderate uterine hemorrhage. She refused any remedy, even bleeding. In this situation, she lay eight days, without the aid of any remedy. I was then again called, & found every hydropic symptom removed. Her breathing though quick was free. The uterine hemorrhage still continued; and I had to use every art to restrain it, which was successfully done, by an astringent infection,[19] which has never failed, after the phlogistic action is removed." Med. Museum. v. 2. p. no1.[20]

---

[19] Astringent infection suggests the obsolete usage of the word "infection" as a process of affecting or impregnating something with another substance; in this case, the use of an astringent that draws together or contracts soft organic tissue. (OED) and J. Worth Estes, *Dictionary of Protopharmacology* (Canton, MA: Science History Publications, 1990), 21.

[20] James W. Wallace, "An Account of Two Cases of Dropsy, Cured by the Loss of Blood, Extracted from a Letter from Dr. James W. Wallace of Faquier County, in Virginia, to Dr. Benjamin Rush. Dated December 16th, 1805," *Philadelphia Medical Museum* 2, no. 4 (1806): 401–403.

In the course of my practice, I have met with many cases of atonic dropsies, after the subsidence of fevers, where the feet & legs swelled to a considerable degree, and sometimes the swelling extended to the bowels. In such cases, friction, tonic medicines, diuretics and bandages, were successfully employed.

Would that as good success had attended the treatment of another species of dropsy, which, at times, has occurred in my practice, viz <u>hydrocephalus</u> or internal dropsy of the brain.

History of a fatal case of Hydrocephalus. By Dr Harris of Kingston, Jamaica.

"Nothing tends so much to the advancement of medical knowledge as a faithful record of cases.

M. K. Harris, in her 26th month, a healthy child, on the 20th of October 1802, became more inactive than usual. She took 2 grains of calomel at night, and brought up some curdled milk in the morning. On the 22^d she was dull & heavy, took an emetic, which ejected some green stuff, but the drowsiness remained. She passed a **119** restless night, with an incessant short cough. This gave the idea of cold & indigestion being the cause of her illness.

23. She took castor oil, followed with an antimonial.

24. She took two does [sic] of calomel, which operated three times.

25. drowsy all the day, with a troublesome cough. She was put into a tepid bath; without any good effect.

26. cough incessant; an emetic of ipecac given on the 27th.

28. The stupor increased; a blister was applied between the shoulders, and assafœtidic glysters were used. In the evening gave 5 grains of calomel, followed with two table spoonfuls of castor oil: Sinapisms applied.

29. The stupor continued; pulse below the natural standard. A blister was now applied to the epigastric region and wine with food given.

30. her head was shaved and a blister applied. Mercurial friction was adopted; and calomel repatedly [sic] given. The pupils much dilated; pulse fuller and more frequent, with heat in the extremities.

Nov. 1^t. pulse irregular, heavy sighs & deep groans.

2. pulse 116. she has not spoken since yesterday. Calomel repeated, so as to affect the mouth.

3. pulse 132. 4th pulse 112. 5th 152. calomel continued.

6th. All the left side affected with spasm. At 11 o'clock pulse 200. She expired at 9. in the evening!

Upon opening the head, the bloodvessels appeared much distended; but there was no extravasation of serous effusion between the membranes. On removing the membranes, the fullness of the vessels on the surface of the brain, exhibited their ramifications in a most beautiful manner; and on cutting through the corpus callosum there were found about four ounces of a pure limpid fluid. This was sufficient to account for the death of the child, without going further."

"From these appearances, we may reasonably presume **120** that, had the disease been suspected in its first stage, there might have been some probability of success, from lessening the quantity of blood in the head, either by leeches, arteriotomy, or cupping, and by the early use of blisters & setons, accompanied by the powerful effects of mercury."

"Although this disease has been very correctly described by several eminent authors, it appears that it has been too often overlooked in practice, on account of the similarity of symptoms with other diseases incident to children. I am induced, from this case, to look back with regret on several cases in which I might have overlooked the disease."

"Happy would it be for mankind, if each individual would profit by the consideration of the error he has committed either in theory or practice."

Museum vol. 2.[21]

"Having, for many years, says Dr Rush, been unsuccessful in all the cases, except two, of internal dropsy of the brain, which came under my care, I began to entertain doubts of the common theory of this disease, and to suspect that instead of its being considered as an idiopethic [*sic*] dropsy, the effusion of water should be considered only as an effect of a primary inflammation or congestion of blood in the brain."

Med. Ob. vol. 2.[22]

In 1790, and in succeeding years, Dr Rush, having adopted this theory, successfully treated a number of cases of dropsy of the brain, with repeated bleeding and cathartics of Jalap & calomel. Since which, other physicians, in the Union, have been equally successful, by adopting a similar mode of practice, when seasonably employed.

Improper indulgencies in diet, producing diseased action of the stomach & bowels, are considered as predisposing causes of this disease. I never saw a case of hydrocephalus among the poor, except when occasioned by

---

[21] Dr. Harris, "History of a Fatal Case of Hydrocephalus. By Dr. Harris, of Kingston, Jamaica, in a Letter to Dr. Farquhar, Dated July 30th, 1805," *Medical Museum* 2, no. 1 (1806): 384–91.

[22] Benjamin Rush, *Medical Inquiries and Observations*, 4th ed., 4 vols. (Philadelphia: Johnson & Warner, 1815), vol. 2, 127.

concussion. Habitually wetting the feet, has, in some instances, produced the disease among young females; also stove heated rooms.

121

In August 1786, Mrs Bangs of Gorham, aged about 30, an habitual & violent dancer, among the Shakers, complained of pain just below the pit of the stomach which extended to the left side, where an oppressive load was felt, and the addomen [sic] soon became enlarged with a sense of soreness to the touch. After enduring these complaints about three weeks, I was called. At this time the bowels were swelled to a considerable degree, and she was very costive, pulse full & rather tense. I drew a pint of blood and gave repeated doses of aloes as a cathartic. No relief, however, was afforded. On a second visit three days after, finding that the pain and swelling had increased, I drew another pint of blood and gave Jalap & calomel in large doses, which operated freely, but to no apparent advantage. Soon after, Dr Rea was called in consultation, who considered her as labouring under <u>ascites</u>, and recommended tapping. But the patient would not consent. The swelling of the abdomen gradually increased, with pain, distress & great anxiety. Aleotic and mercurial cathartics were occasionally used, as she continued very costive. Opiates were sometimes given to alleviate distress & procure sleep. She continued in this way, about two months from the attack, when death closed the scene.

I opened her body, by permission, the next day, assisted by Dr Rea. The liver was found considerably enlarged and inflamed; the surface of which was beset with numerous hydatids containing from an ounce to half a pint of water. The gall bladder was enlarged and contained a glutinous substance. The biliary duct was obstructed by similar matter. The spleen was greatly enlarged, and contained dark grumous blood, though sound in texture. **122** From these appearances, we were induced to believe that if copious bloodletting and drastic cathartics, had been seasonably employed, together with a mercurial salivation, her complaints might have been removed.

In May 1787, I was called to a woman in Standish, who had labored under painful hemorrhoids, with external tumors, several months. Having seen the good effects of a mercurial salivation in phagedenic ulcers, an ounce of unguent. Caml. was left with directions to have it rubbed on the tumors. The ointment was soon used, and a copious salivation took place, which continued about a week. Her complaints were then removed, and a radical cure was effected.

In succeeding years, I have met with many very similar cases, and found that they generally yielded to similar treatment, tho in some cases calomel was given, in order to produce a salivation.

Two cases will be particularly related.

In Nov. 1807 a lady in Portland aged about 50, labored under painful hemorrhoids, without external tumors. She was also troubled with bad digestion, and her appetite had become very much impaired. Being consulted, I left 24 pills each containing one grain of calomel, made up with flour paste, which was boiled, and the pills having been made several weeks, were very hard. Two of these pills were taken night & morning. In one week a salivation was produced, and the hemorrhoidal complaint was greatly alleviated. A few days after, she took a dose of Flor. Sulph, and all the pills were voided by stool, as hard as when swallowed; and to appearance undiminished in size; as the patient informed me. She was then alarmed on account of the quantity of mercury, which had been so long retained in her stomach or bowels, and sent for Dr N. Coffin, who led **123** her to understand that there was no danger. He prescribed some suitable stomachic and her digestion became good. Since which she has enjoyed uniform health.

In May 1812, Capt. Jones, of Falmouth was greatly afflicted with hemorrhoids, which had troubled him, in a greater or less degree for more than a year. At this time I was consulted, when he complained of much pain & anguish with tenesmus. A mercurial salivation was prescribed. Two grains of calomel were taken night & morning. In ten days a copious salivation was produced. His complaints were then removed. Soon after, the salivation ceased, he went abroad and was exposed to inclement weather, which excited febrile disturbance with pain in the groin. A tumor soon arose to the size of a hens egg, which was very hard, and would not yield to discutients. It continued much in the same state, and very painful about three weeks, when Dr Cummins of Portland was called and introduced a seton through the middle of the tumor. This produced some discharge, and it gradually subsided. His health was then restored and he has continued free from hemorrhoidal affection.

Before I adopted the plan of salivating for this disease, a case occurred which seemed to throw some light on its nature. A gentleman of the law, in the County of Plymouth, Massts was sorely afflicted with hemorrhoids, for which various means were used, by physicians & others, such as Flor. Sulph, crem. tart &c, which only afforded some temporary relief. In 1760 he took passage for London and consulted physicians; but to no advantage. He returned home greatly emaciated, and tortured with the disease. He died soon after his arrival. On examining the rectum, by dissection, it was found inflamed, ulcerated and corroded.

124

It does not appear to me that hemorrhoids essentiall differ from tracheal consumption, save in their seat; and this disease has been removed by a mercurial salivation, in a number of cases, which will hereafter be related.

In the course of my practice I have met with many cases of bleeding piles; without pain or injury to the constitution, tho of several years continuance, except when the hemorrhage happened to stop; then fever & severe pain in the rectum ensued, which required repeated bloodletting & oily enemas, also large tents of tow, covered with tallow or hogs lard. Injections of cold water have also been used to advantage in such cases.

It is maintained by physicians in Paris, that the blood in hemorrhoids is thrown out by exhalation from the arteries, as in epixtaxis [*sic*], hemoptysis &c and that the difference of these hemorrhages consists in the parts affected.

125

Chap. 9. (marked Chap. 8.)

Influenza or Epidemical Catarrh.

THIS DISEASE HAS been known from the days of Hippocrates; and prevailed frequently in England during the last century.

In North America, according to Mr Webster,[1] it appeared in 1647, 1655, 1697, 1732, 1737, 1747, 1756, 1761, 1772, 1781, 1789 & 90, and 1802. ——It also prevailed in 1807 & 1816.

It appears, by Mr Smiths records,[2] that this disease was prevalent in Maine, in the winter & autumn, of 1758, called an "Epidemic cough," which was very severe, especially among children.

Except this visitation of the Influenz, [*sic*] we have no account of its appearing in Maine, till the autumn of 1789. At this time, it prevailed in New York & Philadelphia, and, "in the course of a few months, says Dr Rush, pervaded every State in the Union, extending to the West Indies and the ensuing winter, to South America."

The symptoms which ushered in the disease, were chills succeeded by febrile heat, an irritating cough, sneezing, hoarseness, sore throat, hawking, with expectoration of thin sharp mucus; pain in the head, chest & limbs, thirst and a furred tongue; pulse tense & frequent. The fever usually declined in 5 or 6 days; but the cough & expectoration continued two or three weeks, when it commonly subsided, tho it sometimes continued to increase, and the disease terminated in pulmonary consumption. I met with no case of this

---

[1] A reference to Noah Webster (1758–1843) and the chapter in his book "Of the Influenza or Epidemic Catarrh." See Noah Webster, *A Brief History of Epidemic and Pestilential Diseases with the Principal Phenomena of the Physical World Which Precede and Accompany Them and Observations Deduced from Facts Stated*, 2 vols. (Hartford: Hudson and Goodwin, 1799), vol. 2, 30–37.

[2] Barker again cites the diary of the Reverend Thomas Smith.

disease under puberty. My own wife, aged 40, who had been troubled with a slight catarrh many years, was attacked in November. The cough continued to increase through the winter. In March, she felt some pain in the side, raised a little blood with purulent matter, a moderate hectic attended, and she died in June following.[3]

[Here is interleaved a four-column newspaper page with a handwritten note across the top of the page, "A present from George Parkman M.D. of Boston to Dr Barker for his history of diseases in Maine, &c 1822." It begins with "Nothing exceeds the pleasure of relieving distress but that of preventing it" and is all about methods of disease prevention. It favors exercise but avoid dancing, alcohol, and gossiping. Several paragraphs are numbered. No reference given.]

126

Several other cases occurred, in healthy people, which terminated in phthisis pulmonalis. The chief means used were demulcents; for physicians were seldom called, in season; the disease being considered by many as a common cold.

The ~~disease~~ Influenza subsided in the winter, and returned in March 1790, when it appeared to be more inflammatory. A woman, aged 50, of a spare habit, was attacked in April. On the third day a copious hemorrhage from her lungs took place, in a fit of coughing, which greatly reduced her strength, but the fever readily subsided and the cough ceased. She soon recovered, by suitable nutriment, without any medicine. This case induced some, seasonably to send for physicians, and solicit bleeding. Good success attended the practice.

"In several pregnant women, says Dr Rush, the Influenza, at that time, produced uterine hemorrhages & abortions. In some, the nose discharged streams of blood, to the amount, in one case, of twenty ounces." Med. Obser.[4]

Wonderful are the efforts of nature, in many instances, to alleviate human misery; and are they not worthy of imitation?

An account of the Influenza, as it appeared in 1807, & 16, with some dissections, will be given in the sequel.

From 1790, to 1793, general health prevailed, save consumptive complaints.

---

[3] Abigail Gorham Barker, Jeremiah Barker's first wife, died at age forty in Falmouth June 29, 1790. She was born to Abigail and David Gorham Esq. of Barnstable, Massachusetts, on March 5, 1749. Her brother was Judge William Gorham of Gorham, District of Maine. Ruth Gray et al., *Maine Families in 1790* (Camden: Maine Genealogical Society, 1988), vol. 4, 18–19. See also Hugh D. Mc Lellan, *History of Gorham, Maine* (Portland: Smith and Sale, 1903), 396–98.

[4] Benjamin Rush, "An Account of the Influenza," in *Medical Inquiries and Observations*, 4th ed., 4 vols. (Philadelphia: Johnson & Warner, 1815), vol. 2, pp. 265–73.

In Jan. 1793, Mr James Cobb, of Falmouth, aged 45, of a gross habit, walked to Portland, distant six miles. On his return, in the evening, after walking three miles, he perspired very freely, when he was taken into a sleigh and rode home. **127** He had a restless night; but he rode out the next day, when he was attacked with chilliness, followed by febrile heat, pain in the head & back, with loss of appetite. I was called the next morning, when his pulse was frequent & rather tense. I drew a pint of blood and evacuated his stomach & bowels. The fever continued twenty days. After the tenth day, he was attended with low delirium. The means used were occasional cathartics, blisters, antimonials, and a liberal use of cold water, which he earnestly craved. He recovered, without any recollection of his complaints. His family consisted of an aged mother, a brother, two sisters and a hired man. The sick room was 15 feet square, 7 high, and plaistered, which was kept warm by a fire night & day. In the latter part of his fever, all the rest of his family, save his mother, were attacked with a similar fever, and treated much in the same manner, the duration 20 days. They all recovered. One of those patients was confined in the same room; the others in adjoining rooms, equally tight & warm.

Several watchers,[5] particularly those who removed the stools, were invaded with a very similar fever, and some died. This fever was called, by some, <u>contagious</u>. But might it not, with more propriety, be called <u>infectious</u>, propagated by noxious air in the sick rooms. Since which & before, typhous fever[6] has often occurred in my practice, and when sick rooms have been properly ventilated, and cleanliness particularly observed, the disease has not often been communicated. Large unplaistered rooms, among the poor, have been found much more comfortable for the sick, and much safer for their attendants. All these precautions, however, would not secure a person against <u>contagious</u> fevers, as the small pox and measles.

---

[5] This refers to the neighbors, relatives, and possibly lay healers who kept a vigil at the sickbed and helped with necessary tasks.

[6] Typhous fever: see Glossary entry. Associated with confined, poorly ventilated dwelling places, it was also called jail or camp fever when epidemic in those situations. By the early twentieth century it was known to be a louse-borne rickettsial disease characterized by fever, skin eruption, and central nervous system involvement. For more details see James Thacher, *American Modern Practice* (Boston: Ezra Read, 1817), 176–78; Dale C. Smith, "Medical Science, Medical Practice, and the Emerging Concept of Typhus in Mid-Eighteenth Century Britain," in *Theories of Fever from Antiquity to the Enlightenment*, ed. W. F. Bynum and V. Nutton (London: Wellcome Institute for the History of Medicine; Medical History, Supplement No. 1, 1981), 121–34; D. Raoult, T. Woodward, and J. S. Dumler, "The History of Epidemic Typhus," *Infectious Disease Clinics of North America* 18, no. 1 (2004): 127–40.

128

In Jan. 1794, E. Libbe, aged 24, after a hard day's labour, on a cold damp day, rode several miles, in the evening, in a sleigh, without a great coat. On his return, he was suddenly attacked with convulsion fits, and loss of reason. A physician was called, who let blood, and directed paragoric elixir, which was repeatedly given; but the fits recurred, once in about half an hour, with great violence, and continued to attack, about 24 hours. I was then called and gave three grains of opium every half hour for two hours, when the fits began to abate in violence & frequency. Another dose making 15 grains removed the fits entirely, without inducing sleep, and his reason was restored, with a full pulse which before taking the opium could scarcely be felt.

In Feb. 1794, Mrs Trichey, aged 40, complained of indigestion & pain in the stomach, which was relieved by 40 drops of laudanum. As the spring advanced she became infeebled, and began to enlarge in abdominal size, with difficulty of breathing and paucity of urine. In July she became as large as a woman nine months in pregnancy, with great tension & elasticity of the abdomen. At times she was troubled with flatuency, nausea & vomiting; sometimes a slight diarrhœa; catamenia more frequent than natural. During these months she was under a course of aromatic bitters, squills & digitalis; but to no sensible benefit. Dr Watts was called in consultation who advised to an emetic, which operated freely each way; but to no advantage. The swelling continued to increase with great oppression at the stomach, so that she could not lie down in bed. Dr Erving **129** was then called in consultation, who advised to aromatic bitters, digitalis & squills. This course was pursued two weeks, without producing any change; her size continuing to increase with nausea & total loss of appetite. She then laid aside all means, and her case was considered as irremediable.

About a week after this, being in great distress at the stomach, she sent to me for something to afford relief, in her dying moments. I sent a mixture of Laud. & bals. traum[7], equal parts, directing forty drops twice a day. The first dose gave some relief. In less than a week the swelling had sensibly decreased. In a fortnight, the swelling was reduced about one half. In four weeks she was reduced to nearly her natural size, increasing the dose of laud. & b. traumat. one third after the first week. In two months she was restored to health.

This was probably a case of Tympany, owing to confined air, between the intestines, and the membranes which line the muscles of the abdomen; for

---

[7] Laudanum and balsamum traumaticum: see Glossary.

the means did not operate as a diuretic. How they produced the desired effect, I do not pretend to understand.[8]

130

In the spring of 1794, Mr Moses Plumer of Scarboro, aged 60, a farmer, perceived several small tumors in his face, attended with heat & itching. As the summer approached they became painful, and discharged a corrosive humor. Physicians were called who considered them to be cancers. Some were extirpated with the knife; and mercury was used both externally & internally; as well as cicuta, with a view of correcting this humor, and of disposing the sores to heal. The sores, however, would not heal on this plan. Indeed the humor increased in degree of virulency & corrosive power, notwithstanding that the external applications were reinforced with vitriols, lead, various unguents, and even <u>arsenic</u>.

He then laid aside all means, and remained in this forlorn condition, till May 1795, considering his disease as irremediable. At this time I was consulted when the cancerous tumors had enlarged and become open ulcers, attended with much pain.

I then directed a strong lixivium of hard wood ashes to be applied. This readily stopped the progress of the corroding humor, and alleviated his the pains. By this means the cancerous humor was subdued and rendered harmless; so that in a short time the ulcers were cleansed and healed; and a radical cure was effected.

This lixivium is made by boiling a gallon of common ley down to a pint. A dossil of lint, impregnated with this ley, and applied to the cancerous tumor, soon alleviates the pain and converts it into a black lump, which by a common digestive poultice, readily seperates from the sound flesh, with fibrous roots, or is easily extracted with a pair of forceps. The **131** sore then heals by a simple dressing.

Mr Plumer gave me only three dollars for my visit and directions, having been at considerable expense the year past, for medical advice from others. He then proclaimed that he was in possession of a certain remedy for cancers; and many patients thus affected resorted to his house, who were successfully treated. His fee was four dollars exclusive of boarding.

Mr James Larey of Falmouth, one of his patients, having received a cure, purchased the art, of M. Plumer, of making this ley, for fifty dollars, and removed to Hebron, forty miles north of Portland, where he has successfully treated many cancerous cases, in an extensive practice; while I remained

[8] Thacher, *American Modern Practice*, 561–62.

unknown as being Mr Plumers physician, excepting by a few of his neighbours, for some years; so that my practice in cancers, was comparatively small.

In 1800, Mr Plumer proposed applying to Congress for a Patent, pretending that he made his ley with five different sorts of wood, which were peculiarly efficacious as curative means. This he kept a secret. One of his children, however, informed me that the ley was made out of the ashes of oak, Elm, Alder, ash & corn cobbs.

Being informed of his project, I sent his case to Dr Mitchill, which was published in the 4. vol. of the Medical Repository, observing that a strong solution of pot-ash had been found to be equally efficacious in eradicating cancers. Hence it appeared probable, that the pus of an ulcerated cancer absorbed oxygen from the air and acquired an <u>Acid</u> quality. See Med. Repository, vol. 4. p. 297. & 415.[9]

132

In the course of my practice, in Maine, from 1780 to 1795, I met with many cases of cancer, which proved fatal. A few will be related.

In the spring of 1781, Mrs Butler, of Gorham, aged 40, apparently of a good habit, perceived a small tumor on her neck, near the clavicle, attended with heat & itching. In Autumn it had increased to the size of a pea and was painful. In December I was consulted. No means had been used but a carrot poultice.[10] I advised her to consult some experienced physician in Boston. In April 1802, a Journey was performed, and Dr Loyd[11] was consulted, when it had increased to the size of a small nutmeg, tho not ulcerated. He adviced her to have it cut out. But to this she did not consent. The tumor soon discharged

---

[9] H. C. Kunze, "Experiments Proving the Acid Quality of the Pus, or Matter Formed on the Surface of Veneral and Cancerous Ulcers," *Medical Repository* 4, no. 3 (1800–1801): 297–98; Jeremiah Barker, "Use of Alkalies in Cancer. Extract from a Letter of Dr. J. Barker to Dr. Mitchill, Dated Portland (Maine), March 12, 1801," *Medical Repository* 4 (1801): 415–16.

[10] "Poultices of raw carrots, grated and moistened, have superceded those formerly made of hemlock, and they are said to produce as much ease and diminish fœtor more powerfully." Thacher, *American Modern Practice*, 517.

[11] Dr. James Lloyd (1728–1810) apprenticed under Dr. Sylvester Gardiner and Dr. James Clark, both of Boston, and then attended lectures at Harvard College and studied at Guy's Hospital, London. He was one of the leading physicians in Boston, particularly interested in surgery, and was apparently the first in America to introduce the use of ligatures rather than cautery. See James Thacher, *American Medical Biography: Or Memoirs of Eminent Physicians Who Have Flourished in America. To Which Is Prefixed a Succinct History of Medical Science in the United States, from the First Settlement of the Country* (Boston: Richardson & Lord and Cottons & Barnard, 1828), 359–76; Howard A. Kelly and Walter L. Burrage, *American Medical Biographies* (Baltimore: The Norman, Remington Company, 1920), 710; and Martin Kaufman, Stuart Galishoff, and Todd Lee Savitt, *Dictionary of American Medical Biography*, 2 vols. (Westport, CT: Greenwood Press, 1984), vol. 1, 450–51.

a corrosive humor, which corroded the flesh on the breast with great torture. In about three months, the flesh was corroded to such a degree that the matter passed into the chest, and deprived her of life.

Soon after, Mr Mussey of Portland, while shaving himself, cut off a small pimple from the lower part of his face. Soreness with heat & itching was soon felt, which could not be remedied by common means. The sore became ulcerated, and extended its effects to his throat; so that in about a year he could swallow nothing but liquid food. In this way he continued some time, when swallowing was wholly impeded and he died by starvation.

Mrs Small of C. Elizabeth, was troubled with a small painful tumor on the side of her neck, which proved cancerous and extended its effects to her throat; that in about one year, she was unable to swallow, and died.

133

In August 1782, Andrew Crocket of Gorham,[12] aged 50, had a small tumor in his under lip, of a years standing, which was slightly ulcerated. I cut it out and it soon healed. In August 1783, it grew again and extended its effects to the throat. He died the following spring.

In 1790 E. Chick, of Falmouth, perceived a small itching pimple in his under lip which gradually increased in size till 1800, when it became as large as a hens egg, and ulcerated. It soon extended its effects to the throat & proved fatal.

Were it necessary I could mention many other very similar cases of cancer, which terminated fatally under the use of common means. Some tumors had been cut out of a few months standing, before ulceration took place, and were radically cured by a simple dressing; but seldom after they became ulcerated cancers.

"Died at Sullivan, Maine, Sept. 12, 1818, of a cancer, Mrs Esther White, aged 66. The cancer commenced in her upper lip, about 17 years ago. Ulceration began about 10 years since. In its progress it destroyed the whole of the face, skin & muscles; as well as bones, except about half the lower jaw. For six months previous to her death she had become a moving spectacle of horror, her bodily health being perfectly good; but totally blind, deaf & speachless. She prepared her own food, after it was cooked, and with a spoon or her fingers, put it into the esophagus, or passage to the stomach. After destroying the

---

[12] Andrew Crockett (or Crockit) was born circa 1732, married, and bought land in Gorham in 1764, where he was a schoolmaster in 1771. He served as a second lieutenant in the Revolutionary War in 1777 and was a Gorham selectman in 1777 and 1780. McLellan, *History of Gorham, Maine*, 225, 374, 452–59.

eyes, it made its way into the brain, and she died without pain or a struggle, with a full reliance on the promises of the Gospel and resigned to the will of God."   Portland Gazette[13]

Dr William Steward, of Canaan, Maine, in his Botanical Dictionary,[14] printed in 1812, says "I have had opertunities to inform myself of the nature, operation and progress of cancers, having travelled upwards of sixteen thousand miles, through the Northern States of America, within nine years past; during which time I have extracted 47 cancers, without using the knife. Some **134** as they informed me had been affected with them 30 years. Some of these cancers, at first exhibited the appearance of small tumors; others originated from a natural mark; others from a scab, wart, and ulcers. These cancers were formed in different parts of the body; many on the neck, face, nose, upper & under lip, and in the roof of the mouth. The symptoms of a Cancer, in the first stage, are so trifling, that they are apt to be neglected. I have seen some with their eyes eat out, others with the flesh on their arms consumed, also a part of the head, some with their breasts eat off. Those cancerous tumors which form in a womans breast are attended with light pains at first; as they increase there will be a hot, darting, stinging & painful sensation. After they ulcerate, the patient will feel cold & shivering. In this stage of a cancer, rapid progress is often made to a fatal termination."

The means which he used to extract cancers were plaisters of verdigris, vitriol, arsenic & corrosive sublimate, seperately or combined. Previous to their application, in plethoric habits, bloodletting was practiced.

In the course of my practice, in the southern parts of New England, from 1770 to 1780, I met with very few cases of cancer, and these proved fatal. I was informed of three cases of cancerous breasts, which terminated fatally; and one which was cured by a drawing plaister.

---

[13] *Portland Gazette*, October 6, 1818, 3.

[14] Dr. William Steward "utilized the oil of rattlesnakes for deafness, and the grease, sizzled out of dead cats, for the shingles and allied skin diseases." James Alfred Spalding, *Maine Physicians of 1820; a Record of the Members of the Massachusetts Medical Society Practicing in the District of Maine at the Date of Separation* (Lewiston: Lewiston Print Shop, 1928), 42. William Steward, *The Healing Art, or Art of Healing Disclosed, by a Professed Botanist. Being Alphabetically Arranged, It May Be Termed a Botanical Dictionary* (Ballston Spa, NY: James Comstock, 1812). Barker has excerpted section C, "Of a Scirrhous and Cancer," Steward, William. The Healing Art, or Art of Healing Disclosed, by a Professed Botanist. Being Alphabetically Arranged, It May Be Termed a Botanical Dictionary . . . (Ballston Spa, NY: James Comstock, 1812), 6–13.

Since 1780, I have met with several cases of scirrhus[15] tumors, in the breasts of females, which have been removed by a liberal use of <u>cicuta</u> internally & externally. The extract recently made was taken, and an embrocation of the herb in a strong decoction was externally applied. In one case the tumor was as large as a hens egg, and very painful. In others the tumors were numerous and of the size of nutmegs.

135

I have been informed of several cases of scirrhus tumors in female breasts and seen some, in Maine, which have been neglected till they became ulcerated cancers, and which have been amputated, by Surgeons, tho seldom with success.

The following case, related by D[r] Colebrook of London, affords instruction. ——Ann James, aged 55, had for some years complained of a pain, and hard lump in each breast. In Sept. 1762, my advice was requested, when I found a very hard scirrhus, in each breast: that in the left breast, had the mamillary glands indurated & knobbed like ramifications; towards the axilla, a little adhesion to the pectoral muscle. The tumor was as large as a turkeys egg; that in the right breast not so large. She complained of excrutiating pains in both breasts, with total loss of appetite, and inability to do any work. I directed fifteen grains of green hemlock, viz <u>cicuta</u>, three times a day, minced with parsley, to disguise the taste, to be eaten with bread & butter; and that her constant drink should be lime water & milk; keeping her body open with rhubarb or magnesia, that she should have an issue on her arm; and lose about half a pint of blood, once in six or eight weeks, if the pain continued. The cicuta agreed with her stomach and eased her pains, tho it caused a tingling to her fingers ends. The quantity was increased, and the first of Nov. she had a very large menstrual discharge, which had not happened for many years before. The scirrhus was much lessened, and the pains considerably abated. About the end of Nov. the issue stopped, and a violent humor came round the orifice. Her breast was then more swelled and the pain more acute, with giddiness of the head, and weight over her eyes. She was bled till she fainted,

---

[15] "Scirrhus is a disease, so called from the hardness that characterizes it. It is a state of induration, of a peculiar kind, affecting glandular structures generally, but capable of occurring in other textures. It usually precedes carcinoma, of which it may, indeed, be considered as the first stag. . . . Scirrhus is ordinarily accompanied by violent shooting pains. It is also irregular on its surface; and when cut into has a bluish or grayish white color. When the surgeon is satisfied of the existence of scirrhus, he had better remove it at once. No other treatment seems to possess much advantage." Robley Dunglison, *A Dictionary of Medical Science* (Philadelphia: Henry C. Lea, 1874), 933.

and had fainting fits two or three times in a day, with great sickness at the sto-mach, and sometimes bled at the nose. **136** She had taken a purgative twice a week, since I first saw her; but it was thought proper to suspend the use of hemlock for a few days; and take a decoction of the bark. In a short time the hemlock was taken as heretofore, continuing the lime water, also millepedes, which she had been in the habit of taking.

The last of Dec[r] she had a regular menstruation; her pains were much abated, and the scirrhus was much lessened. From this time to the end of Dec[r] she continuing mending in all respects. In Nov. 1763, I was informed that the tumors in her breasts were not half so large, and continued decreasing; and that she was able to labour as usual, without any great pain. She continues to take half a drachm of dry hemlock twice a day; but takes the green when it can be procured, in larger quantities; that she looked well and was in good spirits."   London Magazine 1764.[16]

"The dried leaves of hemlock, says D[r] Thacher, are less liable to injury from keeping than the inspiciated juice. The leaves should be collected in June or July, when the plant is in flower, and its peculiar smell strong. The drying of the leaves should be performed quickly before a fire on tin plates; and the powder should be kept in phials closely stopped, and secluded from the light; for this soon dissipates the green colour, and with it the virtues of the medi-cine. As no medicine is more variable, and uncertain, in its strength than the extract of cicuta, every prescriber should be particularly attentive to the prep-aration which he employs. That which comes from Europe is of little strength, and seldom to be relied on."   Dispensatory.[17]

137

Professor Halle's method of preventing cancerous degeneration of scirrhus congestion in the breast.

---

[16] Kimber, Isaac, and Edward Kimber. "An Account of a Case in Which Green Hemlock Was Applied, by Mr. Josiah Colebrook." London magazine, or, Gentleman's monthly intel-ligencer, 1747–1783 33, December (1764): 674–76. James Boswell, *The London Magazine. Or, Gentleman's Monthly Intelligencer*, ed. Isaac Kimber and Edward Kimber, printed for R[ichard]. Baldwin, jun. at the Rose in Pater-Noster-Row [1747–1783].

[17] James Thacher, *The American New Dispensatory Containing General Principles of Pharmaceutic Chemistry . . . The Whole Compiled from the Most Approved Authors, Both European and American* (Boston: T. B. Wait and Co., 1810), 111–12. Thacher's book, and the earlier *American Dispensatory* by J. R. Coxe (1806), were based on the *Edinburgh New Dispensatory* series be-ginning 1786. For a detailed study of the Edinburgh Dispensatories see: David L. Cowen, *The Edinburgh Dispensatories* ([s.l.]: Bibliographical Society of America, 1951), 8. Cowan also points out that from the third edition of *The Edinburgh New Dispensatory* (1791) edited by Andrew Duncan, Sr., there was a "full and clear account of the "NEW CHEMICAL DOCTRINES published by Mr. Lavoisier." Cowen, *The Edinburgh Dispensatories*, 10.

"I had a poultice made of linseed meal, sometimes mixed with the pulp of carrots, and moistened with their Juice. To this I added a little lard. At the instant of this application, while hot, I covered it with from half an ounce, to a nounce of the powder of hemlock. This was kept applied six hours in the day, and then renewed. I had it also applied in the evening, to remain on during the night. The pains have always ceased after a few days, and the congestion surrounding the hard centre has disappeared by resolution, unless the humor had become disorganized. I have, in general advised both externally & internally the powder of cicuta, in preference to the extract, not omitting local or general bleedings."   Med. Journal N° 1. vol. 9.[18]

Besides the means used for cancers in the face, lips, &c already described, others have been found to be efficacious, viz olive oil, dock root, and lead. "Olive oil boiled in tin, over a gentle fire; three times in 24 hours resolves itself into the consistence of an ointment. This being constantly rubbed on a cancer in the lip of a young girl in Smirna, effected a cure in 14 days.

Edinburgh paper. Schenectady, N. York.

"In Feb. 1813, a pimple on my tongue, of two years standing became a running sore. From this time to the last of July, means were used by physicians, without success. Dr Sterns of Albany, pronounced it a cancer, and advised to have it cut out. At this time I received the following recipe; and by the first of October, by its use alone, the tongue was cured: Take narrow leaved dock root, boil it in soft water and wash the ulcer, with a strong decoction quite warm. Then bruize the hulk of the root, put it on a gauze, and lay it over the ulcer, dip a linen cloth in the decoction, and put that over the gauze; repeat this three times in 24 hours; taking a glass of the decoction as often. Abraham Othout."

138

In 1807, Capt Crowningsel, of Portland had a cancer on his under lip, of several months standing, which was as large as a nutmeg and ulcerated. He was advised, by a friend, to apply the following means, which in a short time, effected a cure.

Take lead & brimstone of each an ounce, melt them together, and stir the mixture, till the brimstone is consumed, then pulverize the lead in a morter.

These means have been found efficacious in some other cancerous cases; and certain cutaneous diseases. But when cancers are inveterate, painful and

[18] Halle, "Observations on a Means for Preventing Cancerous Degeneration in Schirrous Congestion in the Breast," *The New England Journal of Medicine, Surgery and Collateral Branches of Science* 9, no. 1 (1820): 89–91.

corroding, the ley of ashes is considered more eligible, as it subdues the virulence of the humor, destroys the life of the ramifications, and alleviates the
shooting pains; so that they readily heal.

I never saw, nor heard of the return of a cancer treated with the ley of
ashes, except in one instance, in 1806, where it was seated on the side of the
nose, near the eye of five years standing; so that the bone was diseased. This,
however, was cleansed & healed by this means in fourteen days; and remained
apparently sound nearly a year, when it became sore & open; but by the use
of ley & lead it was kept within bounds, and to this day has not been very
troublesome.

In 1800 I was called to a woman who had a corroding cancer in the cartilaginous partition of her nose, which was chiefly destroyed. Its progress, however, was stopped and the ulceration healed, by the ley of ashes; and it has not
returned.

In 1802, Dʳ Vergnies, of Newbury Port, had a painful corroding cancer on
his cheek; an inch diameter, of some standing, which did not yield to common
means. By noticing my account of Plumers case, in the Medical Repository, he
applied the ley of ashes, which in a short time destroyed the cancer. I saw him
in 1820, with a sound cheek, when he presented me with a valuable book.[19]
139

Operation for cancer, performed by Richerard.[sic][20] The sufferer, who was
a Surgeon, had several times submitted to the entire extirpation of a cancer,
in his left breast, also several applications of fire & caustic; but it always shot
out anew, and put forth more horrid excrescences & offensive discharges. No
chance being left against impending death, but from the excision of two ribs.

---

[19] Probably Dr. Francis Vergnies (c. 1747–1830), who practiced in Newburyport, Massachusetts,
and was elected to fellowship in the Massachusetts Medical Society in 1806. He had a medical degree from Toulouse and received an honorary medical degree from Harvard in 1817. In
1821 Vergnies donated 180 medical books to the Massachusetts Medical Society library. Walter
L. Burrage, *A History of the Massachusetts Medical Society* (Norwood, MA: Plimpton Press,
1923), 401–402. He died in 1830 at the age of 83. "Plumer's case" is cited earlier; see MSS p. 130
and Barker, "Use of Alkalies in Cancer. Extract from a Letter of Dr. J. Barker to Dr. Mitchill,
Dated Portland (Maine), March 12, 1801," *Medical Repository* vol. 4, 414–16.

[20] "Among the isolated French contributions of importance are Richerand's resections of the
fifth and sixth ribs (1818)." Fielding H. Garrison, *An Introduction to the History of Medicine*,
4th, reprint ed. (Philadelphia: W. B. Saunders, 1929), 493. See also M. Le Chevalier Richerand,
*Account of a Resection of the Ribs and Pleura Read before the Royal Academy of Sciences of the
Institute of France, April 27, 1818*, trans. Thomas Wilson (Philadelphia: Thomas Town, 1818).
Richerand's biography can be found in J. L. H. Peisse, *Sketches of the Character and Writing of
Eminent Living Surgeons and Physicians of Paris*, trans. Elijah Bartlett (Boston: Carter, Hendee
and Babcock, 1831).

The pleura, underneath, being found much diseased, it was also cut off, in a quadrilateral space of eight inches square. On the 27th day, after the operation, the patient was perfectly cured, retaining a leathery plate on the scar, being tender. Thus Richerard has proved that for very important purposes the cavity of the thorax may be opened for excision of the ribs, and of the pleura. In case of a great lesion of a lobe of the lungs, a part may be cut off with impunity. It was discovered, by this operation that the heart & pericardium are insensible, the last being so transparent, as to shew all the motions of the former; that like the mirror of the eye it becomes opaque only by death. This case occurred in Paris.

New York Evening Post. Sept. 1^{t} 1818.[21]

140

From 1793, to 1795, no epidemical diseases appeared in Maine, nor, as far as I could learn, in any other part of New England.

On the 6th of August 1795, a quarter of veal was brought to my house, from some distance, which had been tied up in a bag, 24 hours, and exposed to the heat of the sun the preceeding day. On examining the meat, it was found highly tainted, and to smell very sour. I then directed it to be put into some brine of common salt, in a cask, to see if it could be purified. But, through mistake, it was thrown into a barrel containing soft soap, where it remained till the next day, when it was taken out, washed in cold water, and found to be entirely free from sourness & fœtor. It was then roasted and eaten with palatableness.

This accidental experiment was repeated with some variation. I procured a tainted quarter of veal, which had a very similar smell, and was condemned in the market. This I immersed in an aqueous solution of pearl ash, which restored it to sweetness. Soon after, a quantity of highly tainted hides were brought in to a tan yard, nearby, and produced much alarm. The tanner, however, soaked them in a lime pit, and the stench was removed.

Now, it appeared to me, highly probable, that if these materials had remained much longer unalkalized, the extricated azotic air, would have acquired such a degree of virulent acidity as to produce pestilential & malignant fevers; and that alkalines were proper remedies. **141** Also, that fresh meat

---

[21] This article appeared in the *New York Evening Post* on September 7, 1818, 2, rather than on September 1, 1818. A similar article about Richerand's surgery was in at least three other newspapers in New York and Massachusetts between August 29, 1818, and September 17, 1818.

taken into the stomach, when the digestive process was impaired, particularly in hot weather, would be liable to undergo putrid fermentation, and evolve a poisonous acid productive of the same effect.

About the middle of August, 1795,[22] William Knight, a seaman, was attacked with fever in Philadelphia, and took passage for Falmouth, Maine, his native place, where he arrived on the 23^d day. He was lodged in a decayed house, containing nine in family. He died on the 11th of September, attended with black stools and a yellow skin. Two weeks after his death, a sister aged 13 years, was seized with vomiting, pain in the head &c succeeded by low delirium. The disease continued 30 days, when an eruption of small boils took place on the skin and suppurated. She recovered. During her sickness, a brother aged 7 years was attacked with fever. A hemorrhage from the nose, took place, in the 2^d week, with black stools, he died on the 14th day. A sister, aged 18 years was seized with fever, and died in 8 days. A profuse hemorrhage from the bowels, took place two hours before death, without pain, while able to walk the room. The mother, aged 49 years, was then seized and died the 9th day, attended with black stools.

They were attended, by a French physician, who gave some gentle evacuants, and prescribed wine with elixir vitriol, "to stop putrefaction," as he said.[23] This account was given by the Father of the family. Three days before the death of the mother, a daughter, aged 25 years, was seized with fever. I was called on the 6th day, when her eyes were suffused with redness; skin of a pale yellow; stools loose, bottle green and very fœtid, pulse low & frequent, **142** tongue dry & dark colored, unable to sit up. She had taken an emetic, and several doses of rhei & calomel. I then made a liberal use of aqua calcis, and volatile alkaline salts. In four days, the fœtor was removed, and the stools became natural. She soon recovered, without any other means. Soon after a youth sickened with fever. I was called on the 3^d day. He complained of nausea, head ach, & thirst, bowels rather loose, stools greenish, pulse 90. After evacuating the stomach and intestines with ipecac & calomel, I directed lime water and pearly ash. His complaints were removed in one week, and he recovered. The sick rooms were then washed with soap suds and the walls

---

[22] Webster wrote, "I never experienced a state of air so debilitating and unfriendly to animal spirits, as the month of August 1795" in Philadelphia; bills of mortality showed double the usual number of deaths. Bilious fever (yellow fever) was present in 1795. Webster, *A Brief History of Epidemic and Pestilential Diseases (Hartford, 1799)*, vol. 1, 312–15.

[23] Barker's 1806 casebook (unpaged) names "The late Dr, Drizio, a French physician."

were whitewashed with lime. Three of the family escaped the fever, and none of their visitors, which were numerous, were invaded.

In Autumn, several cases of fever occurred, in the course of my practice, which evidenced that the stomach & bowels were primarily affected; owing as was supposed, by some, to too great indulgence in fresh meat, by others, to a vitiated atmosphere. The disease was sometimes ushered in with vomiting & purging, or febrile disturbance with a high degree of excitement of a longer or shorter duration, and the stools were black & very fœtid, so that the disease was called "putrid fever." When a seaman arrived from the West Indies, and changed his diet for fresh meat, happened to be thus invaded, the distemper was called "yellow fever," and thought to be imported; but, more probably, it was engendered in his stomach, after his arrival.

143

After suitable depleting and evacuating means, I made a liberal use of al-kaline salts & lime water, which were found congenial to the stomach, and to remove the fœtor of the stools; so that the intestinal discharges soon became natural. But when alkaline remedies were neglected or too sparingly used, the putrefactive process, in the alimentary canal increased and the disease proved fatal, tho other means were used.

In September, a middle aged woman was attacked with fever, to whom I was called the third day, when she complained of nausea, & thirst, with loose and very fœtid stools, of a greenish colour. After an emetic of ipecac, and a dose of calomel, I prescribed an aqueous solution of pearl ash which was liberally used. In one week all her complaints were removed, and health was soon regained.

A young man in the family, was invaded with fever of a higher grade, attended with nausea & vomiting, thirst for water & heat in the stomach. I drew a pint of blood on the 2^d day, gave an emetic & cathartic, and prescribed lime water. A gallon was taken in ten days, and he recovered without any symptoms of putrescency.

Soon after, a young woman, in the family, of a good habit, was seized with similar complaints. I was called on the 2^d day, when depleting & evacuating means were used. I then left a pound of lime which I had procured, and directed it to be put into a gallon of water, and given as in the preceeding case. On the 5th day, she complained of a burning heat in the stomach & nausea. Castor oil & sal. **144** Glaub. were then given, and blisters were appli[ed?]. On the 7th day her stools were black & very fœtid, bowels tense, thirst great. On the 10th she expired.

Greatly disappointed at this event, I enquired whether the lime water had been duly taken; and being informed, by her nurse, that she had given about two quarts, I was induced to examine the remainder, and found that the lime had not been calcined, so as to slack, or afford any taste to the water.

While I was accusing myself of neglect in not attending to the preparation of the lime water, It was reported, by certain empirics, that I had destroyed this patient with lime, when to my sorrow she had taken none. I was also accused of using alkalines in "putrid fevers," which had been considered by some physicians, as tending to promote putrefaction and dissolve the blood!

In August & September I met with a number of cases of cholera among children, and adults. Alkaline salts & earths were the chief means which I employed and they were attended with salutary effects. Injections of lime water impregnated with alkaline salts with and olive oil were very useful.[24] Opiates were beneficial when the patient was much exhausted, particularly in adults; but neutralizing the virulent acid generated in the stomach required the greatest attention. When this was effected the patient generally recovered. Rice was most con[g]enial in the convalescent state. Relapses sometimes occurred in consequence of eating fresh meat with animal broth, which often proved fatal.

145

Believing that I had made some improvement in the treatment of fever, which might be of public utility, in Feb. 1796, I communicated my ideas of the nature of fever, together with some practical observations in 1795, to Mr William Payne, Secretary of the Humane Society in New York,[25] a gentleman formerly of my acquaintance, requesting that they might be submitted to the consideration of some of the Faculty in that City, who had been more conversant with malignant fevers, particularly the year past.

In the summer & autumn of 1796, I attended several cases of malignant & puerperal fevers, in which alkalines were very efficacious, after proper evacuants. But such a deep rooted prejudice existed in the minds of some against these means, that I was obliged to pursue their use amidst great opposition, particularly by those who were in the habit of using spiritous stimulants in fevers.

---

[24] Here injection probably refers to enema or clyster; see OED injection, enema.
[25] The Constitution of the Humane Society of the State of New York dated July 12, 1794, shows William Payne as secretary and lists Drs. Samuel Mitchill and Elihu H. Smith as medical counselors. This document is found in the *Evans Collection of Early American Imprints* 1794, Evans number 47079 and, for 1795, Evans number 29202. Barker's letter to Benjamin Rush on September 22, 1806, states, "In Jan. 1796, I communicated the result of my observations on fevers as they appeared in 1795 to Mr. Payne Sec of the Society in New York, a Gentleman formerly of this state; the only acquaintance I had in the middle states" (Rush letters at the Historical Society of Pennsylvania).

I was consulted in several cases of fever of a high grade, where wine & brandy were the chief means employed, when, on giving a cathartic, black and very fœtid stools were voided. In these cases alkalines were substituted to great advantage, for the putrid fermentation was quelled, and the fever soon subsided.

In Nov. I attended several cases of typhous fever,[26] in which after suitable depletion, sulphate of soda, and the carbonate of potass, were successfully employed, without much nervous affection. But when spiritous stimulants were used, stupor & delirium supervened, which were sometimes happily removed by hemorrhages from the nose or bowels, particularly when bloodletting had been neglected, or too sparingly employed.

146

The last of Nov. 1796, I received a letter from the Secretary of the Humane Society of New York,[27] who informed me that my medical observations met with the approbation of Professor Mitchill, who favored me with his "Remarks on the Gaseous oxyd of azote, explanatory of the phenomena or fever," printed in August 1795.[28] In this I found that there was a coincidence of sentiment, respecting the febrile cause, tho without any communication of ideas. But as the Professor had closed his treatise without entering into the practical consideration of the subject, I had still to pursue the use of alkalines in fevers amidst increased opposition, till May 1797, when a New York Magazine was sent to me, by Dʳ Mitchill containing his letter to Dʳ Percival of Great Britain, dated January, 1797, in which he recommends the use of

---

[26] See Glossary entry. "Typhous" here, used as an adjective, refers to a febrile illness in which stupor and severe debility develops. It is also one of Hippocrates four types of fever. In epidemic form typhous had many names, including jail-house fever and ship-fever. Separation of typhous from typhoid, both febrile illnesses with rashes, would not occur for almost a century. Lester S. King, *Transformations in American Medicine: From Benjamin Rush to William Osler* (Baltimore: Johns Hopkins University Press, 1991), 93–116. See also Raoult, Woodward, and Dumler, "The History of Epidemic Typhus," 127–40.

[27] In a letter dated January 12, 1797 (MHS Col 13), Barker thanks William Payne for obtaining a "valuable collection of books" including Mitchill's theory on fever and contagion. The material helped Barker write on fevers, including his own practical remarks in addition to Mitchill's theories; he promises to hold himself responsible for a "faithful narrative."

[28] Samuel L. Mitchill, *Remarks on the Gaseous Oxyd of Azote or of Nitrogene, and on the Effects It Produces When Generated in the Stomach, Inhaled into the Lungs, and Applied to the Skin: Being an Attempt to Ascertain the True Nature of Contagion, and to Explain Thereupon the Phenomena of Fever. / by Samuel Latham Mitchill, M.D. F.R.S.E. Professor of Chemistry, Natural History and Agriculture in the College of New-York* (New York: T. and J. Swords, 1795).

Alkalines in fevers. See Med. Repos. v. 1. p. 253.[29] This letter was perused by physicians; as well as others, and served to reconcile some of my opponents to the use of alkalines in fevers. Since which alkaline salts & lime have been more generally employed in Maine for medicinal purposes, and found to be an excellent class of medicines, in fevers, particularly of the gastric and intestinal forms; also in cancer, scrofula, and many other diseases of the external surface.

The beneficial effects of alkalines, in the hands of physicians, in different part of the United States, in the treatment of fevers, improvement in the police of Cities; and in the naval department, are particularly stated in the Medical Repository; as well as in other American publications.

---

[29] Samuel L. Mitchill, "Concerning the Use of Alkaline Remedies in Fevers, and the Analogy between Septic Acid and Other Poisons; in a Letter to Thomas Percival M. D. &C of Manchester, from Dr. Mitchill, Dated New-York, January 17, 1797," *Medical Repository* 1 (3rd ed.), no. 2 (1798): 253–78, see 253.

Chap. 10. [marked 9] May 30th. 1798

TO SAMUEL L. MITCHILL M. D. &c, Professor of Chemistry, in New York. on the febrifuge virtues of Lime, Magnesia & Alkaline salts in Dysentery, Yellow fever and Scarlatina Anginosa.

Dear Sir. I have perused your letter to Dr Percival, with particular attention, as well as the other books, and acknowledge myself to be furnished with many new, as well as very important ideas, relative to the proximate cause of fever. Several of my brethren have also read them, and are persuaded of the truth of the doctrine. But there are some among us, who still consider the phenomena of fever to depend on a redundant quantity, or acrid quality of the bile. Their views, therefore, are chiefly directed to emptying the intestines of this <u>mischievous liquor</u>, as they term it. Of what importance is it then that medical prejudices should be combated, and a new order of things established?

For nine months past epidemic fevers have been very prevalent in this northern climate lat. 43°43'[1] and attended with considerable mortality. Having been pretty constantly engaged in practice, I have had an oppertunity of making accurate observations, and have been very particular in noting them.

An account of these distempers, as they have appeared among us, together with the mode of practice which has been pursued, will be related.[2] [This letter represents a portion of the first page of an article Barker published in the *Medical Repository*]. [See Figure vol.1.10.1]

1. 43°43' North latitude today is Falmouth, Maine. In 1786 citizens of Falmouth Neck, a part of Falmouth, separated into what today is called Portland, which is 43°39' North latitude. See William Willis, *The History of Portland*, facsimile ed. (Somersworth, New Hampshire Publishing Company and Maine Historical Society ed. 1972; Portland: Bailely & Noyes, 1865), 579–87.

2. Volume 1 of the manuscript ends here. The complete four-page letter from Barker to Samuel Mitchill is in the Spalding collection at the Maine Historical Society. It was published as Jeremiah Barker, "On Febrifuge Virtues of Lime, Magnesia and Alkaline Salts in Dysentery, Yellow-Fever and Scarlatina Angiosa. In a Letter from Dr. Jeremiah Barker, of Portland, (Maine) Dated May 30, 1798," *Medical Repository* 2, no. 2 (1798): 147–52. (in the *Medical Repository* in 1799, vol. 2, no. 2).

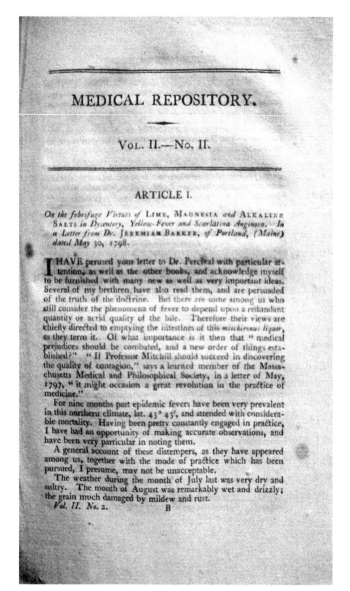

FIGURE VOL.I.10.1. Title page of a Jeremiah Barker article. The title page of one of Barker's articles published in the *Medical Repository*, "On Febrifuge Virtues of Lime, Magnesia and Alkaline Salts in Dysentery, Yellow-Fever and Scarlatina Angiosa. In a Letter from Dr. Jeremiah Barker, of Portland, (Maine) Dated May 30, 1798." *Medical (The) Repository* 2, no. 2 (1799): 147–52.

VOLUME 2

The Jeremiah Barker Manuscript

Consumption

[Introduction]

Kennebunk Decr 20 1831

MY DEAR SIR

I have carefully perused your manuscript with great pleasure, particularly relating to Consumption. The work is calculated to do much good and exactly corresponds with my practice. There are many living witnesses to the truth of your theory, which I have conversed with since the book has been in my possession, and I wish sincerely that it might be printed, as also my brethren who have seen [the] "work." Several patients have been examined, post mortem, who died of pulmonary Consumption under my care and shew the most unequivocal evidence of the propriety & necessity of copious & repeated bleeding, in the early stage of the disease, and, I doubt not, that many might have been saved by adopting your practice of salivation & the cooperative means who have fallen victim to this inveterate disease.

Accept, dear Sir, my sincere thanks, for the perusal of your truly valuable book, and believe me to be, with high respect and esteem, your friend &c.
Dr Barker.   Samuel Emerson[1]

---

[1] Dr. Samuel Emerson (1765–1851), born in Hollis, New Hampshire, was a fifer in the Revolution at age eleven, graduated from Harvard College in 1785, and studied medicine under Dr. Oliver Prescott of Groton. He began his practice of medicine in Kennebunk, District of Maine, in 1790 and kept a case book recording approximately three thousand lying-in patients. He was a member of the Massachusetts Medical Society when he placed a notice in *The Eastern Argus* December 19, 1819, calling for a meeting to form a Maine Medical Society to begin when Maine attained statehood. The first meeting took place in 1820, and the Society was legally incorporated in 1821. James Alfred Spalding, *Maine Physicians of 1820; a Record of the Members of the Massachusetts Medical Society Practicing in the District of Maine at the Date of Separation* (Lewiston: Lewiston Print Shop, 1928), 5–8; Samuel T. Worcester, *History of the*

C2   Medical History continued.   Vol 2^d

A History of Consumptive Diseases of different kinds, reserved for the concluding part, as they have appeared in Maine, and some other parts of New England, since 1768, in my own practice, as well as that of others. Containing also a great variety of extraordinary cases, collected chiefly from Medical Records in different States and Nations, from the days of Hippocrates, viz. 360 years before the Christian Era, to the present time, which serves to show that in the past centuries many things inexplicable for want of post mortem examinations, relative to Consumption and hectic fever, as well as many other diseases, have been, chiefly by these instructive aids, in the present century, clearly investigated, so that good success has attended scientific physicians, when proper means have been <u>seasonably & duly employed</u>.

"The great desideratum in the case of pulmonary consumption is the removal of hectic fever. RUSH.

By Jeremiah Barker F.M.M.S.

C3

An
Inquiry into the causes, nature,
increasinged prevalency, and treatment
of CONSUMPTION. which is
maintained to be curable, if proper means
are seasonably & duly employed.

By Jeremiah Barker Esq. F.M.M.S.
"Nature is the first physician."
Hippocrates

C4

Did all our young physicians record the history of the diseases they meet with, and the effects of remedies on them, they would find their Journals and common place books, more useful to them, in the evening of life, than any of the books which belong to their medical libraries. RUSH.

C5   Introduction.

Among the writings of professional men, in the former part of the 18th century, we find but few observations relative to consumption; the disease, at that time, making up only about one tenth part of the bills of mortality. At the close of the century, however, it appears that they made up one fourth part.

Town of Hollis, New Hampshire, from Its First Settlement to the Year 1879 (Boston: A. Williams & co., 1879), 290.

The increasing prevalency & fatal tendency of this disease have been subjects of very particular inquiry, by learned & experienced physicians, both in Europe & America since the middle of the last century, who, by their diligent researches, have made many valuable discoveries and improvements, relative to its causes, nature and treatment.

Still as few persons, excepting professional men, have attended to these important discoveries & improvements, by far the greater part of mankind, consider the disease termed Consumption, as being incomprehensible in its nature and necessarily fatal in its issue! — On this account I have long wished that multiplied observations might be made, by experienced physicians, explanatory of the nature & tendency of this disease, **C6** in such a manner, as would be intelligible to those who are destitute of medical knowledge, so that the hurtful powers & imprudent habits which induce it might be avoided, or such necessary means as are best calculated to remedy the disease when present, should seasonably be employed.

Since the beginning of the 19th century, European writers, upon consumption, have been numerous. These are particularly noticed by Thomas Young M. D. &c. Physician to St. George's Hospital, in his "Practical & Historical Treatise on Consumptive diseases, deduced from original observations; and collected from Authors of all ages." London, printed 1815.[2]

In this work, the Author has endeavoured, as he says, to comprehend every fact of importance, which he has been able to observe or found recorded, with respect to the nature & cure of the diseases, belonging to a single genus.

---

[2] Thomas Young, *A Practical and Historical Treatise on Consumptive Diseases, Deduced from Original Observations, and Collected from Authors of All Ages* (London: Underwood, 1815), 397. Young cited Lyman Spalding and Jeremiah Barker on page 397: "We have also an account of the beneficial effects of alkalies, by Spalding and Barker; a teaspoon of soda was taken for a dose, and alkalies were mixed with all the food . . . the authors imagine [the alkalies] had neutralized some poisonous acid, that preyed on the fibres of the body." Young's reference for the above quote is Lyman Spalding, Barker, Jeremiah, "Beneficial Effects of Alkalis in Consumption of the Lungs," *Medical Repository* 5, no. 2 (1802): 220–21. The two pages include one case by Spalding and one by Barker. Thomas Young (1773–1829) was a brilliant physician, scientist, and humanist who apparently read at least seven languages before the age of fourteen. In addition to advancing a theory of color vision, he made important contributions to deciphering the Rosetta Stone. See also Thomas Young, *An Introduction to Medical Literature, Including a System of Practical Nosology . . . Together with Detached Essays, on the Study of Physic, on Classification, on Chemical Affinities, on Animal Chemistry, on the Blood, and on the Medical Effects of Climates* (London: Underwood and Blacks, 1813); John H. Talbott, *A Biographical History of Medicine* (New York: Grune & Stratton, 1970), 402–404.

Besides his own, it contains the practical observations of more than 300
physicians in Europe, who have written on consumption, **C7** since the days
of Hippocrates; selected chiefly from Ploucquet's collections of references to
Authors, and the library of the Medical & Surgical Society.[3] He also made
selections from D[r] Rushe's [sic] works and the New York Medical Repository
relative to this disease.

From D[r] Young's researches, it appears that many of the Ancient physicians
were well acquainted with some of the most efficacious remedies for consumption, and successfully employed them.

While the Faculty of foreign nations have been thus laboriously engaged
in investigating the nature of this disease, professional men in America have,
by no means, been negligent in their researches, nor destitute of success; so
that, by their mutual exertions, great good has been derived to mankind; and
in proportion as a knowledge of these important discoveries & improvements
should be disseminated, their beneficial effects may probably, be extended.

Towards the close of the last, and since the commencement of the present
century, several **C8** learned & experienced physicians in North America
have favoured us with truly valuable observations on Consumption, though
chiefly in the middle & Southern States. I have, therefore, presumed to offer
to the public, the results of my inquiries & observations, relative to this disease, as it has appeared in the northern & eastern parts of the Union, having
been pretty constantly engaged in the practice of Medicine for nearly half a
century, both upon the sea coast and in the interior parts of the country.

My principal aim in this attempt, is to aid the efforts of my medical
brethren, in eradicating medical prejudices & disseminating useful knowledge; in engaging the mind to greater solicitude for the enjoyment of life &
health; in exposing & suppressing empirical impositions, which rapidly increase; and finally in rendering the Science of Medicine more respectable &
important in the view of mankind.

To the better accomplishment of this arduous undertaking; and with a
view to engage **C9** greater attention, I shall occasionally avail myself of
such observations of learned and experienced physicians, in different states
& nations, as may tend to aid my endeavours to illucidate the subject; and to

---

[3] Wilhelm Gottfried Ploucquet (1744–1814), *Wilhelm Gottfried Ploucquet realis sive repertorii
medicinae practicae et chirurgiae* in eight volumes was published 1793–1797 with supplements
in 1803 and 1813. This work represented the "first important classified bibliography of medical
literature covering both monographic material and current periodicals" according to Leslie
T. Morton, *A Medical Bibliography (Garrison and Morton)*, 4th ed. (Aldershot, NH: Gower
Publishing Company, 1983). entries 6750, 6750.1, 6750.2.

check the progress of this formidable disease; which is so much the dread & scourge of the human race.

In the course of my investigations I have paid particular attention to those maladies, in which cures have been effected, by what are called, by some, "the efforts of nature"; by others, the "Author of Nature"; as well as to those diseases, which have yielded to the means employed by professional men: — wishing to "Render unto Cæsar the things which are Cæsar's; and unto God the things that are God's."

Chap. I.

THE WORD CONSUMPTION is derived from the Latin <u>consumere</u> to waste or consume. This insidious disease invades the body under various forms, in consequence of its diversified causes; and is distinguished by different names, according to its seat or origin.

When the trachea or windpipe is particularly affected, the disease is called <u>tracheal</u> consumption. When it is manifested in the lungs, it is termed <u>phthisis pulmonalis</u>, or pulmonary consumption.[1] When a morbid condition of the stomach and digestive organs, give rise to this disease, it is denominated <u>atrophy</u>, requiring, in some respects, a different mode of treatment.

A general description of the organs of respiration, will serve to facilitate an explanation of two of the forms of consumption which have been mentioned.

The respiratory organs of the human species are the trachea, with its various branches; the lungs; the pulmonary system of blood vessels, or the arteries & veins of the lungs. **Cıı** The trachea is a tube composed of cartilaginous rings, connected by ligaments and lined with a mucous membrane, which extends to the lungs. It is plentifully furnished with blood vessels; and the membrane is beset with nerves, which come in contact with the air; so that it is rendered exquisitely sensible & highly excitable. The upper end of the windpipe which commences in the throat is termed <u>larynx</u>, from

---

[1] "Consumption" and "phthisis" (Greek for wasting or decay) are terms used through the seventeenth, eighteenth, and early nineteenth centuries; the term "tuberculosis" entered in the mid-nineteenth century. The disease has been known since ancient times; skeletal deformities typical of consumption (tuberculosis) have been found in Egyptian mummies dating to 2400 BC. Hippocrates (460–375 BC) described it as a generally fatal disease. "The Genuine Works of Hippocrates," ed. Francis Adams (Baltimore: Williams and Wilkins, 1939), 99–100, 130–31. Galen (AD 130–200) described the symptoms as hectic fever, sweating, coughing, and bloody sputum. For a short overview of the history of tuberculosis, see I. Barberis et al., "The History of Tuberculosis: From the First Historical Records to the Isolation of Koch's Bacillus," *Journal of Preventive Medicine and Hygiene* 58, no. 1 (2017), E9–E10. For a more comprehensive history, see Lester S. King, *Medical Thinking: A Historical Preface* (Princeton, NJ: Princeton University Press, 1982), 16–69; Helen Bynum, *Spitting Blood: The History of Tuberculosis* (Oxford: Oxford University Press, 2012).

whence it discends [*sic*] into the chest, where it divides into two branches, which communicate with the two divisions of the lungs. Each of these is subdivided into smaller branches called <u>bronchia</u>, and, at length, terminate in air cells, constituting the principal portion of the lobes of the lungs, which are seperated from each other, by a membraneous expansion of the pleura, called mediastinum, and inclosed in appropriate cavities, entirely without communication; so that one lung may perform its office sufficiently for the purposes of life, if the other should be destroyed, as dissections have shown.

C12

The membrane lining the bronchial vessels and air cells of the lungs, is estimated by Dr Hale & others, to be many times more extensive than the surface of the whole body; and these cells are connected together by a quantity of cellular substance, which divides each lobe or lung into several lobules, forming a surface for the innumerable & minute branches of blood vessels, which are dispersed over them.

The blood vessels of these organs are formed by branches of the pulmonary artery & veins. The trunk, from which proceed the branches of the pulmonary artery, arises from the right ventricle of the heart, whose alternate & successive dilatations, receive and propel all the circulating blood through the arterial branches of the lungs, which are larger & more numerous than the veins. The blood is then reconducted, by the pulmonary veins, to the left ventricle of the heart and carried by the aorta or great artery and its branches, to the remotest parts of the body, from whence it is returned by corresponding **C13** veins, to the right ventricle of the heart, to be again distributed through the lungs, after discharging carbonic acid gas, and receiving vital air.

"The blood vessels of the lungs, says Dr Cullen, are more numerous than those of any other part of the body of the same bulk. These vessels of the largest size, as they arise from the heart, are more immediately, than in any other part, subdivided into vessels of the smallest size; and these small vessels spread out near the internal surfaces of the bronchial cavities, are situated in a loose cellular texture, and covered by a tender membrane only; so that considering how readily & frequently these vessels are gorged with blood, we may understand why an hemorrhage from them, is, next to that of the nose, the most frequent of any; and particularly why any violent shock, given the whole body, so readily occasions an hemoptysis."

First lines. hæmop.[2]

---

[2] William Cullen (1710–1790), William Cullen, *First Lines of the Practice of Physic with Supplementary Notes, Including More Recent Improvements in the Practice of Medicine by Peter*

"It requires but small acquaintance with the structure & economy of the lungs, says Dʳ Reid, to be sensible that any considerable discharge of blood from these organs, must be consequent upon rupture of a large number of minute vascular ramifications."[3]

C14

By taking into consideration the particular structure of the respiratory organs, the great delicacy & exquisite sensibility of the membrane lining the windpipe, and air cells of the lungs, together with the many accidents to which these organs are exposed, from various causes, it must be a matter of surprise that they do not oftener become diseased; and that pulmonary consumption is not of more frequent occurrence.

It is a general observation that the ravages of this disease are much greater among females than males. This is ascribed to the greater delicacy of constitution and susceptibility of impression, which characterize the female sex, together with their peculiar fashions, customs, modes of life, &c, all which predispose them, in an especial manner to pulmonary consumption.[4]

In 1809, according to Dʳ Nathan Noyes, bill of mortality of Newbury Port, 110 died in that town; twenty-six of consumption; twenty of which were females![5] —— It was observed that ladies went abroad **C15** in January, with fewer clothes, than a gentleman would wear in July!! not considering that cold applied to the skin, when thinly clad, contracts the perspiratory vessels; so that the blood is accumulated in the lungs, producing distention of

---

Reid, two volumes in one (Brookfield, MA: E. Mirriam & Co. for Isaiah Thomas, 1807), 301. Written between 1778–1789 with numerous editions.

[3] John Reid, *A Treatise on the Origin, Progress, Prevention, and Treatment, of Consumption* (London: Phillips, 1806), 71–72.

[4] From the Statistical Tables of Paris, 1830: of 9,542 cases of phthisis, 5,582 were females and 3,960 males. From the Birmingham Dispensary in 1829, of 86 cases of tubercular consumption, 48 were female and 38 were men. P. C. A. Louis, Henry I. Bowditch, and Charles Cowan, *Pathological Researches on Phthisis* (Boston: Hilliard, Gray, 1836), 464. The issue of gender and consumption is discussed later in this volume, but in 1817, a standard medical textbook concludes, "our fashionable young females, accustomed to a warm apartment during the day, often brave the elements in the evening, and resort to the theatre, or ballroom, with uncovered breast and neck, naked arms to the shoulders, and thin shoes; by such imprudent exposure, who is surprised that colds are contracted, and that so many young persons are consigned to the grave in the bloom of life?" James Thacher, *American Modern Practice* (Boston: Ezra Read, 1817), 432.

[5] Nathan Noyes (1777–1842), Nathan Noyes, "Bill of Mortality for Newburyport, Massachusetts, for A.D. 1809, the Facts Collected and Arranged by Nathan Noyes, M. B.," *Newburyport Herald*, January 16, 1810, 3, col. 3–4.

their vessels, inflammatory action, morbid secretion, cough & expectoration, which unless seasonably relieved will pave the way for this formidable disease.

These observations are equally applicable to the conduct of people in the ~~District~~ State of Maine, in the 44. degree of north latitude⁶ where the mercury in Fahrenheits thermometer, sometimes falls several degrees below zero; and seldom rises much above the freezing point, in the winter months.

That consumption is much more frequent in both sexes, than in former years, and more rapid in its progress is apparent to aged and observing physicians; as well as others. But if the generality of mankind pass heedlessly on, without noticing the hurtful powers & unsalutary habits, which occasion this **C16** devastation among the human species, it is incumbent on medical men, earnestly to exert themselves, in pointing out the various causes of this formidable disease; and in explaining their tendency and destructive effects, in such a manner, if possible, as to induce mankind, especially invalids, to avoid the paths which lead to this disease, and seek for those which guide to health.

In attempting to discharge my duty, relative to this arduous task, the history of the symptoms which characterize the different forms of ~~this disease~~ consumption, will be particularly delineated; the various causes pointed out; and the nature; as well as treatment of the disease described, which will serve to show that the ill success so frequently attending professional men, at this day, is more owing to neglect & delay, on the part of the patient, than to deficiency of skill, on the part of the physician, for diseases, like vices, generally speaking, **C17** become irremediable, only in consequence of a want of consideration, cherishing their sources, and procrastination.

"The progress of sin, says Dʳ Hunter, is like that of certain diseases, whose first symptoms give no alarm, to which a vigorous constitution bids a bold defiance; and treats with neglect; but which, through neglect, silently fix upon some of the noble parts, pray, unseen, unobserved, on the vitals; and the man finds himself dying, before he apprehends any danger! — It was but a slight cold, a tickling cough, a small difficulty of breathing; but it imperceptably [sic] becomes an extenuating hectic; under which nature fails, the nails bend

---

⁶ Maine extends from Kittery in the south, 43°05' to Fort Kent in the north at 47°14; North Latitude. Portland is 43°4' and Bangor 44°10' North Latitude. For reference, Toulouse in Southern France is 43°6' North Latitude. Note that this section or sentence was edited by Barker after March 15, 1820, the date the "District of Maine" separated from Massachusetts, becoming "the State of Maine."

inwards, the hairs fall off, the legs swell, the eyes sink; and the cold hand of death stops the languid current at the fountain."

"Thus the giddy sallies of youth, the mistakes of inconsideration; the errors of inexperience, through neglect, presumption & indulgence, become, before men are aware, habits of vice **C18** and constitutional maladies; by which manhood is dishonoured, old age becomes pitiable, and death is rendered dreadful beyond expression."   Sacred biography.[7]

The following questions have often been asked, whence it is that Consumption is so much more prevalent, in both sexes, in New England, ~~how~~ than in the days of our forefathers? — Must this be charged to a change of our climate or mode of living & dress? If we attend to the mode of living, we shall find a far greater change between that of our hardy ancestors, and the present generation, than ever was known in any climate for ten centuries.

The mode of living & dress is now as different from what it was in the days of our Ancestors, as simplicity is from luxury. Consumption was then of rare occurrence, and it is well known that milk & farinaceous substances composed a great part of their food. Besides spiritous liquors, which inflame the blood and destroy the digestive powers, were little used, by our temperate **C19** Ancestors; and their dress was calculated to ward off the inclemencies of the weather. Of late years, spiritous liquors have become a fashionable drink among both sexes; and very little attention has been paid to suitable cloathing inconsiderately apeing [sic] the fashions of those who reside in warm & temperate climates.[8]

"D[r] Barton of Philadelphia, in his M. S. lectures, says D[r] Comstock of R. Island, has canvassed the question of why the people of New England are so much more frequently visited with Consumptions, than those living only a little more southerly, as in Pennsylvania. He thinks that its being somewhat

---

[7] Henry Hunter, *Sacred Biography—or, the History of the Patriarchs to Which Is Added the History of Deborah, Ruth & Hannah Being a Course of Lectures Delivered at the Seots [Scotch, Scotts, Scots] Church* (Boston: J. White, Thomas & Andrews &c., 1794), vol. 2. Lecture 17, 228–29. Henry Hunter (1741–1802) held a Doctor of Divinity from the University of Edinburgh and was a minister in the Church of Scotland, with congregations both in Scotland and later in London. He began his seven-volume *Sacred Biography* in 1784. See "Hunter, Henry," by Gordon Goodwin revised by Anita McConnell, in H. C. G. Matthew and Brian Harrison, eds., *Oxford Dictionary of National Biography: In Association with the British Academy: From the Earliest Times to the Year 2000*, new ed. (Oxford: Oxford University Press, 2004).

[8] An 1835 treatise on consumption by another New Englander makes all the points made in the Barker manuscript, including female predisposition and dress as well as diet and intemperance. William Sweetser, *A Treatise on Consumption* (Boston: T. H. Carter, 1836), 43–46, 106–108, 115–16. In New England there was a focus on cold weather dress and consumption, whereas in Paris in 1836, the question was raised as to whether women wearing stays contributed to the development of consumption. At least two authors tended to doubt the association. Louis, Bowditch, and Cowan, *Pathological Researches on Phthisis*, 445–46.

colder here, than there, is not the cause; and finally that as Consumption is an heriditary [*sic*] disease, its frequency here is owing to the New Englanders, being almost exclusively the descendants of the inhabitants of Old England; whereas the inhabitants of Pennsylvania are mostly descended from the Germans." "But I suspect, says D^r C, that this difference is more owing to diet than any thing else; for the descendants of the Germans make use of milk, cheese, and other articles, raised on their farms, to the almost total **C20** exclusion of tea, coffee; and what is still more pernicious <u>spirituous liquors</u>. This supposition is confirmed also by a very impressive fact, viz. that in the State of Ohio, although a great mass of the population went from New England, consumptions are rare. Of this I have been assured by an eminent physician of Cincinnati; and also by an honourable member of Congress from that State. Now it is very well known that the people there, live very much upon milk; and use comparatively little tea & coffee."

"Had I the eloquence of Demosthenes & Cicero, or could I speak with the tongue of an Angel, I would say to the weakly & consumptive inhabitants of our country. Keep warm in stove heated rooms & flannel dresses, and let your diet be chiefly milk."

"I esteem a warm air in the cold season of the year, and even a fire in the summer season, in the cool part of the day to be a principal remedy, to which other means of cure ought to be considered as auxiliary. But to obtain the benefit of warm air, I by no means think removal to a warm climate necessary; a thing inconvenient for most, **C21** and impossible for many. By making a warm climate of the sick persons room, by means of a stove kept properly heated, day & night, every advantage of a warm climate may be obtained."

"The writer of the present article has had experience in the plan of treatment here recommended. But at the same time, never trusted wholly to an artificial warm climate, without giving medicines adapted to the state of the system; nor, in his opinion ought the use of any one remedy, entirely to supercede the use of others; for in order that remedies should be successful, they must be varied according to different constitutions, and different states of the system."

"It is to me perfectly clear that no management can have much effect, while the cold changeable air of our variable climate is suffered, at every breath, to enter the weak lungs of the consumptive." "I feel this to be a matter of very great importance, for I cannot conceive of the **C22** most judicious treatment, being successful, in many cases of consumption, without paying attention to keeping the cold damp air from irritating the lungs."

Rhode Island American.[9]

[9] "Remarks on the Treatmant of Consumption by Joseph Comstock," *Rhode-Island American,* published as *Rhode-Island American, and General Advertiser,* January 24, 1817, p. 2.

"It is difficult to deny, says Dr Young, the hereditary transmission of actual disease, if we admit with Dr Thomas Reid of London, that children are sometimes born with cough & emaciated; die within the month, evidently of confirmed consumption."

Essay on Consumption.[10]

I [Barker] have lost two children, born of consumptive mothers, one in three weeks, the other in six months, both with the usual symptoms of pulmonary consumption; and I have seen many instances of children, born of consumptive mothers, who, sooner or later, in life, were invaded with a similar disease. In the relation of cases, I shall have occasion to describe several of this kind, which required more powerful means to eradicate the disease, than those who were born of healthy parents.

C23

The hereditary transmission of consumption is an alarming consideration and persons born of parents infected with this disease, even in a moderate degree, should pay much greater attention to the management of their constitutions, with respect to food, cloathing &c than those who are otherwise circumstanced. Prudence, discretion & regularity, however, are required of all, if health is considered as the greatest temporal blessing.

Between the 18th and 36th year of life is a period in which the human body is most liable to pulmonary consumption; and in which much less attention is paid to the constitution, than in the former or latter periods of life. In the former or puerile stage, children are generally under the particular inspection of their parents or masters; and their health of body is, for the most part, in proportion to the care, power and influence, which are exercised with respect to their appetites, passions, exercise & cloathing. After this period is passed, the ambitious youth, still of **C24** immature judgement, often neglects a regular mode of living, and eagerly engages in excessive exercises of the body & mind in pursuit of business or pleasure; or inconsiderately forms an attachment to such extravagant amusements and irregular habits, as tend to induce inordinate action of the bloodvessels, inflame the vital organs, and pave the way to consumption. But when man has arrived to the meridian of life; and managed his constitution with prudence & discretion, his habit becomes

---

[10] Thomas Reid, *An Essay on the Nature and Cure of the Phthisis Pulmonalis. By T. Reid, M.D* (London: printed for T. Cadell, 1782), 2–3.

firm, and his judgement mature; so that his appetites & desires are conducted with more uniformity & regularity; and, like a full grown plant, is better able to resist or ward off those hurtful powers, and natural evils, which so constantly surround us, than in **C25** the preceding stages of succulency, and great instability of fibre. [written between other lines] ~~great activity on a milk diet, twenty five years. He then made use of animal food which in a short time, destroyed his life!~~

~~English Malady~~

~~Dr Fisher, my fellow physician, when about 25, was to be [illegible] and known to be consumptive.~~

[The rest of page 25 is crossed out and is fragmentary.]

Chap. 2.

Tracheal Consumption.

THE UPPER PART of the trachea called larynx sometimes becomes irritated & inflamed, which produces a soreness of the throat, cough, and discharge of mucus or purulent matters, often mixed with blood, without inducing any morbid affection of the lungs, constituting a local disease, which in some, continues for several months or even years, with little or no fever while in others, the disease is rapid in its progress to death.

Besides the symptoms already mentioned, hoarseness and loss of voice, sooner or later supervene. Indeed hoarseness has often been a primary symptom, with heat & anguish in the throat. The fits of coughing are very tedious, and the discharge from the windpipe profuse, especially in the morning, tho the chest is free from pain; and the breathing, as well as pulse, continue to **C27** be natural, excepting in the last stage of the disease, when they become accelerated, but unattended with rigor or febrile paroxysms.

The feet & legs sometimes swell in the advanced state of the disease, and there is, for the most part, a rapid failure of strength. The appetite for food is seldom impaired, till the body has become greatly exhausted. The tongue is generally natural, tho it is sometimes covered with a whitish fur in the morning. By depressing the tongue the throat appears very red; and is commonly beset with small ulcers, covered with a yellowish matter. These ulcers are very sore, and the patient sometimes complains of a soreness, extending some way into the trachea, with a fullness in the larynx, and great difficulty of swallowing. These last symptoms presage a speedy dissolution.

Cold & dampness applied to the body when thinly clad, particularly in the evening, often give rise to this morbid affection of the trachea. The venereal disease, sometimes **C28** contributes to the production of tracheal consumption, by ultimately depositing its baneful poison in the throat, which corrodes its delicate fibres, like a canker worm up on tender foliage; reminding some of those wretched abodes, "where their worm dieth not and the fire is not quenched."[1]

Having thus described this form of consumption agreeably to my own observations, I shall proceed to the relation of a few cases.

In April, 1804, Mrs Martha Hall of Falmouth, of a slender habit, aged 25 years, applied to me for advice, in care of a morbid affection of the throat, which she had laboured under for six months. Considerable inflammation could be discovered in the throat, which was beset with small ulcers, called "canker sores," attended with a hecking cough, and great difficulty of swallowing, so that very little solid food could be taken, and she was much emaciated; pulse weak & quick. She was considered, by her friends, as being incurably consumptive, and all means were laid aside. Two grains of calomel were then **C29** given night & morning. On the third day a salivation took place and continued about ten days, still using the calomel, until she had taken 18 grains. The disease was then entirely removed. Her health was soon regained by nutriment, and has continued ever since unimpaired.

Several very similar cases were soon committed to my charge, and the disease was removed with equal facility, by mercurial salivation. In one case there was a large scrofulous tumour on the neck, which did not yield to the mercury. This, however, was subdued by repeated embrocations of volatile alkali, which I had often found effectual in dispersing scrofulous tumors.

In March 1806, Mrs Stephens, aged 30 years, complained of a cough, sore throat & expectoration of mucus matter. As the spring advanced she became much enfeebled. Various means were used; but to no advantage. In July I was consulted when calomel was given so as to produce a salivation. Her cough was then removed; but in two weeks it returned. Patent cough drops were then **C30** resorted to; but her complaints increased.

In March 1807, her cough became still more distressing, the throat was very sore, and the matter discharged was pus like with some febrile action. She then wished to give the mercury another trial. Two grains of calomel were given night and morning, and an ounce of mercurial ointment was applied to the neck on a flannel bandage. A copious salivation took place in one week, and an eruption up on the neck with great inflammation. The cough & expectoration

---

[1] Canker worm: A caterpillar that attacks buds and leaves (OED). The source of the quotation is biblical; see *Holy Bible: The Washburn College Bible, Oxford Edition, King James Text, Modern Phrased Version*, Washburn College Bible, Oxford edition, King James text, modern phrased version (Oxford: Oxford University Press, 1980), Mark 9:44.

then ceased, and the salivation continued three weeks. Stimulating plaisters were then applied to the neck, and she gradually recovered; so as to enjoy a comfortable state of health, till 1816 excepting, that, at times, she was troubled with a slight cough, when exposed to cold & dampness.

Mr John Quinby, a merchant in Falmouth, when at the age of 33, was troubled with a soreness of the throat and hawking of matter which at times was tinged with blood.[2] **C31** His father, a brother & a sister had died of consumption. A troublesome cough supervened, and, in every returning spring, a considerable quantity of blood was discharged from the windpipe, tho he felt no uneasiness in his lungs, and was a man of great activity in business, altho he was exercised with these complaints for several years. In 1800, he had recourse to Opium which moderated his cough, and he enjoyed comfortable health, in other respects, till April 1806, when he discharged heavy pus like matter, by cough, every morning, yet his appetite was good, and no febrile disturbance attended. As the summer approached he became more enfeebled his feet swelled. In June, a a hoarseness came on, so that he could only speak in a whisper, saying that his throat seemed to be filled with ulcers. In July he was confined to his house, being scarcely able to walk, and doubted whether he should live a month, as his appetite had failed. Under these circumstances he requested me to salivate him. One grain of calomel was given three times a day, and in six days a salivation took place. The good effects of which far exceeded our expectations. His windpipe was in a great measure, relieved of its **C32** oppressive load; thin mucus only being discharged, with little cough, and that with ease. His appetite returned and he recovered such a degree of strength, as to walk the streets, ride out of town, and transact business. He regretted that he had not employed this remedy before, believing that if he had taken it sooner, the disease might have been eradicated. He lived till

---

[2] John Quinby (1758–1806) was born in Falmouth, Maine, to a prosperous family of shipbuilders. He married, had six children, and, with a partner, bought a parcel of land and mill rights in Stroudwater in 1783. They later built a two-story shop and dwellings at that property. In addition to operating a shop that sold various foods, cigars, rum, fish, etc., Quinby was a ship owner and surveyor of lumber. He died on Saturday, September 27, 1806, of the illness described in Barker's text. An undated letter marked "Monday morning" to John Quinby's son Moses discusses his father's illness and symptoms as well as the family history of consumption, and requests permission to perform an autopsy to delineate the pathology and possibly help the remaining family deal with their future medical needs. Permission was apparently not given, as Barker does not mention findings in the manuscript. John Quinby Papers, MS–186, Research Library, Maine Maritime Museum, Bath Maine. The letter to Moses Quinby: B MS misc. Barker, Jeremiah at Countway Library of Medicine, Boston.

the last of September, in a much more comfortable state, without being confined to his bed a single day.

In June 1816, Mr Hugh Woodbury of Westbrook a black smith, aged 40 years, after being long engaged in grinding scythes, in a wet place, complained of hoarseness, which increased, so that in August, he could only speak in a whisper, attended with cough & expectoration with difficulty of swallowing, tho he continued to work in his shop till November, when I was consulted, and advised to a salivation. His pulse was natural and his appetite good. One grain of calomel was given night & morning and mercurial ointment was rubbed on his neck. In ten days his glands were affected, and some relief was afforded. But his friends, wishing to **C33** expedite the cure, sent for a patent Doctor who gravely observed that mercury was a cold & useless article; and that, as his disease was caused by cold, heating means must be given. Accordingly, a liquid, impregnated with cayenne pepper was substituted! —— The inflammation in his throat rapidly increased and febrile disturbance took place; so that swallowing was soon impeded, and he died in a few days.[3]

Were I to describe the injurious effects of red pepper, used by empirics, in inflammatory diseases, I could fill many pages; but they are too well known to need a description; and such impostors are viewed, by discerning people, as dangerous members of society.

In 1796, I was informed, by Dr James Folsome of Durham, that he once saw a person inspected who died of tracheal consumption, where the upper part of the windpipe was inflamed ulcerated & corroded, but no marks of disease were discovered in his lungs.

C34 "Sometimes, says Dr Rush, the whole force of the consumptive fever falls upon the trachea, instead of the lungs, producing in it, defluction a hawking of blood, which are often followed by ulcers, and a spitting of pus. I have called it a tracheal, instead of a pulmonary consumption. Many people pass through a long life, with a mucus defluction upon the trachea, and enjoy, in other respects, tolerable health. In such persons the disease is of a local nature."

Dr Spence of Dumfries, in a letter which I received from him in June 1805, describes a case then under his care, of this form of consumption. He calls it, very properly, "phthisis trachealis." "I have met with two cases of death from this disease, in which there were tubercles in the trachea. The patients

---

[3] Hugh Woodbury (c. 1766–1816) was born in Cape Elizabeth July 5, 1766, died December 23, 1816, at age fifty, and is buried at Saccarappa Cemetery, Westbrook, Maine.

breathed with great difficulty, and spoke only in a whisper. One of them died
from suffocation. In the other, **C35** the tubercles bursted, a few days before
his death, and discharged a large quantity of fœtid matter." Med. Obs.[4]

"While we lament the great proportion of deaths by consumption, says D[r]
Pascalis[5] of Philadelphia, which our weekly bills of mortality present, we naturally attribute the frequency of phthisis pulmonalis to the severity of our climate and changeableness of our seasons. But this is not all; and there may be
other causes. For one of them, I feel fully satisfied may be traced to ulcerated
tonsils. It is the <u>phthisis laryngis</u>, the ultimate effect of an ulceration which
has progressively extended to the pharynx & œsophagus, to the epiglottis,
and at last, has reached the larynx and trachea. My practice has offered six
cases of <u>phthisis laryngis</u>, within the last twelve months, which always proved
more rapid and more irremediable than the consumption of the lungs. Other
practitioners have undoubtedly witnessed its frequent occurrence, if they
please to recollect its characteristic symptoms of extreme hoarseness and even
of destruction of the voice, the great difficulty of swallowing, which really
subjects the patient to starvation. This complaint is unconnected with any affection of the lungs; and I have seen it existing often, without any symptom of
phthisis pulmonalis. Perhaps the cough is not so frequent, and it takes place
by paroxysms, chiefly in the night; but the patient raises great quantities of
purulent matter, often tinged with blood. This matter is easily thrown off
from the extensive surfaces through which it is secreted. Hence it happens,
that, different from phthisis pulmonalis, in which the matter is confined in
deep recesses of the bronchia, absorbed and mixed with circulating **C36**
fluids, and creating hectic fever; the phthisis laryngis offers the remarkable
circumstance of a natural pulse, although febrile, in its most advanced stage.
The lying posture is not much subject of inconveniency, nor does the patient

---

[4] Benjamin Rush, *Medical Inquiries and Observations*, 4th ed., 4 vols. (Philadelphia: Johnson
& Warner, 1815), vol. 2, 62. The fourth edition used, four volumes in two, was owned by S. G.
Barstow and he numbered the volumes, No. 10 and No. 11. The first volume (Rush's volume
one and two) was printed for B. & T. Kite and the second volume (Rush's volume 3 and
4) was printed for Johnson & Warner. Griggs & Dickinson printed both volumes as well
as 1815 editions for M. Carey and S. W. Conrad. Robert B. Austin, *Early American Medical
Imprints: 1668–1820* (Arlington, MA: The Printers' Devil, 1961), 175. Benjamin Rush had died
in April 1813.

[5] Felix Pascalis (c. 1750–1833), born in Provence, France, was a graduate of Montpellier who
practiced in France until driven out by the French Revolution. He moved to Philadelphia
and later to New York City. He published papers and at one point he was coeditor of the
Medical Repository. Howard A. Kelly and Walter L. Burrage, *American Medical Biographies*
(Baltimore: The Norman, Remington Company, 1920), 894.

require to have the head & thorax erect. The progress of debility and exhaustion is nevertheless more rapid, owing to want of nourishment.

Before I terminate these remarks, I must express my regret at not being able, as yet to point out the causes which concur to produce this ulceration of tonsils among children, who are not exposed to the dangers which might account for them in adults. The next and still more interesting object would be to establish both preventive & curative means. I must leave to time and more fortunate practitioners the desideratum of rescuing children from this baneful evil, or of removing it, as soon as it is found to exist.

Gentle & repeated emetics cause a retroversion in the affected parts, and prove to be the best means for cleansing those ulcers. Small doses of calomel induce a greater degree of irritation in the mouth, which should, therefore, be depended on to soften indurated glands on the edges of the ulcers; but, above all astringents, gargles, injections into the cavities, with a small curved syringe, scarifications, and caustic applied with all necessary caution, remains the best resource which we can derive from the most practical doctrines of surgery."

Med. Repos. vol. 13. 1809.[6]

C37

Besides the beneficial effects of a mercurial salivation in this disease, I have met with many cases in which a deep seated Seton between the shoulder has expedited the cure in stubborn cases by diverting putrid action from the parts affected, as well as by the drain of humors, worn for a considerable time, and removed when the stimulus of the sore ceases. I have also found that the use of lime water freely taken has been productive of salutary effects, as a corrector of the fluids & humors. Likewise, a mixture of olive oil and lime water equal parts, taken into the mouth & throat, repeated, has been as congenial to the sores & ulcers in these parts, as it has to scalds & burns on the external surface. The salutary effects of which is well known to physicians & surgeons, in expediting cures.

C38

In January, 1812, Mrs Eunice Mosier,[7] of Gorham, Maine, aged about 35, of a good habit, after exposure to cold & dampness, in a thin dress, five months

---

[6] Felix Pascalis, "Observations on the Ulcerated Tonsils of Children," *Medical Repository* 3rd hexade, vol. 1, no. 1 (1809): 19–25.

[7] The Mosier or Mosher family were among the first settlers in Gorham, circa 1739. Eunice Elder married Nathaniel Mosier November 15, 1795, and died July 29, 1852, aged seventy-five. Hugh D. Mc Lellan, *History of Gorham, Maine* (Portland: Smith and Sale, 1903), 685–87.

advanced in pregnancy, was seized with oppression at the breast, and a dry hecking cough; attended with such a degree of hoarseness that she could speak only in a whisper, and that with difficulty. These symptoms continued without any alleviation, till June following, when I was consulted, about three weeks after parturition, when she was much enfeebled; but not febrile, neither had any expectoration taken place. In addition to her first complaints, she was troubled with great heat and soreness of the throat, which extended some way into the trachea, also difficulty of breathing, so that she was obliged to be bolstered up in bed; and had very restless nights. The chief means which had been taken used were squills, and, at times, a mixture of gin & molasses. I then prescribed two grains of calomel, three times a day. After taking twelve grains, a salivation took place, when the hoarseness was removed, and her voice restored. But, her other complaints remaining, she continued the calomel, till she had taken twenty four grains. The salivation continued three weeks, without much inconvenience. All her complaints were then removed. Since which she has enjoyed good health.

A few years after, another woman, nearby, was attacked in a similar manner, in the pregnant state, as I have been informed. She was advised, by her friends, to be salivated; but a prejudice against mercury prevented its being used. Common means were taken, but the disease terminated fatally, about four months after parturition.

Chap. 3.

Phthisis Pulmonalis, or pulmonary consumption.

THE WORD <u>PHTHISIS</u> signifies a consumption or wasting; and denotes a morbid affection of the lungs, which has been supposed to depend up on an ulcerative state of these organs, especially if purulent matter is expectorated, and attended with hectic fever; and this fever has been supposed to be "created by matter absorbed and mixed with the circulating fluids."

The ancient notion that "in every instance of an expectoration of pus, there is an ulceration of the lungs," has had a very unfavourable influence on the human mind, inducing a belief in some, that, on this account the disease was incurable, so that the only resort was to the exercise of patience & resignation; in others, that if curable, simple means, which possessed but little power, were the **C40** most eligible, or if powerful means should be resorted to, they ought to be used in a very sparing manner.

Unhappy consequences have formerly attended this view of the disease, and cautious timidity, in my own practice; as well as that of others; so that physicians have been wrongly accused of using "<u>too powerful medicines in consumption</u>." The truth is, that means possessing <u>too little power</u>, have for the most part, been employed, or powerful remedies too sparingly used, and the disease, in most cases, has bid defiance to the instruments of medicine, while committing its ravages uncontrolled.

It is by no means strange that the mind of man should have been occupied with such misconceived ideas, relative to the nature and **C41** treatment of this disease, when we consider that the ancients, from whom we derived medical instruction, were, in great measure destitute of anatomical knowledge.

"As late as the 16th century, says Dr Ramsey,[1] Charles the 5th called a council of Ecclesiastics to consider of the lawfulness of dissecting human bodies. It is said by the biographers of William & John Hunter,[2] both of whom were born & died in the 18th century, that they were the first in England who opened a proper anatomical school, in which the arts of injection, dissection, and of making preparations of different parts of the human body, and of surgery, were systematically taught.

Within the last hundred years, thousands of human bodies have been dissected, and every part minutely examined, and its functions, uses, **C42** connections & relations accurately ascertained. This increase of anatomical knowledge has produced the most beneficial consequences; it has given new light by which physicians have been enabled to explain the animal functions and deduce rational theories of diseases."   Century oration.[3]

That the lungs, in some cases of consumption, have become ulcerated, morbid dissections have shewn. It has also been found, by examining the lungs of others who have died of this disease, that these organs have been free from ulceration or organic lesion, altho, hectic fever, pain in the chest, and copious expectoration of purulent matter, were attending symptoms.

D^r De Haen and Dr John Hunter have maintained & proved that purulent matter is secreted from the extremities of the arteries, in consequence of certain **C43** diseased actions, where there is no ulceration.[4] —— That pus may be plentifully secreted from the vessels of a membrane, is evident in opthalmia [sic], or an inflammation of the eyes, where the adnata, or common membrane, is often covered with purulent matter, where no lesion or ulceration exists. And as purulent matter has often been expectorated when the

---

[1] David Ramsay (1749–1815) was born in Pennsylvania and, after graduating from Princeton College, studied at the medical department of the University of Pennsylvania. A physician, politician, and historian, he moved to Charleston, South Carolina, where he practiced and wrote for the rest of his life. Howard A. Kelly and Walter L. Burrage, *American Medical Biographies* (Baltimore: The Norman, Remington Company, 1920), 954–55.

[2] There is a great deal of literature on the Hunters, but for a brief overview, see John H. Talbott, *A Biographical History of Medicine* (New York: Grune & Stratton, 1970), 255–61.

[3] David Ramsay, *A Review of the Improvements, Progress and State of Medicine in the XVIII Century: Read on the First Day of the XIXth Century, before the Medical Society of South-Carolina, and in Pursuance of Their Vote, and Published at Their Request* (Charleston: W. P. Young, 1801).

[4] Anton de Haen (1704–1776), of Dutch origin, studied in Leiden under Boerhaave and then at the University of Vienna, where he practiced, taught, kept careful case notes, and performed many postmortems. John Hunter (1728–1793), Scottish experimental surgeon, anatomist, teacher, and medical scientist, spent most of his years in London. Talbott, *A Biographical History of Medicine*, 258–61.

lungs, as well as liver, have been found, by dissection, to be in a sound condition, while the membrane lining the bronchial tubes, was besmeared with purulent matter, we have sufficient evidence that inflammatory irritation, in this vascular & very excitable surface, must have given rise to the purulent secretion.

When ulceration does take place in the substance of the lungs, it must be an ultimate effect of this inflammatory **C44** irritation, which sometimes exists for several months, before these organs become ulcerated; so that sufficient time is afforded of diverting & removing this morbid action, so as to prevent organic lesion or ulceration, and this salutary change has frequently been effected, either by the use of certain means, or by the providential occurrence of some other disease, as will hereafter be shown, even when the lungs have been labouring under diseased actions, for a considerable length of time; and attended with the usual train of hectical symptoms.

"Hewson,[5] like other anatomists, says Dr Reid, ~~in 1802,~~ has often found pus contained in the pericardium and cavity of the pleura, without any mark of ulceration. The hectic of consumption is certainly not **C45** occasioned by any irritation derived from the pus, which is often mild & healthy. The hectic fever occurs before the appearance of any symptoms which indicate the presence of matter, and long before expectoration."

Treatise in Consumption 1782.[6]

The symptoms of Pulmonary Consumption, usually commence & progress in the following order. viz. irregular flushes in the face, and a burning heat in the palms of the hands, with an accelerated pulse, increasing in the evening, together with languor, restlessness & dryness of the skin. To these succeed a short hecking cough, tightness across the breast with oppression in breathing, which are increased by unusual exertion, or exposure to the evening air. Pain in some part of the chest, commonly in the side, which sometimes wanders, generally supervenes; with a pulse quicker than **C46** natural, and a greater or lesser degree of tension & fullness. A throbbing of the arteries of the neck is often observable, especially in young females of delicate habits. Sometimes a spitting of blood, and an expectoration of frothy mucus occur, with a sense

---

[5] William Hewson (1739–1774) was British physician, surgeon, anatomist, and early researcher in hematology who trained at St. Thomas and Guy's in London, but also at Edinburgh and Paris, later working with John Hunter. Talbott, *A Biographical History of Medicine*, 311–14.

[6] Thomas Reid, *An Essay on the Nature and Cure of the Phthisis Pulmonalis* (London: printed for T. Cadell, 1782).

of soreness in the chest, particularly under the sternum or breast bone; as also heat & irritation in the vitals, from throat to the pit of the stomach; extending, at times, to the back part of the chest, especially when in bed, preventing quiet repose, and natural sleep.

These are the common symptoms, which constitute the first stage of the disease;[7] and they sometimes continue for several weeks & even months without exciting much alarm; so that they are often neglected or treated with stimulating heating things; the idea of a common cold being suggested to the mind; not considering that cold applied to the body induces heat & inflammation.

C47

If the morbid action or inflammatory irritation, on which these symptoms depend, is not counteracted by proper means & measures, the disease, in a longer or shorter time, assumes a more formidable aspect, and the second stage commences. —— In this stage febrile paroxysms or fever fits occur, twice in 24 hours, with great regularity. The first invades about noon, and remits in three or four hours; but recurs, in the evening with a greater degree of violence, beginning about eight or nine o'clock, and does not abate till after midnight. These paroxysms are preceded by rigors which are sometimes severe; feeling as tho cold water was running over the skin, as they express themselves; and sometimes the feet & legs are very cold. The evening paroxysms are most severe and followed by sweating; pulse quick & tense. As the disease **C48** advances, the fever, cough & difficulty of breathing increase; and the pain in the chest becomes more distressing, especially up on laying down in bed. Mucus and purulent matters are now freely expectorated, sometimes mixed with blood; at other times clear blood is discharged from the windpipe. The morning sweats become profuse, particularly about the chest; and the flesh decays; tho the appetite for food and muscular strength are but little impaired; the patient often being able to walk, ride and trasact [sic] business, with a pulse from 100 to 120 strokes in a minute. The tongue, which is for the most part clean, acquires a preternatural redness; as well as the fauces as far as can be seen by depressing the tongue, yet there is seldom any thirst. The face is commonly pale; but during the fever fit, a crimson spot appears on each cheek; and such a degree of animation is felt, as to inspire the **C49** patient

---

[7] Stages of consumption. First stage: cold, languid, difficulty breathing, increased respiratory rate, occasional cough. Second stage: increased pulse, night sweats, hectic fever, increased cough with expectoration of pus, then blood, emaciation. Third stage: includes diarrhea but some combination of stages one and two. Thomas Young, *A Practical and Historical Treatise on Consumptive Diseases, Deduced from Original Observations, and Collected from Authors of All Ages* (London: Underwood, 1815), 21–23.

with a hope of recovery, even when far advanced in the disease; and dispair seldom occupies the mind.

These are the most prominent symptoms of the second stage, which in some continue for several months, without much apparent alteration, excepting the loss of flesh. In others, where the degree of pulmonic irritation & inflammation is considerable, the disease is more rapid in its progress; and attended with great arterial excitement, called a galloping consumption, which unless arrested in its career, terminates fatally in two or three months. But when this more active inflammation does not exist; and the ordinary symptoms of hectic still continue unrestrained; the functions of the body become greatly impaired; and the third & last stage, in different periods of time, takes place.

C50

In this stage the pulse looses that tension which marks its progress through the second, and becomes weak & frequent. The disease then bears a near resemblance to typhus or the slow fever, and the patient often remains much in the same state for a considerable length of time; so that hope of recovery still predominates, while able to walk or to sit up; and sometimes, after being wholly confined to the bed.

As the disease progresses the flesh rapidly wastes, and the strength fails; the feet swell, the nails curve inwards, the eyes sink, and assume a pearly whiteness. The morning sweats increase to an alarming extent, in a manner deluging the whole surface. Accumulated matters in the lungs are tumultuously poured out, in abundant profusion, sometimes alternating with a colliquative diarrhœa. The stomach **C51** at length, becomes unfit for the reception of food; and the respira-[tory] organs incessantly labour to perform their office; while the vital flame hovers over them, like the glimmering taper of a lamp, whose oil is nearly consumed. The organs of speech are no longer attuned to harmony; giving utterances only to hoarse whispers. the skin shrinks, as it were, to the very bones; and looses that pliancy, sweetness and bloom, which so beautifully characterize the healthy state. —— A pale, decayed & extenuated frame is now presented to view; and a speedy dissolution is threatened. —— Death soon closes the scene!

This truly melancholly detail of human misery, has made a deep impression up on my own mind, having **C52** so often seen it exemplified, in the course of my practice. And should it equally impress the minds of others, it may, possibly, induce them to use their best endeavours to avoid those hurtful powers; and to abandon those unsalutary habits & imprudences, which occasion this distressful train of morbid affections; or, if invaded with this insidious disease, to seek relief before the vital organs are too greatly injured, or the lamp of life is too much exhausted.

Thus, I have described the symptoms of this form of consumption as they have ordinarily occurred, within my own observation. And few physicians, I believe, have been more induced to make accurate & particular observations, than myself, relative to the onset & progress of this formidable disease, as well as the effects of medicine, having lost three wives, by its destructive **C53** ravages; besides many other patients; so that, in former years, when the nature of this disease was "involved in obscurity," and few means, or such as possessed little or no curative power, were employed, I was called, and not with impropriety, "an unskilful and unsuccessful practitioner in consumption." ——But if my ill success has induced me to pay greater attention to the subject, and to use more powerful, as well as efficacious means in this disease, it is hoped that by its being made known it may prove to be of public utility; for I shall be more particular in narrating fatal cases, than those which have terminated favourably not hesitating to expose my own defects & errors of inexperience, in the hope that others may avoid them.

C54

The symptoms of pulmonary consumption do not always commence & progress with that regularity, which has been delineated. Difference in constitution, and diversity of causes, sometimes occasion considerable variation in the symptoms; as also the intervention of some other disease, which will appear by the statement of cases.

Pain in the chest, rigors and expectoration of matter & blood are sometimes absent, where the morbid action or inflammatory irritation of the lungs is in a moderate degree; yet in process of time, suppuration has taken place, as dissections have shewn which serve to show the insidious nature of this disease; as well as the danger of neglect & delay.

A slight catarrhal cough has sometimes existed for years as a solitary symptom, increasing during the winter & spring, and decreasing on the approach of summer, exciting no alarm, the patient being **C55** otherwise in health. But, in process of time, through neglect & delay, the usual train of hectical symptoms have supervened, and sometimes proved fatal.

Hemorrhages from the lungs, nose &c, as also diarrhœa have occurred in the primary stages of this disease, and the hectic fever has subsided; the cough expectoration & night sweats have also been removed by these efforts of nature and the patient has readily recovered.

Hemorrhages, however, which sometimes take place in the last stage of the disease have not been productive of salutary effects; neither has diarrhœa.

A mercurial salivation in the first & second stages of pulmonary consumption, of several months standing, has removed the most formidable symptoms of hectic fever, after suitable depletion, and health has been restored, in a great variety of cases. But in the third stage, bloodletting is improper, and mercury is **C56** generally ineffectual; neither is there any great prospect of success, in this stage, from any other means.

The accession of mania, rhumatic pains, and erysipelatous eruptions have caused an abatement or cessation of pulmonary affection, by diverting morbid action from the labouring parts, and happily broken the chain of hectical symptoms.

Pregnancy taking place in this disease has arrested the hectical symptom by diverting morbid action from the lungs. But after parturition, if depleting and other means have not been used, the symptoms generally recur & prove fatal.

Dispair of recovery, in pulmonary consumption, and resignation to death, in the second stage, of several months standing, have diverted morbid action from the lungs, and prevented the recurrence of rigors & febrile paroxysms; so that health was readily regained, in cooperation with other means, and rendered parmanent [*sic*].
C57

Aphthous ulcers, in the mouth & throat, sometimes take place, in the last stage of this disease; but they more commonly occur in the tracheal form; and hoarseness much oftener happens in the latter than in the former.

The suppression of customary evacuations, particularly in young females, tends readily to produce hectic fever & its train of symptoms, which often proves fatal. But when restored to regularity, the fever generally subsides, & health is regained.

This disease usually invades those who are in the bloom of life, and of irritable inflammatory habits. Persons of a fair complexion, florid cheeks, rosy lips & delicate make, with an accelerated pulse, are much more liable to pulmonary consumption, than those of a different description.

This disease commonly invades in the spring months, when the weather **C58** is extremely variable.

Exposure to evening air, in the parade of parties, and the ball room, clad in <u>cobwebb muslin</u>, has laid the foundation for consumption in many fashionable young females, and consigned them to an untimely grave!

Persons subject to bleeding at the nose, and spitting of blood, are liable to its attacks; for in such cases depletion is generally neglected.

Phthisis Pulmonalis frequently takes place in consequence of neglected Pneumonia, Influenza & Measles. Instances of this kind have often occurred in the course of my practice which will afford a variety of cases; in the statement of which, many other causes will be noticed.

Chap. 4.

IN THE RELATION of cases, I shall begin with those that occurred in my pupilage, which will not only serve to show defective practice, but the progressive state of medical knowledge succeeding years.

In the spring of 1768, a female in Scituate, of a spare, slender habit, aged 21 years, was troubled with some of the symptoms of hectic fever. She had irregular flushes in the cheeks & hot palms, with palpitation of the heart, after any unusual exercise, a coated tongue, and irregular appetite; but no cough. As the summer advanced, febrile disturbance & night sweats took place; so that she was considerably reduced. During the fall & winter months, she was confined to her chamber, and part of the time to her bed. In the mean time tonic & restorative means were used; but to no apparent benefit; for the sweating increased; and little or no hope was entertained, by her physicians, of her recovery.

In the spring of 1769, Dʳ Lincoln, my preceptor, was consulted, who described her pulse as being "quick & sharp," from acrimony, as he supposed in the blood. The other symptoms he ascribed to weakness, and bad digestion.

The means prescribed were tonic bitters & the vitriolic acid, together with a daily use of sallop. A profuse uterine hemorrhage soon took place, attended with great pain; so that her strength was reduced. The means were more freely given, and the night sweats lessened. At the expiration of three months, she was again attacked with a profuse painful hemorrhage. The tonic & restoratives means were continued; and the sweating ceased; as well as her other complaints. Her health was gradually restored, and she continued a vigorous active woman to the age of 70 years, when she was attacked with hemiplegia and died, after two years confinement.

It may be proper to observe, that from the years of puberty she had never menstruated oftener than once in two or three months, and then but sparingly.

The recovery of this patient enhanced the Dʳˢ medical reputation; for the cure was ascribed wholly to the means employed!

Soon after, he was called to several patients, in that town, recently attacked with the common symptoms of pulmonary consumption. Gums, balsams & restoratives were used; but they all died. One patient was advised, by some of the vulgar, to eat a piece of the liver, of a person dead of this **C60A** disease, as a curative mean! This, however, was not done; but if the lungs had been examined probably some marks of inflammation might have been discovered, which would have indicated a more eligible mean.

On the 13th of March 1771, Mrs Cushing of Hingham, a middle aged lady of good habit, after exposure to cold & dampness, was attacked with the usual symptoms of pneumonia. On the 15th Dr Lincoln was called with whom I attended, and noted the case. At this time she complained of acute pain in the left side, a dry cough & difficulty of breathing; pulse frequent full & laborious. Half a pint of blood was drawn; and the bowels were evacuated with six grains of calomel & 20 of Jalap. The blood when cold was buffy, and the crassamentum was dissolved. On this account further bleeding was judged improper. A large blister was drawn upon the pained side; and Cal. ammon. with squills were given. 16th the pain moderate and expectoration of purulent matter mixed with blood took place. The next day the fever & pain increased, and she complained of oppression & great difficulty of breathing, with delirium at night. Neutral salts & castor oil were freely given. **C60B** The fever continued 15 days, with copious expectoration, when she appeared to be convalescent. But, on the first of April she was attacked with chilly fits followed by febrile paroxysms, and night sweats; pulse quick & weak, cough tedious & expectoration profuse. These symptoms continued till the last of the month when diarrhœa took place. The cough & expectoration then ceased. She died on the 2^d of May.[1]

In many other cases of pneumonia where a pint of blood was drawn and sometimes repeated, and where mercury was used as an alterative [sic], with other means, the disease terminated favourably.

Hectic fever independently of pneumonia, was of frequent occurrence in different seasons of the year, tho it took place for the most part, in the winter or spring. Its duration was from six to twelve months; sometimes longer.

My preceptor, in his private lectures, described this fever, as arising from obstructions in the lungs from acrimonious fluids derived from impure chyle, generating an ulcer, and the absorption of purulent matter, which was

---

[1] Hannah Cushing, born in Weymouth, Massachusetts, circa 1736, was the wife of Benza Cushing, probably a distant relative of neurosurgeon Harvey Cushing, whose family moved from Hingham, Massachusetts, to Cleveland, Ohio, in the nineteenth century.

considered as giving rise to the hectical symptoms. **C61** His mode of practice was to use deobstruents, or gums, & balsams, combined with argent. viv; also demulcents with elixir vitriol & paragoric; together with sago, sallop, bitters, &c as restoratives.

Cases of consumption & hectic were numerous; but I had not the pleasure of recording only one during my pupilage, which terminated favourably, and this has already been related.

In 1770, Dʳ Ezekiel Hersey of Hingham departed this life, aged about 70 years. He was an admirer of the medical works of Dʳ George Cheyne of London; and in the main, adopted his mode of practice, particularly in his dietetric [*sic*] rules; and in the use of mercury. Dʳ Hersey commanded an extensive practice, and his medical fame was proportional. A few months before he died, he was consulted by a Mʳ. Shaw of Abington, aged 21 years, in case of a periodical hemorrhage of blood from his lungs, of a years standing; and which recurred at every full moon, in a considerably [*sic*] quantity. **C62** Various means had been used, but to no advantage. He advised to a mercurial salivation, which effected a permanent cure.

Dʳ Hersey will ever be held in grateful remembrance, by the friends of medical science; for he bequeathed one thousand pounds Lawful money, and his widow, at her decease, a like sum, to be applied for the support of a Professor of Anatomy & Surgery in the University of Cambridge [Harvard College].

In 1772, Dʳ Bela Lincoln was invaded with Atrophy, for which he took various means; but to no apparent benefit. Soon after, he relinquished his practice, and undertook a sea voyage; but a remedy was not to be found. When I had finished my studies, he gave me a recommendation as being qualified to practice physic. But, at parting, he observed that the Science of Medicine was, as yet, involved in great obscurity, and that many things were unknown, in the healing art, particularly concerning the nature and treatment of Consumption & hectic fever, **C63** which needed to be discovered; and that as I had his shoulders to stand upon, he hoped I would study diligently, keep exact records of cases, as they should occur in practice, whether fatal or otherwise; open dead bodies, when permitted, note appearances, and labour to make improvements in Medical Science.

He died in 1774. aged 45.[2]

---

[2] Bela Lincoln (1733/4–1774) actually died at age forty. Clifford K. Shipton, *Biographical Sketches of Those Who Attended Harvard College in the Classes 1751–1755; Sibley's Harvard Graduates*, vol. 13 (Boston: Massachusetts Historical Society, 1965), 455–57.

In 1775, I took up my residence in Barnstable, Mass. and married a daughter of David Gorham Esq. aged 25. who was troubled with a slight catarrhal affection, which gradually and almost imperceptably increased for fifteen years, when a rupture of the blood vessels of her lungs took place, and about a gill of blood was discharged, for which salt was given, and half a pint of blood was drawn. The hemorrhage recurred three mornings in succession in like quantities and then ceased. Hectic fever readily supervened, tho in a moderate degree, with cough & expectoration of mucus, and, in a few weeks, of purulent matter. Common means were used. But she gradually declined, and died in three months. **C64** This case will serve to show the insidious nature of this disease; as well as the danger of neglect and delay.

Here, I formed an acquaintance with Dʳ Abner Hersey,[3] who had been engaged in the practice of physic, forty years. From him I hoped to gain instruction relative to the nature & treatment of consumption. But I found that his views of the disease were very similar to those of my Preceptor.

Although Dʳ Hersey was successful in other diseases, even in Pneumonia, he mentioned no successful case of pulmonary consumption, in his practice, excepting his own. He informed me that he had been troubled with consumptive complaints many years, during which time, he had often expectorated purulent matter, particularly after exposure to inclement weather, and undergoing great fatigue; that he was frequently attended with febrile disturbance & hectical flushes; sometimes night sweats, which had considerably reduced his flesh & strength; **C65** but not so as to disable him from riding.

The means used were occasional doses of calomel as an alterative & expectorant; sometimes as a cathartic. A diet consisting chiefly of rye hasty pudding & milk; sometimes chocolate sweetened with honey. A very sparing use of meat; and an entire disuse of spirits of every kind; or any other stimulating articles; riding, for the most part, in a close carriage, to ward off noxious air; keeping himself well covered with flannel; and avoiding night practice. —— By these means, he had kept the hectic fever in subjection, moderated his cough; as well as expectoration; and, in the main, led a tolerably comfortable life.

He was held in great estimation, throughout the County; and was a very useful physician. He also did great good, by distributing religious books

---

[3] Dr. Abner Hersey was born in Hingham in 1721, moved to Barnstable in 1741 to study medicine under his older brother, James, and continued practicing there until his death in 1787. Dr. Ezekiel Hersey was another brother.

among the people, particularly the works of Drs Doddridge & Watts.[4] ——He continued **C66** in both these modes of practice, till 1786, when he died of pulmonic affection, aged 70. In imitation of his brother Ezekiel, he willed £500 Lawful money, towards establishing a Professor of Anatomy & Surgery at Cambridge [Harvard College]. Also the income of his real estate, having no children, for the benefit of Ministers of the Gospel; as well as the people of the County, by large supplies of religious books, annually to be distributed.

In 1818, a case of consumption, which occurred in the latter part of Dr Herseys practice was communicated to me, by a relative of the patient, which serves to show that he was improving in the treatment of this disease.

In 1780, Mrs Lucy Garrett of Barnstable aged 40, of a slender habit, was attacked in the spring with febrile disturbance, some pain in the side & cough. In September, at the vernal equinox, her complaints increased, and she discharged about half a pint of blood from the lungs. The D^r then drew as much from her foot, and directed very similar means & measures to those used **C67** in his own case, respecting diet, medicine, & cloathing as well as avoiding night air. She continued pretty comfortable till the next equinox, when her complaints returned, and another half pint of blood was discharged, by cough from her lungs. She was bled again and the means were continued.

Every year, about the same time, the premonitory symptoms, and discharge of blood from the lungs, recurred for six years; and she was bled as often, continuing the use of means, able, for the most part, to perform domestic business, altho she at times complained of a burning heat in the vitals, and palpitations of the heart, upon unusual exertion; sometimes with chills, fever fits & morning sweats. She was also troubled with canker sores in the throat, but no expectoration of matter.

During this period, she was fully apprehensive of her danger, and resigned to the will of God, expecting every returning year, that the disease would prove fatal. On the return of the seventh year, the bleeding did not recur, neither was the lancet called into aid. She died.
C68

Do we not perceive a cooperation with the Author of Nature, in this case, somewhat analogous to the laudable conduct of this physician, in many other respects? —— Again, may we not suppose, that, if the mercury, taken by this patient, had produced a salivation, as it did in the practice of Dr Rush in 1800, in a consumptive case, her complaints might have been removed?

---

[4] Both were British nonconformist ministers and thinkers. Philip Doddridge (1702–1751) was a prolific author and hymnwriter, as was Isaac Watts (1674–1748).

In Dec. 1773, I was consulted by the Rev. John Hall of Yarmouth,[5] a native of Conn. and missionary to the Indians, who inhabited certain small villages on Cape Cod. He was in the bloom of life, aged 25, but had complained of febrile heat, with oppression at the breast, a hecking cough & hawking of phlegm, some-times tinged with blood, for two months, tho he preached every Sabbath sev-eral miles distant; pulse quick & tense. He had taken various means; but to little advantage; such as gums, balsams, squills & liquorice, with opiates. I prescribed a few additional means, as taught by my Preceptor. But the routine of hectical symptoms increased, sometimes with a moderate discharge of blood from his lungs, especially after preaching. **C69** In the spring a diarrhœa took place, which afforded some relief. But he continued to decline till the following August, when he died, greatly lamented by his friends, particularly the poor Indians.

In the fall of 1774, M[r] Samuel Gilbert, aged 24, educated at Dartmouth College, put himself under my tuition in the study of physic. He also preached to the Indians, in different villages.[6]

In the course of two years, he became affected with the usual symptoms of phthisis; and, finding the common means ineffectual, ~~he~~ entered on board of a privateer, as a Surgeon, destined for the West India coast. There he became so diseased that he quitted his station, and took up his residence at St. Croix, where he soon died.

~~Several~~ A few other fatal cases of consumption will ~~now~~ be described, which occurred in my practice in the State of Maine. These will serve to point out some of **C70** the shoals & rocks on which I have been shipwrecked, in the hope that others may avoid them. Some of these cases were distressing beyond expression; for while the nearest relatives & dearest friends were in the greatest danger, and sinking around me, the arm of flesh was interposed in vain![7]

---

[5] Barker had not yet moved to the District of Maine. This refers to the Cape Cod town of Yarmouth, Barnstable County, Massachusetts, incorporated in 1639.

[6] Samuel Gilbert may not have attended Dartmouth College, according to alumni records and personal communication with Dartmouth College, Rauner Special Collections Library. Given the fact that he "preached to the Indians," we may assume he had attended the Indian Charity School, later called the Moor's Charity School, that had moved from Lebanon, Connecticut to Hanover, New Hampshire, when Eleazar Wheelock moved there circa 1770. George T. Chapman, *Sketches of the Alumni of Dartmouth College, from the First Graduation in 1771 to the Present Time, with a Brief History of the Institution* (Cambridge: Riverside Press, 1867), 7–8.

[7] Jeremiah 17:5. "Thus saith the LORD; Cursed *be* the man that trusteth in man, and maketh flesh his arm, and whose heart departeth from the LORD," suggesting it is poor judgment to put one's confidence in human ability or to rely on one's own natural strength rather than to rely on God. *Holy Bible: The Washburn College Bible, Oxford Edition, King James Text, Modern*

In Decr 1790, I married a daughter of Mrs Garrett,[8] whose case has been related, aged 21, who had enjoyed good health till the preceeding November, when, after exposure to cold & dampness, in a thin dress, she was attacked with chilliness followed by febrile heat, and inflammation in the throat. These complaints, however, soon subsided, by gentle means, tho her former vigour was not restored, and she was liable to febrile disturbance with a hecking cough, upon exposure to inclement weather.

In July 1793, she had a daughter which she nursed three months, when **C71** the symptoms described in the first stage of phthisis, took place, without much alarm, and continued till January 1794. Daily rigors & paroxysms of fever then supervened, together with the other symptoms of the second stage. In April the third stage commenced, and she declined, with its distressful train of symptoms, till June, when death closed the scene!

In 1798 [actually 1795], I married Miss Eunice Riggs, of Falmouth,[9] aged 25, of a florid countenance, and apparently in good health. In 1795 [1798], while lifting a heavy piece of furniture, she was seized with an hemoptysis, and considerable blood was discharged from her lungs, for which, tonic means, as I was told, were used. Her health, however, was soon restored, excepting that a soreness was felt, under the upper part of the sternum, on exposure to cold & dampness.

In the winter of 1799, being pregnant, **C72** she was troubled with some oppression in the vitals, febrile heat, and a hecking cough. As the spring advanced, her complaints increased, with swelled feet, tho she was able to ride out daily, and her appetite was good. ——Strange to relate, no depleting means were used, nor even suggested to the mind!

In August, 1799, she was delivered of a son, which was soon attended with cough, and the usual symptoms of hectic fever. It died in six months. The mother declined and was attended with laborious breathing together with profuse expectoration of purulent matter, till November, when she expired!

Were it necessary, many other fatal cases might be mentioned, which would serve to show that, in their treatment, many things were left undone, which ought to have been done.

Phrased Version, Washburn College Bible, Oxford edition, King James text, modern phrased version (Oxford: Oxford University Press, 1980), 1023.

[8] Susanna Barker's mother, Lucy Garrett, had also developed symptoms of consumption, coughed up blood yearly beginning in 1780, was treated, and died circa 1787.

[9] Here Barker had his dates reversed. He married Eunice Riggs in 1795, and her symptoms began in 1798. She died in November 1799. Hugh D. Mc Lellan, *History of Gorham, Maine* (Portland: Smith and Sale, 1903), 398.

Under the delusive notion that debility was the cause of pulmonary consumption, tonics, and spiritous stimulants were the chief means employed, even in the primary stages of the disease!

At this dark & doleful period, I was infected with the Brunonian doctrine;[10] and am sorry to say that I was not the only physician, who had been drawn into its fascinating and very dangerous vortex.

It is sincerely hoped that this practice will be imputed to ignorance; for I verily thought that my views were correct, while they were extremely **C73** erronious. This, however, is by no means, a sufficient excuse, as I might have known better; for in 1793, Dr Rush had thrown light on the nature and treatment of this disease.[11] But my mind was not then divested of prejudice in favour of preconceived opinions. Besides, his mode of treatment respecting the use of the lancet, met with great opposition, by many of my respectable brethren, which kept my mind in suspense, respecting its utility in phthisis pulmonalis, and such was our negligence, that the lungs had never been examined, in any fatal case, which had occurred in my own practice, nor in the practice of those physicians with whom I was acquainted.

In 1800, Dr Rush was providentially taught the efficacy of a mercurial salivation in this disease, and the success which has attended the practice, in the hands of many physicians, is generally known; so that prejudice & opposition have almost wholly ceased.

Passing over the many unsuccessful cases of consumption, which have occurred in my own practice, as well as in that of others, in the last century, the present happily affords a great variety of successful cases, not only **C74** in my own practice; but in the practice of numerous physicians, in different parts of the United States; as well as in other parts of America, and among European nations.

As the following case, which was communicated from Dr Tracy of Norwich, Conn. to Dr Mitchill of New York, in 1802, served to show the salutary effects of plentiful bleeding in Phthisis Pulmonalis, and to remove a

---

[10] "Brunonian" refers to the theories of John Brown (1735–1788), a student of William Cullen of Edinburgh, whose theory consisted of two kinds of disease: *sthenic*, caused by excessive excitement, or *asthenic*, caused by deficient excitement. This simplified therapeutic decisions— one should allay excitement for diseases thought to be *sthenic* and stimulate diseases thought to be *asthenic*. See Lester S. King, *The Medical World of the Eighteenth Century* (Huntington, NY: Robert E. Krieger Publishing Co. Inc. (reprint 1971), 1958), 143–47. See also Lester S. King, *Medical Thinking: A Historical Preface* (Princeton, NJ: Princeton University Press, 1982), 232–33; Lester S. King, *Transformations in American Medicine: From Benjamin Rush to William Osler* (Baltimore: Johns Hopkins University Press, 1991), 50–51.

[11] King, *Transformations in American Medicine*, 49–58.

prejudice, which existed in my own mind, as well as in the minds of others; against the use of the lancet in this disease, it will be particularly related; for, few physicians in Maine, as far as I can learn, are in possession of the work [the *Medical Repository* of 1802] in which it is contained.

"In April 1801, I was requested to visit Miss B. aged 17 years, who had been, for some time previous, in a debilitated state of health, which, rather from its continuance, than apparent formidableness, had created some anxiety in the minds of her friends, who now had **C75** become solicitous for my advice. On visiting the patient, I found her of a delicate organization, with a clear skin & florid complexion, narrow chested with elevated scapula, light blue eyes, and pupils largely dilated, with that pearly transparency of the cornea, which is usually observed in consumptive habits. On examining her complaints, I found she had been for some weeks previous, affected at turns, with slight fever, a hecking cough, and pain in her right side, often extending to the shoulder point, and erratically affecting the thoracic region. Her respiration was quick, and much accelerated by exercise. The pulse was frequent, with that shortness of stroke which so peculiarly characterises a hectical diathesis. On initial examination of all the symptoms attending the case, I became fully convinced that it was an incipient phthisis pulmonalis; probably arising from a tuberculous state of the lungs, which would terminate fatally. **C76** Under this impression, I suggested to her friends my opinion of her case, and its probable issue. At their request, tho with little confidence that any system of treatment I could adopt, would obviate its fatal tendency, I undertook the charge of the patient.

The practice I adopted was repeated tho small bleedings; a mild mercurial deobstruent course, combined with a nutritious, bland diet, with gentle exercise and mild opiates at night. This method was pursued for two months, with regularity; but without any apparent benefits; the patient evidently lost ground; and, at the expiration of this period, discovered the most unequivocal evidences of a fully established pulmonary consumption. Her cough had become urgent, and very distressing at night, unless suspended by opiates. She now had daily rigors followed by exacerbations of fever, and colliquative night sweats. Her evening paroxysms of fever, were attended with that circumscribed, tho highly oxygenated tynge of the cheek, which is so peculiarly **C77** characteristic of a fully established hectic. Her respiration was short, with increased quickness & tension of pulse, and great prostration of strength. With symptoms so portentous, but small hopes of restoration could be indulged. Wishing however, to gratify my patient & her friends by making every additional medical effort, that might be safely adopted, I omitted the former practice, and adopted the use of <u>digitalis</u>, in the form of a saturated tincture. This she used some weeks; but no apparent good effect arising; and as it excited great nausea,[12] with a vertiginous affection of her head, I was induced to omit its further use. In the room of which I substituted the <u>kali sulphuratum</u> combined with carbone, agreeably to the direction of Dr Garret. This, on being used some time, failing of producing any good effect; and being very offensive to her stomach, was omitted. The routine of <u>hectic symptoms</u> still continued, and clearly evidenced **C78** the second stage of the disease, to be fully established. She, by this time, had become much emaciated, and so weak as to require assistance in walking. I now, with her friends abandoned all hopes of her recovery, and recommended a more palliative practice, consisting of opiates with cordials & mild stomachic's.

At this period, when hope, the usual tho insidious attendant of the complaint, had deserted her, an Haemorrhage from the nose took place, which continued, with little intermission, for sixty hours, notwithstanding every medical effort was made to check it; and which finally seemed alone to yield to the great exhaustion of the vital fluid. ——The patient, at a very moderate computation, must have lost, at least, six pounds of blood, during the continuance of the hemorrhage, exclusive of one pound drawn from the foot, in the mean time. So great a loss of blood, necessarily produced an extreme increase of debility, with constant <u>deliquium animi</u>, or fainting, **C79** on attempting to arise in bed, for several days, and seemed to portend a speedy dissolution.

Under these new & threatening symptoms, I was convinced that the tonic & stimulant medicaments had become necessary, and I adopted a liberal use of the bark, with elix. vitriol & wine, combined with animal diet. Here I ought to premise, that, at the termination of the bleeding, the tense pulse which had marked the case, during its former progress, had remarkably subsided, and become softer, with less frequent vibrations. The respiration was also fuller & performed with much more ease, than in the antecedent state, with a material abatement of cough. This mode of practice was steadily persisted in, with the most promising prospects. The rigor & fever fits subsided, the nocturnal sweats diminished, and the cough wholly disappeared. And altho the patient for several months continued very languid, still a gradual amendment was visible, with a steady abatement of the hectic **C80** symptoms. —— At this

---

[12] Nausea is a common side effect of digitalis (foxglove) excess or toxicity.

time, the subject appears in good health; and is as capable of undergoing fatigue, in domestic concerns, as is usual for young females to practice.

Aware that many cases of <u>chlorosis</u>,[13] in young females, which have terminated happily have been mistakenly pronounced, by their attending physicians, to be true cases of <u>Phthisis</u>, I have been more minute in describing the leading symptoms which attended this case; and trust it will appear, to every well informed mind, that the <u>diagnosis</u> of an exquisitely formed <u>hectic</u>, decisively marked the complaint; and I feel it incumbent to add, that the essential symptoms of <u>chlorosis</u>, at no period existed, during her sickness.

How justifiable an imitation of this violent, tho salutary <u>effort of nature</u>, might be, in similar cases, which so usually baffle our art, is a question that merits mature consideration. But on this subject, might it not be admissible to adopt the sentiments of an ancient Father in physic, when he says, <u>melius est anceps remedium quam nullem?</u>"[14]   Med. Repos. vol. 6.[15]

C81

The first of December, 1806, Miss L. A. of Falmouth, Maine, of a slender & delicate habit, aged 25, after being exposed to cold & dampness, thinly clad and wetting her feet, was attacked with a cough which, at times, had troubled her since she had the measles, in 1803. I was soon called when she complained of some oppression at the pit of the stomach, and febrile heat, with great weakness of body; pulse small & about 90. The stomach & bowels were gently evacuated, and demulcents directed. Two days after, about a gill of blood [approximately 4 fluid ounces] was discharged from her lungs, in the morning, by a harassing cough; and this quantity continued to be thrown up, about the same time, for ten days in succession. During this period, there were exacerbations of fever, twice in 24 hours, preceded by chills, with morning sweats and inability to sit up more than two hours in the day. In the course of the day & first part of the night mucus & frothy matters were expectorated. The chief means employed were sal. sodæ in an infusion of chamomile, and

---

[13] See Glossary. Chlorosis was subsequently found to be severe iron deficiency anemia in young women, but in a 1926 German study, 64 of 143 women with chlorosis had histories suggesting tuberculosis (consumption). Isadore Olef, "Chlorosis," *New England Journal of Medicine* 225, no. 10 (1941): 358–64.

[14] *Anceps remedium est melius quam nullum*—"A doubtful remedy is better than none." Henry T. Riley, *Dictionary of Latin Quotations, Proverbs, Maxims, and Mottos, Classical and Mediaeval: Including Law Terms and Phrases: With a Selection of Greek Quotations* (London,: H.G. Bohn, 1859), 21.

[15] Dr. Tracy, "Remarkable Case of Phthisis Pulmonalis, Wherein a Profuse Spontaneous Hemorrhage Seemed to Be Useful: In a Letter from Dr. Tracy, of Norwich, (Connecticut) to Dr. Mitchill, Dated July 16, 1802," *Medical Repository* 6 (1803): 256–58.

occasional doses of paragoric elixir. At the expiration of ten days, the bleeding
C82 of the lungs ceased; and blood was copiously discharged by stool,
without pain. —— Calomel in small doses was then conjoined.

At this time, I desired that one of my medical brethren might be called in
consultation. Dr Kinsman was called, who concurred with me in opinion, that
there was little or no hope of her recovery, believing her to be far advanced
in pulmonary consumption. The hemorrhage from the rectum, probably
from the hemorrhoidal vessels, recurred once in 24 hours, in the midnight
paroxysm of fever, for eight days. A considerable quantity of blood appeared
to be discharged each time, with some feculent matter, nothing passing her
bowels at any other time. The patient was not apprised of this discharge of
blood, neither was she apprehensive of danger. She often asked how long it
would be before her "measly cough," as she called it, could be removed. As the
bleeding continued, her fever & morning sweats gradually abated, and at the
expiration of eight days, her stools became natural.
C83

At close of the month, after taking 96 grains of calomel, she was seized with
pain in her teeth & Jaws, to which succeeded a gentle salivation. The cough &
expectoration of matter then ceased; and her appetite soon returned, particularly for animal food, of which she sometimes ate to excess.

The middle of Jan. 1807, after dining on roasted goose with pickles, a profuse discharge of blood took place from her bowels, without pain. I was then
called; but prescribed nothing, except moderation in eating. The next day,
she had a natural stool. Her flesh & strength soon increased, by the use of
suitable food, and a bitter decoction, without spiritous stimulants, so that
she could sit up the whole of the day. The last of Feb. she rode out, and now
enjoys better health than before her sickness, free from cough, or any other
complaint, excepting that I neglected to bleed her. But the providential operations of Nature, abundantly supplied the defect; and my negligence was
Justly exposed.
C84

The beginning of February 1807, Miss L. B. of Windham, aged 23, of a delicate constitution, who had been troubled, in months past, with erisipelatous
eruptions on the extremities, and which had disappeared, was seized with a
short dry cough, and oppression at the breast. Pain in the left side, and an
expectoration of frothy mucus, sometimes tinged with blood, soon took
place. Medical aid, however, was not called till the first of May, when I was
consulted. At this time she complained of daily paroxysms of fever, preceded
by chills, oppression at the breast, increased pain in the side, especially on

exertion; a harrassing cough and considerable expectoration of mucus, which she said was constantly flowing into her throat & mouth, tho she had taken no medicine. There were circumscribed spots on the cheeks, hot palms, night sweats, and emaciation of body; pulse small, tense and 90 strokes in a minute.

Thus, this young lady had languished for nearly three months, being considered, by her friends, **C85** as labouring under a confirmed & irremediable pulmonary consumption. But she could not be reconciled to an untimely death, believing that it was in the power of medicine to cure her; and earnestly requested that the most effectual means & measures might be employed.

Fully persuaded that "the dictates of Nature form, for the most part, the safest directory for the conduct of the physician," to use the works of Dr John Reid of London,[16] on the first of May, I drew 12 ounces of blood, which was buffy; directed her to take one grain of calomel, once in six hours; to lodge in an airy room; and to abandon her feather bed & curtains.

I visited her on the 7th, and found her so anxious for life, that she had doubled the mercurial doses, which to her Joy, had inflamed her mouth.

The febrile paroxysms still continued with oppression at the breast, pain in the side, night sweats, cough and frequent spitting of bloody & pus like matter. I then drew a pint of blood which was equally buffy, and directed the increased doses of calomel **C86** to be continued, as they produced but little effect on the bowels.

12th. She had taken 60 grains of calomel which produced a copious salivation, and the cough ceased. The next day, her nurse gave a table spoonful of Flor. sulph.[17] which operated several times, as a cathartic, and produced great prostration of strength. She was then visited by the Rev. Mr Smith, who believed that death was at hand. —— I was sent for in haste, when she complained of heat & disturbance in the stomach; pulse 100 & small. Sal. absynth. & magnesia were then directed, with an infusion of chamomile of which she made a liberal use and found them congenial.

17th. Salivation still copious, febrile paroxysms, oppression & sweats continued, pulse 90 & tense. I then drew 12 ounces of blood, which was still buffy; the alkaline solution continued; febrile disturbance & night sweats abated. **C87**

20th. febrile disturbance &c returned in some degree; pulse 80 and less tense. 8 ounces of blood were drawn, which was nearly free from buff. The

---

[16] John Reid, *A Treatise on the Origin, Progress, Prevention, and Treatment, of Consumption* (London: Phillips, 1806), 121.

[17] Flores of sulphuric, see Glossary.

fever then subsided and the night sweats ceased. Blisters which were drawn, produced a great discharge. The mouth was very sore, and she was unable to sit up; yet her hope of recovery was great, as well as her confidence in the means employed.

24th. the fever & oppression at the breast returned with some pain in the side, when half a pint of blood was drawn at the patients request, by Esq. Payne, a respectable physician in that town; and her complaints subsided.[18]

29th. the pain & oppression returned in a lesser degree. I then drew 8 ounces of blood, which afforded relief; continuing the alkaline solution.

At the close of the month, she could **C88** walk the room, and sit up the chief of the day; appetite for animal food considerable, tho but little was allowed; for she still complained of febrile flushes in the evening & hot palms.

June 5th. She felt some oppression at the breast, pain in the side and raised a little blood. D[r] Payne was then so obliging as to draw half a pint from her arm; and her complaints were removed.

I visited her on the 8th. of June, when she stepped into my chaise, with little assistance; rode two miles, and dined on animal food.

On the 14th she rode three miles and attended public worship with a grateful heart.

Her flesh & strength rapidly increased by suitable nutriment & exercise; without any tonic medicines or spirits. Since which, she has enjoyed good health; entered into the married state; and been made the mother of several children.

C89

"In the first stages of Pulmonary consumption, says D[r] Rees, Cyclopedia vol. 10. N° 1.[19] while the character of the complaint is almost exclusively inflammatory, bloodletting, to a very considerable extent, is found absolutely necessary. This is the case, whether the habit of the patient be delicate or robust, with this precaution, that in delicate habits, the bleeding ought to be less copious, and more frequently repeated. Bloodletting manifests its good effects, in easing pain, removing fever, moderating the cough, diminishing expectoration, and night sweats; as well as preparing the system for mercury,

---

[18] Dr. James Paine (Payne) moved to Windham from Limerick, Maine, in 1797, practiced there until he became ill in 1818, moved to Portland, and died there February 22, 1822. Thomas Laurens Smith, *History of the Town of Windham* (Portland ME: Hoyt & Fogg, 1873), 84.

[19] Abraham Rees, *The Cyclopædia, or, Universal Dictionary of Arts, Sciences, and Literature* (Philadelphia: Published by Samuel F. Bradford and Murray, Fairman and Co., 1805), vol. 10, "Consumption," unpaged.

and other remedies. More than 100 ounces of blood have been drawn, in a variety of cases, with evident advantage, in the space of a few weeks, from persons of very delicate habits, and debilitated frames."

"Some practitioners, presuming that the hectic fever, and the whole series of complaints, were dependant on debility alone, have recommended the use of tonic medicines, in a state of confirmed **C90** consumption. But abundant experience has taught us, that all stimulating or corroborant medicines & food, tend to increase the cough & expectoration; as well as the hectic fever, and, therefore, to accelerate the destruction of the constitution, even in the last stages."

In November 1806, Gideon Wakefield, a seaman, of a spare habit, aged 40, returned from the West Indies, to Falmouth, troubled with some cough, feverishness, and general weakness, as his wife informed me, who requested my advice. I prescribed some demulcents & restoratives, without seeing the patient. He was able, as I was informed, to perform some labour till March 1807, and that very few means had been taken, though his cough & febrile disturbance continued.

On the 7th of March, he complained of a <u>hoarse</u> cough, increased fever, and pain in the chest, after undergoing considerable fatigue, on wet ground, in driving an ox team. In the evening, he drank some warm spirit & water, believing that he had taken a bad cold. —— He was now attended by Dr Folsome of Gorham & myself. On the 8th a pint of blood was drawn by D^r **C91** Folsome, and the pain was removed to his loins. A cathartic of jalap & calomel was given. Two grains of calomel were given, once in six hours; an ounce of mercurial ointment was rubben [*sic*] in, and blisters were applied. On the 10th another pint of blood was drawn, when the pain left his loins, and he complained of pain in his heart; which palpitated considerably. His pulse was small, frequent & tense, before bleeding, afterwards full & soft. The tongue was white, and he was thirsty. On the 12th his pulse intermitted; the pain in his side was tedious, and his breathing was difficult. Another cathartic was given.

14th we found the patient labouring under great pain in the left side, and his respiration was laborious; cough dry & hard; pulse tense. Another pint of blood was drawn, which removed the pain and alleviated his breathing. The blood was sizy & buffy, as in the preceeding bleedings.

15th the pain had not returned. He could now walk the room & converse with more ease. His chief complaints were heat & oppression in his vitals; pulse full & laborious. I left him at 2. PM. setting on the side of his bed, begging for relief. **C92** But none could be afforded. ——He expired at 9 in the evening; and his pulse continued to beat forcibly, as his nurse since informed me, till the breath left his body. He had taken 60 grams of calomel; but his mouth was not affected.

The next day, at 4. PM. I repaired to the house of the deceased, with a pupil; and obtained permission to open his body. Dr Folsome arrived soon after.

On removing the sternum, we found the right lobe of the lungs in the natural state. A portion of the pleura, on that side, near the diaphragm, was suppurated; as also of the mediastinum. The left lobe was highly inflamed, particularly on the back part; and crowded with blood; the forepart was interspersed with small black spots. The heart was much inflamed on its left side; and the coronary vessels were greatly distended. On being punctured, dark blood was discharged with considerable force.

On opening the abdomen, the stomach appeared in a natural state, and contained no offensive matters. The intestines discovered no marks of disease, neither did any part of the abdominal viscera. The spleen, however, was greatly enlarged, **C93** and distended with blood, tho sound in texture.

In this case we are led to see the insidious nature of hectic fever, altho moderate, when treated with neglect, and suffered to run for several months unrestrained, eating & drinking the common way, with inordinate exercise. Judging from appearances, it seems probable that had blood been drawn, at an early period, and mercury given, with regular living, the morbid action of the blood vessels & cough might have been removed; so as to have prevented this fatal disorganization. The spleen did its office, by draining off as much blood as it could hold. But the lancet was not called into aid till it was too late, when it acted only as a palliative.

In the course of my practice, I have met with many very similar cases, where the inflammatory irritation was so moderate, that no danger was suspected, till a short time before death, so that recourse was not had to bloodletting nor mercury, yet on dissection, disorganization has been found in the vitals; sometimes an accumulation of blood, in the pulmonary system, when it appeared, by the pulse and **C94** great bodily decay, that there was not much blood in the vessels; and none to spare!

In October 1807, Dr Aaron Kinsman of Portland, aged 40, of a good habit, tho rather inflamatory [sic], was seized with the Influenza, attended with ophthalmia, coryza & cough; but in so slight a degree that few means were used; and he continued to practice till the last of December, when his cough was tedious and attended with some expectoration of purulent matter. He had slight chills & fever fits, with night sweats. But he did not think his complaints required bleeding; as he was not exercised with pain. In Jan. 1808, he began to suspect some danger, and had recourse to small doses of calomel, with a view of raising a salivation; but it was not productive of the desired effect. —— He died in May 1808.

In April, profuse hemorrhages repeatedly took place from his lungs & nose, which afforded some relief. He then told his wife, as she has since informed me, that he was now fully persuaded of the necessity of seasonable bloodletting in his case, and greatly regretted that it had been dispensed with. And his **C95** friends as deeply regret the loss of this useful & benevolent physician.

In the winter of 1809, the Rev. Asa Rand of Gorham,[20] aged 25, of a slender habit, tho his countenance was florid, complained of pain in the left side of his breast about two inches above the extremity of the sternum, with some cough; complaints which had troubled him, at times, for more than three years; to remedy which, he had occasionally used blisters; and these afforded temporary relief.

The middle of March 1810, after being exposed to cold & dampness, and wetting his feet, the pain in his side returned and increased to a considerable degree, with febrile disturbance & cough. Dr Folsome was then called, who gave evacuants, and prescribed a mercurial salivation. The mercury, however, was not taken, but it should interfere with an intended Journey. In April, the pain continuing troublesome, a large blister was applied to his side, which excoriated deeply, discharged freely, and was beset with "canker sores," as they are called. The pain, however, did not yield as heretofore. **C96** He was then bled, by Dr Folsome; and some relief was afforded. The last of May, the pain in his side, febrile disturbance & cough increased, when some opium was taken; but it was not productive of the desired effect.

The beginning of June, Dr Folsome, being absent, a physician advised to the tincture of the bark, and Island Moss. on account his weakness. These were taken, but the febrile disturbance increased; his strength failed, and the pain in his side, as well as cough grew worse; so that he was considered, by his friends; as well as several physicians, who saw him, as being incurably consumptive.

On the 10th of July, four physicians met at the house of this faithful & useful Minister, viz Drs Folsome, Howe, Thorndike & myself,[21] in order to give our best & most friendly advice.

---

[20] Asa Rand (c. 1774–1861) was born in Rindge, New Hampshire, graduated from Dartmouth College in 1806, and was ordained in Gorham, Maine, in 1809. He resigned his ministry June 12, 1822, because of ill health and failing voice. He moved to Portland, Maine, founded a religious newspaper, the *Christian Mirror*, and later edited the *Boston Recorder*. He died August 24, 1861, at eighty-eight years of age. Mc Lellan, *History of Gorham, Maine*,1903, 193.

[21] Drs. Folsom(e), Thorndike, and Barker were all practicing on Gorham at this time. The fourth physician named may be Dr. Ebenezer Howe (1773–1841) of Standish.

The patient, at this time, was considerably emaciated; his countenance pale, tho, at times, it was said to be highly flushed; and morning sweats had taken place. His cough was very tedious, with some expectoration of mucus; and the pain in his side was so excrutiating **C97** especially after a fit of coughing, as to excite bitter groans; pulse weak and 90, in a minute.

We endeavoured to convince him that inflammatory irritation of the respiratory organs, gave rise to his complaints, which, by continuing, would endanger a fatal disorganization of the lungs. We were unanimously of opinion that a mercurial salivation was eligible; and that it might be instrumental of diverting morbid action from the labouring parts; so as to remove his complaints. The patient then consented to use this means, tho not with any expectation of being benefitted, as he said, thinking it too late; but merely to gratify his friends. Accordingly, a pill composed of 2/3 of a grain of calomel & 1/3 of opium was prepared & given, by Dr Folsome, night & morning. Besides, half an ounce of strong mercurial ointment, was applied to the pained part. —— In ten days, a salivation took place; and the discharge, which was copious, continued fifteen days, tho he took only sixteen grains of calomel.

C98

When the salivation took place, his cough ceased, and in five days the pain yielded; gradually abating under the salival discharge. As the salivation increased, the febrile disturbance decreased; and his pulse became natural. His flesh & strength were soon regained, by suitable nutriment, without the use of any stimulating medicines.

In a few weeks, he was able to attend public worship; and on the first Sabbath in September, assisted in performing divine service; the 116th Psalm, Dr Watts' version, composing a part, which is descriptive of his <u>mental</u>, as well as bodily affections.[22]

---

[22] From the Project Gutenberg ebook of The Psalms of David, by Isaac Watts. *The Psalms of David imitated in the language of The New Testament and applied to The Christian State and Worship* by I. Watts D.D. Psalm 116:1. First Part. Recovery from sickness.

1 I love the Lord; he heard my cries,
And pity'd every groan:
Long as I live, when troubles rise,
I'll hasten to his throne.

2 I love the Lord; he bow'd his ear,
And chas'd my griefs away;
O let my heart no more despair,
While I have breath to pray!

The day following, he set off on a Journey, in a chaise, and rode to the western part of the state. He returned in October, having preached several times, in his absence. In succeeding years he continued in the work of the ministry, and laboriously performed parochial duties; but finding that public speaking was injurious to his health, he asked dismission in 1822, and editied [*sic*] the *Christian Mirror*.

C99 Had he pursued his intended journey, while this inflammatory state of the lungs existed, we may naturally suppose that it would have been injurious, and increased his complaints, as has often been the case with patients laboring under pulmonic affections; and paved the way for a fatal termination of the disease. But after the morbid action of the blood vessels is removed by bleeding, salivating &c exercise, in riding or sailing, is eligible and often beneficial.

Peter Thacher Esq. of Gorham,²³ aged 30, in the study & practice of law, of a tall & slender make, great instability of the arterial system, evidenced by an accelerated pulse, and occasional flushes in the face, complained, in the winter of 1808, of a troublesome hecking cough, especially on exposure to cold & dampness; with some oppression at the breast, and febrile disturbance.

In March I was consulted, and advised to bleeding & a mercurial salivation; pulse 90 & tense. But he could not be reconciled ****C100**** to the use of

---

3 My flesh declin'd, my spirits fell,
And I drew near the dead,
While inward pangs, and fears of hell
Perplex'd my wakeful head.

4 "My God," I cry'd "thy servant save,
"Thou ever good and just;
"Thy power can rescue from the grave,
"Thy power is all my trust."

5 The Lord beheld me sore distrest,
He bid my pains remove:
Return, my soul, to God thy rest,
For thou hast known his love.

6 My God hath sav'd my soul from death,
And dry'd my failing tears;
Now to his praise I'll spend my breath,
And my remaining years.

²³ Peter Thacher, son of Judge Thacher, read law with William Symmes, Esq., of Portland. In 1804 he began his law practice in Saccarappa (from the Indian name for the Presumpscot River falls), a village later to become Westbrook, Maine. After five years he returned to his home in Gorham, Maine, where died of consumption in January 1811.

these means, and would consent to use nothing but demulcents, as liquorice, flaxseed, honey &c.

In April his complaints were more troublesome, for which he took Turlingtons balsam of life. In May & June, they were less tedious, and few means were taken in succeeding months, feeling no increase of his complaints till March 1809, when they increased to a considerable degree. At this time, I was again consulted, and my former advice was given; but he would not consent to take any means, excepting such as were simple, viz squills, liquorice &c. In September, finding that his health had become much impaired, he requested me to lend him some medical books, descriptive of his complaints, with medical prescriptions. I then put into his hand Dr Rushs medical observations,[24] and the Medical Museum.[25] These books were perused; but a prejudice existed in his mind against the lancet and mercury, having imbibed an idea from a Brunonian, that debility was the cause of his complaints, and that stimulating **C101** and strengthening means were indicated in his case.

In Feb. 1810, my advice was particularly requested, when he informed me that wine & cordials, which had been prescribed, by a physician, were not congenial; and that he had substituted cyder & water.

At this time his cough was tedious, and he complained of oppression & stricture of his breast, with running pains in the chest, shortness of breath, and diffusive heat, especially after exercise. His pulse was 85 & tense, with a flushed countenance; and his appetite for animal food was unimpaired. I again advised him to be bled & to take calomel. But he could not be persuaded that his case could with propriety be called <u>pulmonary consumption</u>. He believed

---

[24] "Observations" probably refers to Benjamin Rush, *Medical Inquiries and Observations*, 2nd ed. Philadelphia, J Conrad and Company. Barker wrote to Rush in Philadelphia on September 22, 1806, "Last week, I procured from the Portland Book-store, your four volumes of *Medical Inquires and Observations*, previously to which I was in possession only of your 2nd & 3rd volumes, excepting in review." Historical Society of Pennsylvania, Rush MSS vol. 2, p. 28.

[25] Medical Museum refers to the *Philadelphia Medical Museum* (1804–1811), the second medical journal published in the United States. (The first was the *Medical Repository*, 1797–1824, New York City.) Barker's letters and articles are found in both publications. For information on early US medical journals, see J. S. Billings, "Literature and Institutions," in *A Century of American Medicine: 1776–1876*, ed. Edward H. Clarke (Philadelphia: Henry C. Lea, 1876); Victor Robinson, "The Early Medical Journals of America Founded during the Quarter Century 1797–1822," *Medical Life* 36, no. 11 (1929), 533–88; Joseph E. Garland, "Medical Journalism in New England 1788–1924," *Boston Medical and Surgical Journal* 190 (1924), 865–79; R. J. Kahn and P. G. Kahn, "The Medical Repository—The First U.S. Medical Journal (1797–1824)," *New England Journal of Medicine* 337 (1997), 1926–30.

that his complaints were owing to weakness. Respecting mercury, he thought it too powerful; and bleeding, he imagined would weaken him, so as to hinder his attending to the business of his profession. Some other means, must therefore be devised to remove his complaints.

C102

On the 10th of July, I called to see him, when he had become much emaciated; cough tedious with some expectoration of mucus, and shortness of breathing. He complained of slight chills, followed by febrile heat & morning sweats, pulse 90 small & tense. At this time he was able to ride & transact business as usual; fearless of any danger.

I then took much pains to convince him that he laboured under the symptoms of pulmonary consumption, which had progressed to the second stage, and that bleeding, as well as salivating were highly expedient, observing, that his Pastor, whose complaints were pretty similar, had consented to undergo a salivation. He did not believe that mercury would benefit his Pastor, for he viewed him as being incurably consumptive; and lamented the loss which the town would sustain by his death. With respect to his own case, he still expressed a belief that debility was the cause and that invigorating means were the most suitable.

C103

The use of appropriate remedies was therefore urged in vain, and no means were used, after this time, as far as I could learn, excepting patent cough drops, and other secret nostrums, which load our newspapers, with alluring encomiums, greatly to the injury of consumptive invalids; for these compositions consist of heating & stimulating ingredients, evidenced by their effects; so that the inflammatory action of the blood vessels, is thereby increased and the lungs become subjected to engorgement and disorganization!

Why then do legislators, who, in general are acquainted with the nature of diseases, countenance such empirical impositions, when every College of Physicians, and every Medical Society, in the United States, bear testimony against them, knowing that most of their nostrums are injurious or feeble, and tend to preclude the use of proper means, which ****C104**** should only be prescribed or administered by experienced physicians, according to the varying state of the system, when labouring under disease.

During the autumnal months, the inflammatory irritation of the vital organs of this patient, and attending train of hectical symptoms continued to increase, yet he was able to ride on horseback till the beginning of winter, and his strength of body was such that he could sit up the chief of the time

and transact business; both of a public & private nature, till the day before his death, which took place on the 25th of Jan. 1811, having lost his consort, his parents; his brothers & his sisters; eight in number, all of whom died of pulmonary affections! And their minds were equally irreconcileable to the lancet and to mercury. But we trust, <u>they</u> were reconciled to the will of God.
C105

The memory of this young man will doubtless be held in grateful remembrance, by those who are destitute of the light of the Gospel; for he has left a considerable donation to the Missionary Society, in the District of Maine.

In the fall of 1809, Dr Charles Kitteridge of Portland, aged about 30, of inflammatory habit, evidenced by an eruption on his face, and a florid countenance, was attacked with cough & oppression at the breast, attended with febrile heat. He continued, however to ride & practice till the winter, when his complaints increased and an expectoration of mucous, deeply tinged with blood took place for which he made a liberal use of Island moss. But he continued to split blood for 20 days in succession, as he informed me. Yet he could not be reconciled to the use of the lancet, in his case, believing that his complaints, depended upon a debilitated state of the lungs.
C106

He then relinquished his practice and undertook a long Journey.

In the spring of 1810, he returned to Portland and resumed his practice, in tolerable health, excepting a slight cough & some expectoration of mucus. In May, he informed me that he had not been bled nor taken any mercury; but was making a liberal use of the Lichen, which he found to be nutritious & restorative.

In July, he was again attacked with raising blood. About a gill, as he said, was discharged every morning for eleven days, which afforded some relief.

He was a physician who was prejudiced against the use of the lancet, in most cases. But the "fortuitous operations of nature," in his case, as he expressed himself, induced him to believe that bloodletting might be more liberally employed, than he had imagined. Soon after, he took passage for the West Indies and died of pulmonary consumption.[26]

These two last cases afford additional evidence of the dangerous and unhappy effects of the Brunonian doctrine.

---

[26] *Portland Gazette*, September 14, 1812: "Doct. Charles Kittredge, late of Portland." Jacob Kittredge was administrator of the estate.

C107

"Mr Tracy, of Connecticut, says Dr Rush, informed me, ~~that~~ in the spring of 1802, that he had been bled 25 times, in six months, by order of Dr Sheldon, in the inflammatory state of consumption, and ascribes his recovery chiefly to this frequent use of the lancet."

"I bled a Methodist minister, in the inflammatory state of this disease, 15 times in the course of six weeks, in February & March. The quantity drawn was not less than eight ounces, and it was at all times covered with a buff. By the addition of country air and moderate exercise he recovered his health, in the ensuing spring, so perfectly, as to discharge all the duties of his profession, for many years; nor was he ever afflicted afterwards with a disease in his breast."

"To these cases, I might add many others, who have been perfectly cured, by frequent, and of many whose lives have been prolonged, by occasional bleedings. But I am sorry to add, that I could relate many more cases of consumptive patients, who have died martyrs to their prejudices against the use of this invaluable remedy."

"From many years experience of the efficacy **C108** of bleeding, in this species of consumption, I feel myself authorised to assert, that where a greater proportion of persons die of consumption, when it makes its first appearance in the lungs, with symptoms of inflammatory diathesis, than die of ordinary pneumonies, provided exercise be used afterwards, it must, in nine cases out of ten, be ascribed to the erronious theories of physicians, or to the obstinacy or timidity of patients."

"A salivation has lately been prescribed in this disease with success. It is to be lamented that in a majority of cases, in which the mercury has been given, it has failed of exciting a salivation. Where it affects the mouth it generally succeeds, in recent cases, which is more than can be said of any, or of all other remedies, in consumption. In its hectic state a salivation often cures; and even in its typhus or last stage, I have more than once prescribed it with success. It should never be advised, till the inflammatory diathesis of the system, has been, in a great degree reduced by bloodletting and other depleting remedies."

Med. ob.[27]

"It will possibly be thought a rash practice, says Dr Mead, vol. 3. to draw blood in hectic fever, when the patient is much wasted in his flesh, and very weak. But it is better to try a doubtful remedy than none; and a temporary

---

[27] Benjamin Rush, *Medical Inquiries and Observations*, 4th ed., 4 vols. (Philadelphia: Johnson & Warner, 1815), vol. 2, 69–72.

C109 lessening of his strength is of service, when attended with a removal of a part of the cause, which would weaken the body more & more every day. Wherefore if the lungs be ulcerated, and the fever run high, it will be proper to take away as much blood as the patient can bear, at proper intervals; so as to allow the body time to recruit. I have seen cases judged almost desperate, where this method of practice succeeded well. But if it happen otherwise, the physician is not to be branded with the death of the patient, whose viscera had become so corrupted that it was impossible to save him. It is, therefore, of the utmost consequence, to attempt the cure of this dreadful disease <u>early</u>; and as it arises from inflammation, it requires, not only one; but several bleedings."[28]

"The neglect of venesection in catarrh, says D[r] Reid,[29] is mentioned as a cause of consumption, in the reports of Professor Frank of Hague, 1808, who confesses that he was formerly too much influenced, in his opinions & practice by the imaginary theories of D[r] John Brown.

[28] Most of this quotation is in Richard Mead, *The Medical Works of Richard Mead* (Dublin: Printed for Thomas Ewing, 1767), 360.

[29] Reid, *A Treatise on the Origin, Progress, Prevention, and Treatment, of Consumption*, 131–34. And Reid earlier referred to Cullen's four "different affections capable of producing ulcerations or confirmed consumption of the lungs . . . hemoptysis, catarrh, pneumonia, and tubercles." Reid, *A Treatise on the Origin, Progress, Prevention, and Treatment, of Consumption*, 70.

Chap. 5.

HAVING THUS FAR, endeavored to establish the efficacy chiefly of bleeding & mercury, in <u>Phthisis</u> <u>pulmonalis</u>, we shall now proceed to point out, the beneficial effects of certain cooperative means, and examine their respective advantages, viz. emetics, cathartics, alkalines and digitalis; also dispair of recovery & fear of death. Likewise epispastics, issues, setons & cauteries; opiates, tonics, suitable diet, and salubrious air, with exercise.[1]

The circumstances under which, each of these, have been found useful, will be deduced mostly from cases, which will be related, in illustration of their effects, not only in my own practice; but in that of others, both in Europe & America.

The first of Nov. 1809, Mr Thomas Pierce of Falmouth, a mason, aged 40 ~~years~~ who had been troubled, at times, for several years, with rheumatic pains in the limbs, complained of some oppression at the breast, a sore throat & cough, after exposure to cold & dampness, working in clay morter. He continued, however, to labour till the middle of the month, when growing worse, he was bled, by Dr Hunt,[2] and an emetic & cathartic were given, which afforded considerable relief.

On the 6th of Dec. Dr H. being sick, I was called, when he was troubled with a very hoarse cough and expectoration of mucus. His throat was inflamed & beset **C111** with apthæ. His body had become emaciated; and

---

[1] Thacher's treatment of pulmonary consumption begins with three pages on diet and regimen as being more important than "all the drugs and medicines that can be prescribed by the most skillful physician." James Thacher, *American Modern Practice* (Boston: Ezra Read, 1817), 436–46.

[2] Dr. Jacob Hunt (1778–1846) was born in Loudon, New Hampshire, on February 8, 1778, and graduated from Dartmouth Medical School in 1806. In 1808 Barker had married Judge William Gorham's widow and moved back to Gorham from Stroudwater. In 1815 Hunt would purchase Barker's Stroudwater house, today often called the Barker/Hunt house. Jacob Hunt died August 18, 1846. M. K. Lovejoy, E. G. Shettleworth, and W. D. Barry, *This Was Stroudwater: 1727–1860* (Portland, ME: National Society of Colonial Dames of America in the State of Maine, 1985), 199–205; *Dartmouth College and Associated Schools General Catalogue 1769–1940* (Hanover, NH: Dartmouth College Publications, 1940), 838.

his feet swelled; pulse quick and appetite irregular. I directed a quarter of a grain of corrosive sublimate, dissolved in an infusion of digitalis, three times in 24 hours. His throat was gargled with lime water impregnated with pearl ash; a draught of which was often swallowed. Epispastics were applied, and cathartics occasionally given.

The fever continued, with paroxysms & remissions twice in 24 hours; pulse 100. A.M. 120. P.M. with red spots on the cheeks, and morning sweats. His hope of recovery, however, was great; and he was offended at the suggestion of his being consumptive, tho his flesh rapidly decayed, and he was unable to sit up more than half of the day.

On the 10th Dr Cummins of Portland, was called in consultation, who pronounced his case decidedly hectical, and viewed him as being near the last stage of consumption. He advised to a continuance of the means, tho with little or no expectation of a recovery.

On the 12th being considered by his friends, as hopeless, he was visited by the Rev Mr Bradly,[3] who seriously reminded him of his dangerous situation; and advised him to think of another world. —— Fear of death then occupied his mind; and it seemed to operate as a sedative. The activity of his pulse readily abated when the stimulus of hope was removed. A salivation then took place; and the urinary discharge greatly increased; so that his fever was much reduced; and his cough, as well as expectoration, **C112** moderated. By the last of the month, persisting in the use of the alkaline solution alone, his appetite became regular, and his pulse natural. A decoction of the bark was then given, with lichen.

Animal food was taken with moderation, and friction over the stomach as well as limbs was used, before his meals. In this way his health was gradually restored. Since which he has been a laborious man, free from disease, and says that he enjoys better health than before his sickness.

The beneficial effects of alkalines, in slow fevers and epidemics, about the close of the last century, induced me to give them a trial in hectic fever and I am persuaded from repeated trials, that their efficacy, in this disease, is much greater than is generally imagined. For several centuries these means have been considered by medical writers, as febrifuges; but they have been directed in so sparing a manner, that their efficacy has not been fully known; and their being generally neutralised with acids, has tended greatly to lessen

[3] Reverend Caleb Bradley (Bradly) was ordained at the Stroudwater Congregational Church in 1799 and the Westbrook Congregational Church until 1829, and was scribe to the Cumberland Association of Congregational Ministers from 1807 to 1823; he died in 1861.

their power. Some have considered them as unsafe in fevers, supposing that they tended to promote putrefaction, others that they were not sufficiently powerful to deserve much attention.

C113

The following cases will serve to show that alkalines are not only safe, even when liberally given, and their use continued, but that they possess considerable power & efficacy in hectic fever.

In May 1800, a Portland lady, of a slender habit, tho florid countenance, aged about 20 years, was at my house on a visit, when she complained of some oppression of the breast, hurried breathing, after exercise, and a hecking cough, which took place in February preceeding. I advised her to avoid the evening air, and to substitute wollen for muslin. The lancet & mercury were seldom used, at that time, by any physicians, among us, in phthisis pulmonalis.

Febrile paroxysms, preceeded by chills, commenced in June following, as I was informed, followed with other hectical symptoms. Few means were used in the summer, excepting blisters & expectorants. In the fall she took some pills of digitalis, each containing one fourth of a grain; but as they produced vomiting, they were soon omitted. After this elix. vitriol was given, which was offensive to the stomach. Tonic bitters were then substituted, but they excited the fever, and increased her other complaints, so that they were also laid aside.

C114

In Jan. 1801, she was unable to walk, and could sit up only a few hours in the day. Her symptoms were quick pulse, febrile paroxysms, flushed cheeks and redness of the tongue, with apthæ; some pain in the side, cough & expectoration of mucus; sometimes mixed with blood & yellowish matter; morning sweats and impaired appetite.

At this time, I was requested to visit her, and prescribed alkaline salts, which accorded with the views of Dr Erving, her attending physician. These means were congenial and often taken. The consequence was that her febrile & other complaints gradually abated, and her appetite mended.

Her confidence in <u>alkalines</u> was such, that she had them mixed with almost all her food; and took very little medicine of any other kind, while using them, until the fever had subsided, when tonic bitters were conjoined to advantage.

In April she menstruated, after several months suspension; and in May she was attacked with a diarrhœa, for which I prescribed the chalk Julep.

In June she was able to walk and to ride in a carriage. In July she rode to Gorham eight miles, where she spent the summer, and made a liberal use of milk, with few complaints.

It appeared, from calculation that in the course **C115** of six months, she had taken, at least, a pound & a half of pearl ash, and four ounces of sal. sodæ. —— Great attention was also paid to her food, which consisted chiefly of oily & mucilaginous articles, as milk & its preparations with Indian meal, salop, jelly of calves feet, eggs &c.

In Sept. she returned to Portland, and had evidently gained flesh. I then called to see her; and found her pulse natural; and she made no complaint, excepting some degree of debility.

The recovery of this patient to such a measure of health, served to enhance the reputation of alkalies, in consumption & hectic fever.

Such was the delicacy of her habit, and susceptability [sic] of impression, that on the approach of the following winter, she was again invaded with pulmonary complaints; and she declined till the next August, when she died. —— What means were employed in her last sickness, I have not been informed, excepting that the warm bath was used. Would not stove heated rooms, recommended by Dʳ Comstock, be useful for such invalids?

Dʳ Lyman Spalding of Portsmouth, informed me, in a letter dated August 1, 1801, that he had made a liberal use of soda & lime water in Phthisis, and that they had removed hectical symptoms, where he did not promise much relief; so that he viewed them as being very efficacious in consumption &c. His common dose of soda was a tea spoonful.

C116

The first of September 1801, Mʳˢ Skilling, of Cape Elizabeth, aged 18 years, who resided in low marshy ground, near a fresh pond, was attacked with Typhus mitior, five months advanced in pregnancy. I was then called and drew a pint of blood. The stomach & bowels were evacuated, and antiphlogistics given. The fever terminated in 14 days; but it left her with a cough & expectoration of mucus, which gradually decreased during gestation.

The beginning of Feb. 1802, she was put to bed, after ~~considerable~~ an easy travail; and nursed her infant one month when her milk failed. Her cough & expectoration then increased. Febrile paroxysms preceeded by chills, soon took place, with night sweats. Her stomach was often nauseated on the approach of the chilly fit, so as to eject her food, and she felt running pains in the chest. By the last of April, she was reduced so low as to be confined to her bed. On the first of May, I called to see her; and obtained the preceeding account, since her delivery. I found that her friends viewed her as being in an irrecoverable consumption, and had advised her not to apply to physicians of the body. Her symptoms at this time, were cough & expectoration of mucus & pus like matter, pain the left side, tho not stationary, daily paroxysms of fever, preceeded by chills, night sweats, great emaciation of body, and swelled feet, irregular appetite and total inability to sit up; pulse 100 and weak. My opinion of her case was asked. I readily denominated the case consumptive, and gave very little encouragement as to her recovery. **C117** But advised to the use of means. Her friends objected to my advice, and said that I ought rather to warn the patient of her near approach to death! This office I declined. Soon after, the Rev. Mr Lancaster[4] of Scarborough was requested to visit her, who informed the patient & her friends, that recoveries had been effected, by the use of proper means, in apparently hopeless cases of consumption; and advised them to consult a physician.

The next day, I was requested, by Mr Skilling, to attend to his wife's case, and prescribe as I should judge proper. In the first place, I gave an emetic of ipecac 15 grains, sal. absynth 20 grains, which operated five times, following each ejection with an aqueous solution of alkaline salts. Much ropy matter of a greenish hue was ejected, and a cathartic operation was produced. The chilly fits did not invade her on that day; and the febrile paroxysms were very slight. But the next day, these symptoms recurred as heretofore. Twenty grains of sal. absynth. were then given, twice a day in the febrile paroxysms. Lime water was also occasionally used. Friction with a coarse flannel wetted with lixivium of wood ashes, was directed twice a day, on the approach of the chilly fits, particularly to the extremities, and over the region of the stomach; strong enough to inflame the skin, and to produce vesication. The friction was then omitted for a time; and renewed when the inflammation subsided. Adhesive plaisters, impregnated with mustard, were applied. Occasional doses of laudanum were given to moderate the cough and pain in the chest.
C118

On this plan, the chilly fits, as well as febrile disturbance gradually lessened, her appetite mended, and the stomach became retentive of food, which consisted chiefly of milk, porridge, rice & chocolate. The last of May, she relished animal food, particularly pork & salted fish, which were taken in small quantities at a time. She now could sit up half of the day, and was much less feverish. The night sweats, cough, expectoration & pain had gradually abated; pulse 80, and stronger. By the middle of June the swelling of her

---

[4] Reverend Thomas Lancaster, a graduate of Harvard College, was ordained in 1775 and served as the seventh pastor of the First Congregational Church of Scarborough for more than fifty years. He died in 1831 at the age of eighty-seven. Cumberland Association of Congregational Ministers, *The Centennial of the Cumberland Association of Congregational Ministers, at the Second Parish Church in Portland, Maine* (Portland ME: B. Thurston, 1888), 22–23.

feet had nearly subsided; and she could walk without assistance. Her appetite & digestion now became good, and she could bear considerable food. All medicines were laid aside. By the first of August, her flesh & strength were regained. In Autumn, she became robust, and attended to domestic business.

In succeeding years, she had several children, attended with laborious & tedious travails; so that recourse was had to copious bloodletting, followed with an emetic & cathartic, which served to moderate the pains and relax the system; so as to facilitate labour and prevent puerperal fever. Thus treated, she was not confined to her bed, but a few days, and nursed her children.

This mode of practice I have pursued with good success, and little detention, in such cases, since **C119** the memorable year of 1784, when many women died of puerperal fever, where these means were neglected or too sparingly used, at least in my own practice.

In preceeding years, I had frequently seen tedious travails, happily terminated, by a <u>spontaneous vomiting</u>. This salutary effort of nature, induced me to consider emetics as eligible in such cases when vomiting did not occur; and I am happy to find that many of my obstetric brethren, in different parts of the Union have used & recommended these means in laborious parturient cases; as well as depletion with the lancet, in order to lessen violent pains, remove rigidity, facilitate labour and prevent fever, convulsions, rupture of the uterus & blood vessels, noticed by various writers, both in Europe & America; and which have often taken place in consequence of torturing pains in plethoric habits; for which, suffering patients, have, to my knowledge, been treated, by female accouchers, <u>solely</u> with spiritous liquors! —— The injurious and dangerous consequences of which, are too well known to need a description.

This practice is imputed to their ignorance of the nature of diseases and appropriate remedies.

C120

Since 1800, I have made a liberal use of alkalines, in Phthisis pulmonalis, particularly where the lancet and mercury have either been omitted or sparingly used; and they have evidently been attended with salutary effects, by reducing the hectic fever, and correcting morbid degeneracy of the humours; not omitting blisters & setons, which tend to remove local affections by counterirritation, and diverting morbid action from labouring parts.

"Alkalis, says Dᵣ Young, though not very powerful in their operation, are in some measure useful, in many cases of consumption. Sal Sodæ has been given with apparent advantage, in pretty large doses, at all periods of the disease; and some benefit was derived, in my own case, from the long continued use of the supercarbonate of potass, or artificial seltzer water. I cannot help being persuaded that there was an incipient formation of tubercles, from the difficulty of breathing and hectic symptoms. I was bled only twice. In my own case a small blister was kept open, more than a year; and it was occasionally, for a short time, exceedingly painful."[5]

"External applications, whether blisters or caustics, are often highly useful, in relieving the pain and other symptoms of inflammation; and probably, also in promoting the absorption of tubercles."[6]

C121

With regard to digitalis, I have made use of it in several cases of Phthisis; and when it operated as a diuretic, good effects were experienced. But merely, by retarding the circulations, it was not productive of the desired effect, unless bloodletting had been premised, sufficiently to liberate the distended and engorged vessels of the lungs; otherwise, the oppression & stricture of the breast remained, tho the pulse was reduced to 40, in a minute, when torpor and anxiety took place, bordering up on suffocation. I have most always prepared it by infusion; else it seldom produces its diuretic & depleting effect; so as to moderate fever and relieve the lungs.

D[r] Spence of Dumphries, Virg. in a letter to D[r] Mitchill of N. York, Med Repos. vol.5th [7] has favoured us, with an interesting case of Phthisis, in which the conjoint aid of bloodletting, blistering, cooling, purges, a low diet, chiefly of milk & vegetables, horehound tea, digitalis, and gentle exercise, were instrumental in removing very formidable symptoms, which entirely destroyed the patients hope of recovery. He was bled three times; and the last time, when the disease was considerably advanced, being "attacked with sharp pains in his side, and a severe spitting of blood, he was <u>copiously</u> bled, and expectorated a great deal of blood, during the succeeding night, followed by a vast quantity of corruption, of a most offensive nature."

C122

About this time, the saturated tincture of digitalis was given, beginning with 30 drops, and increased to 110. which, in one week reduced his pulse to

---

[5] Thomas Young, *A Practical and Historical Treatise on Consumptive Diseases, Deduced from Original Observations, and Collected from Authors of All Ages* (London: Underwood, 1815), 67–68.

[6] Young, *A Practical and Historical Treatise on Consumptive Diseases, Deduced from Original Observations, and Collected from Authors of All Ages*, 68.

[7] John Spence, "A Case of Pulmonary Consumption Cured by the Use of Digitalis Purpura: In a Letter from John Spence, M.D. Of Dumfries (Virg.) to Dr. Mitchill and Dated January 26, 1801," *Medical Repository* 5 (1802): 13–17.

45. The patient then observed that "he made a great deal of clear water." As he was costive, opening pills were frequently taken, and he indulged freely in ripe fruits, besides milk & vegetables.

The consequence, of this judicious depleting & antiphlogistic plan, was, that the fever subsided, together with his other complaints. He was then directed to ride out every morning, to avoid all bodily exertions, to continue his vegetable diet, and to take the drops sparingly, which were soon laid aside. Animal food was then taken; and his health was restored.

"Previous to the use of digitalis, says Dr Rand,[8] if there is any pain in the chest, or an hemoptysis; if the pulse is hard & the respiration difficult; and the patient not advanced in life, venesection will be necessary. A blister should be applied to the side, between the shoulders, or over the sternum in the course of the mediastinum; and the bowels gently evacuated. The tincture of digitalis may be given three or four times in a day, beginning with 12 drops and increasing each dose one drop, till the number of pulsations of **C123** the artery is diminished to 50 or 60; and continued at that number, till the disease is removed. I have increased them to an 100, four times in a day. At night, when the cough has prevented sleep, I have generally given one grain of opium."

"The haustus salinus, in the intermediate time, I have experienced beneficial, cooperating with the general intention of the digitalis. All the neutral salts retard the circulations and diminish the irritability of the heart, by their action on the stomach."

"The physician should pay the strictest attention to the state of the pulse; the respiration; the state of the stomach & appetite. Should the digitalis have a very sudden effect in depressing the circulations; and inducing an intermission of the pulse, sickness at the stomach with languor & faintness, we must immediately suspend the use of it, lest sudden death ensue. The physician should see his patient, at least every day, as few persons are so conversant with the state of the pulse & respiration, as to enable them to judge of the propriety of continuing or suspending the medicine."

C124

"Mr R. Crocker, aged 32; a founder & artist in fine brass, constitutionally healthy, but for some years since, has had a difficulty of breathing and dry cough. Many months previous to his confinement in Feb. last, he was obliged

[8] Isaac Rand (1743–1822) of Boston, trained under his father and Dr. James Lloyd; he later practiced obstetrics. Howard A. Kelly and Walter L. Burrage, *American Medical Biographies* (Baltimore: The Norman, Remington Company, 1920), 955–56.

to relinquish his business. On the 29th of the month I first saw him. He was then afflicted with a severe cough, attended with a copious purulent expectoration, difficult respiration, hectic fever, night sweats, inappetency, nausea, and was emaciated to a skeleton. His legs were œdematous; pulse 100 to 110 in a minute. He supposed his case remediless; and only to gratify his friends, consulted a physician. With only the hope of smoothing his pillow in death, I prescribed, after obviating some difficulties of the bowels, I prescribed the tincture of digitalis, as above directed. The third dose of 15 drops relieved his breathing, and reduced his pulse to 75 in a minute. Three days after, the pulse fell to 60, then to 50. I continued to increase the drops; till he had attained to 100, four times a day, when nausea was produced, and an intermittent pulse. I then suspended its use for a day or two; and directed a strong infusion of camomile flowers, which obviated the disagreeable effect of the tincture. He soon returned to the use of the medicine; pulse 55 in the morning and 60 **C125** to 65, in the evening, till his recovery. When the stricture of his breast & difficulty of breathing were removed, to which the perpetual blisters contributed, he began to take the bark in decoction, three times a day, and opium at night. The digitalis rendered his body soluble.

His diet consisted of animal food, oysters, and Madeira wine; a bottle was his daily quantity. His residence being in a dirty alley, and the weather from February to the middle of May, unfriendly to his health, he could not take fresh air till the last of April. The expectoration however, gradually lessened, and assumed a better colour, till the cough and expectoration ceased, which was the beginning of May. He has recovered his flesh and strength; and thinks himself in better health than he had enjoyed for many years. He desisted from the use of medicine the first of May. His pulse is now, June 1, 1804, regular, and at 75 or 80 in a minute."

Observations on Phthisis. Boston. [9]

C126

Case of Phthisis, in Philadelphia.

Eleanor Wells, aged 40, was admitted into the almshouse, on the 15th of Feb. 1800. The history of her case, which she gave was the following. At the commencement of the winter season, she was attacked with pleurisy, for which she was bled twice, and took some medicine, tho not with entire

---

[9] Isaac Rand, *Observations on Phthisis Pulmonalis, and the Use of the Digitalis Purpurea in the Treatment of That Disease: With Practical Remarks on the Use of the Tepid Bath. Read at the Request of the Massachusetts Medical Society, June 6, 1804* (Boston: Printed at the Repertory office, 1804), 12–14.

relief; owning, as she supposed to her being obliged to spend much of her time in a damp cellar; so that she was constantly harassed by a cough & pain in her breast. In this state she remained; till eight weeks previous to her admission, when all the symptoms were greatly increased. When Dr Wilson saw her, she complained of a fixed pain under the sternum, had a bad cough, with copious expectoration of pus like matter; great heat of the palms of the hands and soles of the feet; with profuse night sweats; flushed cheeks in the afternoon, chills & fever. When Dr Church visited her, soon after her admission, he believed that she laboured under genuine phthisis; and ordered her to take a grain of the powdered leaves of digitalis, three times a day, and a blister to be applied to the breast. After the use of these remedies for a few days, she was much relieved. The medicine was, therefore, continued, and the dose gradually increased to two grains, three times a day, beyond which it was not carried, for the sickness induced by it was so distressing as to forbid more. The medicine was continued till the latter end of March, when she no longer complained of pain of the breast. Her cough & night sweats were **C126A** gone, and in short every unfavourable symptom had disappeared, and she only remained debilitated, for which she took a decoction of Peruvian bark; was allowed a little wine and animal food, which completely restored her to health; and she was discharged cured on the 14th of April following.

It must be remarked, that the above mentioned woman lost about twenty ounces of blood at three bleedings, during the taking digitalis, and took occasional laxatives. These powerful remedies, no doubt aided the digitalis in effecting the cure.

This woman said that her parents and several of her relations died of consumption."

Moore on Digitalis.[10]

Much observation has induced me to believe that in every case of Phthisis Pulmonalis, more or less blood ought to be drawn, unless a diarrhœa or some other plentiful evacuations attend the disease; so as sufficiently to reduce morbid action and inflammatory irritation of the blood vessels.

---

[10] John Moore et al., "An Inaugural Dissertation on Digitalis Purpurea, or Fox-Glove: And Its Use in Some Diseases: Submitted to the Examination of the Rev. John Ewing, S.T.P. Provost; the Trustees & Medical Faculty, of the University of Pennsylvania, on the Thirty-First of May 1800, for the Degree of Doctor of Medicine" (MD, University of Pennsylvania, 1800).

Dr John Warren, in his "view of the mercurial practice in febrile diseases," has recorded an extraordinary case **C126B** of Phthisis, in which a profuse diarrhœa seemed to be a substitute for bleeding.

"In 1805, I visited a lady, who, for several weeks, has laboured under a severe cough, with slight pain in her side. On examination, her pulse was found small & irregular, about 100, in a minute, with short & difficult respiration, stricture over the chest, night sweats, extreme debility; and most of the common symptoms of deep pulmonary affection. Expectoration of matter of a purulent appearance; constant diarrhœa, extreme emaciation designated the extreme hazard of this case.

She was from home, when she these complaints first came on, and had taken no medicine till I visited her.

As her countenance was of a yellowish cast, I gave the first day, an emetic of ipecac, and an opiate at night. I then gave the usual expectorant medicines; but, for several days the symptom increased rapidly; and I considered her case as almost desperate.

Her diarrhœa & cough continuing, I ordered a pill of one grain of ipecac and two of calomel to be given every twelve hours. On the third day, after having taken six pills, the mouth, **C127** to my astonishment, became suddenly sore; and, on examination I found her breath strongly affected with a mercurial fœtor. The pills were then discontinued. For several days the salivation continued to increase; the ulceration, in the mouth became extremely troublesome; the breath intolerably offensive; and the gums, tongue & fauces, so much swelled, as to occasion great distress, and almost to threaten suffocation. The most powerful doses of opium procured little rest at night.

From this time, her cough abated; the night sweats were less profuse; her pulse daily became slower; and by the time the salivation had subsided, which was not till at the end of the fourth week; all her symptoms had completely disappeared. She has had no complaint of any kind since, has recovered her strength & flesh; and, at this time, is in perfect health."

Reviewers remarks:

"The introduction of mercury, in the treatment of pulmonary diseases, after allaying inflammatory action, by venesection, and other evacuants, may be deemed **C128** one of the most important innovations, in modern practice. In directing the attention of practitioners to the use of this remedy, in a disease which, upon a moderate computation, must be supposed to augment the whole number of deaths, in the United States, at least, one sixth, Dr Rush deserves the tribute of of gratitude."

"We shall only add, that our own success, in several recent cases, has tended very materially to strengthen our opinion, in favour of mercury, in the treatment of Phthisis, after the removal of the symptoms, which more particularly characterize its inflammatory stage."

New England Journal vol. 4. N. 2.[11]

Origin of mercurial salivation, in Phthisis pulmonalis.

An account of the salutary effects of a salivation, in pulmonary consumption, in two letters, from Dr Rush, to Dr E. Miller.[12]   Med. Repos. vol 5th.[13]

"Dear Sir. On the 17th of Dec. 1800, William Kains, a sailor, aged 26, was admitted into the Pennsylvania Hospital, in the second stage of pulmonary consumption. Several of this man's relations had died of this disease. As his pulse was active, I ordered eight ounces of blood to be **C129** drawn; and the same quantity to be taken five days after. I directed him to live chiefly upon milk & vegetables, and to take a medicine known in our Hospital, by the name of "antimonial powder," composed of 15 grains of nitre, one sixth of a grain of tart. antim, and half a grain of calomel, three times a day. Contrary to my ~~expectations~~ intentions, 16 doses of this powder brought on a salivation. The effects of which were as unexpected, as they were agreeable. It suddenly put a stop to his cough, and removed every other symptom of his pulmonary disease. The salivation continued, without any additional doses, for ten days. I looked, with a good deal of apprehension, for a return of his consumptive symptoms, after the spitting had ceased; but happily, without finding them.

---

[11] "A View of Mercurial Practice in Febrile Diseases. By John Warren, M.D, President of the Massachusetts Medical Society and Professor of Anatomy and Surgery in the University of Cambridge. Boston, T.B. Wait & Co. 8vo. Pp195, 1813," *New England Journal of Medicine and Surgery* 4 (1815): 175–81.

[12] Edward Miller (1760–1812) was born in Dover, Delaware. His preceptorship was followed by an M.D. from the University of Pennsylvania, and he remained friendly and generally agreed with his mentor, Benjamin Rush. Miller practiced in Maryland and Delaware before moving in 1796 to New York City, where, with Samuel Mitchill and Elihu Hubbard Smith, he edited the *Medical Repository* for many years. Horrocks, Thomas A. "Miller, Edward (1760-1812), physician and teacher." American National Biography. 1 Feb. 2000; Accessed 20 Apr. 2020. https://www-anb-org.ezproxy.library.tufts.edu/view/10.1093/anb/9780198606697.001.0001/anb-9780198606697-e-1200618.

[13] Benjamin Rush, "An Account of the Salutary Effects of a Salivation, and Tonic Remedies, in Pulmonary Consumption: In Three Letters to Dr. Edward Miller, by Benjamin Rush, M.D., Professor of the Institutes of Medicine and of Clinical Practice in the University of Pennsylvania," *Medical Repository* 5 (1802): 5–10.

In a week after, his mouth & throat recovered from the mercurial disease, and he was discharged as cured, on the 10th of Jan. 1801."

On the 17th of Jan. 1801, William Poole, aged 23, was admitted into the Hospital, in the third or apparently last stage of the disease, which has been mentioned. His cough was distressing, especially in the nights. He was much emaciated and had frequent chills, with constant sweats. His pulse forbad bleeding. Incouraged by the accidental cure first related, I prescribed for him the antimonial powder, and ordered mercurial ointment to his sides & breast, in order **C130** to excite a salivation. In a few days, I was highly gratified; by hearing him complain of swelled gums, and great pain in his teeth. From this time, his cough, fever, chills & sweats left him.

To obviate the weakness & want of appetite, induced by his disease, I ordered an infusion of columbo root with elix. vitriol; and to drink wine & porter with his food; from which he found great benefit. The salivary glands were not affected by the mercury, in this patient, an effect, experience has taught me, not essential, in all cases, to its salutary operation in abstracting disease from internal & vital parts of the body. He was discharged cured, on the 2^d of May last."

"It was not in the winter of 1801, that I first combated pulmonary consumption with mercury. Many years ago, I had frequently attempted to cure it, by a salivation; but without being able to excite it. The failure was probably owing to the mercury being given before the morbid action of the blood vessels was reduced by bloodletting, and low diet, or 2dly after the suppurative ~~action~~ action in the lungs, was so far advanced as to prevent the action of the mercury predominating over it. Perhaps a third cause of failure may be derived from the mercury being given after all the excitability of the system, on which medicines **C131** act, had been wholly expended, or 4^ly from its not being given with some other medicine, calculated by its previous or accompanying stimulus, to prepare the system for its impression, on the mouth or salivary glands; or, lastly, from its not being given in a form, as in the antimoniac powder, in which it is diffused through the mouth; in the act of swallowing it."

"I have said nothing of the state of the lungs, in the above patients; previously to the healthy change induced by the salivation. It is probable they were affected with tubercles or ulcers; both of which I believe have been cured by other remedies, besides mercury. But if those consequences of pulmonary consumption did not exist, such a preternatural secretion, and excretion of morbid matter had taken place, in the lungs, as would have produced death as certainly as tubercles or ulcers, when not opposed by medicine."

"There is no more reason why a salivation should not be prescribed as generally, in diseases of all the internal & vital organs, than that bloodletting should not be used, in diseases of great morbid action, in every part of the body."

"I have only to add, to my letter, that a patient should not be considered as safe or free from danger, after the removal of the cough, fever, **C132** and other symptoms of consumption by means of a salivation. The general weakness which predisposes to it should be obviated by Journeys, sea voyages, a long course of tonics, and a total abstraction of all its remote & exciting causes.

From, dear Sir, your sincere friend,

Philadelphia, March 18th 1801.   Benjamin Rush.

Letter 2.[d]

Dear Sir,

Soon after writing the above letter, an event occurred which made it necessary for me to delay sending it. William Kains, whose case I have related, in his passage down the Delaware, in February, caught a severe cold, from being detained several weeks by the ice. He was sent back to our Hospital, on the 2[d] of March, where he died on the 29th of April following. D[r] Parke,[14] who succeeded me in attending the Hospital, politely attempted to relieve him, at my request by a salivation; but without success. If the death of this man should lead physicians to be more careful in enjoying their patients, after the cure of a pulmonary affection, to obviate the return **C133** of it, by avoiding all the remote & exciting causes of a relapse; and to use such remedies as are best calculated to remove the remaining debility of the system, it will not have occurred in vain. I have lately seen <u>Poole</u>, and was delighted to find him in good health, and fine spirits. He has gained not only flesh, but fat.

Within the course of the present month, I have arrested this formidable disease, by gently touching the mouth with calomel, in two young ladies in

---

[14] Thomas Parke (1749–1835) was a graduate of University of Pennsylvania and on the medical staff of Philadelphia Hospital from 1774 to 1779. Charles Lawrence, *History of the Philadelphia Almshouses and Hospitals from the Beginning of the Eighteenth to the Ending of the Nineteenth Centuries . . . : Showing the Mode of Distributing Public Relief through the Management of the Boards of Overseers of the Poor, Gaurdians of the Poor and the Directors of the Department of Charities and Correction* (Philadelphia: Charles Laurence, Superintendent, 1905), 393. Between 1792 and 1817, perhaps longer, Parke was on the medical staff of Pennsylvania Hospital. He was also a director of the Library Company of Philadelphia from 1778–1835. Thomas G. Morton, Frank Woodbury, and Pennsylvania Hospital, *The History of the Pennsylvania Hospital, 1751–1895* (Philadelphia: Times Printing House, 1895), 84, 442.

our city, who were affected with alarming catarrhs, which had supervened previous debility of a long standing. They are both now riding in the country, by my advice, in order to remove the debility from their systems, which was the forerunner of their disease.

Dr Stewart, an intelligent young physician of this city, has lately put into my hands, the history of a case of a Mrs Cornvil, a woman, aged 25 years, whom he had cured in the spring of 1799, of a confirmed **C134** pulmonary consumption, by means of a salivation of five weeks continuance. The salivation, he remarks, was sometimes interrupted by a diarrhœa, and by great morbid excitement in the blood vessels; but was always restored by checking the former, by means of laudanum, and reducing the latter, by means of bloodletting. The Doctor concludes his letter, which is dated May 12th, of the present year, by saying, "Mrs Cornvil is now free of all pulmonary complaints, and has, since her cure, become the mother of a healthy child." Dr Physick informs me, he has salivated two patients in consumptions, with success, and has hopes of curing a third, now under his care, by the same remedy. Thus, have we made one more impression on a most formidable & distressing disease. Let us not dispair; and when we speak of an incurable disease, let us always remember, that we only express the imperfection of our knowledge in medicine.

From, dear Sir, your friend,

Philadelphia May 20th, 1801.   Benjamin Rush."

Chap. 6ᵗʰ

I SHALL NOW proceed to relate a number of the most extraordinary cases of pulmonary affections, which have occasionally occurred, in the course of my practice, in Maine; and in that of some others, bearing a near resemblance to Phthisis pulmonalis; and some, perhaps, may come under this denomination.

These cases will serve to show the great varieties of the disease, and diversity of causes, which it is hoped, will tend to throw some further light on the nature and treatment of pulmonary diseases.

Case I.

The middle of March 1788, the Rev. Peter T. Smith[1] of Windham, aged 55, of a spare habit, who had been troubled with erisipelatous eruptions on his legs, complained, at this time, after their subsidence, of some oppression at the breast, pain in the left side, febrile disturbance, cough & difficult breathing. I was then called and finding his pulse frequent & hard, I drew a pint of blood which was buffy. His complaints were then moderated. A cathartic of Glaubers salts was given. Two days after his complaints increased with expectoration of mucus tinged with blood. A like quantity of blood was drawn, another cathartic given and a blister applied to his side. The fever continued 14 days, when it subsided, together with the pain and difficulty of breathing.
During the fever, gums & balsams, impregnated with argent viv. were given, as expectorants.

When the fever had subsided, he complained of an oppressive load, in the inferior part of the chest. An emetic & cathartic were then given, but no relief was afforded. Pectorals & tonics were used, without any beneficial effect. His cough & expectoration continued, with slight febrile paroxysms; pulse quick

---

[1] Rev. Peter T. Smith of Windham (1731–1826), son of Rev. Thomas Smith, graduated from Harvard College in 1753, taught school briefly, and in 1755 moved to Windham and settled in the ministry. William Willis, *Journals of the Rev. Thomas Smith and the Rev. Samuel Deane . . . With Notes and Biographical Notices and a Summary History of Portland* (Portland: Joseph S. Bailey, 1849), 370, 376.

& weak. In the latter part of April, his feet & legs swelled, and night sweats took place, with inability to sit up, only a few hours in the day.

The beginning of May, Drs Coffin & Louther were called in consultation, who readily concurred with me, in an opinion, that there was little or no hope of a recovery; and this opinion was not concealed from the patient, who with Christian fortitude, calmly resigned himself to the will of Providence; and means were chiefly laid aside. He continued to decline till the middle of June, attended with expectoration of purulent matter, hectic flushes & night sweats. His body was now greatly emaciated, tho the swelling of his feet & legs had increased. An infusion **C137** of digitalis was given, which operated as a diuretic. The swelling then abated and friction was used.

On the 20th of June, he complained of pain in the left side, just above the midriff, to which an adhesive plaister was applied. A small, red tumor then arose, which I opened with a lancet, when about two quarts of matter were discharged, resembling cream, and free from fœtor. He laid on the left side, during the night, and the matter continued to flow, in considerable quantity, as appeared by his bedding.

The weight in his chest was then removed, and the febrile disturbance ceased; as also the cough, expectoration & sweats.

A sponge tent was introduced to enlarge the orifice, from which matter was freely discharged, several times in a day, on removing the tent, and this discharge did not wholly cease, till the expiration of three months.

In the mean time, his flesh & strength were gradually regained, and he was restored to health, which he still enjoyed free from any complaint, excepting old age. He died, Oct. 1826, aged 96. **C138** Had twice the quantity of blood been drawn in the disease, and mercury been used, so as to produce a salivation, it is probable this Empiema might have been prevented. But the time of such an improvement, in the treatment of pulmonary affections, had not arrived!

Case II.

In May 1795, Joseph Noyes Esq. of Falmouth[2], aged 50, of a corpulent habit, who had been troubled with a dull pain in his left side, on any unusual exertion, complained of an increase of the pain in his side, after considerable fatigue, in surveying low wet land, with a cough, oppression at the breast,

---

[2] Joseph Noyes (1745–1795) served as Falmouth town treasurer and selectman before and during the Revolutionary War. In 1776 he was sent to Boston with Jedidiah Preble, Samuel Freeman, and John Waite to serve in the Massachusetts House of Representatives. William Willis, *The History of Portland*, facsimile ed. (Somersworth: New Hampshire Publishing Company and Maine Historical Society, 1972; Portland: Bailely & Noyes, 1865), 541, 827, 861–62.

and febrile disturbance. The idea of his having taken a cold, suggested to the mind of his nurse, the use of warm teas. The fever & pain increased, and his cough was tedious, tho he attended public worship under the exercise of these feelings, and his face appeared very florid.

He was attended by Dr Coffin & myself.

On the 3^d day from his attack, when medical aid was first called, a pint of blood was drawn, which was buffy; his bowels were evacuated, and cooling means were directed, a blister was applied to his side, and common expectorants were given. Some ease was afforded; but on the 4 day, the pain & fever increased, and his breathing was difficult. Another pint of blood was drawn, which was equally buffy, very little ease was afforded. His pulse was full, **C139** slow, and intermitting, cough dry & hard, with little expectoration; and he complained of heat; as well as distressing pain in his side, tho he could walk the room, and converse as usual. On the 5th day, 12 ounces of blood were drawn; but no ease was afforded. He died on the 14th day, setting in his chair; for he could not lie down in bed.

The next day, we opened his body; and found that the left lobe of his lungs was partially suppurated, and adhered to the pleura. No other morbid affection was discovered.

In 1794, Mr James Folsome of Gilmanton, N.H. aged 25, of a florid countenance, put himself under my tuition, in the study of physic.

In May 1795, while undergoing some fatigue by running after a horse, he was attacked with hemoptysis, in a slight degree. In May 1796, after some fatigue in walking fast, he was attacked in like manner. The following August, he pursued the practice of physic in Durham, where he was exposed to the air of a fresh river, when some cough & febrile disturbance took place. The latter part of the month, he was attacked with hemoptysis, and discharged about two gills of blood when opium & spirits, were taken. The beginning of September, he rode to my house, distant 30 miles, ~~when he was~~ being troubled with cough & expectoration of mucus.

C140

At midnight, he complained of heat in the vitals, & febrile disturbance, preceeded by chilliness. About a gill of blood was then discharged in a fit of coughing. A drop of laudanum in brandy was taken and he rested quietly. The next day at 12 o'clock, he was attacked with cough and discharged another gill of blood from his lungs. Another dose of laudanum was taken. In two hours, the cough & bleeding recurred as usual. The following day at 12 o'clock he discharged another gill. A cathartic was then taken, and the bleeding ceased.

He then proceeded on his Journey to Gilmanton, 80 miles on horseback, and his health appeared to be restored. In Autumn, he returned, and took up his residence in Windham, where he practiced physic, till the next spring, when the usual train of hectical symptoms took place. He then returned to N.H. where he declined, &, in Autumn, expired.

This bright & promising young man had been reading the Medical Elements of Dʳ John Brown; and, like many others, both in Europe & America, was "too much influenced by his imaginary theories," myself not excepted. **C141**

In Feb. 1804, Hon. William Gorham³ of Gorham, aged 61, of an inflammatory habit, and who had been troubled with rheumatic pains in his limbs for some a considerable time, complained of some cough with expectoration of mucus. Issues, which had been on his legs, now discharged blood instead of pus.

On the 20ᵗʰ of March, he rode to Portland, in a sleigh, which, on entering the town, upset, and his clothes were wet. He rode home in the evening when the weather was disagreeable. In the night he was attacked with a chilly fit, followed with fever; yet he went out the next day, and attended public business.

On the 23ᵈ he complained of oppression at the breast and his cough was tedious. An emetic & cathartic were given, and a blister was applied to his chest. On the 26ᵗʰ I was called in consultation, when his pulse was frequent & full, cough troublesome, saline cathartics & demulcents were given. He continued in this way till 5' of April, when profuse sweats took place.

On the 8ᵗʰ he expectorated some blood. His physician was then called who drew half a pint. The next morning he discharged about a gill by cough. I was then called with his physician, when his pulse was quick & full, skin hot & dry, cough & expectoration considerable. Laud. & vin. antim. were given. **C142** At 5 o'clock P.M. he discharged about a gill of blood. The next day, he left his bed, in search of papers to transact some business, when he threw up about half a pint of clear blood.

At this time, three physicians were consulted. One, viz. Dʳ Harding, advised to let blood, as his pulse was full & active. But we could not agree to the

³ William Gorham (1743–1804) studied law with his father, who was Register of Probate for the county of Barnstable, Massachusetts. He arrived in Gorham in the District of Maine in 1760 at age eighteen and became Judge of Probate in 1782 and then Judge of the Court of Common Pleas from 1787 to 1804. Judge Gorham was a delegate to the Portland convention that considered separation from Massachusetts. He died in Gorham on July 22, 1804, survived by his second wife, who later became the fifth wife of Dr. Jeremiah Barker. Hugh D. McLellan, *History of Gorham, Maine* (Portland: Smith and Sale, 1903), 520–23.

measure, lest it should weaken him! He continued to raise a little blood once in two or three days, for some time, when it ceased. Laud. & restoratives, were the chief means used. After this, he so far recovered as to ride out, and transact public business. —— Hectic fever, however, supervened; and he gradually declined till 25th of July when he expired, greatly lamented by his friends, tho reconciled to the will of God.

In the winter of 1805, the Rev. J. Noyes[4] of Gorham, aged 25, a zealous preacher of the Gospel, and laboriously engaged in parochial duties which exposed him to much fatigue, was occasionally attacked with spitting of blood, and some cough; for which he used no means, save smoking segars! My advice was then asked concerning their use, which I reprobated, as tending to induce consumption, **C143** and his pulse was then considerably accelerated. As the spring advanced, his complaints rather increased, and he expectorated mucus & yellow matter, tho he continued his labours, as usual. In the summer, his face & hands were sometimes observed to be very pale, at other times, they glowed with redness.

In Autumn, he undertook a journey of 100 miles, on horseback; during which he often raised blood from his lungs; and he grew worse in other respects. He returned in a chaise; but was never able to preach again; for the usual train of hectical symptoms supervened; and he declined in a rapid manner till March, when he died, tho he rode out in a sleigh the day before his death.

The chief means used on his journey was elix. vitriol, as he informed me on his return; and few means were employed, in his declining state, excepting palliatives. —— He was greatly lamented, by all who knew his fidelity & usefulness.

C144

Case of recovery from apparent Consumption, communicated to D[r] Adams, Editor of the Medical Register, by Eliphalet Lyman MB. of Fryburg, Maine, dated Nov. 1806.[5]

---

[4] Jeremiah Noyes (1778–1807) was born in Newburyport, Massachusetts, on April 7, 1778; graduated from Dartmouth College in 1799; and was ordained at the Congregational church in Gorham on November 16, 1803. He died January 15, 1807. McLellan, *History of Gorham, Maine*, 192; Charles Franklin Emerson, *General Catalogue of Dartmouth College and the Associated Schools 1769–1910, Including a Historical Sketch of the College* (Hanover, NH: Printed for the college, 1911), 208. Barker states that Rev. Noyes died in March.

[5] Lyman, Eliphalet. "Case of Recovery from Apparent Consumption." [In English]. *The Medical and Agricultural Register, For the Years 1806 and 1807*; 1, no. 13 (1807), 196–97. Lyman (1781–1858), who graduated from Dartmouth College in 1803 and received an M.D. in 1814, was a physician and farmer who practiced in Connecticut and Massachusetts. He died in 1858 at seventy-seven years of age. *Dartmouth College and Associated Schools General Catalogue*

"T. H. aged 15 years, of a slender habit, after riding a journey in the rain, in July last, was attacked with a violent cough & difficulty of breathing, pain in his right side & fever. In this situation he remained for a number of weeks, before medical aid was called. After a thorough examination, I was fully persuaded that the disease termed <u>Phthisis Pulmonalis</u>, was seated on him; and had made such ravages on his lungs, that he must soon fail. The symptoms grew more & more aggravated, for a number of weeks, expectoration was very copious, debility very great, hectic fever quite regular, together with diarrhœa, swelled legs & feet, and sunken eyes. In short, the last symptoms of that terrible disease were notorious to all who saw him; and death was hourly expected to close the scene.

But remarkable as it may be, his cough ceased, almost instantly, respiration became less laborious; and the emaciated youth began to mend; and, by slow degrees, he gained an **C145** entire & perfect state of health, even better than he ever enjoyed.

No symptoms were wanting in this case, that usually appear, in <u>Phthisis</u>; no symptoms uncommon, excepting the fixity of pain in his right side. The remedies applied were those commonly used in such cases.

Until within a short time previous to his convalescence, he was obliged to lie wholly on his right side. This induced us to believe that there was an adhesion of that part of the lungs, on the right side of the mediastinum, to the plura. —— Immediately before the cessation of his cough, he expectorated very large quantities of matter, resembling the substance of the lungs, mixed with pus. The pain in his side then ceased, sometime previously to this copious discharge.

Quere, may this be properly termed a case of <u>Phthisis Pulmonalis</u>. If so, must we not conclude that a portion of the lungs was wholly destroyed; and that the remainder are left entire? ——Was the whole of the right lobe destroyed, or in part?"   Eliphalet Lyman.

1769–1940 (Hanover, NH: Dartmouth College Publications, 1940), 837. Dr. Daniel Adams (1776–1830), an apothecary, was also a Dartmouth graduate of 1797, A.B. in 1799, and M.D. in 1822. He practiced in several New England states and was living in Boston circa 1806 while editing *The Medical and Agricultural Register*. There were two Daniel Adams, M.D., in Keene, New Hampshire, apparently not related to each other. Emerson, *General Catalogue of Dartmouth College and the Associated Schools 1769–1910*, 837; Simon Goodell Griffin, Octavius Applegate, and Frank H. Whitcomb, *A History of the Town of Keene from 1732, When the Township Was Granted by Massachusetts, to 1874, When It Became a City* (Keene, NH: Sentinel Print. Co., 1904), 555, 557.

C146 "

The usual weight of the lungs, in health, says Portal,[6] of Paris, is from one pound to a pound & a half. In Consumption, they sometimes weigh 5 or 6 pounds. Sometimes they are much reduced in bulk; and leave a "vacant space," in the chest."

"Mudge, says Dr Rand, in his treatice on the Catarrh, relates the case of a man, who laboured under Phthisis pulmonalis, who expectorated such quantities of pus, with fever, night sweats, and every concomitant of this disease, that death seemed inevitable, as the disease eluded every method of cure. After some time, however, to his surprise, the expectoration lessened, the cough subsided, his appetite & digestion increased, he acquired flesh, and was restored to his usual health. He died some time after, of an acute disease, the small pox. Upon inspecting, his thorax, he discovered that the phthisis pulmonalis was cured by the absorption of the whole right lobe of the lungs. One side of his chest was deficient of its lobe; and that part of the trachea, to which the lobe appended was closed up. In this case, we discover the curative process was ****C147**** conducted and finally accomplished by the absorbents removing the diseased part. The digitalis, had it been employed, might have contributed to their curative exertions."[7]

In the Medical communications, to the M.M.S. N°.2. part 2. p. 52.[8] a dissection is described, where it appears that the right lobe of the lungs was entirely obliterated, in Phthisis, yet the patient recovered, and enjoyed health, for six years, when he died of the stone.

If the lungs, in consumption, have been found to weigh several pounds more than in health, their vessels must have been greatly distended, and overcharged with a proportional increased quantity of blood. Hence we may account for the oppression, stricture & load, so often complained of, in the vitals, when labouring under this disease; as well as pain in the chest, febrile disturbance, difficulty of breathing, &c, while the pulse is small & often weak;

---

[6] Antoine Portal (1742–1832) was a French anatomist, physician, and medical historian. Antoine Portal, Gaspare Federigo, and Georg Friedrich Mühry, *Observations Sur La Nature et Le Traitement De La Phthisie Pulmonaire*, *Ed. rev. et augm. par l'auteur, avec des observations et des remarques par Murhy sic . . . qui a traduit cet ouvrage en allemand, et avec celles de Gaspard Fédérigo . . . qui l'a traduit en italien*, 2 vols. (Paris: Collin, 1809).

[7] Isaac Rand, *Observations on Phthisis Pulmonalis, and the Use of the Digitalis Purpurea in the Treatment of That Disease: With Practical Remarks on the Use of the Tepid Bath. Read at the Request of the Massachusetts Medical Society, June 6, 1804* (Boston: Printed at the Repertory office, 1804), 8.

[8] Josiah Bartlett, "Article IX a Case of Calculus of the Bladder," *Medical Communications and Dissertations of the Massachusetts Medical Society* 1 (1813): 52–55.

so that recourse has frequently been had to stimulants & heating medicines, which increase the accumulated mass in the lungs, and velocity of the blood.

This fluid sometimes pervades the extreme terminations of the arteries, at their junction with the veins, or passes through by rupture; producing hemoptysis, or spitting of blood, so that the vessels are **C148** unloaded and relief is afforded, which is often salutary, tho this mode of depletion is attended with great hazard, as appears in some cases that have been related, and not unusually lays the foundation for pulmonary consumption, when proper means are neglected; or those which are improper are used.

Furthermore; if one lobe of the lungs, in this disease, can be absorbed, in a state of purulency, into the circulating mass, with impunity & advantage, most certainly, the opinion, which has been advanced by some writers, that "the absorption of matter from ulcerated lungs, and admixture with the circulating fluids, creates hectic fever," must be exploded. Of course, the fever must be accounted for in some other way. We shall, in the sequel, attempt to describe the proximate or immediate cause of hectic fever, independently on organic lesion, ulceration or absorption of purulent matter; which will serve to explain the nature of this insidious disease, and its ravages on the blood vessels of the whole system, noticed by increased arterial action, pain in the chest & diffusive heat from the lungs to the extremities, with redness at the face &c, and by examining the inflamed state of the arteries & veins, after death. **C149**

Salutary effects of profuse hemorrhages, from the lungs, in pulmonic affections.

In April 1785, Mr John Cash, of Raimond Maine, aged 30, of a slender make, after exposure to cold & dampness, was seized with chilliness, to which succeeded febrile heat, oppression at the breast, cough and pain in the side. I was sent for on the 3^d^ day; but could not attend till the 4th, when I found him free from fever pain & cough, able to walk the room. —— A few hours before my arrival, as I was informed, blood was forcibly & freely discharged from his wind pipe in a violent fit of coughing. About a quart was supposed to be thrown up, in the course of half an hour. He soon recovered, without any purulent expectoration, or the use of means. Since this event, he has been accostomed to hard labour, and is now in the enjoyment of health. viz. 1829.[9]

---

[9] "viz. 1829" appears to have been written in at a later date with a tremulous hand and a different pen.

New York Dec. 28th 1809.

"I George Hunter of this City; front street, N° 150, do certify & declare, upon every thing that is sacred; and hundreds can testify to the **C150** same, that for several years past, I have been afflicted with an affection of the lungs, and, through the colder seasons of every year, have been exercised with a severe and almost incessent [*sic*] cough, with a discharge of large quantities of phlegm and mucus, alternately thrown off. But in the hot season of every year, my cough has been somewhat abated, till the last past, which continued till the month of August, with unabating severity. At length, I bled profusely from the lungs; and continued so to do, for four days, with intervals of abatement, until my life was dispaired of, by two eminent physicians of this City.

I was then induced to try Dr Roger's vegetable pulmonic detergent;[10] a few doses of which checked the bleeding; and a few cakes of it restored me to the enjoyment of a very good degree of bodily health, which continues to this day." —— In this case, the cure was ascribed to a little resin & elecampane, verifying an old proverb, "None are so blind, as those who <u>will not</u> see." **C151**

In Jan. 1801, Mrs Ann Conner of Falmouth, aged 68, who had been afflicted with the dry or spasmodic asthma, many years; and which was of frequent occurrence, especially on exposure to easterly winds, was attacked with a violent paroxysm of this disease, attended with tightness across the chest, wheezing and cough, when blood was profusely discharged from her lungs. I was then called in haste; and found her so exhausted, that the pulse could scarcely be felt; and death appeared to be depictured in her countenance, tho her breathing was easy.

Wine & spiceries were given, and she gradually recovered to her pristine state of health, which, in other respects, appeared to be good. From this time, she was free from asthma, the remainder of her days, and enjoyed comfortable health. She died in 1817.

No one will suppose that the cordials, which were taken, were the curative means in this case. **C152**

A young woman in Falmouth, after exposure to cold & dampness, in husking of corn, was attacked with chilliness, to which succeeded febrile

---

[10] The 1816 issue of *Beers' Almanac* includes an advertisement for Dr Roger's Vegetable Pulmonic Detergent, an example of an early nineteenth-century proprietary medicine "for Coughs, Consumptions, & Asthmas." Dr. Rogers used testimonials to inform readers of his "twenty years experience." Thomas A. Horrocks, *Popular Print and Popular Medicine: Almanacs and Health Advice in Early America* (Amherst: University of Massachusetts Press, 2008), 99.

heat, oppression in the vitals, and a spitting of blood. The usual train of hectical symptoms ensued. In about a month I was called, and prescribed such medicines as were commonly used; but she continued to decline, about a month longer, when she met with a fright, and a copious discharge of blood took place from her lungs. The hectic fever was then removed with her other complaints, when tonic means were used, and she recovered.

"I have seen two cases of inflammatory consumption, says Dr Rush, attended by an hemorrhage of a quart of blood from the lungs. They both recovered. I ascribed their recovery wholly, to the inflammatory action of their systems, being suddenly reduced by a spontaneous discharge of blood. These facts, I hope, will serve to establish the usefulness of bloodletting, in the inflammatory state of consumption, with those physicians who are yet disposed **C153** to trust more to the fortuitous operations of nature, than to the decisions of reason and experience."

"I have always found this remedy to be more necessary in the winter and first spring months, than at any other time. We obtain by means of repeated bleedings, such a mitigation of all the symptoms, as enables the patient to use exercise with advantage, as soon as the weather becomes so dry and settled, as to admit of his going about every day."

"As an ignorance of the quantity of blood, which has been drawn by design, or lost by accident, has contributed to encourage prejudices against bloodletting; so an ignorance of the rapid manner in which blood is regained or regenerated, when lost or drawn, has helped to keep up prejudices against the lancet."   Med. Obser. vol. 2 & 4.[11]

C154

An account of the good effects of copious bloodletting, in the cure of an Hemorrhage from the lungs; in a letter from the Rev. Dr Samuel S. Smith, President of the College of New Jersey, to D^r. B. Rush.

Princeton March 19th, 1798.

Dear Sir,

As the science of medicine is established on an induction of facts, well attested histories of the successful treatment of diseases must be singularly useful. It is with a view to add one case more to your useful collection, that I have been induced to give you an account of an uncommon hemorrhage with which I have been afflicted myself; and of my perfect recovery.

---

[11] Benjamin Rush, *Medical Inquiries and Observations*, 2nd ed., 4 vols. (Philadelphia: J. Conrad & Co., 1805).

A certain weakness of breast, and tendency to hemorrhage, was hereditary on my mother's side of the family, whom I was supposed to resemble in constitution & countenance. Shortly after I was licensed to preach, I was thrown into a situation which required unusual exertions. I had often to address very large assemblies, at least three times in the week, and frequently every day. In consequence of these efforts, at the end of about **C155** three years, I began to raise small quantities of blood, at the close of each discourse. This symptom continued to increase; and during nearly four years more, though I moderated my exertions, and made them much less frequent, I raised some blood at the end of almost every sermon that I delivered; and sometimes in considerable quantities. The spitting often continued in a less or greater degree, for several days afterwards.

I was at length obliged to intermit preaching entirely for the space of eight months, during which time, I spent part of a season at the Sweet Springs in Virginia; and recovered a tolerable though a delicate state of health. At this period, I was removed to Princeton, where speaking to small assemblies, and in a Chapel happily accomodated to favour the voice, I continued to preach, and to attend my other duties in the college, during two years, with increasing health & vigour.

In the autumn of 1782, I suddenly broke **C156** a blood vessel in my breast, as I was walking. A considerable quantity of blood issued from the wound; but by bleeding copiously at my arm, the flux from my breast, at that time was stopped. Nearly about the same time, the next evening, I felt my pulse quicken, and an unusual tension growing on all my nerves, and, in a few seconds, the blood began to spout with great velocity through my mouth & nose. I was again bled largely twice in the course of the evening, from my arm & foot.

The following evening a similar paroxysm returned; and the blood again spouted with great force from my mouth. The physician was sitting on my bed side at the time; and when I perceived the quickening of my pulse, and that strange stricture coming, as it seemed to my feeling, on the whole system of the nerves, I gave him notice of it, and requested him to bleed me. He refused, and said so much bleeding would only tend to bring on an habitual hemorrhage by debility. I told him I ~~had~~ would rather die bleeding from the arm **C157** than from the mouth. At last, when he saw the force with which the blood issued, and, in consequence of my earnest solicitations, he bled me again. —— I requested him to leave me his lancet, and I would be answerable for my own life. This he reluctantly consented to do. At this time two other physicians were called in, who bled me twice more the same evening, before they could effectually stop the flux from my mouth. Next day, I expectorated nearly a pint of clotted blood that had been lodged somewhere in the cavities of the lungs.

Being now in possession of a lancet, and apprised, by experience, of the symptoms that preceded the return of my disorder, I determined to anticipate it; and, when the physicians were not present, to open my own veins. This I did accordingly, whenever I perceived the symptoms I have already mentioned, which now recurred more frequently for four or five days. After that period they subsided. But I continued bleeding at the arm, two, three and four times in the day, till the tenth day. My intention was to take off the impulse **C158** of the blood from the wounded part, to prevent inflammation, and to give it time to heal. I may, perhaps, have bled myself oftener than was necessary. After pursuing this course, however, the flux of blood no more discoursed itself from my breast. Two & thirty times I was bled, in the space of ten days, in my arms & feet, besides what flowed from my mouth. And it was computed, from the dimensions of the vessels in which it was received, and other circumstances, that I lost, in that time, at least two gallons of blood. Even in this reduced state, so great was my apprehension of the hemorrhage in my breast returning, I continued to bleed at the arm, twice in the week for some time, afterwards once in the week, and finally, once in a month, during several months, though not in large quantities at each time.

After the hemorrhage was entirely stopped, my flesh wasted away for want of its proper nourishment in the blood, till not a muscle could be perceived on any of my limbs. The **C159** skin appeared to be drawn almost close to the skeleton. I spoke only in a whisper. And I was not sensible of having forgotten myself for a moment in sleep during six weeks. My complexion was tinged with a yellowish hue, and an acid so prevailed in my constitution, that, with my tongue, I have frequently curdled a small bowl of milk. For more than three months I could not use bread, nor any vegetable substance in my diet. I lived chiefly on beef liquor, soups, and white meats. I drank a little weak wine & water frequently; but after many trials, I found porter as a drink agree best with my stomach; and at the end of some months, I used it freely & constantly. As soon as I could bear the motion of a carriage, I took gentle exercise in that way. Afterwards, when I could sit on a horse alone, I was helped into the saddle, and every day rode a small distance, increasing it gradually, till I rode from twelve to fifteen miles in a day. Here my recovery was at a stand for some months, when I resolved to try the effect **C160** of a long journey on horseback. I rode first into Connecticut, and afterwards to Boston, in which journeys, I laid the foundation of that good health, which I have now enjoyed for more than ten years, and my voice, particularly, is clearer & stronger than it ever was. ——A habit that required frequent aperient medicines, was greatly increased by the loss of blood; and for more than seven years, I was obliged to have recourse to them. It is now upwards of three years since I have used them at all. A pint of beer or of cyder, at any time, sufficiently answers the purpose.

I believe it would be dangerous for an indolent and inactive person to be reduced so low by bleeding as I have been, or one who had not equal resolution to make the exertions necessary to recover him from that state. Activity in duty, and firmness of mind are often among the best medicines.

I am, Dear Sir, with the greatest
respect, your obedient humble servant.
Samuel S. Smith.[12]
Medical Museum. vol. 2.[13]

C161

Many other cases of spontaneous haemorrhages, will be related, in the sequel, which have been considered as the Providential operations of nature, and afforded instruction. Also of the beneficial effects repeated & copious bloodletting, which by diminishing the quantity of fluid, diminishes the diameter of the vessels, and disposes to <u>adhesive</u> instead of suppurative inflammation, and thereby give the ruptured vessels an oppertunity to heal and become sound. Likewise where profuse effusion of blood, prevented its ever recurring, by removing plethora, phlogistic diathesis, and actual inflammation.

---

[12] Samuel Stanhope Smith (1751–1819) graduated from the College of New Jersey in 1769 (established in 1746; renamed Princeton University at its sesquicentennial celebration in 1896). He developed consumption circa 1773, married Ann Witherspoon, daughter of the president of the college in 1775, and became professor of moral philosophy in 1779. After the death of President Witherspoon in 1794, Smith became college president in 1795. Though some trustees were concerned about Smith's emphasis on scientific instruction, he continued in that position until he resigned in 1812. Lach, Edward L. "Smith, Samuel Stanhope (1751–1819), clergyman and college president." *American National Biography*. 1 Feb. 2000; Accessed 20 Apr. 2020. https://www-anb-org.ezproxy.library.tufts.edu/view/10.1093/anb/9780198606697.001.0001/anb-9780198606697-e-0900704. Edward L. Lach, "Smith, Samuel Stanhope (1751–1819), Clergyman and College President," in *American National Biography* (New York: Oxford University Press, 2000).

[13] Samuel S. Smith, "An Account of the Good Effects of Copious Blood-Letting in the Cure of an Hemorrhage from the Lungs; in a Letter from the Rev. Dr. Samuel S. Smith, Prefident of the College of New Jersey, to Dr. Benjamin Rush," *The Philadelphia Medical Museum, Conducted by John Redman Coxe, M.D. (1805–1810)*, February 1, 1806, 1–6.

C162

In March 1811, Mr S. Lobdel, a merchant in Falmouth, aged 25, was seized with the usual symptoms of a common cold, for which an emetic was given, by a physician, followed with cathartics, sudorifics & expectorants. His complaints gradually abated; so that, in a few weeks, he went out and transacted some business. But his flesh & strength decreased, tho tonics & restoratives were taken.

In July, hectic fever, with its usual train, made its appearance; and preyed on the vital organs, unrestrained, till the middle of August, when he put himself under my care. His pulse was then 90 & tense; and he was much enfeebled. —— A pint of blood was drawn, which was buffy. Two grains of calomel were given night & morning, together with an aqueous solution of corrosive sublimate, till the last of the month. No change, however, was perceived. I then drew another pint of blood, which was equally buffy. Paleness then appeared, and he fainted. The means were continued, with half a grain of opium at night, to quiet the cough. After taking eighty grains of calomel, and eight of sublimate, a salivation was produced. The fever then subsided, with his other complaints, and his health was soon regained, by suitable nutriment and gentle exercise.

C163

"It would be happy for mankind, says Dr Reid, if the term cold, when considered as a disease, should be expunged, and the term heat substituted. What is denominated catching a cold, ought rather to be called catching a heat." [14]

Again, "When a person barks once, always suspect a thief within," which he denominates "inflammatory irritation." —— This destructive invader invites an undue quantity of blood, into the vessels of the lungs, and commences its ravages, by inflammatory action. How then is this thief to be expelled? —— Not by soothing, flattering words, and cordial treatment, as tho harmless & innocent; but by the point of the lancet. Otherwise, it will bid defiance to medicine, and proceed to rob the patient of his life; as has, unhappily, been the case, in thousands of instances, from time immemorial!

Happily, however, the time has arrived, when this subtle invader has been detected, by inspecting dead bodies, and its disorganizing ravages have been exposed to public view. ——

---

[14] John Reid, *A Treatise on the Origin, Progress, Prevention, and Treatment, of Consumption* (London: Phillips, 1806), 112–17.

Of what importance is it then, that physicians should unitedly and <u>harmoniously</u> combine, in drawing this mischievous agent from its lurking place; as well as in giving such directions, as might tend to prevent its future admission. **C164**

In August, 1811, Mr Amos Mason, of Falmouth, aged 30, of a vigorous habit, who was much engaged by day, in the mowing field, and by night, in rafting boards down a fresh river, when the weather was foggy & rainy, complained of oppression at the breast & febrile heat, to which succeeded cough & expectoration of mucus, tinged with blood. He also complained of wandering pain in his chest, which inclined to settle in the left side.

During the month of September, he was unable to labour, tho not confined to the house. Few means were taken, as he informed me, except bilious pills.

On the 6th of October, I was consulted, when he complained of heat in the vitals, cough, pain in his side, and febrile disturbance in the night, so that he was deprived of quiet sleep; pulse 90 & full. I then drew a pint of blood, which was buffy, and gave a cathartic of Jalap & calomel, also furnished him with a number of pills each containing one grain of calomel, and directed him to take two night & morning, with a diet chiefly of milk & vegetables. He then visited his friends, in a distant town, where he met with an Empiric, who reprobated the lancet, and advised him to lay aside the mercurial pills. Instead of which, **C165** he directed him to take a spirituous tincture of certain pungent heating articles.

This plan was pursued for some time, but he sensibly grew worse; as the fever had increased with the pain in his side; and morning sweats had taken place, with an increase of his cough & expectoration; so that, at the close of the year, his strength was considerably impaired, and his flesh waisted. He then began to be alarmed, fearing, with his friends, that unless some remedy could be obtained, he should soon become incurably consumptive.

On the 3^d of January 1812, he went to Portland, and consulted Dr Cummins, who sent him to Dr Hunt of Falmouth, his neighbour, with a letter, in which he gave it as his opinion, that "unless Mr Mason was bled & salivated, he would soon die of pulmonary consumption." Dr Hunt declined taking charge of him; and he brought the letter to me, wishing that I would attend to his case, after relating what had occurred in his absence, and lamenting that he had been subjected to empirical impositions, to the neglect of proper means. **C166**

His pulse, at this time, was 90 and tense; the pain in his side severe, on any unusual exertion; cough tedious with expectoration of purulent matter, often tinged with blood; and his night sweats had increased.

I then drew a pint of blood, which was buffy, and gave one grain & a half of calomel night & morning; a large blister was also applied to his chest.

On the 4th a seton was put into his side.

On the 8th remaining much the same, another pint of blood was drawn, and an ounce of Unguent. hydrarg. was applied to his neck by friction, continuing the calomel, which operated cathartically.

On the 13th no abatement of his fever nor pain; another pint of blood was drawn, and another ounce of the unguent was applied.

On the 21^t he complained of distress in the region of the liver. I then gave 15 grains of calomel with as much aloes, and another ounce of Unguent. was applied; as also on the 26th.

28th, no alleviation of his complaints; the hectic paroxysms still recurred with regularity, twice in 24 hours, with red spots on his cheeks, preceeded by chills. I then drew twelve ounces of blood, and gave a grain of opium at night, as his bowels were loose, and he slept but little. At this time he could sit up the chief of the day.

C167

On the 30th his salivary glands were slightly affected, and there was some discharge. But the febrile action & pain continued much the same; so that he became very impatient & fretful, on account of his expenses and loss of time; for he wished to make an addition to his farm.

Drs Cummins & Hunt, then called to see him; but gave no encouragement of a recovery. The patient wished to know my real opinion of his case. —— I told him that as the means did not appear to have the desired effect, and as a sufficiency had been supposed to have been used, there was little or no hope of his recovery; and advised him to prepare for death, —— to send for the Minister, request his prayers, read the Bible; and cease to think of adding to his temporal interest. ——He did so; and appeared to be greatly alarmed at the thoughts of exchanging worlds, which had never before entered his mind!

The consequence of this reduction of mental stimulus, and dispair of recovery, cooperating with the depleting means, was such, that the hectic fever rapidly subsided; the salivary glands now discharged very freely, and **C168** the cough abated, together with the pain in his side. His pulse also became natural, and calmness ensued. He soon recovered without the use of tonic or stimulating medicine; so that, in a few weeks, he was able to visit his friends, as well as the Sanctuary. Since which he has enjoyed health of body, and a Christian temper.

In March 1811, Miss Eliza Barker of Falmouth,[15] aged 24 years, small in stature and of a slender habit, after riding 30 miles in an open sleigh, on a damp cloudy day, facing an easterly wind, was seized with oppression & stricture of

---

[15] Elizabeth Barker was the fifth child of Jeremiah and Abigail Barker, born January 29, 1787.

the breast, a hecking cough, ~~and~~ febrile disturbance, and opthalmia. A pint of blood was then drawn, and ten grains of calomel with as much Jalap were given. Her complaints were ~~then~~ alleviated; but soon returned, by exposure to inclement air, when another pint of blood was drawn, and relief was afforded.

She enjoyed comfortable health, till the next November, when she walked out, on a rainy evening, in Boston. She was then attacked in a similar manner, when application was made to a physician of our acquaintance, who prescribed a pil composed of one grain of calomel and one of opium, every night, with antimonial wine, and a blister was applied to the chest. In one week, her salivary glands were slightly affected, and temporary relief was afforded.
C169

Being informed of her illness, I advised, in a letter, to bleeding. But she did not comply with my advice, for the following reasons, assigned in her answer.

Boston, Nov. 29th, 1811

"My dear father, I received your letter last evening, and am happy that it is in my power to relieve your anxiety, by informing you that I am much better. Your plan of bleeding, I have no doubt is often very beneficial; but as other means have been made instrumental in removing my complaints, I have cause for gratitude. I have a particular aversion to being bled so often; owing to my being nervous."

Her complaints, however, as I was informed, in a succeeding letter, returned; so that she was obliged to be confined to the house, and was considered, by her friends, as labouring under the symptoms of pulmonary consumption; also by her physician, as not being a subject of bleeding.

The last of January, 1812, she rode to Portland, in a stage sleigh, in two days, & underwent considerable fatigue. I then called to see her, and found that she was troubled with oppression & stricture of the breast, a hecking cough, and some expectoration of bloody matter, attended with running pain in the chest, pulse 90 and tense. —— I drew 12 ounces of blood, by her consent, which was buffy. The next day, the matter expectorated was more deeply tinged with blood and her countenance was florid. A **C170** pint of blood was drawn, which was less buffy; paleness then ensued, with faintness. The next day, the matter expectorated was free from blood; and her complaints were, in some measure, alleviated. She then rode to Falmouth, three miles, in a chaise. But the oppression & stricture continued, and there was a very constant hecking cough, with febrile disturbance, so that she was much enfeebled, and her flesh decayed.

One grain of calomel was then given night & morning, and an ounce of Unguent. hydrarg. was applied to her side, which was at times pained. In one week a salivation was produced, and the mercury was omitted. The salivation continued three weeks, discharging about a pint by day; and, as she supposed, as much by night, without much inconvenience.

During this course, the morbid action of the blood vessels was much lessened, the cough ceased, and the oppression of the breast was removed.

When the salivation had ceased, she walked into a cold chamber, to call her nurse, which produced some chilliness, succeeded by febrile disturbance, with heat in the vitals & hands. The stricture & oppression of the chest returned, rigors & fever fits recurred daily with regularity; pulse quick and rather tense. I then gave the digitalis a trial. Twenty drops of the saturated tincture were given, three times a day, and gradually increased to 100, when nausea was produced. **C171**

Under this course, the pulse was reduced from 90 to 40. —— The rigors and febrile paroxysms abated. But, the heat in the vitals, stricture & oppression of the breast continued, with torpor & anxiety of the praecordia. When the drops were omitted, the pulse became quick & tense as usual, and the oppression abated, so that she could breathe with more ease.

Disappointed in this attempt, Crem. tart, tamarinds, castor oil, and alkalines were freely given; and some relief was afforded, by an abatement of the febrile heat. Lichen was also liberally used.

The beginning of March, however, the hectical symptoms increased, and clearly evinced the second stage of the disease. Daily rigors & exacerbations of fever, with red spots on the cheeks, occurred, with cough & oppression, stricture & heat in the vitals. But the patient was not discouraged, a strong hope of recovery prevailed; and this I believe produced such a degree of excitement in her mind, as to keep up an increase the morbid action of the blood vessels, in cooperation with the stimulus of the febrile cause.

On the 9th of March I drew 16 ounces of blood, which afforded some relief, as to the stricture and pain in the side. Still the chills and fever fits recurred every day; but no **C172** night sweats followed. A little blood was raised every morning with mucus & yellow matter. Blisters were con continued on the chest, which were very sore; and pediluvium was used, as her feet were cold on the approach of the rigor. On the 15th of the month, I drew a pint of blood, and further relief was afforded.

From this time, to the 28th the fever gradually declined; the cough & expectoration lessened; pulse 80. But on the 28th, the rigors & febrile paroxysms recurred with greater violence than heretofore, pulse 90 & tense. At this time the weather changed to an easterly storm. Bloodletting was again proposed. But the voice of my friends, and some physicians, was against me; so that I was accused of unprecedented and rash practice. The patient then requested me to send for Dr Samuel Ayer of Portland,[16] whose education had been completed in Philadelphia. The D^r readily came, and after examining her case, with much deliberation, advised me to continue the use of the lancet, in the febrile paroxysms; according to the urgency of the symptoms, as the most probable means of removing the fever and preventing disorganization of the vital organs, together with other antiphlogistic means; and to keep a perpetual blister on the sternum.

C173

On the first of April, twelve ounces of blood were drawn from her arm, and repeated three times, in like quantity, besides once from her foot, by the middle of the month, without producing any visible change, excepting temporary relief. By depressing the tongue, her throat appeared very red; and there was some hoarseness. The balsam of honey was sent, by a friend, for her cough; but it produced heat & irritation. The food most congenial, was milk, with bread or rice. The fever, however, continued to rage uncontrolled, with stricture oppression & heat of the vitals, especially in the evening paroxysm; so that little hope was entertained of her recovery, fearing that disorganization had taken place, as the morbid action of the blood vessels had been of so long continuance, and such powerful means were used to so little purpose.

At this time, she was visited by the Rev. Asa Rand. His prayers, in her behalf, were solemn & importunate; and that a blessing might attend the means employed.

In the evening, the paroxysm of fever returned as usual. But the heat & oppression **C174** in her vitals was such, that she could not lie in bed. At midnight, I was called up, when she requested me to bleed her again, saying that the heat extended through her lungs, to the back; and that her distress was insupportable!

I waited a short time, in great perplexity of mind; the fever continuing to rage; pulse 100 and tense. Twenty one ounces of blood, which was

---

[16] Samuel Ayer (1786–1832) was born in Concord, New Hampshire, graduated from Dartmouth in 1807, and spent two years with Dr. Nathan Smith (Professor at Dartmouth, and later at Yale, University of Vermont, and the Medical School of Maine). Ayer received an M.B. degree in 1810 and then went to Philadelphia for an M.D. degree. He practiced in Portland and Eastport, Maine. James Alfred Spalding, *Maine Physicians of 1820; a Record of the Members of the Massachusetts Medical Society Practicing in the District of Maine at the Date of Separation* (Lewiston: Lewiston Print Shop, 1928), 11–15.

weighed, were drawn from a large orifice, in a recumbent [*sic*] posture; besides some spilt on the bedding. But no immediate change was produced. —— I then dispaired of her recovery. She also considered her case as remediless; and resigned herself to the will of God, in the hope of Celestial happiness, through the merits of the Redeemer. Under these exercises of the mind, her complaints gradually subsided; but sleep had departed.

She then requested me to send for Miss Sarah Emmons of Portland, an intimate associate, to attend, in her dying moments; believing that the next paroxysm would terminate her life. This pious Christian conversed on the subject of religion; and prayed with the hopeless patient, as one preparing to depart!

C175

Contrary to our expectations, the rigor did not invade her as usual, neither did a paroxysm of fever recur. She was able to sit up, the latter part of the day; and had a quiet nights rest, for the first time, as she said, since she sickened in Boston.

The next day, her pulse was natural; the redness had left her throat; and the respiratory organs were at ease.

By the use of a milk & vegetable diet, without any tonic, save lime water, a gill of which was taken three times a day, her strength was regained, so that, in three days, she walked out of the room, and, the beginning of May, rode two miles, in a chaise.

In June, she married the Rev. Daniel A. Clark, of Weymouth, and rode to that town, distant 120 miles, without much fatigue. Her health was soon restored. Since which she has enjoyed this invaluable blessing, free from pulmonary affections; and is now the mother of six children, viz. 1831.

Her mother died of consumption, from catarrh, of many years standing, when this child was three years old.

C176 A son of mine,[17] born of this consumptive mother, six years before her death, was troubled in early infancy, with a catarrhal defluction on his lungs, producing cough, and, an times, a spasmodic stricture across the chest, for which stimulants, both external & internal were used; but to no advantage, except, that opiates afforded some temporary relief.

---

[17] David Gorham Barker, M.D. (1784–1830), son of Jeremiah and Abigail Gorham Barker, was born March 7, 1784. He practiced in Durham and Sedgwick, Maine, and died April 15, 1830. James Alfred Spalding, "After Consulting Hours: Jeremiah Barker, M.D., Gorham and Falmouth, Maine, 1752–1835," *Bulletin of the American Academy of Medicine* 10 (1909), 242–65.

As he grew in years, these complaints increased; so that he gradually declined, and his growth was impeded. At the age of 16, I sent him to Virginia, by water, where he resided several months, in the summer season, and was free from pulmonary complaints. He also increased rapidly in stature. On his return, however, the disease soon recurred, and at times, molested him severely, till 1807, when, at the age of 23 years, he was violently attacked with the Influenza, which then prevailed, for which he was repeatedly bled, and deeply salivated. Since which, he has been laboriously engaged in the practice of physic, in Maine; and, for the most part, enjoyed health. Sometimes, when much exposed to inclement weather, he has been attacked with his pulmonic affection, in some degree; but found that **C177** it was readily removed, by the use of the lancet and mercurial cathartics. In 1818, he informed me, that, in the course of the last seven years, he had bled himself more than a dozen times, and seldom drew less than a pint of blood, tho of a slender habit, yet he was able to undergo great fatigue in practice by night, as well as by day, with increasing strength and vigour.

A communication from Dr John R. Lucas of Mecklenburgh, Virginia, published in Ritche's Enquirer,[18] printed at Richmond, relates a remarkable instance of the violence & obstinacy of acute inflammation. The patient was captain James Niblett, of the same county, aged 30 years, of a full & plethoric habit, when in health, and accostomed [sic] to daily exercise on foot, of a bilious aspect. "His complaint was an inflammatory affection of the lungs. Dr Lucas visited him, at intervals, from the 29th of May last, to the 8th of August 1809; during which period, blood letting was almost the only remedy prescribed. Emollient means were given, during the time; but merely for the purpose of harmonizing the state of the bowels and preventing costiveness. Depletion seems to have been from first to last, relied on by Dr Lucas; and the result of the lancet's reiterated application afforded the most ample testimony of its efficacy. The loss of blood sustained by Mr Niblett was truly astonishing; and we subjoin an account of it in the words of Dr Lucas himself, from the

---

[18] It is likely that Barker found this reference in "Blood-Letting to the Amount of Fifty-Seven Pounds Troy," *Medical Repository* 3rd hexade, vol. 2, no. 3 (1811): 295–96. "Ritchie's Enquirer" refers to the *Richmond Enquirer* that Thomas Ritchie (1778–1854) bought in 1804 and edited for the next forty-one years. Ritchie had read medicine and law and was a schoolteacher and bookseller before beginning his newspaper career. Silbey, Joel H. "Ritchie, Thomas (1778–1854), newspaper editor and Democratic party activist," in *American National Biography*. 1 Feb. 2000; Accessed 20 Apr. 2020. https://www-anb-org.ezproxy.library.tufts.edu/view/10.1093/anb/9780198606697.001.0001/anb-9780198606697-e-0300419. Joel H. Silbey, "Ritchie, Thomas (1778–1854), Newspaper Editor and Democratic Party Activist," in *American National Biography*, online (Oxford University Press, 2000).

C178 28th of May to the 26th of July. Captain Niblett, observes Dr Lucas, lost by measurement 600 ounces of blood, and by weight 688 ounces six drachms. or 57 pounds troy; the largest quantity, it is presumed, ever drawn from the veins of any human being, in the same length of time, by medical advice; and for the person to bear it and do well. He was bled fifty different times, and the blood, every time, was covered with a thick strong white coat, and he lost from 4 to 20 ounces each time. He was cupped, and had leeches applied daily for seven weeks, exclusive of bleeding at the arm and the discharge from a seton."

The following melancholly case, will serve to show the highly inflammatory nature of pulmonary affection, under certain circumstances.

"On Fryday the 8th of June 1804 departed this life, at Hager's Town, Maryland, John R. Young, M.D., a young man of uncommon talents and great industry.

He had completed his medical education under the direction of Professor Barton and graduated with more than an ordinary share of reputation, in June 1803; after which he returned to the place of his nativity, and succeeded his **C179** father, in a very extensive practice. The fatigue which he was obliged to undergo in the discharge of professional duties, was more than his delicate constitution could long support. He had an hereditary predisposition to phthisis pulmonalis, but as he never had been warned of its approach by any premonitary [*sic*] symptoms, his friends had reason to hope, that his judgement & skill would be sufficient to obviate the fatal disease. About the middle of April, during several days of cold damp weather, he underwent very great fatigue in the exercise of his profession, and contracted a slight indisposition. On the 17th, after having rid all the morning in a cold mist, he returned at noon, and ate a hearty dinner, but felt some oppression at his breast, with cold extremities, and an inclination to sleep. He had sat by the fire but a few minutes, when a universal glow of heat was felt, and an irritation of the trachea which excited a slight cough. A profuse hemorrhage from the lungs immediately commenced, and syncope succeeded. Upon **C180** reviving, the hemorrhage again appeared. Repeated venesection was used; and large quantities of muriate of soda administered. The hemorrhage gradually subsided; and on the third day entirely disappeared; but his pulse remained very full and elastic. He was bled ten times in as many days, and took digitalis without producing much effect. He had regular exacerbations of fever after the tenth day; during the paroxysm his pulse indicated great irritability of the arterial system, was elastic & full, tho not very frequent. In the apyrexia, debility was extreme. The intermission being complete, the bark was used; but without producing any good effect. He now complained of a pain in the left lobe of his lungs; for which he again had recourse to phlebotomy, without any obvious benefit. Digitalis reduced the pulse for a short time, but a more violent arterial action always succeeded. Mercury was used, but no ptyalism could be excited, tho it relieved the pain in his breast. His fever continued with regular exacerbations, and a pulse indicating the highest grade of irritability, to **C181** the last, notwithstanding the means used to overcome it. He died after violent spasms of an hours duration, without ever having expectorated more than ordinary.

He was the only son of an aged & venerable parent." Med. Repos. vol. 8th.[19]

Case of Haemoptysis. By D[r]. Anson Smith, of Kingston, in Upper Canada.[20]

"In Feb. 1810, a young gentleman of this town, aged 23, was attacked by an alarming pulmonary hemorrhage.

Feb. 27. Lethargic indisposition; slight febrile symptoms, pulse about 70 in a minute; not full nor hard, and free from cough or pain.

28. took cathartic pills, which operated gently; saliva to day, occasionally streaked with blood.

March 1st The hemorrhage commenced last evening at 10 o'clock, and recurred at 4 in the morning; loss of blood about 12 ounces. I saw him at 11 A.M. and bled him 20 ounces. Hemorrhage at 2 P.M. 6 ounces; at 9, 12 ounces.

2[d] At 3 o'clock A.M. hemorrhage 6 ounces; pulse full & strong, about 76. Venesection 16 ounces. At **C182** 3 P.M. hemorrhage 5 ounces; at 9 o'clock 7 ounces.

3[d] Hemorrhage at 3 A.M. 3 ounces, and at 7, 3. pulse 110, and near deliquium animi. At 6 A.M. hemorrhage 2 ounces; pulse 80 and irregular.

4th hemorrhage ceased.

From this statement it will appear that the loss of blood, by natural & artificial bleedings, during about 60 hours amounted to more than 90 ounces. His pulse, from the 4th to the 12th was pretty regular and about 60. But there were daily occasional symptoms which indicated a return of the hemorrhage, viz. a flushing of the face; and a peculiar sensation of heat across the chest,

---

[19] "Obituary," *The Medical Repository of Original Essays and Intelligence, Relative to Physic, Surgery, Chemistry, and Natural History* 2 (1805): 340.

[20] Anson Smith, "Case of Hemoptysis; to Which Is Subjoined Some Sketches Respecting the Use of Digitalis in Haemorrhagic Affections," *Medical Repository* 3rd hexade, vol. 2, no. 3 (1811): 223–26. The obituary notice of the death in Boston of Dr. Anson Smith, aged forty, of Kingston, Upper Canada, formerly of Burlington, appeared in *The Christian Visitant (Albany, NY)* 1, no. 19 (Saturday, October 7, 1815): 150.

which, as they had always ushered in the hemoptic paroxysm, were considered as the harbingers of its recurrence. There was also a kind of jerking or throbbing of the pulse.

The means used during the hemorrhage, were epispastics to the chest; cold water to the back of the neck & spine; diluted sulphuric acid, and muriate of soda, with mucilages; keeping the room at the temperature of the freezing point. After the 12ᵗʰ of March, from one to two grains of the digitalis were given daily; and cathartics of the sulphate of soda, so as to produce copious stools, were occasionally taken. He soon recovered.

C183

This case serves to show the good effects of of plentiful bleeding and powerful cathartics, with cooperative means, in order to remove plethora & inflammatory action of the lungs. In Dʳ Youngs case the lancet seems to have been too sparingly used, and cathartics were neglected, among which sal. Glaub — has been found to be the best.

In a natural state of the lungs, the exhalents exercise the office of secreting and throwing out a mucous serous fluid. By becoming diseased their capacity is lost and blood passes through their patulous mouths unaltered. When cold & dampness are applied to the extremities & surface of the body the blood is propelled to the lungs in such a manner as to destroy the equilibrium of the pulmonary system of bloodvessels and the general system.

C184

These two circulations, as described by Dʳ Ware,[21] are placed in opposite scales, and balance one another, and although one is more extensive and widely diffused than the other, yet they are so adapted, by their peculiar arrangement as to maintain an equilibrium. Hence, any derangement in either of these systems, will affect the circulation of the other. Consequently any circumstance which shall cause a less quantity of blood to exist in the general system, will produce an engorgement of the vessels of the lungs and inflammatory action. When the lungs become thus overcharged & inflamed, the blood often finds a passage through the mouths of the extreme vessels, dilated

[21] John Ware (1795–1864), born in Hingham, Massachusetts, was a teacher of medicine, writer, and editor. He graduated from Harvard College in 1813 and Harvard Medical School in 1816. Practicing in Boston, he taught, was physician for the Boston almshouse, and was an editor of the *New England Journal Medicine and Surgery* from 1824 to 1827. In 1828, with the establishment of the *Boston Medical and Surgical Journal*, he became its first editor. Ware succeeded Dr. James Jackson as professor of medicine at Harvard Medical School and was president of the Massachusetts Medical Society from 1848 to 1852. Howard A. Kelly and Walter L. Burrage, *American Medical Biographies* (Baltimore: The Norman, Remington Company, 1920), 1190–91.

by the efforts of nature to liberate their gorged state. Were it not for this wise provision of nature to emit superabundant blood from the lungs, their small vessels would be in danger of being ruptured; for the vital organs, from their structure, are fuller of blood than any other parts. The different functions of these organs, and of the rest of the body are constantly throwing into them, **C185** an unusual quantity of blood with which they become gorged, when cold & dampness are applied to the surface, and in public speaking.

The discharge of blood from the lungs, in such cases, is not attended with much danger, unless the inflammation which attends is so great as to endanger suppuration, and the subject is predisposed to consumption by hereditary taint. Still every attempt should be made to prevent its recurrence, lest it should injure the lungs and prove an exciting cause of pulmonary consumption, which begins with inflammatory action and sooner or later terminates in suppuration & ulceration unless proper means are seasonally & duly employed.

These observations refer only to active hemorrhage, where the life of the part is vigorous & full of blood, in passive, the vital powers & quantity of blood are both diminished and occur in the lungs in the advanced stages of chronic diseases of those organs, and of phthisis pulmonalis, **C186** in consequence of their want of power to retain the vital fluid. In such cases tonics and restoratives are indicated, tho with little or no prospect of success. See prize dissertation, 1818.[22]

In order to prevent a recurrence of hemoptysis, great attention should be paid to suitable cloathing, so as to prevent cold & dampness from propelling the blood from the surface, and extremities to the lungs; also to avoid violent exercise of the body or voice. Gentle exercise by walking, moderate labour and riding on horseback, so as to equalize the circulation, with a nutritious diet, chiefly of milk & its preparations have been found to be the best preventives and most conducive to health.

In some cases, however, of a periodical and habitual recurrence of the disease, a mercurial salivation, or the intervention of some other disease, have produced such an alteration in the general system, and vital powers as to prevent its ever returning, and a vigorous constitution has been uniformly enjoyed.

---

[22] John Ware, *Medical Dissertations on Hemoptysis or the Spitting of Blood, and on Suppuration, Which Obtained the Boylston Premiums for the Years 1818 & 1820* (Boston: Cummings and Hilliard, 1820), 13.

C187

As in phthisis pulmonalis, morbid action and inflammatory irritation often subsist for a considerable length of time before organic lesion or ulcers are formed, oppertunities are afforded of calling into aid a variety of useful means according to existing circumstances. In some cases the morbid action has been removed solely by bleeding, salivating cathartics, digitalis, and external stimulants. In others, the conjoint aid of all these means are required in order to remove the complaints. But when the disease is far advanced & neglected, the most appropriate remedies, are for the most part ineffectual; and this is the case with all other diseases; so that under these circumstances, **C188** there is no propriety of calling any of them incurable. Does any one say that typhous fever, pneumonia or apoplexy are incurable, because many die of these diseases? Surely not. But if proper means were not seasonably & duly employed, they would terminate life much more rapidly than consumption.

When a person is attacked with pneumonia, the idea of inflammation is readily entertained, so that a physician is called without delay; and if depleting cooling means are duly employed, the disease generally terminates favorably, in about one week. But when the symptoms of phthisis pulmonalis invade, the idea of cold & weakness is suggested to the mind, and heating stimulants are taken with avidity, such as ardent spirits, cayenne pepper &c. In this way, the inconsiderate patient often continues for some time; and, for the most part, consults an empiric, who ascribes the complaints to cold, and encourages the use of such means, together with sweating materials, till inflammatory action has **C189** induced such a morbid state of the lungs, that the situation of the patient is nearly hopeless. A physician may then be consulted; but if he suggests that depleting means are indicated, he is often opposed by the prejudices of the patient and his friends; and the prospect of success is then rendered so doubtful that he is unwilling to take charge of the case, for if the patient should not recover, however judiciously treated, he is in danger of being accused, by empirics, of killing the patient! —— Were it necessary I could relate numerous cases of consumption, treated in this way, by thoughtless patients, and daring imposters, which terminated fatally. The preposterous treatment of such cases is too well known to need a description and may be considered as a principal cause of the increasing prevalency, as well as fatal termination of this disease.

Patent Doctors, as they are called, are numerous, among us, who are in the habit of selling their boasted skill, to the ignorant & illiterate for a few dollars, and equal confidence is placed in these, by many equally ignorant, so that their mischievous **C190** practice rapidly increases, among the vulgar, and fills our grave yards with untimely deaths! But what is still more melancholly, certain strolling irregular preachers, have of late undertaken to practice on this inflaming plan, which, in addition to their stimulating discourses, to live as we list with impunity, tend to destroy the soul, as well as body.

It is a matter of regret that many people, of good understanding, and carefulness of every thing, save that which relates to bodily health, are so negligent & imprudent, when labouring under any complaint which endangers a consumption.

In March 1780, Mrs M. P. a lady in Cambridge, aged 25, of a good habit, left her chamber about two weeks after parturition, passed through a cold entry and received company, in the parlor. In a short time, she was seized with chilliness, to which succeeded febrile health, pain in the side and cough. The idea of having taken a cold was suggested to the mind, and heating cordials were taken, which afforded some temporary relief. The pain, however, returned with increasing violence, for which aleotic pills were taken and elixir paragoric. A moderate hectic supervened, and she gradually **C191** declined. In May following, she rode to Barnstable, in a chaise, distant 75 miles, when I was consulted. I found her considerably emaciated, pulse 100 and weak, cough troublesome with expectoration of mucus. The journey, tho slowly performed, aggravated the fever & pain, and she sensibly grew worse in every respect. Aloe pills & paregoric elixir were the chief means which had been used, and which afforded temporary relief; so that a hope of recovery was entertained, for she was able to ride, and her appetite was pretty good. Viewing her case as hopeless, palliatives were only prescribed. On the 8th of July she rode a few miles, in a chaise, returned in the evening and drank tea with the family. She then walked to the door, and, in a fit of coughing, a large quantity of purulent matter was discharged from the windpipe. She expired at eleven o'clock.

Had proper means been seasonable & duly employed, her complaints might probably have been removed.

In the course of my practice, I have met with many very similar cases, thus managed, which proved fatal. On the contrary, I have seen many cases of this kind differently treated, that terminated favourably.
C192

In April 1790, a lady in Portland, aged 40, who had been troubled, for some years, with a slight catarrhal cough, walked to Church with kid shoes, and in a thin dress, when the ground was wet. The next morning, her cough was worse, and she expectorated bloody mucus which recurred three mornings in succession, discharging about two ounces of blood each time. Salted butter &

mucilages were the chief means employed. A moderate hectic, with its usual train ensued, and she died in July following.

Soon after, a lady, in the bloom of life, rode ten miles in a chaise, covered with a muslin gown, in a damp evening air. The next morning, she awoke with hoarseness; and pulmonary consumption ensued, which terminated life in a few months. A physician, ironically, called this a <u>muslin</u> consumption. No depleting means were used!

The following observations on Phthisis Pulmonalis, by Doctor Young of New York, are considered applicable & instructive. "As the <u>prevention</u> of this destructive disease is preferable to the best methods of curing it, it is of importance to point **C193** out some of the causes which produce it, especially with respect to females. The first I shall mention is a combination among the shoemakers, who appear to have resolved that as the ladies gowns have no <u>bodies</u>, their shoes should have only the semblance of a <u>sole</u>; but so narrow that half an inch of the vamp comes to the pavement at every step, and admits the water very freely. Secondly, I must mention the pernicious effects of their <u>bodyless gowns</u> without <u>sleeves</u>. When a lady rises in the morning, she dresses comfortably, probably in a gown with long sleeves, but Mrs A. receives the following polite card, from Mrs B. —– "Mrs B. presents her most respectful compliments to Mrs A. and, having invited a few select friends, requests the pleasure of her company to spend a social evening." The weather is cold & damp, but Mrs B. cannot think of entertaining company in the common room; and, about half an hour before the visitants are expected, a fire is kindled in the best parlor, which had been well scrubbed in the forenoon; and to have all things compleat, the carpet is **C194** laid down before the floor is dry. The time draws near. Mrs A. retires into a cold room to dress, and as a suitable substitute for the warm morning dress, adopts thin book or cambric muslin,[23] with short wide sleeves, and other corresponding articles of dress! The neck and breast are bare, or covered with very thin gauze, and the arms naked almost to the shoulders. If the breast is left open to facilitate the entrance of Cupid's <u>darts</u>, it affords a more certain <u>mark</u> for the <u>envenomed shafts</u> of the <u>grisly king of terrors</u>. A muff or a tippet may be worn in the street, but are laid aside before the room gets warm. Mrs A. is bedecked in a suit much better adapted to the month of August than December. She looks out of the window and observes that it has rained, and that the streets are very wet, but no matter; the walks are pretty dry, and it is but a step. Madam sets off, and

---

[23] Book muslin was a thin white muslin used in ladies' dresses. Cambric muslin was a fine cotton cloth made to imitate linen cambric.

gets her feet wet. When she arrives, the fire just begins to blaze, the room is cold & damp; but off goes the muff & tippet. Her <u>feet</u> are <u>wet</u> & <u>cold</u>, but politeness **C195** will not permit her to dry them; she sits shivering until the fire has warmed the room. The company having all arrived, the warm tea is served about; which with the <u>heat</u> of a crowded room, opens the pores and produces a copious perspiration. At length the company breaks up, and the visitants return home through the damp night air, and find many of their fires extinguished, and the rooms cold; they go shivering to bed, and are awakened in the morning with a most violent cough & hoarseness!!"

"The Deity has mercifully adapted the human constitution to bear very considerable extremes of <u>heat</u> & <u>cold</u>; but the changes from one condition to the other must be gradual; as all sudden changes either from <u>heat</u> to <u>cold</u>, or from extreme <u>cold</u> to <u>heat</u>, are attended with imminent danger. When a warm morning gown, with long sleeves & a shawl, is exchanged for a thin <u>muslin</u> without <u>sleeves</u>, and a gauze handkerchief, the change is too great and too sudden to be born with impunity, **C196** and any person who considers the circumstances can be at no loss to account for the frequency & fatality of consumptions. Here is <u>fashion</u> exhibited on one side, attended with disease, death, and desolation; and common prudence on the other side, promising health, pleasure and longevity, submitted to the choice of rational beings."

Med. Repos. v. 12.[24]

In the course of my practice, I have met with many cases of pulmonary consumption, brought on by very similar imprudences, among females. Some had recourse to cordials, and patent cough drops, which, by their stimulating quality, increased the inflammation of their lungs to such a degree as to produce suppuration, with an extenuating hectic, and the disease proved fatal. Others applied to physicians, who, by pursuing a different course, removed plethora and inflammatory irritation from the vital organs, before they were too greatly injured, and health was restored.

---

[24] Joseph Young, "Observations on Phthisis Pulmonalis, or Consumption of the Lungs," *The Medical Repository of Original Essays and Intelligence, Relative to Physic, Surgery, Chemistry, and Natural History* 6 (1809): 241–46. Choice of clothing as a public health issue is discussed in James Thacher, "Of Clothing," in *American Modern Practice* (Boston: Ezra Read, 1817), chap. 8, 135–39. Bynum discusses the relationship between consumption and dress in the early nineteenth century and suggests, "the cultivation of adult female delicacy began in childhood." Helen Bynum, *Spitting Blood: The History of Tuberculosis* (Oxford: Oxford University Press, 2012), 77–81.

C197

It has often been said that when Phthisis pulmonalis has become seated or confirmed, means are ineffectual. This requires explanation. It is well known that this disease often exists for several months, with the usual train of symptoms, in the first and second stages, without producing organic lesion or ulceration; for under these alarming symptoms many have recovered, by the use of the lancet, mercury, and other cooperative means when they appeared to be hopeless.

Hence we infer that the disease may with strict propriety be said to be seated and confirmed, in these stages, for death would generally take place unless such means were used, as appear by the **C198** fatal cases already related, where appropriate remedies were neglected. It is in the third stage only that this disease may, with any degree of propriety be said to be incurable by the use of means, where from neglect & delay, a lesion of organs has taken place, with suppuration or abscess. Yet, under these last circumstances, cures have been affected, by the efforts of nature, throwing off one lobe of the lungs by expectoration. But such favourable termination of the disease, at this late period, should by no means encourage procrastination, for they rarely happen. As well might a man defer repentance, till far advanced in life, or when threatened with the approach of death. Even in the last stage of Phthisis pulmonalis, when it has proved fatal, dissections have shewn that organic lesion does not always occur. Extreme debility, in consequence of a protracted hectic, with night sweats &c have left the patient so exhausted, after the inflammatory stages are passed, that death has taken place from mere <u>inaction</u> of body & mind, and neglect of exercise with restorative means, the only time, in this disease, in which these remedies are eligible, as long experience has taught me, as well as others.

C199

The following case, communicated to me, from a learned physician, in Mass^tts will be adduced as an example.

"A middle-aged man, was invaded with the usual symptoms of Phthisis pulmonalis and was carried through the primary stages, by the use of depleting & antiphlogistic means, so that the hectic fever subsided. But he became so feeble & inactive that little or no hope was entertained of his recovery. His physician then reminded him of his danger, and advised him to make his will and settle his temporal business, as his strength was so greatly exhausted. —— Anger was then excited, and he declared that he would live, in spite of his predictions to the contrary. He then called for his horse, and, with difficulty was seated on the saddle. After riding a few rods, he returned, and was brought into the sick room, where he made use of restorative means. The next day, in an angry tone, he again called for his horse, and rode a little further. This he practiced daily, till in a few weeks, he has able to perform a long journey and recovered"

I have known this passion to be raised, in the primary stages of Phthisis when it so excited the fever as to produce heat in the vitals **C200** and a spitting of blood. I have also found that in these stages, fear of death & dispair of recovery have reduced the excitement, so as to be productive of salutary effects.

We are taught, from high authority, that "To every thing there is a season, and a time to every purpose under Heaven." Eccles. 3^d.1st. There is a time to fear, and a time to be angry, if we sin not; a time to exercise, & a time to rest.

Case of Pulmonary Consumption related by Dr Rush.   Me. Ob. vol. 2.[25]

"In 1785, I attended a young lady, who had complained of a pain in her right side, and had frequent chills, with fever of the hectic kind. They all gave way to frequent & gentle bleedings. In the summer of 1786, she was seized with the same complaints, and as she had great objection to bleeding, she consulted a physician who gratified her, by attempting to cure her by recommending exercise and country air. In Autumn she returned to the city much worse than when she left it. I was again sent for, and found her confined to her bed, with a pain in her right side, but without the least cough or fever. **C201** Her pulse was preternaturally slow. She could lie only on her left side. She sometimes complained of acute flying pains in her head, bowels & limbs. About a month before her death, which was on the 3^d of May 1787, her pulse became quick, and she had a little hecking cough; but without any discharge from her lungs. On my first visit to her, in the preceeding autumn, I had told her friends that I believed she had an abscess in her lungs. The want of cough & fever, afterwards, however gave me reason to suspect that I had been mistaken. The morning after her death, I received a message from her father, informing me, that it had been among the last requests of his daughter, that the cause of her death should be ascertained by my opening her body. I complied with this request, and in company with Dr Hall, examined her thorax. We found the left lobe of the lungs perfectly sound; the right lobe adhered to the pleura, in seperating of which, Dr Hall plunged his **C202** hand into a large sac, which contained about half a pint of purulent matter, and which had nearly destroyed the whole substance of the right lobe of the lungs.

---

[25] Benjamin Rush, "Pulmonary Consumption," in *Medical Inquiries and Observations*, 4th ed., 4 vols. (Philadelphia: Johnson & Warner, 1815), vol. 2, 49–99.

I have met with only two other cases of consumption, in which there was an absence of a quick pulse. In both of these the pulse was regular to the last day of life."

This case serves to show the impropriety of exercise, in pulmonic inflammation, as also the propriety of repeated bleedings, which probably might have removed her complaints on the second attack, as they did at first.

In July 1806, Mr D. Chenery of Falmouth, aged 30, of a good habit, was seized with pain in the left side, after great exertion in loading hay. He continued, however, to labour through the season, tho the pain was, at times, very tedious, for which a variety of patent medicines, of a stimulating inflaming nature were taken.

The 7th of Jan. 1807, he applied to me for advice. He then complained of pain in the side, particularly on any exertion, a harrassing cough, **C203** with expectoration of matter tinged with blood, flushed cheeks, febrile paroxysms, and night sweats, pulse 90 and rather tense. I prescribed bloodletting & a mercurial salivation. The former he objected to, lest it should weaken him, tho he was able to walk out and do some labour. The latter he complied with. After taking two grains of calomel night & morning for two weeks, a salivation was produced; as also a diarrhœa. His cough & expectoration then ceased, and his other complaints were mitigated.

The last of Jan. he was exposed to inclement weather, and his cough returned, with some pain in his side, tho no particular attention was paid to his complaints, till the 2^d of March, when I was again called. I found him able to walk out and pay some attention to business, pulse 100 and tense, with pain in the side. I then drew a pint of blood, gave a mercurial cathartic and applied an ounce of mercurial ointment to his pained side. His salivary glands were soon affected, and his complaints were alleviated.

On the 20th of March, he made an ox plow, in **C204** an open shed, exposed to cold & dampness. He was then seized with great pain in the side, a dry cough & difficulty of breathing; pulse hard & labouring. I was then soon called and drew 24 ounces of blood, which was buffy & cup form.[26] An ounce of Glaubers salts was given, and a blister applied. The fever & pain then abated, with his other complaints; and his pulse became natural.

The first of April, he was seized with the Influenza, attended with pain in the side, cough and soreness in the chest; pulse 90 & rather tense. I then drew

---

[26] Cup form refers to the raised edge and central depression of the buffy coat or crusta phlogistica; see "buffy/buffy coat" in the Glossary and a discussion of "sizy and buffy" in chapter 3 of the Introduction.

12 ounces of blood, gave a cathartic and applied blisters. —— His complaints were soon removed, and he was able to go abroad.

On the 28th, when I saw him last, he had suffered no return of his complaints, and his pulse was natural. He said his lungs felt perfectly well, tho he complained of some oppression at the stomach, having dined freely on veal, &c.

On the 30th, after setting up late in the evening, in social conversation, he complained of oppression at the breast, and suddenly expectorated a large quantity of purulent matter, when he shortly expired. —— Probably, for want of timely care, an abscess had formed in his lungs.

C205 In the course of my practice, I have met with many very similar cases, which have terminated in like manner, when stimulating means were used, and depleting remedies neglected. Sometimes an Empyema was produced, and the disease terminated favorably. But when bloodletting & purging with cooperative means were seasonably & duly employed, pulmonic inflammation was not followed by an abscess or ulceration of the lungs.

"An abscess in the lungs, says Dr Rush, is generally the consequence of a neglected or half cured pneumony." A similar observation might be made, relative to a neglected or half cured phthisis, that is, where depleting means were either neglected or used in too sparing a manner, as has often been the case, in my own practice, while ignorant of the inflammatory nature of the disease, and the most appropriate remedies. Obstruction & debility were then thought to be the primary & principal causes of pulmonary consumption. Therefore, **C206** deobstruents, so called, and stimulants were the chief means employed, while inflammatory action, unnoticed and of course unrestrained, was ravaging the lungs! Hence we may easily account for the frequent occurrence of abscesses, ulcers & tubercles, as natural effects of continued inflammation in the respiratory organs.

Chap. 7*th*

By consulting d^r Young's "Practical & Historical treatise on consumptive diseases,"[1] we find that many distinguished physicians, among the Ancients, made a liberal use of the lancet as well as cathartics, in pulmonary affections, and were attended with success.

A number of their practical observations will be extracted, as they are replete with instruction, and the work is in the hands of but few physicians among us.

"Hippocrates has enumerated, in different parts of his works, 360 years before the Christian era, several varieties of consumptive affections, including the consequences of some other pulmonary diseases; as well as atrophies, arising from different causes. He notices the short dry cough, with which genuine consumption usually begins and subsequent **C208** expectoration, the pain in the chest, temporary flushes of heat, diarrhœa, falling off of the hair, curvature of the nails, &c. The remedies which he recommends are caustics, cathartics & bleeding, with a diet chiefly of milk. He also advises to many simple vegetables of little efficacy."

"Celsus, who lived 20 years before Christ, has briefly recorded the practice of the most celebrated physicians & surgeons of the earliest ages. Hemoptysis is considered as one of the causes of purulent expectoration, for which bleeding may be performed several days, in succession, if the symptoms require it."

"The nature of hectic fever, as independant of consumption, is fully considered by Galen in various parts of his voluminous works. The indications to relieve the cough are bleeding occasionally; and evacuating the bowels with aloes, scammony &c. All that are curable are cured by bleeding & purging."

---

[1] Thomas Young, *A Practical and Historical Treatise on Consumptive Diseases, Deduced from Original Observations, and Collected from Authors of All Ages* (London: Underwood, 1815).

"Thessalus[2] is zealous for bleeding in hemoptysis. Benneverius,[3] says Shenk, has known Consumption to be cured by bleeding alone." Med. Obser. 1609.[4] **C209** "Our countryman Bennet, [5] 1654, may be considered as the earliest writer, on the subject of consumption, that can be quoted with perfect confidence. His experience of the disease, in his own person, gives additional authority to his own observations."

"With respect to the symptoms, he observes that a sound in breathing, like the ticking of a watch, is a mark of its commencement. The juices appear to be rendered unfit for nourishment by the excessive heat of the hectic fever. The lungs were sometimes found reduced to a state like mud or clay. In one case the lungs appeared softened, but otherwise sound. Indeed a decline without any organic disease, is very common in England, and generally fatal. The disease, when hereditary, tho incurable, is slow in its progress."

"Consumption is sometimes prevented by moderate bleeding at the nose, returning periodically. In one case an ounce or two flowed daily, and when it ceased for a season, the phthisical symptoms succeeded and continued till the bleeding was restored."

"In the hemoptysis, which often leads to consumption, he depends chiefly on bleeding, and the application of warmth to the extremities. After bleeding in the arm, if the symptoms continue, he bleeds in the foot."

---

[2] Thessalus (fl. 375 BC) was a student of Hippocrates and, according to Galen, was a Dogmatist incorporating speculative material into the Hippocratic teaching. Cecilia Charlotte Mettler and Fred A. Mettler, *History of Medicine; a Correlative Text, Arranged According to Subjects* (Philadelphia etc.: Blakiston, 1947), 329.

[3] Benneverius, probably Antonio Benivieni (Benivenius) (c. 1440–1502), used dissection to show normal and pathological anatomy. Mettler and Mettler, *History of Medicine; a Correlative Text, Arranged According to Subjects*, 249–50.

[4] Here Barker cites the medical observations of Johannes Schenck: Johannes Schenck von Grafenberg, *Paratereseon, Sive Observationum Medicarum, Rararum, Novarum, Admirabilium, &Amp; Monstrosarum, Volumen, Tomis Septem De Toto Homine Institutum. In Quo, Quae Medici . . . Abdita, Vulgo Incognita, Gravia, PericulosaqUe, Circa Humani Corporis Anatomen &Amp; Fabricam, Ejusdemque Morborum Causas, Signa, Eventus, &Amp; Curationes Accidere Compererunt, Exemplis Ut Plurimum &Amp; Historiis Proposita Exhibentur*, ed. Johann Georg Schenck (Francofurti: Rhode, 1609).

[5] Christopher Bennet (1617–1655). The *Bibliotheca Osleriana* entry 2010 refers to the DNB (*Dictionary of National Biography*) regarding the first edition of Bennet's book, *Theatri tabidorum vestibulum seu exercitationes dianoeticae cum historiis et experimentis demonstrativis* (London: Thomas Newcomb, 1654). "Its most valuable feature is the constant reference to cases observed and to dissections, not to authority." *Bibliotheca Osleriana* entry 6642 refers to William Osler's complete set of the DNB, a gift to him at a dinner in 1898 honoring him on his election as Fellow of the Royal Society: "after speeches a small hand-car was wheeled in with the 56 volumes of this work."

C210 "Neither salted nor dried meat, nor spices, should be admitted; and fasting should be, occasionally, enjoined, avoiding all violent exertion of the voice."

"Gideon Harvey,[6] 1672, London, mentions in his Morbus Anglicus, two cases of hemoptysis, cured by copious bleeding; and says that bleeding was successfully employed in consumption by Hippocrates & Galen. Colds & coughs, he says, are cured by bleeding and cathartics."

"Sydenham[7] recommends bleeding, with mild cathartics & pectorals, in confirmed consumption. He also prescribed daily riding, where there is no fever nor ulcer in the lungs."

"Stahl,[8] 1704, forbids balsams, and the antihectic poterii. He depends chiefly on bleeding, as the mode of treatment is to be principally directed to the cure of the hectic."

"Hofman[9] says, half of the cases of consumption originate in hemoptysis, and care must be taken not to stop the bleeding too hastily. Small bleedings often relieve the breathing in advanced cases; the reverse in earlier stage."

---

[6] Gideon Harvey (c.1640–1700), Gideon Harvey, *Morbus Anglicus, or, a Theoretick and Practical Discourse of Consumptions, and Hypochondriak Melancholy: Comprizing Their Nature, Subject, Kinds, Causes, Signs, Prognosticks, and Cures: Likewise a Discourse of Spitting of Blood, Its Differences, Causes, Signs, Prognosticks, and Cure* (London: William Thackeray, 1672). One medical historian described Gideon Harvey as "a pompous English physician who considered himself something of a leader of medical opinion." Mettler and Mettler, *History of Medicine; a Correlative Text, Arranged According to Subjects*, 74–75.

[7] Thomas Sydenham (1624–1689) has been referred to as the "designer of modern clinical medicine." Thomas Sydenham, Samuel Johnson, and John Swan, *The Entire Works of Dr. Thomas Sydenham, Newly Made English from the Originals: Wherein the History of Acute and Chronic Diseases, and the Safest and Most Effectual Methods of Treating Them, Are Faithfully, Clearly, and Accurately Delivered. To Which Are Added, Explanatory and Practical Notes, from the Best Medicinal Writers* (London: Printed for Edward Cave, at St. John's Gate, 1742), 613–14. For an overview of Sydenham, see John H. Talbott, *A Biographical History of Medicine* (New York: Grune & Stratton, 1970), 125–28; David Riesman, *Thomas Sydenham, Clinician* (New York: P. B. Hoeber, Inc., 1926).

[8] George Ernst Stahl (1660–1734) developed a system of medicine and chemistry in Germany. Georg Ernst Stahl, *Medicinae Dogmatico-Systematicae Partis Theoreticae Sectio I [&II]* (Halae: Orphanotrophei, 1707).

[9] Friedrich Hoffmann (1660–1742) was from 1694 professor at the University of Halle and an iatrochemist; that is, a person seeking to provide chemical solutions to various diseases. He was a friend of the English chemist and physicist, Robert Boyle (1627–1691). William Cullen was influenced by Hoffmann, particularly his neural concept of disease with changes in normal tone altered by the nervous system. Arturo Castiglioni, *A History of Medicine*, 2nd ed. (New York: Alfred A. Knopf, 1947), 584–86; Andrew Wear, "Medicine in Early Modern Europe, 1500–1700," in *The Western Medical Tradition: 800 B.C.–1800 A.D.*, ed. Lawrence I. Conrad and Wellcome Institute for the History of Medicine (Cambridge; New York: Cambridge University Press, 1995), 358–59, 93.

C211

Boerhaave[10] observes that people of a consumptive habit, are liable to sweat during their sleep, from any slight cause without the actual presence of hectic fever. Consumption from ulcerated lungs, he says should be treated with a large bleeding every third day, and repeated four times, or till the inflammatory crust has entirely disappeared, together with a very temperate way of living & dieting, to which milk properly belongs. 1701.

"In Dover's Legacy to his Country, 4th edition, London 1733,[11] we find authority for a very active & somewhat hazardous practice in consumption, and some other diseases. It consists in the frequent repetition of bleeding, in small quantities, which, he says, is more beneficial than horse exercise, and he supports his opinion by the relation of several cases; one in which there was a considerable fetid expectoration, & hemoptysis, was cured by bleeding every other day, and the cold bath." ****C212****

He mentions a pleurisy, in which 260 ounces of blood were taken away with success. Another case, in which the patient lost six ounces, every day, for a fortnight, then every other day. Afterwards every third and fifth day. —— A third patient was bled, at least fifty times. They did well."

"Van Sweiten[12] favours the practice of frequent bleedings in Consumption, and says that he knew a lady, who lost several ounces of blood almost daily, and sometimes twice a day, for several years, and survived, tho much reduced."

---

[10] Hermann Boerhaave (1668–1738) was a professor at the Medical Faculty at Leiden, Holland, from 1709 to 1730. He systematized medical knowledge, developed a system of chemistry, and had a great influence on English-speaking medical students. Roy Porter, "The Eighteenth Century," in *The Western Medical Tradition: 800 B.C.–1800 A.D*, ed. Lawrence I. Conrad and Wellcome Institute for the History of Medicine (Cambridge; New York: Cambridge University Press, 1995), 453; Herman Boerhaave, *Boerhaave's Aphorisms: Concerning the Knowledge and Cure of Diseases Translatd from the Last Edition Printed in Latin at Leyden, 1715*, Classics of Medicine Library (London: R. Cowse and W. Innys in St. Paul's Church-Yard, 1715); Herman Boerhaave, *New Method of Chemistry; Including the Theory and Practice of That Art . . . To Which Is Prefix'd a Critical History of Chemistry and Chemists . . . Translated from the Printed Edition . . . By P. Shaw,* (London: J. Osborn and T. Longman, 1727). For a brief overview of Boerhaave, see Edgar Ashworth Underwood, *Boerhaave's Men at Leyden and After* (Edinburgh: Edinburgh University Press, 1977), 1–14; Talbott, *A Biographical History of Medicine*, 170–72.

[11] Thomas Dover (1662–1742) received an A.B. from Oxford in 1684 and an M.B. from Cambridge in 1687, and studied under Sydenham. His major work "was not profound judged by 18th century standards . . . [and might be thought of as a] housewive's medical friend." Talbott, *A Biographical History of Medicine*, 167–70. Thomas Dover and Augustin Belloste, *The Ancient Physician's Legacy to His Country: Being What He Has Collected Himself in Forty-Nine Years Practice, or, an Account of the Several Diseases Incident to Mankind . . . Design'd for the Use of All Private Families* (London: Printed for the relict of the late R. Bradly, 1733).

[12] Gerhard Van Swieten (1700–1772) studied under Boerhaave and then taught in Vienna.

"Stoll of Vienna, 1777,[13] disapproves of balsams & the bark, where there is any inflammatory affection, and considers riding, in such cases, as improper as in a pleurisy. But in Dyspeptic Atrophy, with habitual cough, it may have succeeded.

The best remedies in the former case, are small & repeated bleedings. From a prejudice against bleeding, many colds have been converted into consumptions."

C213

"The works of Dr Cullen[14] of Scotland, 1775, contain some original matter which require the careful consideration of the rational practitioner. Evacuations of all kinds, particularly bloodletting, in consumption, a low regimen, and blisters to the breast or back, followed by issues are recommended, and active exercise discouraged."

"D[r] Mudge's[15] works, London 1779, contain several interesting remarks on Consumption. A person who had recovered from this disease, died of the small pox, some years after and was found to have lost the greater part of the right lung.

For hemoptysis he recommends bleeding. Emetics are sometimes useful by exciting nausea. He employed vapours by an inhaler, in catarrhal cough successfully. But if these remedies fail, he recommends, as in consumption, occasional bleeding; a large scapulary issue, and a diet of milk & vegetables. He was himself cured of a consumption with hemoptysis. He suffered a caustic to be made, nearly three inches in diameter, which contained fifty peas."[16]

---

[13] Maximilian Stoll (1742–1787) studied theology and later medicine, working at the Vienna Clinic. He stressed the importance of the patient's history and daily progress records. Maximilian Stoll, *Rationis Medendi in Nosocomio Practico Vindobenensi* (1777).

[14] William Cullen (1710–1790) of Glasgow and later Edinburgh, taught many of the future leaders of medicine. His teaching and writings influenced many, including Benjamin Rush, William Shippen, and Samuel Bard. Talbott, *A Biographical History of Medicine*, 244–46. William Cullen, *First Lines of the Practice of Physic with Supplementary Notes, Including More Recent Improvements in the Practice of Medicine by Peter Reid*, two volumes in one (Brookfield: E. Mirriam & Co. for Isaiah Thomas, 1807).

[15] John Mudge (1721–1793) worked on innovations in telescope mirrors as well as medicine. John Mudge, *A Radical and Expeditious Cure for a Recent Catarrhous Cough: Preceded by Some Observations on Respiration, with Occasional and Practical Remarks on Some Other Diseases of the Lungs; to Which Is Added a Chapter on the Vis Vitae, So Far as It Is Concerned in Preserving and Reinstating the Health of an Animal; Accompanied with Some Strictures on the Treatment of Compound Fractures*, ed. Edmund Allen (Madrid: Real Colegio de Cirugía de San Carlos, 1779), 63–64.

[16] This is called a "pea issue," that is, a small cut or artificial ulcer made by a physician, into which a pea, or in this case, fifty peas, may be placed to keep the issue open and draining. See Glossary entry for "issue."

C214

"The compendium of <u>Vogel</u>, is an elaborate & useful compilation, 1783.[17] He considers <u>hectic</u>, as no otherwise distinguished from slow fever, than by the greater severity of the symptoms. In almost all hectics, the lungs are sooner or later affected. Bark must be avoided, in hectic fever, where there is any tendency to inflammation, obstruction or biliary derangement; even venesection will not render its use safe in such cases."

"D[r] <u>Percival</u>,[18] 1789, says that "sweats & diarrhœa may tend to relieve a plethora, as bleeding would do; and that rising before the sweat takes place aggravates the fever."

Thus it appears, that the lancet has been liberally used, in pulmonary consumption, by scientific & experienced physicians, in different parts of Europe, from the days of the venerable Hippocrates, to the latter part of the 18th century, or the days of the unfortunate Brown,[19] who, by his excentric notions & heated imagination, spun out a cobweb theory of diseases, which fascinated a considerable ****C215**** number of physicians, both in Europe & America, so that the lancet, and other depleting means were greatly neglected, even in inflammatory diseases, and stimulants, chiefly of spiritous liquors, unhappily substituted, greatly to the injury of mankind, and deterioration of the practice of physic, for a time, viz the closing part of the last century. Indeed the enchantment is not as yet fully broken but continues in a greater or less degree, both in Europe & America, among people, as well as physicians; so that great perplexity & discord often attend consultations, and many greatly suffer, by the disuse of depleting means; ~~and~~ as well as by the use of those which are

---

[17] Samuel Gottlieb von Vogel (1750–1837) was considered the father of the German sea bath. Thomas Young cites Vogel on the bottom of page 319: "S. G. VOGELS handbuch der practischen arzneywissenschaft. About 1783. Ed. 2. Stendal. 1785 . . . II. 141." Young, *A Practical and Historical Treatise on Consumptive Diseases, Deduced from Original Observations, and Collected from Authors of All Ages*, 319–21.

[18] Thomas Percival (1740–1804) was a dissenter who trained at the University of Edinburgh and practiced and taught in Manchester. Barker is probably referring to Thomas Percival, *Essays Medical and Experimental*, 4th ed. (Warrington: W. Eyres, for J. Johnson 1788). Percival is best known for his writings on medical ethics. Talbott, *A Biographical History of Medicine*, 271–74. Thomas Percival and Joseph Meredith Toner Collection (Library of Congress), *Extracts from the Medical Ethics of Dr. Percival* (Philadelphia: Clark & Raser, printers, 1823).

[19] John Brown (1735–1788) trained at the University of Edinburgh and was a student of Cullen. He developed a system of medicine, the once popular Brunonian doctrine, with its disease categories of sthenic and asthenic and its use of alcohol and opiates, discussed elsewhere. Porter, "The Eighteenth Century," 378–79, 95; Talbott, *A Biographical History of Medicine*, 472–74. John Brown, *The Elements of Medicine; or a Translation of the Elementa Medicinae Brunonis* (London: J. Johnson, 1788).

stimulating, not only in pulmonary consumption, & hectic; but in Typhous Fever, which resembles it in many respects; so that experienced physicians have sometimes found it difficult to distinguish hectic from a common slow fever, or typhus mitior. The difference appears to be, chiefly, in the <u>seat</u> of the disease.

C216

"I doubt not, says Dr Prichard,[20] physician to the Infirmary, and to St Peter's Hospital in Bristol, that Dr Armstrong's excellent work on Typhous fever, will be productive of much benefit to the community, by directing the attention of medical practitioners to the most powerful resources which they possess, for arresting the career, or mitigating the violence of that formidable malady. There is, however a deeply rooted prejudice in the public and even in a considerable part of our profession, against the evacuation of blood in continued fever. I ought to observe, that the vulgar prejudice against bleeding in various disorders, is fostered & encouraged, by some medical practitioners, who, to the disgrace of their profession, seek a short lived popularity by coinciding with, and putting themselves on the side of the prevailing notions! An instance of this kind lately fell under my notice, in the case of a gentleman of plethoric habit, labouring under epilepsy, for whom, with the advice of another physician, I prescribed ****C217**** venesection. This man, afterwards went to South Devon, where he resides, and there fell under the care of a physician & apothecary, professing extensive practice, in that district. These persons assured their patient, that drawing blood in epilepsy, is a practice fraught with the most imminent peril; and that the frequent use of bleeding, is a most dangerous innovation on the more cautious methods of the old school; also that the whole tribe of scribblers, who are continually filling the medical journals with such alarming accounts of their sanguinary proceedings, deserve to be hanged up & gibbetted without mercy, as little better than

---

[20] James Cowles Prichard (1786–1848), born to a Quaker family, took an M.D. degree at Edinburgh University and studied at Trinity College, Cambridge, St. John's College, and Trinity College, Oxford. He opened a private practice in Bristol in 1810 and also served as a physician to St. Peter's Hospital, a poorhouse and lunatic asylum, and later at the Bristol Infirmary. He became a fellow of the Royal Society in 1827. He was enthusiastic about the benefits of bloodletting, counterirritation, and trepanning and interested in mental illness. His main interests in addition to medicine included anthropology and ethnology. Augstein, H. F. "Prichard, James Cowles (1786–1848), physician and ethnologist." *Oxford Dictionary of National Biography*. 23 Sep. 2004; Accessed 20 Apr. 2020. https://www-oxforddnb-com.ezproxy.library.tufts.edu/view/10.1093/ref:odnb/9780198614128.001.0001/odnb-9780198614128-e-22776. H. F. Augstein, "Prichard, James Cowles (1786–1848), Physician and Ethnologist" (Oxford: Oxford University Press, 2004).

licensed murderers! ——I have detected many other instances, in which this kind of <u>ruse</u>, has been exercised by crafty persons. But I have generally had the pleasure of observing, that stratagems in medical practice, at length, defeat themselves; and that the fair combatant is ultimately left in undisputed possession **C218** of the field. It is therefore much to be desired, that those physicians, who have had oppertunities of putting their practice to the test of experience, would communicate the results of their observations to the public. The greater the range of facts which shall be set before the faculty, the more speedily will that conclusion be obtained, which sooner or later must necessarily follow, namely, a settled and universal conviction, that bleeding, and other antiphlogistic means, are not less appropriate in typhus fever, than in pneumonia, tho the adoption of them requires greater circumspection, in the former disease than in the latter.

From the 12th of Jan. 1817, to the 12th of May following, 41 cases of typhus occurred in St Peters Hospital. Five, advanced in years, & infirm died. All the rest, were bled, purged & took calomel; within ten days, after the attack, and recovered. The Apothecary was attacked with this fever, and drew two pounds of blood from his arm. On the next day, he was nearly well."

Edinburgh Medical Journal.[21]

C219

About 1788, when Browns Elements of Medicine, first appeared in Maine, they were read by others, besides physicians, so that a conjoint prejudice was formed against the lancet and other depleting means in almost every disease; for debility was considered as the cause; therefore, stimulants were readily resorted to, among which brandy was thought to be the most eligible, and liberally dispersed, to all orders of men & ages, whether sick or well.

Some distinguished characters, among physicians, Lawyers & Divines, soon fell victims to these spiritous potations!!!

Besides the fashionable use of spiritous liquors in our families, which was considered as praiseworthy & commendable, they were used by consumptive invalids, labouring under hectic fever, with its usual train of symptoms, together with beef tea, and an occasional steak, which accorded with the Brunonian school; a mode of instruction **C220** fraught with the most imminent peril; and a very "dangerous innovation on the more cautious methods of the old school," where venesection and other antiphlogistic means were successfully employed.

---

[21] J. C. Prichard, "Cases of Typhus Fever, with Observations on the Nature and Treatment of the Disease," *Edinburgh Medical and Surgical Journal* 13 (1817), 413–27.

The Brunonian mode of treatment, however, was generally pursued, by persons labouring under pulmonary consumption; for they seldom consulted physicians. Indeed few physicians among us, could be found, at that time, who used the lancet, or any antiphlogistic means, in this disease; but preferred the stimulating plan; and advised to such articles as could easily be procured by the patient or his friends, at any retailors shop, who judged themselves capable of administring them without medical advice.

Thus things were conducted by many, till 1798, a term of about ten years, when Dr Rush's "Inquiry into the causes and cure of the Pulmonary Consumption," printed in 1793, was brought to Portland and read by me, as well as by some of my Brunonian brethren. But our prejudice against the use of the lancet, in this disease, was such that very little attention was paid to **C221** the advice of this learned & experienced physician, till the beginning of the 19th century, when Dr Tracy's patient, who was considerably advanced in Phthisis pulmonalis, and considered as hopeless, received a cure from a spontaneous hemorrhage of blood from the nose, whose case has already been related.[22] This unexpected recovery, in consequence of the salutary "efforts of nature," induced us to believe that an imitation of nature, in similar cases, would be justifiable.

Dr Rush's Inquiry was then read, with greater attention, and two cases of spontaneous hemorrhages of blood from the lungs to the quantity of a quart, were found; but to the joy & surprise of the friends of these patients, they both recovered.

About that time, several other cases of spontaneous hemorrhages from the lungs, in consumptive patients, were related to me from physicians and others, in which the disease terminated favourably. ——These events induced us to think on our ways, and acknowledge our folly.
C222

Since the beginning of the 19th century, bloodletting and other cooperative means have been used by many physicians in Maine & elsewhere, in pulmonary consumption, and when "seasonably and duly employed," cures have been effected.[23] On the contrary when appropriate remedies have been

---

[22] Dr. Tracy, "Remarkable Case of Phthisis Pulmonalis, Wherein a Profuse Spontaneous Hemorrhage Seemed to Be Useful: In a Letter from Dr. Tracy, of Norwich, (Connecticut) to Dr. Mitchill, Dated July 16, 1802," *Medical Repository* 6 (1803): 256–58.

[23] For example, in an 1801 letter from Dr. Benjamin Vaughn of Hallowell, Maine, to Benjamin Rush: "Bleeding is now in such repute in our town, that our patients send to the doctor not for his advice, but to be blooded." Manuscript Correspondence of Benjamin Rush UV18, at the Historical Society of Pennsylvania. June 21, 1801 (MSS 55, p. 3).

neglected or too sparingly used, disorganization of the lungs has frequently taken place in a few months, where the constitution was strong, and inflammatory action considerable. In these cases the disease generally proved fatal, unless it terminated either in Empiema, or the loss of a particularly affected lung, by expectoration or absorption.

From 1790, to 1800, when little use was made of the lancet, or other depleting means, in pulmonary affections, I met with more cases of Empiema, than in twice ten preceeding years, chiefly in my own practice, owing I believe to the sparing use which was made of the lancet in pulmonary complaints. **C223**

When the disease terminated in Empiema I was frequently successful in discharging the matter by making an aperture between the ribs; and gained some credid [sic] of curing the patient, while I deserved none; for had depleting means been properly used, the disease would not have terminated in this hazardous manner.

Since 1800, I have met with but one case of Empiema, which originated from a pleuritic affection, treated by a patent Doctor who made no use of the lancet nor any depleting means. He accounted for the disease from <u>cold</u>, and considered <u>heating</u> means, such as cayenne pepper &c, as the most proper remedies!! ——The matter found its way between the ribs, and was discharged without surgical aid, three weeks after the fever had subsided, and his appetite returned. He soon recovered.

In consumptive habits, where proper means have been neglected, ~~in pulmonary consumption~~ the disease has continued, in some instances, months & years, attended with **C224** a moderate hectic, hot palms, stricture across the chest, and a burning heat in the vitals, with occasional pain in the side, cough and expectoration of mucus, pus & blood, particularly in the spring months; but, as the summer approached, there was some alleviation of their complaints, for a time. Yet the disease has at length been eradicated, chiefly by spontaneous or artificial bleedings, repeated cathartics, and a mercurial salivation.

A number of cases of this kind will be related, as they have occurred in the practice of physicians, in different parts of the Union, which will serve to show that the disease is curable, even when "<u>seated and confirmed</u>" properly treated, by scientific physician; and when due attention has been paid to their rules, by patients and nurses.

Chap. 8.

AS THE MEDICAL MUSEUM, as well as the Medical Repository are rare books in Maine, and the former is discontinued, I have been requested to extract some of the most extraordinary cases of consumption, from these voluminous works, which cannot conveniently be purchased, by young physicians.[1]

Case of Phthisis Pulmonalis communicated to Dr Rush, by Dr Harris.

Belle Fort. Sep.20th 1803.

Dear Sir.

It is with heart felt joy, I now have the satisfaction of informing you of the salutary effect of your prescription in pulmonary consumption, the subject of which is myself.

Last spring I was attacked with Phthisis Pulmonalis, from being exposed thoughtlessly to a current of air, when in full perspiration, from exercise in the garden. I was in a great heat & the sweat dripped from me, when I opened my breast, bare to the fresh breeze, then blowing. Its effect was a sudden chill, pain in my breast, wheezing, cough, and soon after expectoration supervened, with copious night sweats, which produced great exhaustion, and wore me down to a mere **C226** skeleton. I had no prospect of subduing the disease, but looked forward for it to end only with my life; when, about three weeks since, I was affected, after being exposed to cold, with a violent peripneumony, from which I had little prospect of recovery. In this situation your letters occurred to me, ~~written~~ published in the Medical Repository vol. 5.th I was then determined, at all events to try the effect. Danger from the violence of the disease

---

[1] This chapter was probably written between 1811 and 1824. The (Philadelphia) *Medical Museum*, the second medical journal published in the United States, survived from 1804 to 1811. The *Medical Repository* (also known as *Mitchill's Repository*), the first medical journal in the United States, was published in New York City from 1797 to 1824. The editor's "Circular Address" in 1797 requested "histories of such diseases as reign in your particular places of residence, at each and every season of the year." *Medical Repository* 1 (1797): ix. Twelve articles by Dr. Jeremiah Barker were published in the *Medical Repository* between 1798 and 1807, most dealing with diseases in the County of Cumberland, District of Maine, during a particular season or year. At least one letter by Barker was published in the *Medical Museum* (1807).

would not admit the gradual process of the calomel. I took it as copiously as I could bear it, and rubbed on the mercurial ointment on my side & thighs; at the same time bled copiously, thirty ounces a day, for several days; blistered the whole breast, depleted in every possible manner, to give the mercury liberty to operate. In 48 hours it answered the purpose; for as soon as my mouth got sore, the pains gradually left me, cough ceased, expectoration abated, and every pulmonary symptom began to disappear. I had expectorated, in some days, nearly half a pint, and **C227** coughed incessantly. Now, I cough, none of any consequence, and do not expectorate more than two or three times in the day, and that with ease; my appetite has returned, and every prospect of health is great.

Whether I should continue the ptyalism or use tonics, I am rather at a loss to know; my debility is very great, not being able yet to walk alone. I can sit up a little. From the violence of the peripneumony in a great measure, I carried the spitting to upwards of two quarts daily, for some time. Now I do not spit more than half a pint, and feel quite well. Should I not get cold, I believe no doubt remains, but that the mercury has conquered the disease, which I believe nothing else yet known could have done; and for the discovery & publication of which, I acknowledge myself indebted to you, for the rescue of my life. May God bless you.

I am with deep gratitude,

Dr Benj. Rush.   William Harris.

Medical Museum, vol. 3.[2]

C228
History of three cases of Phthisis Pulmonalis.
By Dr William Watson of Lewistown, Penn.
Communicated to Dr. John Redman Coxe[3]
"On the 8th of Feb. 1804, I was called to visit E. W. Hale Esq. councellor at law, about 27 years of age, who, a few days before, had been attacked with pneumonia,

---

[2] William Harris, "Case of Phthsis Pulmonalis, Cured by Mercury," *Philadelphia Medical Museum* 3 (1807): 119–20.

[3] John Redman Coxe (1773–1864), born in Trenton, New Jersey, was taught by his grandfather, Dr. Redman in Philadelphia. He continued his studies in London, Edinburgh, and Paris, returning to work with Benjamin Rush. He founded and edited the *Medical Museum*, 1805–1811, and was professor of chemistry and later of materia medica and pharmacy at the University of Pennsylvania. Coxe wrote several books, including *The Philadelphia Medical Dictionary*, (Philadelphia, Thomas Dobson and Son) 1808, 2nd ed. 1817. Howard A. Kelly and Walter L. Burrage, *American Medical Biographies* (Baltimore: The Norman, Remington Company, 1920), 254–55; Martin Kaufman, Stuart Galishoff, and Todd Lee Savitt, *Dictionary of American Medical Biography*, 2 vols. (Westport, CT: Greenwood Press, 1984), 163.

from great exposure to cold. He was able to walk about; but, contrary to his usual appearance, was very much dejected. He complained of lassitude, fever, a hard & dry cough; but without pain in any part of the thorax; pulse small & tense. I conceived his disease to be a bad catarrh; but having suspected, for some months previous, that his lungs were in a very weak state, I felt a good deal apprehensive of the event.

He was bled and took an emetic of ipecac. His blood shew evident marks of inflammation; and his pulse rose after the operation. I left him a few pills of digitalis & opium; and as I lived twelve miles distant, directed him to be bled next morning if the cough & stricture were not relieved. He was bled the next morning and I visited him on the 10ᵗʰ. He had found no **C229** relief from the remedies mentioned; and the indication for bleeding was greater than at any time before. I bled him, and found the blood coated as in pleurisy. I left him some antimonial powders, composed of nitre, tartar emetic & calomel, in the proportion directed by Dʳ Rush. He was to take one every second hour till my return; and also to be bled every day, if the fever & stricture were not abated.

On the 12ᵗʰ he seemed much better; was able to walk about; but as the cough was still hard & dry, with stricture, he was again bled and directed to have the operation performed daily till he could expectorate with freedom. The powders were repeated so as to purge and sweat him. On the 17ᵗʰ he sent for me, I found him much worse: he was unable to leave his bed, fever very high, cheeks efflorescent, and his pulse frequent with tension. I bled him, and the next morning, bled him again. The blood was very inflammatory, but still no pain in the chest. The antimonial powders were continued, which sweat & purged him; but neither the cough, fever, nor stricture were relieved. I visited him on the 20ᵗʰ, when he complained much of **C230** weakness and a distressing tickling cough. His pulse still indicated bloodletting, continuing inflammatory. I gave him a mixture of nitre & spermacetis, in the yolk of an egg, for the tickling cough. The arterial action was now less convulsive; fever much moderated; but the cough and oppression of the precordia continued with much distress. From the outset of the disease, he had expectorated, after coughing, a little thin acrid matter mixed with some blood. I now applied a blistering plaister over each lobe of the lungs, so large as to cover the whole anterior portion of the thorax. While the blisters were rising he sweated most profusely. The blisters rose well and excited severe strangury,[4] which I did not attempt to relieve as long as it could be bourne, having observed, in fevers, the happiest effects from this symptom, in determining excitement from parts

---

4 Cantharides, or Spanish Fly, had been a commonly used blistering agent since ancient times and was known to have a side effect of stranguria, or urinary obstruction, due to irritation and blistering of the urinary system. See also Glossary entry.

more essential to life. The strangury was removed by spiritus nitri dulcis. The cough was now very distressing, and expectoration difficult, and there was a total change in the action of the pulse. It was faltering & thread like; **C231** and the coughing harassed him so much, that I was apprehensive he could not survive many hours. Profuse sweating attended with faintness. Laudanum was prescribed, and to be repeated after short intervals, to prevent the torpor of indirect debility. He took a little Madaira wine frequently and sago gruel for food; with these he was supported for several days. From his cough, hoarseness, stricture, and the matter expectorated, being streaked with blood, I was satisfied the disease had degenerated into phthisis pulmonalis. At this time he was as much emaciated as I had ever known a patient to be in the typhus state of the same disease.

It was then twenty two days from the period of attack, and I had no hopes of a recovery. He was unable to change his position in bed. A severe hectic visited him every afternoon, and he could not speak to be understood. He took wine, laudanum and sometimes bark; but they afforded a very temporary relief.

I had seen, in the Medical Repository, Dr Rush's letters to Dr Miller on the efficacy of mercury in pulmonary consumption; and had attempted to relieve others with this medicine; **C232** but they were too much exhausted before they would submit to its administration. I now began it with Mr Hale, but doubted much whether ptyalysm could be excited. I feared that the excitability was too far exhausted to favour the operation of any remedy.

Half an ounce of strong mercurial ointment was directed to be rubbed into his sides and breast every night; and two grains of calomel, with half a grain of opium to be taken every fourth hour. This prescription was attended to, till the 26th, when I saw him. The mercury had produced no affection of the stomach or intestines. He had become costive. In addition to the other directions, another half ounce of the ointment was to be rubbed into the same parts every morning. On the 28th, two glisters were used, which removed the constipation. The mercury was continued without any evident effect. Four grains of calomel were then directed night & morning in addition, mixed with honey, to be dissolved in the mouth, in order to excite action in the gums & salivary glands.
C233

On the 4th of March, there was no symptoms of mercurial disease, the medicine did not even purge him. The mercury had now been taken for eleven days in the quantities mentioned. He ceased to take in internally; but two ounces of mercurial ointment were directed to be rubbed into his sides, breasts, and thighs, every 24 hours, and Madaira wine with laudanum to be given so as to support the continued excitement of the medicine. They were prescribed with the intention of raising the system to that point, which would favour the salutary operation of mercury; but without effect. The cough & expectoration of pus and florid blood continued and the hectic fever was very high every afternoon.

The vascular system and muscles were in an extreme state of debility. Bark did not agree with his stomach, so that wine, soups and opium were given as substitutes.

On the 14th I consulted Dr Harris, who I had heard was successful in the cure of phthisis with mercury. He advised to use more durable stimulants, as columbo & gentian, **C234** with the application of flannel bandages saturated with mercurial ointment, to the breast & sides, after removing the skin by blisters; and to nauseate the stomach with tartar emetic to excite a new action. The nauseating dose was used and the saturated bandages were applied. Calomel was rubbed into the gums, and mercurial ointment into his throat. The bandages were renewed, once in 24 hours.

On the 26th his mouth & breath indicated the action of the mercury; but his pulmonary symptoms continued with violence.

I visited him on the 4th of April when the salivation had begun.

Thus, after having spent <u>forty two</u> days, in the most assiduous attempts to salivate him, with unspeakable joy, I succeeded, after having prescribed two hundred & twenty two grains of calomel; and thirty ounces of mercurial ointment, composed of two parts of Hog's lard and one part of quicksilver.

8th He salivated about two pints in 24 hours. The cough had abated in frequency & violence. **C235** The saturated bandages were suffered to remain, but the calomel & opium were omitted.

12th The salivation had increased to three pints, the cough easy and the quantity of pus diminished.

16th The mouth & fauces very much swelled, salivation very profuse. The columbo, &c. were with held, and laudanum was directed, with a gargle of borax & honey in water.

19th The discharge of purulent matter ceased, and the cough had entirely left him.

At this time from two to three quarts of saliva daily flowed from his mouth; emaciation extreme, and he was unable to sit up, tho his appetite was good. He now took columbo, in infusion, cordial diet & laudanum. The saturated bandages were removed the first of May. At this time he could walk the room, tho the salivation had not abated. The salivation abated the 11ᵗʰ. of May and ceased the 15ᵗʰ of June. His recovery to health was rapid, and he became more ~~rapid~~ lusty than he had ever been before."

C236 "On the 10ᵗʰ of April, 1804, I was called to visit Mʳˢ Irvine, a married lady of delicate habit, aged 30 years, who had been afflicted with cough & pain of the chest, for 18 months before. She was unable to sit up, much ema- ciated, with incessant cough and purulent expectoration, no appetite, hectic fever in the afternoon, pulse quick & irregular; oppression & dyspnœa, on the slightest motion. She had borne three children, and from the birth of the last, she dated her disease.

I drew a few ounces of blood, gave the antimonial powders, and directed two drachms of mercurial ointment to be rubbed into her sides & breast every night. On the 13ᵗʰ. her mouth became sore, the gums swelled and a salivation took place.

About two o'clock the next morning, I was sent for, in the utmost haste. When I arrived I found the attendants supporting her in bed, in a fainting fit. In her sleep, she had been attacked with menorrhagia, and the discharge was so profuse as to induce deliquium, before it was discovered.

C237

No pulse could be felt, and the hemorrhage continued. I gave her a little lau- danum, and directed one of the attendants to introduce flour into the vagina, and press upon it with the hand. As soon as she could swallow, I gave kino & alum. The discharge, however, did not abate. I was afraid to apply cold water, by reason of the mercury; but I soon saw it must be used or my patient must sink. Cold water was then applied to the abdomen, perineum, &c. The win- dows were opened; and she was directed to drink cold water. The disease abated soon after, and ceased in two or three days. I looked forward with much anxiety for the consequence. On the 15ᵗʰ her throat, fauces, tongue &c swelled astonish- ingly; but her breathing was not much impeded; and I was now relieved from my apprehensions. The tumefaction prevented swallowing; so that for ten days she was supported by injections of broath. The swelling then gave way to blis- tering on the back of the neck, and around the throat, with borax as a gargle.

22ᵈ Salivated about a pint daily; the mercurial frictions were continued. May 1ˢᵗ **C238** Salivation profuse, cough & purulent expectoration much abated. 9ᵗʰ cough & expectoration ceased. 14ᵗʰ mercurial frictions omitted, and an infusion of columbo with wine ~~with~~ and a cordial diet were taken. From this time she recovered strength daily. The salivation left her the 7ᵗʰ of June. By the 1ᵗ of August, her strength was quite restored. She is now more healthy and strong than she has been for several years."

Mrs Lyon, aged 23 years, put her self under my care in May 1804. She had laboured under phthisis pulmonalis about two years, with the usual train of symptoms. Mercury was used both externally & internally, and blisters were applied, as in the case of Mr Hale; but without effect, although continued six weeks. Columbo & opiates were also used to as little advantage, when she died, a lamentable instance of too late application; ——the excitability being exhausted below that point in which mercury will excite its peculiar salutary action."

Medical Museum vol. 2.[5]

C239

An account of the effects of Labour, as an auxiliary, in the cure of Pulmonary Consumption. In a letter from the Rev. Dr Samuel K. Jennings, Virg. to Dr Benjamin Rush.

Dear Sir.

That theory only is to be considered a rational one, which is supported by facts, and will admit of the most extensive practical utility. If the following facts can be of any service to you, it will afford me singular satisfaction to have communicated them.

I myself furnish the first case. My maternal grandmother, my mother, five of my sisters, and four of her brothers, my sister being my mother's first child, and a brother next in succession to me by birth, all of them have been swept off the stage of life, in the course of my recollection, by the fatal disease Phthisis Pulmonalis.

From my youth up to the age of twenty-nine, I was sensible of great debility of the lungs, and was never, during that time, able to call aloud, read or sing, with the ease which **C240** is common to other people. I had generally lived a studious & sedentary life, except that I had been the two last years engaged particularly in the practice of physic. An offer was at that time made me to take charge of an academy. For the sake of gaining more leisure for the purpose of reading & study, I accepted the offer. In the meantime, I had been three years, occasionally employed in speaking publickly on religious subjects. From this last engagement, I considered my lungs to have gained some strength. It followed, however, that study & confinement did less agree with me than formerly. I could perceive a daily declension, and, at length, having been caught in a moderate rain, I was seized with a very severe

---

[5] William Watson, "History of Several Cases of Phthisis Pulmonalis Treated with Mercury," *Philadelphia Medical Museum* 2, no. 1 (1806): 6–15.

& obstinate cough. I was bled again & again to no purpose. After considerable depletion, opium was tried in vain. Debility, the cough, and every inflammatory symptom increased. I had recourse to riding, took a journey of several weeks, and continued to let blood as often as the pains were severe, **C241** but still in vain. In the meantime, I obtained your Inquiries, and immediately turned my attention to the subject which most concerned me. After having read carefully, that part of your work, I pursued the following plan.

I let blood moderately, every third day, especially if affected with inflammatory symptoms, until, with the previous bloodlettings, I had been bled fifteen times, in the course of five weeks. By this time, I was much reduced; but my cough was no better. I then had recourse to the use of the axe and to Labour of the severest kind. I could not at the time repeat ten strokes without rest. It would seem, in the first instance, to increase my cough. The result was, that in two weeks, I was nearly recovered. Finding much amendment, I grew remiss in my labour, and in a few weeks relapsed, and was nearly as ill as before. Two bleedings and similar labour, however, finally ~~recovered~~ restored me to good health; and I can now sing aloud, on a sharp key; can speak two hours together, and consider myself freed from every symptom of that disease.

C242

My wife furnishes a second recent case. Her mother, and one of two only sisters, have died of the same disease very lately. She was in her youth an active industrious woman, and exercised laboriously. But for several years past she has been declining; so that from a fleshy & healthy woman, she became pale, sickly, emaciated, valetudinarian. The last summer, she brought a fine son. By suckling him she declined in an unusual degree; was at length taken with a cough, chills at noon and in the evening, night sweats &c. I bled her as often as I could find her pulse tense; advised her, contrary to her inclinations, to use ~~severe~~ servile labour. She took my advice. Her cough is nearly removed, and I have no doubt but she will recover.

I should not have considered these cases of sufficient importance to call your attention, had it not been for the hereditary circumstances attending them. In my own case they are indeed striking, for not only the persons above named; but a number of my maternal cousins have died of the same disease.

I shall offer a short reflection or two, drawn **C243** from my own case. In the first place, I am persuaded that hard labour, if employed in an early stage, can cure the hereditary predisposition in some cases. Hence I further conclude, that consumptive parents ought never to choose sedentary or light employment for their children.

Secondly, I conclude that although a trotting horse may afford sufficient exercise for many, yet labor will be far more successful.

Lastly, in all cases, the labor should be such as to require considerable efforts on the part of the patient. I labored <u>continually</u>, and rarely with sufficient intervals to refresh myself by rest.

I am sincerely, Sir, your most obedient, Samuel K. Jennings.

October 25th. 1804.   Medical Museum vol. 1.[6]

An account of the successful use of opium, cordial drinks & animal food in Pulmonary Consumption. By Benjamin Rush, M. D.

C244

Eliza Davis, aged 25. was admitted into the Pennsylvania hospital, on the 7th of Feb. 1805, apparently in the last stage of pulmonary consumption, brought on by an attack of fever six months before. She expectorated pus in large quantities, had a diarrhœa, and spoke only in a whisper. She was so weak as to turn herself in bed with difficulty. Still her pulse had a small degree of tension, which I considered as an obstacle to the use of the only remedies indicated in her case. I directed, therefore, four ounces of blood to be drawn, and ordered a blister to be applied to her breast; and small doses of calomel, tartarized antimony with sal. nitre, and a little laudanum every two hours.

On the 12th I found her pulse so much changed into that state of weakness, softness & frequency which characterises thyphus fever, that I directed two grains of opium every night. On the 19th she complained of a sore mouth, and difficulty of swallowing. The calomel was the laid aside, and instead of opium I directed eighty drops of laudanum morning, noon and night.

On the 26th her diarrhœa returned, for which I prescribed the chalk julep, rendered cordial by an unusual quantity of laudanum. It had the desire effect. On the first of March I found her pulse evidently <u>slower</u> & <u>fuller</u> than it had been, and without any tension. Her ****C245**** voice became stronger, her cough was less frequent, and her expectoration less copious than they had been; and she now complained of pains only in her head & back. I considered this change in her symptoms as highly favourable, and in order to secure the advantages thus obtained over her disease, I directed one hundred & twenty drops of laudanum, and a pint of wine in the course of a day, and to live

---

[6] Samuel K Jennings, "An Account of the Effects of Labor in the Cure of Pulmonary Consumption in a Letter from the Rev. Samuel K. Jennings, of Bedford County, Virginia, to Dr. Benjamin Rush," *The Philadelphia Medical Museum* 1, no. 2 (1805): 194–97.

wholly on the most cordial animal food. My tour of attendance at the hospital expired at this time, and she was committed to the care of D^r. Park, who continued the use of my prescriptions; by which means she was rapidly restored to health, and discharged cured on the 9th of April.

On the 6th of August, I saw her in a street, with a full face & rosy countenance, apparently in perfect health.   Medical Museum vol. 1.[7]

C246

Phthisis Pulmonalis, illustrated by dissection and by practice. In a Memoir, by Dr Elias Black, late House Physician to the New York Hospital. Addressed to the Hon. Samuel L. Mitchill, Nov. 1, 1808.[8]

Dear Sir.

According to your request, I examined the body of John Martin, a black, who died yesterday, of Phthisis Pulmonalis. As his dissection presented appearances extraordinary for a defunct,[9] by that disease, I will, if you please, detail the case.

He was a seaman, aged 20, born in the West Indies, of a slender habit, narrow across the shoulders, and had a contracted chest. He was admitted into the Hospital in April, having been sick all the preceding winter, with fevers and slight pulmonic diseases. His complaint, on admission, appeared to be intermittent fever & catarrh, but these soon gave way to all the symptoms of pulmonary consumption. His eyes became pearly, his cough was very distressing, expectoration purulent; the pulse rather smaller than natural & corded; tongue red at the point & edges, with a red list up the middle, bounded by a thin coat of fur; pain ****C247**** in the chest and hectic paroxysms. These symptoms shew the disease to be rapidly advancing, and to my apprehension to depend on membraneous inflammation of the lungs. He was accordingly put on the use of calomel, with the other curative means, as blisters & expectorants. The mercury was continued until his mouth became sore, when all the phthisical symptoms subsided. His expectoration was mucous, and lessened in quantity; his strength so far returned as to enable him

[7] Benjamin Rush, "An Account of the Successful Use of Opium, Cordial Drinks, and Animal Food, in Two Cases of Pulmonary Consumption," *Philadelphia Medical Museum* 1 (1805): 318–22.

[8] Dr. Elias Black, "Consumption of the Lungs, Illustrated by Dissection and Practice. In a Memoir by Dr. Elias Black, Late House-Physician to the New-York Hospital, and Now Physician in the City of Rio Janeiro. Addressed to the Honorable Samuel L. Mitchill. Dated Nov. 1, 1808," *Medical Repository* 1, 3rd hexade, no. 2 (1809): 116–25.

[9] Defunct, here used as a noun, meaning a dead person (OED).

to walk all over the house. These flattering symptoms were preserved during the mercurial action only; for as soon as that subsided, his emaciation being extreme, he relapsed into his former state. The same remedies were again exhibited, but without effect. He sunk under his disease, and became, before his death, typhoid.

On dissection, the following appearances presented. In the abdomen, the liver was rather lighter coloured than natural, and of a bilious tinge; it was also increased in size. Many of the mesenteric glands were enlarged; the bladder **C248** was thickened and distended with urine. The rest of the viscera appeared healthy. In the thorax the pericardium contained rather more fluid than usual, and of a turbid reddish appearance. The lungs were more flabby than natural. On their edges were small air vesicles; there were no adhesions between their lobes nor between them & the pleura. On cutting into them, no traces of organic lesion could be discovered. The presence of inflammation could not be detected, as transudation had taken place; the body having laid 26 hours after death, before it was examined.

From the history of this man's case, I am confirmed in an opinion, which I sometime since formed, that phthisis pulmonalis was not always attended with tubercles and ulcers, and consequently fatal from that cause. I was led to this belief by seeing a number of cases of this disease, yield to calomel, which from all appearances would have terminated in death; had not this remedy been used.

There appears a species of consumption, of **C249** which the above case is an instance, where extensive inflammation of the membrane, lining the bronchia, ushers in the disease; and, for the most part, attends it throughout. This inflammation appears to assist very much, in the production of that peculiar irritability, which, when the formation of pus is perfectly established, gives rise to all the terrible symptoms of confirmed consumption.

W. Oaks, aged 34, was admitted with hemoptysis. This complaint had continued three weeks, during which he raised blood daily. At the end of this time his bloody expectoration ceased, and the symptoms of consumption came on with violence. He expectorated large quantities of purulent matter, and was very hoarse. He complained of pain in the chest, which daily increased; so that he could not lie down. He had taken such a quantity of salt, to check his bleeding, that he could scarcely swallow. His cough & difficulty of breathing were very great, and no hope was entertained of his recovery. In this situation mercurial frictions were used. A Salivation soon came on, and all the unfavourable symptoms left him.

C250

Three cases of conversion of other disease into consumption.

M. S. aged 18 years, was admitted with an inveterate itch of six months standing; his body was completely covered with the eruption. On the use of medicine or from some unknown cause, after he had been in the house about two months; the eruption disappeared, and diarrhœa came on. This was checked by anodynes & astringents. But a second translation of action took place to the lungs; and now his disease put on all the appearances of phthisis pulmonalis, with membraneous inflammation. The disease advanced with alarming rapidity, and it was supposed, by the physician in attendance, that he would not live a fortnight. He was of a sanguine habit, and subject to bleeding at the nose. Calomel was given to six grains a day, with a small quantity of tart. emit. & opium, **C251** until salivation was produced. All the phthisical symptoms soon went off, and the eruption returned to the skin, but with diminished violence.

Two cases of conversion of rheumatism into phthisis occurred last spring. The rheumatic affection had continued a long time; in one ten months. The passive inflammation appeared to leave the parts, which it had so long invested, and to centre on the lungs. All the symptoms of consumption readily succeeded this translation of action. They expectorated purulent matter in very large quanty [*sic*], had distressing cough; hectic paroxysms; and the pulse, as well as tongue, put on all the appearances & character described in John Martin's case. Calomel with tart. emet. and opium were given, and salivation was soon produced. They both recovered of their phthisical complaints; and one of the rheumatism.   Med. Repos. N°. 50.[10]

---

[10] Elias Black, "Consumption of the Lungs, Illustrated by Dissection and Practice. In a Memoir by Dr. Elias Black, Late House-Physician to the New-York Hospital, and Now Physician in the City of Rio Janeiro. Addressed to the Honorable Samuel L. Mitchill. Dated Nov. 1, 1808," 116–25.

Chap. 9.

PULMONARY AFFECTIONS REMOVED by the intervention of some other diseases, also by powerful means, and manual operation.

In March, 1805, Mrs R. of Falmouth, aged 25 years, of a slender habit, was invaded with the usual symptoms of pulmonary consumption. In May she became pregnant, and passed the summer & autumn with few complaints, except a slight cough and erratic pains in the chest.

In Feb. 1806, after parturition her pulmonary complaints increased, morning sweats took place, with febrile disturbance. As the spring advanced she continued to languish with regular paroxisms of hectic fever, attended with cough and expectoration of mucus & pus; increased pain in the chest, and night sweats; pulse weak & quick, so that bloodletting did not appear to be indicated, and the excitability was thought to be too low to admit of the use of mercury. Adhesive **C253** plaisters, and epispastics were largely applied to the chest; but no relief was afforded, and she grew worse in every respect, till the middle of May, when a violent strangury took place, probably from the liberal use of blisters. During the exercise of this new disease her pulmonary complaints decreased and were soon entirely removed. The fever & sweats also ceased. Since which she has enjoyed good health.

In the spring of 1807, Mrs P. aged 20, of a slender delicate habit, complained of a hecking cough, oppression at the breast, and febrile disturbance. These symptoms increased till October, under the use of simple means. At this time she was seized with great pain in the loins, a strangury. I was then called and finding her pulse quick & rather tense, I drew a pint of blood which moderated the pain, a dose of Jalap & calomel was given and the heat in the loins was alleviated.

C254

Three days after the pain & anguish returned with suppression of urine, but her pulmonary complaints were less tedious. 12 ounces of blood were drawn, and calomel was given so as to produce a salivation. As the salival discharge increased the strangury & cough decreased, so that in one week they were removed. She soon recovered to her usual health.

Mrs A. B. born of a consumptive mother, was troubled, at times, with cough & inflammation of the trachea, between the years of 15 & 24, when she entered into the marriage state, and became pregnant. After parturition the usual train of hectical symptoms took place, and continued to increase about one month, when she was seized with exquisite pain in the back & hip, which soon extended to the leg & foot. The whole limb readily swelled with such tension, that it could not be moved without great torture. The limb continued in this condition about ten days, when the pain & swelling subsided. Her pulmonary complaints were then removed.

C255

The means used for this swelling of the limb were mercurial cathartics with occasional doses of laudanum. Strong sinapisms were applied to the leg & foot which inflamed the skin to vesication. After this, she enjoyed good health.

In the spring of 1812, Dr Kidder of Newmarket, N.H. aged 60, of a tall & slender make,[1] was invaded with the usual symptoms of pulmonary consumption, which progressed till December, when he was thought to be far advanced in the second stage and very little hope was entertained of his recovery. At this time, a Carbuncle formed between his shoulders, and was attended with excrutiating pain. During its progress his pulmonary complaints abated and when the carbuncle was cured were entirely removed.

This case was related to me by the Doctor in June 1820.

C256

In June 1822 Dr Lawrence of Hampton, N.H. related a case of Phthisis to me, which occurred in the practice of Dr Cutter of Portsmouth, in which, when the disease was far advanced, the patient was seized with great pain and inflammation in one of his eyes, which progressed to its total destruction by suppuration. During which the pulmonary complaints were removed, and the patient recovered.

---

[1] Make: in the sense of the build or physique of the body (OED).

In Feb 1802, Miss D. of Falmouth, after laboring under the symptoms of Phthisis three months, was seized with a felon on one of her fingers, and the inflammation extended to the shoulder, so that the whole limb was much tumefied. The finger in one week assumed a livid[2] hue & was amputated. The inflammation of the arm, then gradually subsided. During this painful affection, she was free from pulmonary complaints, which never after recurred. **C257** Might not the actual cautery have answered a very similar purpose. This remedy has been highly extolled by Hippocrates, and much used by the Ancients for many obstinate local affections.

We are informed in the Boston Recorder, that the actual cautery has of late been applied to the chest in Phthisis Pulmonalis to great advantage, by European Physicians.[3]

I have been credibly informed that a patient labouring under the symptoms of pulmonary consumption of a few months standing was effectually cured by having the feet & legs badly scalded with boiling water.

"A boy, six years old, says D[r] Ogden, had from earliest infancy a cough with profuse expectoration. At two years, he was epileptic. When six, his clothes caught fire and the skin of the thorax was severely burned, & suppurated. His complaints were removed."

C258

D[r]. Philip Carrigain, of Concord, N.H. began to practice physic in early life, possessed of a very slender constitution, and subject to frequent & profuse hemoptysis. It was not unusual for him, after having ridden several miles, on dismounting to bring up from half a pint, to a pint of blood, as fast as he could expectorate it, but when riding he brought up no blood. Besides frequent bloodletting to obviate plethora, he conceived the idea of the efficacy of breast milk. Of every nursing woman whom he met, he solicited permission to draw her breasts. This course he followed about a year, taking, during that time, little or no other nourishment, except cows milk, when he could not find a supply of breast milk.

At the end of the year, he had become quite free from hemoptysis, but did not recover perfect health & vigor till the natural small pox was taken when 25 years old, and which, tho it nearly destroyed life, completely revolutionized

---

[2] Livid: of a bluish leaden color, black and blue (OED).

[3] *Boston Recorder* was a newspaper that existed from 1817 to 1824. "Grand Surgical Operation," *Boston Recorder*, December 16, 1820, 204.

his constitution; so that he never experienced a recurrence of hemoptysis more than once or twice after wards. He died at the age of 57.

N. England Journal. v.11. N.4.[4]

C259

Jason Fairbanks of Dedham, Mass. had been constitutionally infirm from his birth, always an invalid. His complaints had been pain in the side, cough & frequent hemoptysis, with general weakness, so that he could never labour, nor take any considerable exercise without inducing hemoptysis. From wounds of his body, he sustained the loss of so much blood that he was pale, faint and exhausted to such a degree that he could not walk without staggering. His wounds became gangrenous and his life was dispaired of. At length, however, he recovered, and became possessed of what he never before enjoyed, a state of perfect health, and able to endure great hardships, without injury to his body.   ibid.[5]

D[r]. Pardon Bowen, of Providence, informed me, that his wife, aged 50, complained, in the winter of 1817, of stricture & oppression of the breast, with febrile action, which produced an hemoptysis, recurring about once a week for three months; discharging about half a pint of blood each time. To remedy which he bled her eleven times ****C260**** drawing about a pint, when the symptoms of recurrence were noticed and gave saline cathartics, with a low diet. Her complaints were then removed, and health was restored. I saw her in 1822, active & vigorous.

Case stated by T. Knight Esq. F. R. S.

The patient had been healthy tho delicate from her birth, till she married and had one child. Her appearance then in her 19th year became consumptive, and within a few weeks afterwards, suddenly discharged a considerable quantity of blood from her lungs. She passed the first winter in rooms kept warm and of as equal temperature as was practicable. Blisters & leeches were repeatedly applied by D[r] Philip. In the succeeding summer her health & strength were improved. But at the end of the following winter, she was so much emaciated & reduced by a long continued discharge of blood from her lungs and the effects of her feverish state, that ****C261**** I thought all hope of recovery past. But D[r] P. expressed a belief that if she could be placed in a situation

[4] Richard Hazeltine, "Observations on the Efficacy of Bloodletting in Hemoptysis," *New England Journal of Medicine and Surgery* 11, no. 4 (1822): 337–51; for Dr. Carrigain, see p. 51.

[5] Hazeltine, "Observations on the Efficacy of Bloodletting in Hemoptysis," 346–47.

where she could have the benefit of a climate as favorable as the best part of an English summer, for 18 successive months, she might recover.

A flue of sufficient power, and surrounded by an air chamber was constructed wholly of brick work, space being prepared to receive garden pots to be filled with wetted sand to give to the heated air the requisite degree of humidity; and from the top of this air chamber, pipes of tin, cased with wood, were made to convey a warm current of air to rise through different parts of the floor of every room into which she should have occasion to enter. She was thus given the benefit of a warm temperature of 60 degrees, with a constant & rapid change of air. A summer temperature of 18 months was thus afforded, and she has perfectly recovered her health & strength.

London Medical Journal.[6]

C262

In Autumn, 1816, a young lady in Gorham of a delicate habit, was exposed to damp air, and repeatedly wet her feet, while on a visit from home. She was then attacked with febrile disturbance, oppression at the breast, pain in the side, cough and expectoration of clear blood, which continued to recur for several days. A physician was called, who drew a pint of blood, and the pain was removed to the arm pit, as she says. Repeated doses of jalap & calomel were then given, which operated powerfully and removed the pain. Laudanum was occasionally ~~given~~ used, which moderated the cough.

She was then advised to return to Gorham, and live chiefly on milk & vegetables. But her complaints continued to molest her, in a greater or less degree, particularly in the spring months, when they were worse than at other times. In this way she continued nearly three years, taking very little medicine, for she was considered by her friends and some physicians as being incurably

---

[6] Thomas Andrew Knight, Esq. F.R.S., "An Account of a New Mode of Preserving an Equable and Salutary Temperature of the Air of Rooms for Consumptive Patients," *The London Medical and Physical Journal* 46 (1821): 115–16. Thomas Andrew Knight (1759–1838) was a British botanist and horticulturalist, Fellow of the Royal Society, and second president of the Royal Horticultural Society. Janet Browne, "Knight, Thomas Andrew (1759–1838), Horticulturist and Plant Physiologist," in *Oxford Dictionary of National Biography* (Oxford: Oxford University Press, 2014). Knight's article reported on a patient of Dr. Wilson Philip (1770–1851), who was born in Glasgow as Alexander Philip Wilson, received an M.D. in Edinburgh in 1792, was a Fellow of the Royal Society of Edinburgh, and at some point reversed his name. Philip moved to London in 1817 and was elected a Fellow of the Royal Society of London. He later disappeared, apparently having fled to France to avoid debtor's prison due to injudicious investments. He is thought to have died there and may be the inspiration for Thackeray's Dr. Firmin in "The Adventures of Philip." He was a prolific writer on many medical subjects, including pulmonary consumption. J. F. Payne and Patrick Wallis, "Philip, Alexander Philip Wilson (1770–C.1851), Physician and Physiologist," in *Oxford Dictionary of National Biography* (Oxford: Oxford University Press, 2004).

consumptive. At the expiration of this term, my advice was requested. Her complaints at this time were febrile disturbance, pain **C263** & a burning heat, as she called it, in her vitals, chiefly in the left side, tho at times wandering, cough and expectoration of a purulent matter chiefly in the morning, night sweats with a quick & feeble pulse; tho she was able to sit up the chief of the day and to ride in a carriage. I prescribed a mercurial salivation. Soon after, application was made to Dr Folsome of Gorham, who left twelve grains of calomel, directing two grains to be taken night and morning. Each dose operated powerfully as a cathartic, and were all taken. Her complaints were then much alleviated. A moderate salivation supervened, with a discharge of bloody matter. When the salivation ceased, her complaints were entirely removed, and her strength was soon restored without the use of any means, save suitable nutriments. She then took passage for Boston in a packet, to visit her friends, and continues in the enjoyment of health.

This case serves to show the great length of time that inflammatory irritation and morbid action may sometimes continue in the vital organs & membranes **C264** without producing organic lesion or ulcers, also the beneficial effects of seasonable bleeding, both natural & artificial; as well as cathartics and a low diet, avoiding stimulants of every kind; likewise, the salutary effects of purgative & salivating means, even when the disease is far advanced. But this ought not to encourage procrastination and negligence in the use of means, lest the lungs should become too greatly infused to receive any benefit from ~~proper~~ appropriate remedies. Furthermore, it shows the proper time for exercise on a sea voyage, viz <u>after</u> morbid action is removed. For want of this discrimination many consumptive patients have suffered an increase, instead of experiencing any alleviation of their pulmonary affections.

The following case may serve as an example.

In August 1817, a young gentleman in Portland, of a good habit, bright talents and great activity in business, after exposure to **C265** foggy weather in a thin dress, was attacked with an irritating cough, and some febrile disturbance, which induced languor & depression of spirits. Not thinking that a physician was needed, he took a friend in his chaise, and rode about 40 miles into the country, in order to restore his spirits & usual vigor. But his complaints increased and he became more enfeebled. He was noticed by people on his tour and viewed as a person labouring under the symptoms of pulmonary consumption, tho he was not apprehensive of any danger, believing that he had only a common cold; requiring exercise & cordials!

On his return, his complaints were so increased that he confined himself to his chamber, and then consulted a physician, who found him labouring under the symptoms of pulmonary consumption and prescribed the usual means. Still the disease advanced, night sweats **C266** increased to a considerable degree, and his cough, as well as expectoration continued with febrile paroxysms; so that his flesh wasted and his strength declined.

In October, I called as a friend, and enquired after his health. His wife informed me that he was growing better very fast, and they were not apprehensive of any danger. She wished me to see him, but feared that if another physician should be consulted, he might be alarmed, which would depress his spirits and reduce his strength. I asked her if he had been bled, or taken any mercury. She said he had not been bled, but had taken some mercury, tho it had no sensible effect. ——He continued in much the same, supposed hopeful state, as I was informed, till December, when he was advised by his friends, to take passage, in a ship for a warm climate. Soon after he sailed, his nose occasionally bled, and some relief was afforded. On his arrival **C267** in Charlestown, he bled at his nose repeatedly & profusely, which afforded further relief, and a hope was entertained by his friends & physicians, that it would tend to remove the hectic fever. But, alas! it was at too late a period. ——In January 1818, he took passage for Havana, and was able to sit in his chair on deck, as they entered the harbour, and a hope was entertained by his attendants, that he would recover; his cough having ceased, tho his feet had swelled. He expired the next morning, while sitting in his easy chair, greatly lamented by all his acquaintance; for he was full of benovelence [*sic*] and hospitality, particularly to the poor & needy.

C268 In the spring of 1816, a lady, in Maine, of a florid countenance and good habit, who had taken up her residence near a fresh river, on low ground, complained of oppression at the breast, cough & hoarseness, with some febrile disturbance, hot palms, languor & heaviness. She was then attacked with a spontaneous hæmorrhage from the lungs and considerable blood was discharged. Her complaints were then alleviated, tho the hoarseness continued with some cough.

In the winter & spring of 1817, she felt an increase of her pulmonary affections, and at times raised blood, which again afforded relief, tho her lungs were very susceptable [*sic*] of impression from inclement air, and oppressed on unusual exertion.

In December, her complaints increased on the admission of cold air into the lungs, so that she was confined, for the most part, to the house. In January 1818 her cough was troublesome, and bloody mucous was expectorated. She then complained of great heat in the vitals, with running pains, stricture and an oppressive load.

C269

During the months of January & February she raised blood, once in two or three days; at other times, mucous & yellow matters were expectorated. Febrile disturbance preceded by chills attended, with some pain in the left side; so that she was ~~so that she was~~ confined to the house, the chief of the time till May. Under these circumstances, nauseating doses of ipecac were occasionally given, in order to check the bleeding; and Glaubers salts were liberally used to reduce the fever. Epispastics were also applied to the chest. In April she discharged blood more freely than heretofore, and her complaints were alleviated; so that she was able to pay some attention to domestic business.

I called to see her the first of June 1818, when she related her complaints as above and regretted that she had not been bled; but her physician, who was not then in the habit of reading American authors on phthisis pulmonalis, did not think the lancet eligible in her case, nor mercury. **C270** At this time she complained of some cough and expectoration, with pain in the side ~~with~~ and heat in the vitals on any unusual exertion; also an increased heat in the hands & feet, pulse small & about 90. But the oppression at the breast & hoarseness were much lessened.

In August she complained of inflammation in the throat with imposthumations, which suppurated; for which Glaubers salts were liberally used, with a low diet.

In the winter of 1819, she complained of oppression at the vitals, and a burning heat, when clear blood was discharged by cough, several times; as also mucous & yellow matters. Ipecac, and salts were occasionally given.

In the spring her complaints abated, tho her lungs were irritated when exposed to damp air. In July she complained of a return of heat & irritation in the lungs with running pains in the chest, which were very tedious; as well as her cough. She requested her physician to bleed her, **C271** but he feared it would weaken her, tho she was able to do some domestic labour. Repeated discharges of blood, however, took place from her lungs, greatly to the alleviation of her complaints; and she passed the following summer & winter in comfortable health; so that she could go abroad without any inconvenience, and continues almost entirely free from pulmonary affection.

C272

In 1818, Samuel Whitney, a healthy man, aged 23, removed from Buxton, Maine, to the Province of Canada, by trade a shoemaker.

In the spring of 1819, he was attacked with a catarrhal cough, which was soon followed by febrile disturbance, pain in the side & expectoration of mucus. As no physician was near, he applied to an empiric in the hope of being bled. But he reprobated the lancet, and directed spiritous stimulants; some of which he used. His complaints gradually increased; and, in the summer, purulent matter was expectorated. His fever increased, and, night sweats took place. A physician was then consulted, who advised to a mercurial salivation; but this was not complied with, common means being only used.

In December 1820, he rode from Canada to Buxton, on horseback, and his complaints were aggravated, particularly the pain in his side, and febrile disturbance.

In February 1821, he rode to Gorham, in a sleigh, distant eight miles, without much fatigue, when I was consulted. His complaints, at this time, were pain in the inferior part of the chest, on the right side, over which there was some swelling, cough and expectoration of purulent matter, night sweats, and occasional vomiting after eating, tho his appetite was good; pulse 100, and pretty full, tho not tense, without rigors or paroxysms of fever. I advised **C273** to a mercurial salivation; and to have a seton put into his side. He concluded to take the matter into consideration, and returned to Buxton.

"He continued to decline, as I have since been informed by his nurse, with swelled feet, & loss of flesh, without the use of any means, save a vomit and some gums & balsams, & with common teas."

"About the middle of April, the swelling of his feet increased and extended over the whole body, to a considerable degree, even to his neck, with oppression & difficulty of breathing. On the 20th of May, an hemorrhage of blood took place from his lungs, to the amount of two quarts, which was very sizy & clotted. His breathing then became easy, and relief was afforded for three days, when the difficulty of breathing returned, and continued one week. Another hemorrhage of blood from his lungs then occurred in great profusion, of a pale red colour without siziness. He expired while bleeding; and continued to flow from his mouth & nose, in considerable quantity, for two days, when he was interred."

"He had a craving appetite for animal food particularly fresh meat, till within a few days of his death, and was freely indulged."

– – – – – – – – – – – – "For want of timely care
Millions have died of medicable wounds."[7]

7 John Armstrong and John Aikin, *The Art of Preserving Health* (Philadelphia: Benjamin Johnson [etc.], 1804), 109.

C274

In the summer of 1819, Samuel Gilkey of Gorham aged 30, a labourer, of a spare habit, was attacked with a slight catarrh, and running pains in his chest. In Autumn his complaints increased with pain in the left side, irregular appetite, and frequent vomiting, after taking food; for which pearl ash was taken to advantage.

In December, after exposure to cold & dampness, the pain in his side increased, with his other complaints, so that he was confined to the house, and could sit up but little. I was then called when his pulse was quick & rather tense. I drew a pint of blood and gave several mercurial cathartics; also applied blisters and stimulating plaisters to his chest. Some relief was afforded; but the pain soon returned, when another pint of blood was drawn, and calomel given in small doses; but his mouth was not affected.

In Jan. 1820, he was much enfeebled, and the pain was so severe, at times that he could not sleep without opium, which was offensive to his stomach. As he was unwilling to loose any more blood, or pursue the use of mercury, I put a seton in his side, including a large portion of flesh. This was very sore and discharged freely. The pain then abated, and his health was, in some measure restored.

C275

In the spring, he removed on a farm, distant 100 miles;[8] but was unable to do much labour, and his complaints returned to a considerable degree; so that little hope was entertained of his recovery. In August, he was severely attacked with cholera, and the diarrhœa continued several weeks, which greatly reduced his flesh & strength. His pulmonary affections, however, were entirely removed, and his health was soon restored. Since which he has continued a laborious man; free from complaints.

In Autumn 1819, a middle aged gentleman in Gorham, of a feeble habit, was troubled with a diarrhœa, which reduced his strength to a considerable degree. The first of Nov. after riding in rainy weather, on horseback, he was attacked with pain in his breast, cough & expectoration; with also febrile disturbance. He was bled, by Dr Folsome, and advised to a mercurial salivation. But the patient was unwilling to take mercury, lest it should interfere with an intended Journey. His complaints increased under the use of common

---

[8] There were a number of Gilkeys in Gorham in the late eighteenth century; this Samuel Gilkey was probably the son of Joseph and Phebe Gilkey, born May 25, 1784. He moved to a farm in Troy, Maine, approximately 108 miles from Gorham. Hugh D. Mc Lellan, *History of Gorham, Maine* (Portland: Smith and Sale, 1903), 514.

means, and in the latter part of the **C276** month, he appeared to labour under such a degree of membraneous inflammation in the chest, as endangered organic lesion, for purulent expectoration had taken place. I was then requested, by his physician, to make him a visit, when I reminded him of the danger of his situation and advised him to take mercury, in order to produce salivation. He then consented; and an aqueous solution of corrosive sublimate was given, equal to about one grain of mercury in the course of 24 hours. A sense of heat and irritation was felt in the stomach, after each dose, which, in three days, so affected his mouth that a moderate salivation was produced and continued about one week, tho he took only three grains of the mercury. His complaints were then removed and his strength was gradually restored by suitable food; so that in January 1821, he performed a journey, in a sleigh, of 100 miles, entered into the marriage state and returned.

In some cases of catarrh and pulmonic affection, with loss of appetite, sulfate of copper, blue vitriol, given in small doses, **C277** has been productive of good effects, in diverting morbid action from the lungs and restoring appetite, especially when joined with ipecacuanha.

The following cases were transmitted to me, from Lyman Spalding, M.D. &c of New York, in May 1819.[9]

"Alderman Bracket of N. York, has, for years, been liable to an affection of the lungs, which, he believes, disposes him to pulmonary consumption. He seldom passes a year without a return of his complaints.

In the spring of 1818, he suffered an unusually severe attack, which confined him to the house for many weeks. His symptoms were pain in the side, teasing cough, at first, without expectoration, loss of appetite, night sweats, & hard wiery pulse; but not full, with febrile action. He lost blood twice, which relieved the fever & pain in the side; but **C278** had very little effect on the cough. About a week after the last bleeding, he took Ipecacuanha and sulphate of copper, which acted like a charm in subduing the cough and

---

[9] These four cases were copied, nearly verbatim, from a paper titled "Cases of Supposed Incipient Phthisis Pulmonalis Cured by Sulfate of Copper and Ipecacuanha" by Lyman Spalding. At the end of this paper, now in the Lyman Spalding Collection at The Countway Library of Medicine, is found the following notation in the same hand: "Copied for J. Barker 1819." The few differences between the Barker and Spalding versions appear here in square brackets. The first US Pharmacopoeia was being founded in 1819. Lyman Spalding, one of the five delegates appointed by the committee in Washington, became chairman of the Committee on Publications. This gathering of knowledgeable physicians and pharmacists was trying to rid the United States of "the evil of irregularity and uncertainty in the preparation of medicines" that varied from state to state. Glenn Sonnedecker, "The Founding Period of the U.S. Pharmacopeia: III. The First Edition," *Pharmacy in History* 36, no. 3 (1994): 103–22.

hectic symptoms. A journey to Niagara in the summer, restored him to better health than he had enjoyed for years."

"The 24ᵗʰ of March, 1817, I was desired to visit a sea captain [Captain Abel Arrington][10] of this city, of middle age and of intemperate habits. I found him labouring under a severe cough, with copious expectoration. His pulse was weak & quick; he had distinct febrile paroxysms, morning & evening; night sweats and pain in his side. He had not left his room for many days; and was able to sit up but a few hours at a time. His indisposition had continued for several weeks, and was increasing. He had taken balsams and a variety of remedies usually given in consumption. I prescribed an emetic of sulphate of copper & ipecac, which was repeated on the third day. He also took lichen and a ferruginous preparation. He **C279** became convalescent, immediately after the use of the emetics; went abroad in two weeks, and, on the first of May, proceeded to sea, in good health, taking command of a vessel."

"In Nov. 1818, Mʳˢ Trevell [Mrs. Doctor Trevett] was attacked with an inflammation of the chest, attended with difficulty of breathing, cough & pain in the side. The urgent symptoms subsided after bleeding, blistering &c. But an asthmatic difficulty of breathing remained, attended with a teasing cough.

Feb. 1819. she had a comfortable accouchment, [sic] and was doing well for two weeks, when she was seized with difficulty of breathing, pain in the side, incessant cough, with terrific dreams, from which she awoke with great emotion, struggling for breath. After these symptoms had continued for a week or ten days, she was so much reduced as not to be able to be ~~turned~~ removed from her bed. At this time she began to have cold chills, which, in a day or two, became regular febrile paroxysms, recurring every **C280** twenty-four hours.

The incessant cough, pain in the side, want of appetite, loss of strength and regular chills, succeeded by heat, sweating and a crimsoned cheek, induced a belief that she was disposed to phthisis pulmonalis. —— A large blister was applied to the chest, which procured some relief from the pain; but did not remove the cough, nor interrupt the febrile symptoms. She took six grains of sulphate of copper & twenty grains of Ipecacuanha. The febrile ~~symptoms~~ paroxysms, which had continued in for nearly two weeks, were then suspended, and returned no more; the cough was much relieved. From that time she became convalescent, and the cure was completed by quassia, lichen, &c."

---

[10] Spalding, Lyman (1775–1821) Papers, 1798–1912 (inclusive), 1798–circa 1820 (bulk). Spalding, Lyman, 1775–1821, Cases of supposed incipient phthisis pulmonalis, cured by sulphate of copper and ipecacuanha, A.MS.s.; 3 sides (9 pages), circa 1818. B MS c2 Box 2, Folder 10, Countway Library of Medicine; Harvard University. Accessed February 18, 2019.

"On the 15th of Nov. 1818, I was desired to visit Mrs Sherwood of this city, who, about six weeks before, had returned in good health from a summers residence in the country. She took cold, the beginning of November, and is now **C281** labouring under a violent cough, attended with copious expectoration. She has a constant pain in the side, with a weak pulse and loss of appetite. Soon after twelve o'clock at noon, and at midnight, she has a febrile paroxysm, in which she experiences a sensation of cold, for an hour or more, and then becomes hot & restless, with a flushed face. I prescribed an emetic of tartrite of antimony, and a blister to the side.

Nov. 18th. The symptoms are all aggravated. She does not sit up more than an hour at a time, and cannot walk from her chair to the bed. Her cough is incessant and attended with copious expectoration. The febrile paroxysms return regularly twice in 24 hours. She has night sweats, pain in both sides, and an entire disrelish for food. The pulse is very slow and weak; the tongue is covered with a moist & whitish coat. I directed her child to be weaned, which was eight months old, and prescribed an emetic of sulphate of copper & Ipecacuanha, **C282** and placed a blister on the left side. The emetic relieved the cough and broke up the febrile action; and the paroxysms did not return.

Nov. 23d. The patient has improved much, and now takes squills, lichen, infusion of flaxseed, &c. The pain in the side remaining, a blister was applied.

Nov. 25th. The cough is troublesome; the pain in the side is not yet gone. She has flushes in the face in the afternoon, and sweats at night. I prescribed an emetic of sulphate of copper & ipecac.

26th. The emetic removed every vestige of the disease. The cure was completed by lichen, sulphate of iron, myrrh, etc."

These cases are descriptive of that kind of consumption, in which the digestive organs cease to perform their office, from deficient vital energy, evidenced by loss of appetite, a coated tongue, and in one case, a slow weak pulse, with great prostration of strength. These symptoms do not characterize genuine phthisis, where the patient can walk abroad or **C283** ride, with a tense pulse, from 90 to 120 strokes in a minute, in the primary stages of the disease; and where the appetite and digestive powers are generally unimpaired, till the last, or typhous stage of this disease is fully established; and then there is often a craving for various sorts of food, till near the close of life.

In the former kind of consumption, emetics, among which the sulphate of copper & Ipecac were found to be the best, excite the stomach to action & vigour which influences the whole system; so as to remove other complaints, when the tonic power of lichen, iron, &c are useful means to restore the digestive powers and appetite. But in real phthisis, where extensive inflammation exists in the chest, producing great excitement & morbid action, and where the vessels of the lungs are surcharged with blood, secreting purulent matter, or secerning the vital fluid, besides bloodletting and mercury, <u>cathartics</u> have been found more eligible than emetics, in order to divert **C284** inflammatory action from the respiratory organs, and thereby lessen the secretion of purulent matter; evidenced by the effects of a diarrhœa, which sometimes takes place in the primary stages of phthisis, greatly to the alleviation of the symptoms, as appears by the relation of a number of cases, which induces me to believe that cathartics have been too much neglected, in phthisis pulmonalis, at least in my own practice.

In Pneumonia, where the debility is such as to confine a patient to his bed, every physician employs cathartics, after bleeding, to advantage. But, in the inflammatory state of phthisis, where the energy & strength are found to be greater than in pneumony, purgative means have seldom been used! Neither have they been prescribed, by any medical writers, of modern date, which **C285** I have read, though they have been recommended, by some of the ancients, as has already been noticed.

In June 1820, Dr Fisher of Beverly, aged 70, of a debilitated habit, informed me, that, in the spring, he was seized with a violent pain in his head, which he considered as an effect of inflammation. A translation of morbid action, however, to his lungs readily took place; and the symptoms of phthisis pulmonalis supervened in an alarming manner. A second translation of action to his stomach soon succeeded, and a powerful diarrhœa was produced. His pulmonary complaints were then removed, and his health was soon restored. —— verifying the words of Hippocrates "<u>Nature is the first</u> <u>physician</u>" Ought we not then to imitate nature; and willingly receive instruction?
C286

A son of mine, born of a consumptive mother, whose case has been related, after much exposure to inclement weather, in the spring of 1819, while visiting patients on Islands, ~~adjacent to~~ in the County of Hancock, suffered under a return of his pulmonary complaints, to an alarming degree. Bloodletting, emetics & cathartics, with various other means were used, tho very little relief was afforded; and he continued to labour under the usual symptoms of pulmonary consumption, till August, when he was considered by an experienced physician as being in a hopeless condition.

At this time, a diarrhœa took place, which continued night & day, and became habitual. His pulmonary complaints, ~~however,~~ were soon alleviated, when opiates and tonics were used to check the diarrhœa. This being restrained, his pulmonary complaints returned; so that he was obliged to have recourse to cathartics, in order to reproduce the diarrhœa; and his lungs were again relieved. In this way he continued through the following winter, able to ride, as his strength was not much impaired, and his appetite was good.

In May 1820, he took passage for Portland, by water, and repaired to my house in Gorham, still exercised with a diarrhœa, several times in 24 hours, of that kind, called <u>lientery</u>; for which he had been **C287** in the habit of taking two grains of opium every night, to procure some rest; sometimes brandy & water; but this last was not congenial as his pulse was 120 in a minute and rather full. He had a craving appetite for animal food, particularly fresh meat, which had been freely indulged. I prescribed a milk diet with lime water, and sea bread; also salted fish, which he found more congenial than fresh meat. Still the diarrhœa continued; but his strength was such that he could ride or walk to Portland, distant eight miles and return, in the course of the day without much fatigue; also do some labour in the garden & field.

In August, he took a grain of saccharum saturni night & morning, for a few days, which checked the diarrhœa; but he then complained of tension of the abdomen, flatulency, and oppression of the breast with stricture. At this time Dʳ Rea called to see him, who had laboured under a pretty similar complaint, and advised to a daily use of aloes, in small doses, which he found beneficial in his own case. He pursued the plan, and his diarrhœa gradually abated, till the first of October, when it ceased. His health was soon restored by suitable nutriment, without stimulants, and his pulse became natural. He died in April, 1829.

C288

In 1784, Mʳˢ B. of Barnstable, aged 40, of a slender delicate habit, several of whose relatives had died of pulmonary consumption, was invaded with the usual symptoms of this disease, which progressed to the second stage before medical aid was called, when purulent expectoration had taken place. Her physician Dʳ Hersey, prescribed small doses of calomel & Ethiops mineral. These means operated cathartically in such a powerful manner, that she was considerably reduced, and they were soon laid aside. But her pulmonary complaints were greatly alleviated; so that she expectorated but little, and her appetite mended.

Soon after, she took passage, by water, to Portland, and resided, some time, at my house in Stroudwater, where she put herself under my care. Her complaints then were an habitual diarrhœa, which recurred every morning,

C289 some cough, and slight hectic flushes, with night sweats, tho she was able to ride out, and her appetite was pretty good.

I put her under a course of lime water with one grain of opium at night. Her complaints were soon removed excepting the diarrhœa, which continued to occur every morning, tho at no other time, and without much inconvenience, for twenty years. During this time she was free from pulmonary affections. She made a daily use of opium in small doses, sometimes a little wine. Her diet consisted chiefly of salted provision, with tea & coffee.

After this period, when she had arrived to the age of sixty years, the diarrhœa ceased. Her lungs then became affected as heretofore; her appetite failed and she declined for three months with very little fever when she expired.

C290

"Tuberculous disease of the lungs, By John Baron M.D. London 1822.[11]

A young man, of a delicate frame, had been long affected with frequent cough; at first, without any expectoration; pulse quick & inspiration hurried. He had been in this situation many months, when after a fit of coughing more violent than usual, a small globular shaped mass of tuberculous matter, partly tinged with blood was discharged. This kind of expectoration occurred a great many successive time, at considerable intervals.

I kept him in a regular temperature, stimulated the chest, occasionally with blisters and tart. emet. and confined him to a strictly vegetable diet, with an occasional use of anodynes to appease the cough. I began with the use of Brandish's caustic alkali in tea.[12] After some weeks, I gave the hydriodate of potass. He began with eight drops twice a day; and continued it for three weeks. It was then omitted for two weeks, and resumed, increasing **C291** the dose to 12 drops. The consequence was an almost complete removal of the cough, and entire reduction of the pulse to the natural standard; a healthy state of the stomach & bowels, with increase of flesh & strength; so that he soon became able to ride on horse back. He recovered.

---

[11]   John Baron, *Illustrations of the Enquiry Respecting Tuberculous Diseases* (London: Underwood, 1822).

[12] Joseph Brandish, *Observations on the Use of Caustic Alkali, in Scrofula, and Other Chronic Diseases* (London: T. Reynolds & Son; J. Murray; J. Callow, 1811), 25. The ingredients of the tea included Lixiva (potassium carbonate or potash) and limewater (calcium oxide in water).

A tuberculous condition of the abdomen was also removed by leeches to the abdomen, and an ointment of the hydriodate of potass, rubbed over the abdomen, and the potass was used internally with mild aperients. The swelling & tension of the abdomen was entirely removed, and he recovered.

Dr B. teaches that tubercles arise independant of any original morbid processes, and when ever they occur, either in the liver, mesentery or other parts, there nature is the same. He recommends mercury, when they occur in any parts save the lungs. They can only be remedied in the early stage of the disease. Whatever enfeebles the constitution predisposes to tubercles."

Medical Recorder vol. 7.[13]

C292

Case presented to me, by Dr William Bowen of Providence, in June 1822.

Caries of the 5th & 6th ribs, disorganization of the right lobe of the lungs with a description of an operation. By Dr. Milton Antony of Augusta, Georgia[14]

Elmore Allen, æt 17 years, between two & three years ago, fell from a horse and the sixth right rib was believed to be broken. The pain did not continue severe long. In a few days, little attention being paid to the case, the local irritation and ecchymosis, measurably abated. For two years, he could often walk & ride without much inconvenience. Sundry times irritation and tumefaction in the injured part, from over exertion or accident, made him keep his bed several days, sometimes weeks. Once inflammation was such, that a blister was drawn on the part. Six months ago, the part became **C293** distressful; soon after, pungent severe pain was fixed at the vertebræ and sternal articulations of the rib, hectic fever ensued; pain in the wound ceased; uneasy sense of weight & distention followed.

Mar 3^d 1821, I made by first visit to him. He was in good spirits, considerably emaciated, had not rested at night, for some time, without opium. He showed effort and dilatation of the nostrils at each inspiration. No more

---

[13] Dr. Baron is cited in P. W. Alison, "Treatment of Scrofulous Disease with a View to Their Prevention," *Medical Recorder* 7 (1824): 613–21.

[14] Milton Antony (1789–1839), after an apprenticeship and one year at University of Pennsylvania Medical School, practiced, taught, and was the guiding spirit and first editor of the *Southern Medical and Surgical Journal*. The daring 1821 operation presented here was republished in several countries. See Howard A. Kelly and Walter L. Burrage, *American Medical Biographies* (Baltimore: The Norman, Remington Company, 1920), 33–34, and Martin Kaufman, Stuart Galishoff, and Todd Lee Savitt, *Dictionary of American Medical Biography*, 2 vols. (Westport, CT: Greenwood Press, 1984), vol. 1. 16–17.

respiration appeared on the left side than seemed to result from inflation of the left lobe; the pulse was 120, in a minute, laborious, like a sluggish undulation, full, strong, distinct to the eye, in three left intercostal spaces, giving to the touch, a sensation like that given, when water is in the pericardium, or when it adheres **C294** extensively to the heart. The tumor was from the sternum to the anterior edge of the latissimus dorsi, two inches in width, one inch in elevation, at the highest part, which was several inches immediately over the injured part of the rib. The skin over the tumor was unchanged, except by slight enlargement of superficial vessels.

Dr Pugely, an aged accurate surgeon thought, with me, that an abscess pressed on the right lobe.

At 4. P.M. Allen was placed supine on a table, with his right arm extended by the side of his head, while the left arm & lower limbs were held. I made a free incision from the sternum through the integuments, over the space between the 5th & 6th ribs, to the lower end of the tumor. The fleshy digital origin of the serratus magnus, from the sixth **C295** rib; the interlocking fibres of the origin of the pectoralis major, the intercostal muscles and their vessels had been removed, by the resources of the system. Copious grume and old red coagula were discharged with condensed coagula of fragments of membrane, like lymph. The 6th rib was carious and brownish from its sternal articulation, to the other end of the wound, where it seemed healthy and attached to the surrounding parts. Its anterior half was easily removed, in fragments, by the fingers; the sternum seemed healthy. Two inches of the lower edge of the 5th rib was carious; a section of it, cleared of surrounding parts each way, to where healthy adhesion existed, was removed by a cutting forceps; the intercostal artery was cut & tied. Much of the same sort of matter, removed from within the ribs seemed more homogeneous, more **C296** broken, very dark, greyish, occasionally tinged with crimson. I passed my first and second fingers, three & a half inches in every direction, without more resistance than from the matter, except occasionally from fragments of bronchial tubes. Dr Pugely made full & satisfactory examination to the same effect; no motion of respiration was perceptable [sic] to the fingers. I removed all the disorganized parenchyma of the lungs within the reach of my fingers, between one and two pounds, from between & around the branches of several bronchial tubes. I introduced large pledgets between the cut edges retracted, and covered the wound with plaster, applying a roller to prevent motion of the ribs. During the operation Allen became weak & faint, tho free from pain, except smarting of the edges. He slept badly at night, till he took an anodyne. The next day was very weak and breathed laboriously.

C297

His room was crowded at evening, so that he was depressed, breathed harder and was thought to be dying. The room was ventilated, and he rested well, as also the second & third day, with little fever. I saw him on the fourth, when he was chearful, pulse 96 at the exarcebation [*sic*], natural in fullness, somewhat convulsive. He desired a little weak wine & water occasionally, being sickened by the sent [*sic*] of the wound in dressing. Lint was put two inches within the ribs, and I directed the wound to be kept open, by large pledgets. On the 9th day he was much better, the discharge from the thorax more free, and there was motion of respiration in the side.

11th The wound had closed in the middle by granulation tho open at each end; appetite & pulse good, regular stools and but slight fever. 12th he was raised out of bed & put erect. 13th was very chearful. The bottom of the cavities filled with healthy granulations discharging pus ****C298**** like cream; the motion of the ribs in respiration increased. I enjoined absolute rest.

30th day, he walked the house. 40th he was free from pain & uneasiness. He has had no cough at any period of the case. A livid soft membraneous conical substance protruded from the wound. On its removal a substance escaped like that removed in the last part of the first operation. I could introduce my finger two & a half inches in, down & back. He was sensible of my touch. I removed half a pound of disorganized substance of the lungs, and dressed the wound with a large tent. He remains easy.

64th day. He has the full habit of his ordinary health, walks out with ease. The inferior end of the remaining portion of the lungs seems adhered or healed, so that its respiration is unaffected. The patient grows fleshy & strong, and attended publick worship. After this he was seized with the measles & died.

C299 The foregoing case was published in the New England Journal. vol. 11. N°4, by my consent, at the request of George Parkman, M.D. of Boston.[15]

Cases, something similar, have occurred in Europe.[16] See Journal of Arts and Sciences, N°. 11.50. Also London Medical Repository N°. 10. 235.[17]

---

[15] Milton Antony, "Caries of the 5th and 6th Ribs. Disorganization of the Right Lobe of the Lungs, with a Description of an Operation [Communicated for the New England Journal of Medicine and Surgery by George Parkman, M.D.]," *New England Journal of Medicine and Surgery* 11, no. 4 (1822): 374–76.

[16] An example: "Grand Surgical Operation," 204.

[17] M. Le Chevalier Richerand, "Richerand's Operation of Cutting into the Pleura," *The London Medical Repository, Monthly Journal, and Review* 10 (July–December 1818): 228–36. This is the translated unabridged account that Richerand read to the Royal Academy of Sciences of the French Institute on April 27, 1818. He was Professor of the Faculty of Medicine and Chief

C300

The following case of neglected consumption was transmitted to me by a medical friend, 1822, from the Revue Medicale, a European Journal.

The subject was tall, of a sanguineous habit. His father died of asthma at the age of 32, and his mother was subject to frequent attacks of hemoptysis. At twenty he left a sedentary employment, and entered the army, where he suffered great fatigue. In 1816, he was attacked with cough which threatened consumption, violent pains in the epigastrium & loins. The heart beat with great violence, rigor followed by heat severe headach, fever pulse full strong & frequent, pulsation of the superficial arteries visible, no external heat tho he complained of extreme internal heat, skin pale, appetite for cooling food & fruits. The above symptoms appeared in the course of his disease. ——Leeches were applied to the anus, and his diet was regulated. Under this course the symptoms declined but the least exercise renewed them. He kept his hands often to the epigastrium to relieve pain. **C301** Rubefacients & blisters were applied with some benefit.

In 1818, the disease assumed a very alarming aspect. The pulsation of the arteries & heart were visible, at some paces distant, appetite for food very great. Leeches were again used; but the whole aspect of the patient altered for the worse, with a severe chill followed by extreme heat and a sense of suffocation. He was then largely bled, and venesection was repeated twice with benefit. ——In 18 days after, he had a similar attack with similar treatment & relief. ——He then returned to his occupation, but some journeys on foot, at the beginning of 1819, brought on a return of the disease. Symptoms of effusions in the pleura and pericardium now came on with general anasarca. The visible pulsation at the arteries continued. He died May 6th. Dissection, water in the pleura, pericardium & peritoneum. Tubercles here & there in the lungs in a **C302** state of suppuration. Heart large its four cavities being dilated; its membranes brown, covered with a brown mucous and deep red spots adhering firmly to the muscular structure, destroyed in the places where the red spots existed. Valves, particularly of the right ventricle, filled with reddish mucous.

Surgeon to the Hospital of Saint Louis in Paris. The patient was a forty-year-old male "officer of health" who had recurrent cancer involving his anterior chest wall, ribs, and lung over three years and had had several unsuccessful local excisions, and cauteries. The surgery was performed March 31, 1818, with Professor Dupuytren assisting, and included resection of tumors, involved ribs and pleura, and drainage of pus. The patient was discharged home on the twenty-seventh day. Though everyone earnestly wished that there be no return of the cancer, that was not the expectation; in fact, it was stipulated that should the malady not return, there would be a question as to whether it had been cancer they had been treating (p. 234).

Ascending aorta, carotid, and the branches which go to the face & brain, subclavian tracheal artery, and its divisions, even to the collateral arteries of the fingers, presented an internal tunic, which was thick, hard of a deep red colour, and covered with a white purulent matter. Between the internal and fibrous tunic there existed a layer of serosity of a citron color and considerably dense. The pulmonary veins & arteries presented the same morbid changes. The abdominal aorta, hypogastric and crural arteries were in a similar state. **C303** The appearance of inflammation, however, diminished more & more as the examination proceeded, thro the inferior extremities. The veins of the chest had experienced the same changes. Their internal membrane & valves were thick, red and torn with a slight effort. This was the state of the mucous membrane in its whole extent from the fauces to the termination of the rectum. The liver was much enlarged; the spleen very small. The proper texture of the omentum had undergone changes not dissimilar from those exhibited by the mucous structures.

See New England Journal v. 10. N³.[18]

---

[18] "Intelligence: Revue Médicale Historique et Philosophique; Par MM. V. Bally, Bellanger, F. Bérard, Bestieu, Bousquet, Delpeon, Desportes, Double, Dunal, Esquirol, Gasc, Girandy, Jadioux, Laurent, Nicod. Prunelle, Rouzet. Ire Année (1820.)—Ire Livraison. Janvier," *New England Journal of Medicine and Surgery* 10, no. 3 (1821): 311–15. The same issue of the *New England Journal of Medicine and Surgery* contains the conclusion of a two-part review of R. T. C. Laennec's book on the discovery and use of the stethoscope. "Review, Article VIII [Concluded from Page 156.] De L'auscultation Mediate Ou Traité Du Diagnostic Des Maladies Des Poumons et Du Coeur, Fondé Principalement Sur Ce Nouveau Moyen D'exploration. Par R. T. H. Laennec, D. M. P. Médecin De L'hôpital Necker, Médecin Honoraire Des Dispensaires, Membre De La Société De La Faculté De Médecine De Paris, et De Plusieurs Autres Sociétés Nationales et Étrangères. Tome Second. A Paris, Ches J. A. Brosson et S. J. S. Chaudé, Libraires. 1819," *New England Journal of Medicine and Surgery* 10, no. 3 (1821): 265–93. The reviewers of volume 1 valued the book so highly they were "disposed to promote the translation of it in this country." But without the experience of using a stethoscope, they were "not prepared to give an opinion" on the usefulness of the instrument. "Review, Article III: Laennec, R. T. H. De L'auscultation Médiate, Volume One. 1819," *New England Journal of Medicine and Surgery* 10, no. 2 (1821): 132–56. It is fitting that the last journal issue cited by Barker in his manuscript includes a review article about an instrument that would become symbolic of the new medicine, its diagnosis, and its technology. Therapeutically, the same issue includes a review of the first US pharmacopoeia, "Article IX: 'The Pharmacopaeia of the United States of America.' 1820. By the Authority of the Medical Societies and Colleges. Boston: Printed by Wells & Lilley, for Charles Ewer. Dec. 1820. 8vo. Pp.268," *New England Journal of Medicine and Surgery* 10, no. 3 (1821): 293–310. Finally, the issue includes a notice that the Massachusetts Medical Society had appointed a committee "to consider in what relation those fellows of the society who reside in Maine at the time of separation of that district from Massachusetts, should stand to the society." "Massachusetts Medical Society Report of Annual

This case serves to show extensive inflammation of the blood vessels, and consequent morbid affection on other parts, which probably might have been prevented if blood letting had been copiously and repeatedly practiced in the first & very lengthy stage of the disease, instead of the depending on leeches, or if, by the efforts of Nature, "spontaneous profuse hemorrhages from the nose or other parts had taken place, as has often been the case, [End of Volume 2 MS]

Meeting of the Society, Holden June 6th, 1821," *New England Journal of Medicine and Surgery* 10, no. 3 (1821): 317–17.

EPILOGUE

You have now read over one hundred of Barker's case records and observations, supplemented by those of other physicians from Maine, Massachusetts, New York, Philadelphia, and a few in European centers. The publication of this manuscript, as written, allows scholars, students, and an interested public to use this two-hundred-year-old primary source to study life, death, disease, diagnosis and treatment, preventive medicine, and public health as seen through his eyes and thoughts.

Barker emphasized the treatment of epidemic and other medical diseases because these were the great threat to society in his time. This is true whether one considers the number of deaths per year or the social disruption precipitated by epidemics. His emphasis may also represent a point of view that was not generally available to others: he had almost fifty years of experience practicing in rural northern New England with access to extensive American and European medical books and other sources to strengthen his arguments.

Although he did deliver babies, Barker barely mentioned his obstetric practice other than his discussion of an unusual epidemic of childbed fever in the wider community in 1784–1785. But pregnancy and delivery are normal events, not to be included in a discussion of disease. We do have one interesting newspaper piece from 1800 in which Barker refuted local gossip about a woman who supposedly gave birth to a *"black child*; and that the husband, on this account, sent the infant from home, I think it my duty, as a friend to an injured reputation, thus publicly to certify, that I was the attending physician to the woman alluded to; and that, to my certain knowledge, she was put to bed in October last, with a *white child*, which she has ever since kept with her and nursed; receiving every mark of attention and kindness from her husband. The report, therefore, in my opinion, must have originated from vain jesting or malice, as it does not contain the least shadow of truth, and is entirely groundless. JEREMIAH BARKER. *Falmouth, January 1800."* [*Jenks' Portland Gazette* 2, no. 93 (February 3,1800): 3]

The Barker manuscript gives us a fascinating window into another time, with striking similarities to and differences from our own. He practiced just

at the cusp of the great changes that ushered in modern medicine. His lifelong determination to record the details of his practice enables us to see these
changes evolve. Now that his work is finally published, after two hundred
years of obscurity, may it serve to inform, encourage, and humble us in the
present day.

GLOSSARY

Sources for this Glossary, unless otherwise stated, are listed here.
(Definitions use the spelling and syntax of the original in most cases.)

Coxe: Coxe, J. R. (1817). *The Philadelphia Medical Dictionary*. Philadelphia: Thomas Dobson.

Duncan: Duncan, A. (1805). *The Edinburgh New Dispensatory*. Worcester: Press of Isaiah Thomas.

D: Dunglison, R. (1874). *A Dictionary of Medical Science*. Philadelphia: Henry C. Lea.

Estes: Estes, J. W. (1990). *Dictionary of Protopharmacology*. Canton, MA: Science History Publications.

Goldstein: Goldstein, Daniel A. *The Historical Apothecary Compendium: A Guide to Terms and Symbols*. Atglen, PA: Schiffer, 2015.

Hooper: Hooper, R. (1799). *A compendious medical dictionary: Containing an explaination of the terms in anatomy, physiology, surgery, materia medica, chemistry, and practice of physic: collected from the most approved authors*. London: Printed for Murray and Highley (unpaginated).

Thacher: Thacher, James. *The American New Dispensatory Containing General Principles of Pharmaceutic Chemistry. . . . The Whole Compiled from the Most Approved Authors, Both European and American*. Boston: T. B. Wait and Co., 1810.

Thacher, James. *American Modern Practice*. Boston: Ezra Read, 1817.

OED: Oxford English Dictionary

For a comprehensive review of therapeutics in Colonial New England, see Estes, J. Worth, "Therapeutic Practice in Colonial New England." In *Medicine in Colonial Massachusetts, 1620–1820: A Conference Held 25 & 26 May 1978*, edited by Frederick S. Allis, 289–383. Boston: The Colonial Society of Massachusetts, 1980.

℥ Ounce. ℥ii = 2 ounces (8 drachms or 480 grains) (Estes 125)

Ɜ Scruple. Ɜii = 2 scruples (20 grains) (Estes 125)

Accoucher or accoucheur One who practices the art of midwifery. (D 8) Often a male midwife.

Accouchement Parturition, labor. (D 8)

Adnata The exterior coat of the eye. (Coxe 15)

Agaric A fungal species that grows on a number of different trees and has supposed styptic powers, though Duncan questions its efficacy other than as a sponge to stop bleeding. (Duncan 169)

Ague A fever with regular paroxysms (Thacher, *American Modern Practice* 289–97); an acute high fever with paroxysms marked by shivering, borrowing from the Anglo-Norman and Middle French *ague*. (OED)

Ail Disease; to be sick; from the Saxon. (D 28)

Aleotic A medication capable of causing a constitutional change. (OED)

Aloes The inspissated juice of the *Aloe* (*Aloe perfoliate* or *Aloe barbadensis*). A cathartic that affects the rectum chiefly, works slowly but occasionally causes bloody diarrhea. (D 36, Estes 6–7)

Aloetic pills "Take of Aloes in powder [and] Soap, equal parts. Beat them with simple syrup into a mass fit for making pills." (Duncan 620)

Alterative A medicine that corrects or evacuates foul humors by unexplained mechanisms; it may also alter pulse rate. (Estes 7)

Alum Potassium aluminum sulfate, a powerful astringent that can strengthen the body and decrease excessive evacuations from the mouth, lungs, uterus, or bowels; an antispasmodic, for internal or topical use. (Estes 7, 8) A neutral salt . . . externally applied as a styptic to bleeding vessels. (Hooper)

Alvine That which relates to the lower belly. (D 38)

Anagallis A common European plant; a reputed antispasmodic and stomachic. A decoction of this in beer is said to form an important part of *Stoy's medicine for hydrophobia*. (D 47) Pimpernel, *Anagallis arvensis*. (Estes 10)

Anasarca The accumulation of excess fluid in the body. Commonly, it begins with swelling around the ankles and is characterized by swelling of the limbs and of the soft parts covering the abdomen, thorax, and even the face, with paleness and dryness of the skin, and pitting when any of these (especially the ankles) are pressed upon. (D 49) A dropsical swelling of the skin or cellular membrane. (Coxe 39) See also: Dropsy

Angina A quincy; that is, an inflammation of the throat that may interrupt respiration. (Coxe 42–43) A strangling or choking.

Anodynes Opiates, paregorics, narcotics, hypnotics, drugs allaying pain or producing sleep. (Coxe 45) An analgesic, usually made with opium. (Estes 11)

Antimonii, Antimony, Antimonical The ore of antimony, chiefly the trisulfide and used in various preparations since the seventeenth century. An emetic, cathartic, tonic, diaphoretic, and febrifuge. (Estes 12–14)

Antiphlogistic A medicine used to neutralize fevers. The word is derived from the Greek word *phlogiston*, fire or fire principle. (Estes 14–15) Any medicine or diet that reduces inflammation. (Coxe 49)

Aperient A drug used to open the bowels, to relieve constipation; a laxative. (OED)

Aphthae Roundish, pearl-colored vesicles, confined to the lips, mouth, and intestinal canal, and generally terminating in curd-like sloughs. (D 70) Aphthous: ulcerations in the throat.

Apoplexy A suspension of sense and voluntary motion. (Coxe 53) From the Greek, a striking down; cerebral hemorrhage. (D 73)

Apyrexia Absence or intermission of fever. (Coxe 56) Apyrexia is the condition of an intermittent fever between the paroxysms. (D76)

Aqua calcis Lime water made from fresh burnt lime (calcium oxide) and water. It possesses astringent powers and is also a powerful antacid. It can also be used externally in cancer and chronic cutaneous diseases. (Duncan 413–15)

Aqua fortis From the Latin: strong water. An early scientific name for nitric acid. (D 702, OED) An antiphlogistic, antiseptic, antisyphilitic (Estes 137)

Aqua Fontana "Spring water" used as a diluent. (Estes 84)

Argent viv. *Argentum vivum.* Hydrargyrum (metallic mercury) or quicksilver does not act on the body, when taken into the stomach; but if oxydized, and combined with acids, it acts powerfully. (D 82, 511) See also: Calomel, Corrosive sublimate, Ethiops mineral, Jalap, Mercurials, Turpeth mineral, Unguent. Caml. (abbreviation of Calomel)

Asa fatida, Asafœtida   Asa, a healer; stinking healer, Devil's Dung (Coxe 68) A gum resin native to Persia, *Ferula assafœtida*, used as a stimulant, expectorant, antispasmodic, and antihelmentic; also useful in croup, dyspepsia, amenorrhea, asthma, and hysteria. (Duncan 225)

Ascites   A collection of serous fluid in the abdomen. Ascites proper is dropsy of the peritoneum, and is characterized by increased size of the abdomen. (D 94)

Asthenic   Diminished animal power; extreme debility. (Coxe 72) Lacking strength, infirm, inactive. (D 97) Thus asthenic/sthenic means inactive/active.

Astringent   A medication that should strengthen a relaxed body and decrease excessive evacuations. (Estes 21)

Astringent lotions   Medications applied externally to "contract broken or ulcerated skin." (Estes 21)

Azotic air   In the new chemistry, the name for the basis of atmospheric air, and of ammonia, nitrous acid, etc., azotic gas; mephitic or phlogisticated air; atmospheric mephitis; nitrogene. (Coxe 79) Of, pertaining to, or chemically combined with azote (nitrogen). Azote was the name given by Lavoisier for its inability to support life. (OED)

Balsam of Life, Turlington's   Tinctura benzoini composita. (D 111) Stimulant. Used chiefly to treat wounds and ulcers. The basis of Turlington's Balsam of Life . . . is the Compound Tincture of Benzoin. (D 1039) Patented by Robert Turlington in 1744, it was made of twenty-seven ingredients and was said to cure urinary tract stones, colic, and "inward weakness"; later advertisements promoted it simply as a panacea. (Estes 197) See also: *Balsamum traumaticum*

Balsamum traumaticum   Wound balsam. Same as Turlington's Balsam. See also: Balsam of Life. (Estes 197, Thacher 337)

Bark   When used alone this refers to cinchona. The active ingredient, quinine, was isolated in the early nineteenth century. (Estes 24, 47–49, Thacher 100–106)

Blistering   The application of a plaster consisting of *cantharides* (Spanish fly) or other medication in order to produce vesication or blistering that removes fluid directly from the body, similar to laxatives and cathartics. The term "counter-irritation" is also used for this procedure. (Estes 36–38) See also: Cantharides, Vesication

Book-muslin   A fine kind of muslin owing its name to the book-like manner in which it is folded when sold in the piece. (OED)

Borborigmi   Rumblings of the gut. (OED) A rumbling noise in the intestines caused by wind. (Coxe 91)

Brandish's solution   Impure solution of potash. (Goldstein 88)

Brimstone   Sulfur. Used as a cathartic, diaphoretic as well as applied to the skin. (Estes 30, 186)

Bronchotomy   A surgical operation, which consists in making an opening either into the trachea, into the larynx, or into both, to extract foreign bodies or to permit the passage of air to the lungs. (D 114)

Buffy or buffy coat   *Corium phlogisticum, fibrin coagula, crusta pseudomembranacea,* or *crusta inflammatoria* and in a more specific case, *crusta pleuritica*. The grayish crust or buff, varying in thickness, observed on blood drawn from a vein during the existence of violent inflammation, pregnancy, &c. It is particularly manifest in pleurisy. (D 257) In 1921 R. Fåhraeus noted that blood allowed to flow into a tall, transparent container would, after clotting, form layers . . . nearer the top of the clot, a pale green or whitish layer may be discerned, especially if the subject of the venesection has been ill . . . this is called crusta phlogistica. (Fåhraeus, Robin. 1921.

The Suspension-Stability of the Blood. Stockholm. 3–44; Wintrobe, M.M. 1980. *Blood,*
pure and eloquent: a story of discovery, of people, and of ideas. NY: McGraw-Hill. 3–4)
See also: Cup, Sizy

Calcination   Defined in 1817 as "chemical pulverization; the union of metal with
oxygen by means of heat, air, or other chemical process." (Coxe 99)

Calomel   Mercurous chloride frequently used as a laxative. It was the most widely
used of all the mercurial drugs from at least 1595. Cathartic, diuretic, emetic, sialagogue (promoting salivation), alterative, expectorant, anthelminthic, and emetic.
(Estes 34) Submuriate of quicksilver (mercurous chloride) is a combination of
muriate of quicksilver ground to a powder combined with purified quicksilver. It
increases secretions and is used in chronic inflammations as well as to treat syphilis. (Duncan 459–61) An inorganic mercurial diuretic described by Paracelsus in
the sixteenth century; organic mercurials were used from 1920s to 1960s when
thiazide and then loop diuretics replaced mercurials. Calomel was used as a cathartic, emetic, and sialagogue (to produce salivation) and for many theoretical
reasons. "The Diuretic Action of Calomel," *The Lancet* 136, no. 3499 (1890): 634. See
also: Argent viv., Corrosive sublimate, Ethiops mineral, Jalap, Mercurials, Turpeth
mineral, Unguent, Caml

Cambric   A fine white linen originally made at Cambray in Flanders (also applied to
an imitation made of hard-spun cotton yarn). (OED)

Camomile, chamomile   Leaves of maywood, or wild chamomile, *Anthemis cotula*. In
small doses, tonic, and diaphoretic, emetic in large doses; used for hysteria, spasmodic and flatulent colics (Estes 55, Thacher 79) The name of a Composite plant,
Anthemis nobilis, an aromatic creeping herb, found on dry sandy commons in England,
with downy leaves, and flowers white in the ray and yellow in the disk. (OED)

Camphor   An extract of *Cinnamomum camphora* that can be administered internally and externally usually in a compound preparation. It is an analgesic, anti-
inflammatory, diaphoretic, diuretic, tonic. (Estes 35)

Canker ail   Probably refers to scarlatina anginosa or scarlet fever. Calvin Jones, *A*
Treatise on the Scarlatina Anginosa: Or What Is Vulgarly Called the Scarlet Fever, or
Canker-Rash. Replete with Every Thing Necessary to the Pathology and Practice, Deduced
from Actual Experience and Observation (Catskill [N.Y.]: M. Crosswell & Co., 1794);
Thacher, *American Modern Practice* 400–408.

Canker distemper   Refers to a number of diseases that have in common ulcerations
around the mouth. Distemper is a derangement or disturbance of the humours or
tempers; tempers being a proportionate mixture or combination of elements or
qualities. Disease was considered a disturbance in the bodily humours in mediæval
physiology. (OED)

Cantharides   Spanish fly; a corrosive agent that when applied to the skin as a plaster,
causes blisters full of serous matter to form. "It is considered the most powerful
medicine in the *materia medica*." It relieves inflammatory diseases, as phrenitis,
pleuritis, hepatitis, phlegmon, bubo, myositis, arthritis, etc., . . . but it ought to be
used with much caution. (Hooper) Powdered Spanish fly, *Lytta* (formerly *Cantharis*)
vesicatoria, is prepared from an emerald green beetle in the family *Meloidae* and
functions as a general stimulant to remove fluid from the body directly as "blister
fluid" and indirectly in urine or phlegm. It is thought to be a "counter-irritant"
that "reflexly reduces irritability, especially of the blood vessels thereby altering
the circulation in patients with severe fevers." (Estes 36–38) See also: Blistering,
Epispastic, Vesication

Catamenia Menses. (D180)

Cataplasm A medicine applied externally, under the form of a thick pap. (D 181) A watery fermenting poultice made of flour and yeast. (Estes 42, 81)

Cathartics Purging medicines, or such as increase the number of alvine (excretions from the intestines; OED) evacuations; emetics. (Coxe 117) A medicine that causes vomit or bowel movement.

Catarrh Increased discharge of mucus from the nose [and throat]. *Catarrhus* is the common cold. (Coxe 116, 154)

Caustic A chemical that dissolves or destroys animal matter; sometimes used for skin ulcers. (Estes 43, 79)

Cerate From the Latin *cere*, wax. A composition of oil, wax, or lard with or without other ingredients. (D 193) Beeswax, or an external application with a consistency between those of plasters and unguents. (Estes 44) See also: Turner's cerate

Chalk Julep Chalk or Creta is calcium carbonate, an antacid. Julep is a sweet aqueous medication derived from the Persian word for rose-water. (Estes 56, 107–108)

Chamomile *Chamaemelum* (Roman chamomile) Dried powdered flowers of chamomile. Tonic, diaphoretic, antiseptic, antispasmodic, antihysteric, carminative, digestive, and aperient. (Estes 45)

Chlorosis Green sickness; white fever, or virgin's disease; known by dyspepsia, paleness, weakness, palpitation and retained menses. (Coxe 129)

Cholera An excessive vomiting and purging; the gall flux. (Coxe 129)

Chyle A nutritive fluid extracted by intestinal absorption from food which has been subjected to the action of the digestive organs, of a whitish appearance; the emulsified oil in the intestinal canal. (D 213)

Cicuta The leaves of modern poison hemlock, *Conium maculatum* . . . in small doses a potent . . . tonic, narcotic, and sedative. . . . Poisonous in large doses. (Estes 47, Thacher 111–12)

Cineritious The color of ashes. (D 218) Like ashes, ash-coloured. (Coxe 134)

Clyster A liquid thrown into the large intestines by means of a syringe. (D. 228) An enema. See also: Glyster

Colliquative An epithet given to various discharges, which produce rapid exhaustion. Hence, we say . . . *Colliquative diarrhea*, &c. (D 236)

Coloquintida *Colocynthis* or Bitter apple is grown in the Levant (Eastern Mediterranean, Turkey for example) and is one of the "most powerful and most violent cathartics." Many physicians condemn its use. (Duncan 211, Coxe 142)

Columbo Also, colomba, is the powdered root of *Swertia carboliniensis*. It is a mild tonic, antiseptic, or antiemetic. (Estes 52, Thacher 111, Duncan 203–204)

Confused group A medley, mixture, hotchpotch. (OED)

Consumption *Consumptio*, wasting; consumption of the lungs; decline; decay (Coxe 148); or phthisis, wasting of the flesh. (Coxe 343) "*Phthisis*" is Greek for consumption or wasting. "Consumption" and "Phthisis" are terms used through the seventeenth, eighteenth, and early nineteenth centuries; the term "tuberculosis" entered in the mid-nineteenth century. See also: Phthsis.

Contrayerva Literally, "counter herb" or antidote; an astringent tonic and diaphoretic. The root of *Dorstenia contrajerva*. (Estes 53)

Corrosive sublimate *Hydrargyri oxymurias*. (D 993) It is used as an antisyphilitic that promotes good health in venereal complaints, old cutaneous affections, &c . . . is a good gargle in venereal sore-throat, or as an injection in gonorrhea. Externally it is applied in cases of tetter (Herpes, Impetigo, Eczema, Psoriasis, see D 1029) and to destroy fungus, or stimulate old ulcers. . . . White of egg is the best antidote to it, when taken in an overdose. (D 510) It is the same as *Hydrargyrus muriatus corrosivus* or mercuric chloride and was introduced for the treatment of syphilis in 1750. Used topically or by ingesting; considered highly dangerous. (Estes 55, 99) See also: Argent viv., Calomel, Ethiops mineral, Jalap, Mercurials, Turpeth mineral, Unguent, Caml

Coryza Inflammation attended with increased discharge of the membranes lining the nose and the sinuses communicating with it. (D 265) Catarrh, or increased discharge of mucus from the nose. (Coxe 134)

Costive Constipated. (D 265)

Crassamentum The thick part or deposit of any fluid (crassus: thick, crassamen: dregs). It is particularly applied to the clot of the blood. (D.270) The red globules and coagulable lymph of the blood; dregs. (Coxe 156)

Cream of tartar Powdered sodium potassium bitartrate had originally been obtained from the dregs (called "tartar") of wine casks; cathartic and diuretic used in fevers. (Estes 55) The scum of a boiling solution of tartar; a vegetable alkali, tartaric acid. (Coxe 156, 404)

Croup An inflammation of the trachea. See *Cynache trachealis*. (Hooper) Many other names including *Cynache stridula*, choak in Ireland, hives in the southern parts of the United States, and quincy in many parts of New England. (Thacher, *American Modern Practice* 239)

Cup May refer to a small vessel used for receiving blood during venesection, usually contains about four ounces (D 281), but more likely the raised edge and central depression of the buffy coat or *crusta phlogistica* on blood drawn from a person suffering from an inflammatory process/infection. See also: Buffy, Sizy

Cynanche From the Greek, "I suffocate." Inflammation of the upper part of the air passages or upper alimentary canal. It would include many diseases of the upper airways. (D 286–87) Quincy. (Coxe 162)

Cynanche trachealis The croup. (Coxe 163)

Datura stramonium Thorn apple, a plant native to America, used as a remedy in mania and melancholy. It can be taken internally or externally as an ointment from the leaves, causing external inflammations. (Duncan 217) The leaves, roots, and seeds of thorn apple, or jimson (Jamestown) weed. It has many other common names and was used in mania and as an antiepileptic. Potent narcotic, tonic, diuretic, anodyne antispasmodic, and antitussive. Used chiefly in disorders of the nervous system. (Estes 184) See also: *Stramonium officiale*

Decoction An extract obtained by boiling the raw plant ingredient(s) in water. (Estes 60)

Defluction A discharge of fluid from any part. (Hooper)

Deglutition Swallowing.

Dejections Discharge of excrement by stool. (Coxe 168)

Deliquium, Deliquium Animi Fainting; swooning. (Coxe 168)

Demulcent An agent that prevents the action of acrid and stimulant materials by lubricating the surface exposed to them with a viscid matter. (Estes 60) Medicines supposed to be capable of correcting certain acrid conditions imagined to exist in the humors. Substances of a mucilaginous or saccharine nature belong to this class. (D 302)

Deobstruent A medicine given with the view of removing any obstruction. (Coxe 169)

Despumation The separation of the froth and other impurities, which rise, by the action of the fire, to the surface of any fluid. The expulsion of impure matter from fluids of the body. (D 308, OED)

Desquamation Exfoliation, or separation of the epidermis, in the form of scales, of a greater or less size. . . . This affection is a common consequence of exanthematous diseases. (Coxe 170, D 308)

Detergents Medicines that possess the property of cleansing the skin and wounds, ulcers, &c. (Coxe 170), (D 308)

Digitalis Foxglove; finger-like. (Coxe 176) The leaves of this plant . . . which are indigenous in Great Britain, are powerfully sedative,—diminishing the velocity of the pulse, and a diuretic; . . . Digitalis has been administered in inflammatory diseases, phthisis, active hemorrhage, dropsy, delirium tremens, &c. (D 317) It acts on the kidney as a diuretic that removes abnormal tissue fluids in dropsy. (Estes 68)

Discutient, Discut A medicine that dissipates, dispels, or dissolves morbid matter. (Estes 69)

Dossil Bourdonnet. (D 327) From old French for spigot, plug, tap. A term in French surgery term for charpie, which is old linen unraveled into short ends of thread for surgical dressings (OED) rolled into a small mass of an olive shape, which is used for plugging wounds, absorbing the discharge, and preventing the union of their edges. In cases of deep and penetrating wounds, as of the abdomen or chest, a thread is attached to them by which they may be readily withdrawn and be prevented from passing altogether in those cavities. (D137) See also: Linteum, Pledget

Drachm 1 drachm = 3 scruples = 60 grains = 3.888 grams (Estes 124)

Dropsical Suffering from dropsy, the morbid accumulation of watery fluid in the serous cavities and connective tissue (OED); from the French "hydropisie" from the Greek for water. (OED) See also: Dropsy

Dropsy Also, hydrops: an accumulation of serous fluid such as in the legs or abdomen produced by a number of conditions such as heart, kidney, or liver disease. (D 329, 517–18) See also: Anasarca

Efflorescence From the Latin "to flourish," blooming of flowers, but here meaning redness of the skin. (Coxe 188)

Ejections The discharge of anything by vomit or stool, but more commonly vomiting. (Coxe 188)

Elecampane *Inula helenium*. (D 343) The root *Inula* was formerly in high esteem in dyspepsia, cachexia, pulmonary affections, &c. It is now (1874) scarcely used. (D 553)

Elect. Scordio A pharmaceutical composition of a soft consistence, somewhat thicker than honey, and formed of powders, pulps, extracts, syrup, honey, &c. In the London and American Pharmacopoeias, electuaries are classed under Confections. (D 344)

Elix[ir]. vitriol A sweetened alcoholic solution containing sulfuric acid. (Estes 75, 204–205)

Embrocation A fluid application to be rubbed on any part of the body. It is often used synonymously with liniment. (D 348) Rubbing a part with spirit, etc. (Coxe 192) An ointment or liniment to be rubbed on a painful part of the body. (Estes 75)

Emetic, Emetica A medication that causes vomit. (Coxe 193)

Empyema A collection of pus in the thorax. (Coxe 195)

Encomium A formal or high-flown expression of praise. (OED)

Epiploitis The epiploon is the caul covering the bowels, the omentum (Coxe 201, 319) and epiploitis is the inflammation of this caul. But Coxe also defines epiploitis as the puerperal fever. (Coxe 201)

Epispastic Blister plaster or drawing drugs. (Coxe 201) An epithet for every medicinal substance which, when applied to the skin, excites pain, heat, and more or less redness, followed by separation of the epidermis,—which is raised up by effused serum,—or by suppuration. Now [1874] usually restricted to blisters. (D 370)

Epistaxis Bleeding at the nose. (D 370)

Erysipelas St. Anthony's fire; a diffused inflammation with fever of two or three days, generally with coma or delirium if on the face. (Coxe 203)

Erysipelatous Superficial inflammation of the skin, with general fever, tension, and swelling of the part; the surface smooth and shining as if oiled. (D 374)

Ethiops mineral, Aethiops mineral *Hydrargyri sulphuretum nigrum* or black mercuric sulfide, assumed to have the same effects as calomel though generally ineffective. (Estes 4, 79, 99–100) Black sulphuret of mercury . . . used chiefly in scrofulous and cutaneous affections. (D 24, 511) See also: Argent viv., Calomel, Corrosive sublimate, Jalap, Mercurials, Turpeth mineral, Unguent, Caml

Exanthemata Pleural of exathem, a rash. (D 383)

Exulceration A small superficial ulceration. (Coxe 209)

Factitious Not genuine or natural. (OED) It can also mean that which is made by art, in opposition to what is natural, or found already existing in nature. (D 397)

Farinaceous A mealy substance. (Coxe 210) Having the appearance or nature of farina. Any article of food that contains farina. (D 403)

Farrago A confused group; a medley, mixture, hotchpotch. (OED)

Fatuity Idiocy, imbecility, dementia. "Death is dreadful, and fatuity is more dreadful." Samuel Johnson: Letter to Mrs. Thrale, April 6, 1779. (OED)

Fauces Pleural of faux, the top of the throat. (Coxe 210) A cavity behind the tongue, palatine arch, uvula, and tonsils; from which the pharynx and larynx proceed. (Hooper)

Febrifuge A medicine which possesses the property of abating or driving away fever. (D 406)

Felon Paronychia. A tumour or inflammation of the fingertip that may spread to other parts, with pain and swelling. (D 411, 759)

Ferruginous Rust of iron. (Coxe 212) Resembling iron rust in colour. (OED)

Fixed air Carbonic acid. It is unfit for respiration. (Hooper) This refers to carbon dioxide, which was described in the seventeenth century by van Helmont and studied more thoroughly by Joseph Black in Scotland in the 1750s and Joseph Priestley in England in the 1770s. Chalk is a form of limestone composed of calcium carbonate which, when acid is added, releases carbon dioxide.

Flores of sulphuris "Flowers of sulphur"—usually means sublimated sulphur. Cooling, cathartic, diaphoretic, and resolvent; antagonizes the side effects of mercury and antimony. (Estes 84, 186)

Fœtor A stink; fœtid effluvia from the body or diseased part. (Coxe 216)

Fomentations Warm medicated decoctions applied to the body on flannel, linen, or sponges, or squeezed from a bladder. (Estes 84)

Fomes The focus or seat of any disease. (D 430) "Bilious fomes" refers to morbific matter, meaning disease-causing material.

Fret Chafing, an erosion; Herpes. (D 436)

Friction Friction of the body by a piece of flannel or a coarse linen cloth. Friction is a kind of exercise that remarkably contributes to the health of sedentary persons; it excites and kindles the natural warmth; promotes perspiration, strengthens the fibres, and tends to dissipate stagnant humours. The operation is particularly beneficial to the nervous, debilitated and studious. (Thacher, *American Modern Practice* 80)

Froward Habitually disposed to disobedience and opposition. (Merriam-Webster 2017)

Gamboge, gamb. Gambogia: Cambogia (D 445) named from Cambodia, where it comes from. (OED) Gum resin of *Garcina hanburii*. Introduced in 1603 and promoted in England by the East India Company from 1615. Dangerously potent emetic and cathartic; anthelminthic. (Estes 88)

Gargarism A gargle or wash for a sore throat. (Coxe 223)

Garrotillo Spanish name for malignant sore throat. (Coxe 223) May refer to croup or severe cases of diphtheria that may cause strangulation.

Gibbeted To be hanged, as on a gibbet (synonymous with gallows); refers to putting a man who had been executed on an upright post with a projecting arm as a warning to others. (OED)

Gill One quarter of a liquid pint, four ounces.

Glauber's salts Sulphate of soda. (D 459) Vitriolated soda or sodium sulphate, used as a cathartic and diuretic. It was introduced by Johann Rudolph Glauber of Amsterdam circa 1650. (Estes 90, 205)

Glyster An enema. (D 228) See also: Clyster

Grume, Grumous Clots, clotted. (D 472) Grumus, coagulated blood or milk; a hard white tubercle of the skin resembling millet (small seeds). (Coxe 231)

Guaiacum The resin—*Guaiaci resina . . .*—and the wood—*Guaiaci lignum*—are both officinal [that is, they function as a medicine]. Their odor is slightly fragrant; taste warm and bitter, of the resin more so than of the wood. . . . Guaiacum is stimulant and diaphoretic; and in large doses, purgative. It is administered in chronic rheumatism, gout, cutaneous diseases, and the sequelae of syphilis. (D 472), (Estes104)

Gum arabic Extract of *Acacia senegal*. Demulcent and sedative. Also used as a cheap substitute for *Acacia vera*. (Estes 17)

Gutta Drops. Abbreviated Gtt. or gut. (Estes 127)

Haemoptysis, Hemoptysis The discharge of blood from the mouth. (Coxe 234) Hemorrhage from the mucous membranes of the lungs; characterized by the expectoration of more or less florid and frothy blood. (D 481)

Halter Refers to a rope for hanging: a noose. (OED)

Haustus salinus Haustus is a draught, a liquid form of medicine. (Coxe 237) Salinus is saline (salt). *Haustis salinus* is a liquid medicine which can be taken as a draught and may include potassium carbonate, citric acid, sugar; used in divided doses as to decrease fever. (D 917)

Hectic fever Habitual fever with accessions at noon and evening, generally with night sweats and brick colored urine. (Coxe 237) The name of a slow, continued, or remittent fever, which generally accompanies the end of organic affections, and has been esteemed idiopathic, although it is probably always symptomatic. It is the fever of irritation and debility, and is characterized by progressive emaciation, frequent pulse, hot skin—especially of the palms of the hands and soles of the feet—and, towards the end, colliquative sweats and diarrhœa. Being symptomatic, it can only be removed by getting rid of the original affection. This is generally difficult, and almost hopeless in the disease that it most commonly accompanies—consumption. (D 489)

Hellebore   *Veratrum albus* or white hellebore causes violent emesis and purges but is used in small doses in maniacal cases. (Duncan 321–22) The Eurasian genus *Helleborus* includes approximately twenty species of herbaceous and/or evergreen perennial flowering plants.

Helleborus niger   A drastic cathartic, stimulant of the uterus. Side effects include vomiting, vertigo, abdominal cramps, convulsions, and death. It contains a number of active chemicals including digitalis-like glycosides. (Estes 94)

Hemiplegia   Palsy on one side of the body, plus fifteen other entries, such as *hemiplegia ex apoplexia*, hemiplegia after apoplexy. (Coxe 239) Paralysis of one side of the body. (D 492) See also: Palsy

Hydatids   Clear vesicle of serous dropsical fluid. (Coxe 247)

Hydragogues   Medicines which, by causing watery evacuations, are believed to be capable of expelling serum effused into any part of the body. These are generally cathartics or diuretics. (D 509)

Ichor   A thin, aqueous, and acrid discharge. (Hooper) Any thin acrid discharge from wounds. (Coxe 254) See also: Sanies

Idiot   A fool; a natural; a changeling; one without the powers of reason. (Samuel Johnson's *A Dictionary of the English Language*, 1755 p. 1039) Changeling is often used to refer to a child who is considered undesirable, or who does not resemble his or her family. (OED)

Imposthume, Imposthumations   Abscess. (D 535) A purulent swelling or cyst in any part of the body; an abscess. (OED)

Incarnans   Medicines generating new flesh. (Coxe 237) Medicines that were fancied to promote the regeneration of the flesh. Certain bandages and sutures have also been so called. Incarnation: growth of flesh or granulations. (D 536) To be incarned is to heal, cover with flesh.

Influenza   In the eighteenth century it referred to "any contagious epidemic catarrh," (Coxe 258) but the term itself originally referred to the influence of the stars and naturally occurring phenomena such as earthquakes.

Ipecacuanha   Ipecac or *Cephaelis ipecachuana*. Used for the treatment of dysentery, primarily as a dependable mild, safe emetic. In small doses it is a diaphoretic and expectorant. Suitable for treatment of most fevers and of opium poisoning. It was often combined with opium and called Dover's Powder. (Estes 70, 104, and Thacher 135–36)

Island Moss   *Lichen islandicus, Muscus islandicus*, Iceland Lichen. This plant is inodorous, with a bitter and mucilaginous taste. It is esteemed to be tonic, demulcent [soothing agent], and nutrient. (D 587) Mucilaginous substance derived from the leaves of Iceland moss, edible liverwort, or eryngo-leaved liverwort. (Estes 115)

Issue   "I go out." A fonticulus. (D 559) Fonticulus is a small ulcer produced by art, either by the aid of caustics or of cutting instruments; the discharge from which is kept up with a view to fulfil certain therapeutical indications. The *Pea issue . . .* is kept up by means of a pea placed in it. This *Pea . . .* is sometimes formed of wax. The common dried garden pea answers the purpose. The seton is also an issue. (D 431) Issues refer to incisions or artificial ulcers made for the purpose of causing a discharge . . . of blood or other matter from the body, either due to disease or produced surgically by counter-irritation. (OED) See also: Seton

Jalap The powdered root of *Exogonium purga*, a cathartic and diuretic. (Estes 106) "Dr. Rush's celebrated purgative in yellow fever . . . ten grains of Jalup and ten grains of calomel." (Thacher 113)

Jaundice Icterus. A disease, the principal symptom of which is yellowness of the skin and eyes, with white fæces and high-colored urine. . . . Prognosis is favorable in ordinary cases;—when complicated with hepatic disease, unfavorable. (D. 561, 531) May be due to liver disease such as hepatitis, obstruction of bile ducts, infection such as yellow fever, etc.

Julep Any liquid formula that is clear and sweet. (Coxe 265)

Kali sulphuratum Vegetable alkali, or potash; . . . this plant, when burnt, yields *fossil alkali*. Kali sulfuratum is hepar sulphuris or liver of sulfur. (Coxe 267) Potassium sulfate, which acts as a mild cathartic and diaphoretic; it is also an antidote to a number of mineral poisons such as mercury. (Estes 109)

Kino *Gummi rubrum astringens*; red astringent gum. (Coxe 268) An astringent is a drug that diminishes excessive evacuations such as hemorrhage, spitting of blood, diarrhea, or sweating by condensing or contracting the tissue of which the vessels are formed. Kino is a red extract from *Pterocarpus marsupium*, a powerful astringent for internal and external use. (Estes 21, 110)

Laudanum Tincture of opium, although earlier versions might include non-opiate ingredients. The 1820 U.S.P. formula for laudanum contained about 6% opium. Modern laudanum contains 10% opium, or 1.0% morphine. (Estes 112–13)

Ley (Lye) Lixivium, Lye—Soap, Liquor potassae. (D 586) Potassium hydroxide (Lixiva or Caustic lye or potash) or sodium hydroxide, an antacid. (Estes 117, 119) See also: Absynthum sal., Lixivinum, Potassium carbonate, Sal. Absinth

Lientery Lienteria is the purging of undigested food. (Coxe 277) Frequent liquid evacuations, the food only half digested, a condition always symptomatic of great irritation in the intestinal canal. (D 588)

Limewater Aqua calcis. This is usually made by dissolving quicklime or calcium oxide in water. Commonly used as an astringent with tonic, diuretic, . . . and antacid properties. (Estes. 34, 161)

Limon Juice or rind of lemon. Succ. Limon = lemon juice. (Estes 186)

Linteum Linen or lint. (Coxe 279) Charpie. A soft, flocculent substance made by scraping or unraveling old linen cloth . . . employed in surgery as a dressing to wounds, ulcers, &c., either simply or covered with ointment. *Patent lint* is generally prepared out of cloth manufactured for the purpose and is therefore more uniform in shape and consistence. (D 595) See also: Dossil, Pledget

Lixivinum, Lixivia When used alone, denotes potash or potassium carbonate. After 1790 sometimes also referred to lye or potassium hydroxide. (Estes 117–18) See also: Absynthum sal., Ley (Lye), Potassium carbonate, Sal. Absinth

Lochia The flow of blood or evacuations from the womb after delivery. (Coxe 281)

Magnesia Magnesia Usta. Magnesium oxide. Gastric antacid. (Estes 122)

Marsh rosemary Statice or the root of sea lavender, *Limonium nashii*. Astringent, antiseptic, and expectorant; administered internally and externally. (Estes 182)

Mel Honey. (Estes 127)

Menorrhagia Excessive discharge of the menses. (Coxe 296)

Mentha Piperita Leaves of peppermint. Also, Menth. pip. (Estes 128)

Mercurials Hydrargyrus, Calomel, etc. Possibly used as early as 1140, introduced for treatment of syphilis in 1497. By the eighteenth century is was used as a cathartic, diuretic, emetic, and sialagogue; that is, to produce increased salivation. (Estes

98–99) See also: Argent viv., Calomel, Corrosive sublimate, Ethiops mineral, Jalap, Turpeth mineral, Unguent, Caml

Millepedes   *Millepedæ*, millipedes, wood lice. (Coxe 360) The expressed juice of forty or fifty living millipedes, given in a mild drink, is said to cure very obstinate jaundices. (Hooper) *Onisci aselli* (D 658) had, at one time, a place in the pharmacopoeias. They were considered stimulant and diuretic, and useful in jaundice. (D 724)

Mindererus, Spirits   Nearly the same as aqua ammonia acetate. Introduced by Dr. Raymond Minderer of Augsburg in 1610 as a cathartic and diaphoretic. (Estes 130)

Muriate of soda   *Murias sodae* or common salt. (Coxe 305) Muriaticus sal or sea salt, a warm and dry tonic, antiseptic, digestive, appetite stimulant, cathartic, and emetic. (Estes 133) Sea salt, sodium chloride. (Goldstein 197)

Muriatic Acid   *Spiritus salis marini*, muriatic acid made by distilling sea salt and diluted vitriolic acid. (Coxe 391) An aqueous solution of chlorohydric acid gas . . . the odor is suffocating, taste very acid and caustic . . . possessed of tonic and antiseptic properties. It is used in typhus, cutaneous eruptions, in gargles for inflammatory and putrid sore throats. (D 673) Hydrochloric acid. When appropriately diluted, acts as a diuretic, tonic, and reduces inflammation. (Estes 133) See also: *Spiritus salis marini*

Muslin   Any lightweight cotton fabric; etymologically from Mosul, the name of the city in modern Iraq where muslin was formerly made. (OED)

Myrrh   *Gummi refina*. A gum resin from Abyssinia and the East Indies, a heating and stimulating medicine, used to promote secretions. (Duncan 263–64, 572) A stimulating tonic, antidiarrheal, and expectorant and considered an antiseptic when applied topically as a tincture. (Estes 134)

Nervine   Nervina, neurotics, medicines that relieve disorders of the nerves. (Coxe 310) A medicine that acts on the nervous system. (D 697)

Ol. Amygd.   Amygdala, OL. Oil of bitter almonds. Used internally as a sedative, antispasmodic, and expectorant, and externally as an emollient and to relax tense muscles. (Estes 10)

Omentum   The epiploon, or caul covering the bowels. (Coxe 319)

Oxymel, Oximel   A compound of vinegar and honey. (Coxe 326) Honey and vinegar boiled to a syrupy consistence. . . . It is cooling; externally detergent. Oxymel scillæ, is an expectorant and diuretic. (D 743) An expectorant. (Estes 145) See also: Squill

Palsy   Paralysis—various types include shaking palsy, mercury and lead palsy. (D 749) Loss of the power of voluntary motion in certain parts of the body only; sometimes it is accompanied with a loss of sense or feeling. (Thacher, *American Modern Practice* 1817, 543) Paralysis or paresis (weakness) of all or part of the body, sometimes with tremor. (OED) See also: Hemiplegia

Pan. Antim.   Panacea Antimonialis, and evaporated mixture of Sal Tartari and Antimonium Muriatum. Both formulations are cathartic and emetic. (Estes 147)

Paragoric Elixir   Camphorated tincture of opium. A tincture of 0.2% opium plus benzoin, camphor, root of licorice, oil of anisum (anise), and clarified honey. The adjective "paregoric," means "soothing." Narcotic, antitussive, and antidiarrheal. (Estes 148, Thacher 347)

Parenchyma   The solid and interior part of the viscera; the connecting medium of the substance of the lungs. (Coxe 332)

Parotid glands Situated near the articulation of the lower jaw; secreting saliva. A swelling of the parotid gland is the mumps. (Coxe 333)

Parturient Bringing forth, or about to bring forth, or having recently brought forth young. A *Parturient* or *Parturifacient* is a medicine that induces or promotes labor, as ergot. (D760)

Peccant Morbid. Not healthy. An epithet given by the humorists to the humors when erring in quality or quantity. (D 767) Causing disorder of the system; morbid, unhealthy, corrupt: used esp. in the humoral pathology; also, inducing disease. (OED)

Pediluvium A warm bath for the feet. (Coxe 354)

Peripneumonary Or peripneumonia: inflammation of the pleura [membrane covering the lungs, pleurisy]. (Coxe 337)

Petechial, Petechiae Purple [or red] spots on the skin not elevated, appearing in contagious diseases. (Coxe 339)

Phagedenic Medicines that destroy fungous flesh. (Hooper) *Phagedœnica*, medicines that eat away fungeous, or proud flesh. (Coxe 340) That which rapidly eats away. A phagedenic ulcer is one which rapidly eats and corrodes the neighboring parts. Where the slough extends deeper than the surface, the term *Sloughing phagedaena, P. putris, is* applied to it. (D 783)

Phlogistic *Phlogistici*, inflammatory diseases. (Coxe 341)

Phrenitis Inflammation of the brain, phrensy. (Coxe 342)

Phthsis Consumption, or wasting of flesh; corruption. (Coxe 243) See also: Consumption

Pledget A small compress or *gateau* of lint—the filaments arranged parallel to each other—flattened between the hands after the extremities have been cut off or folded down. It is applied over wounds, ulcers, &c., to preserve them from the contact of the air, to retain dressings in situ, and to absorb the discharges. (D 811) See also: Dossil, Linteum

Pneumony Pneumonia. (D 818)

Polygalia Senega *Polygala Senega* or Senega is otherwise known as snakeroot, rattlesnake root. It is mentioned earlier in the manuscript as Seneka; anti-inflammatory, diuretic, and cathartic. (Estes 155, 176) See also: Seneka, Snakeroot

Porter Cerevisia. [Brewer's yeast] From being drunk by porters. (D838) A strong dark beer containing about 6.8% alcohol. Astringent tonic. (Estes 156) A kind of beer apparently so named because originally it was made for or chiefly drunk by porters and the lower class of laborers. (OED)

Potassium carbonate Same as Lixiva. Deobstruent, attenuant, diaphoretic, antacid, diuretic, and aperient. (Estes 118, 156) Made from potassium hydroxide and carbon dioxide. It is an alkalinizing agent use in cooking and, in the past, for making soap and glass. It was originally made from wood ashes produced in large iron pots; hence "pot ashes." See Morris, *Academic Press Dictionary of Science and Technology.* See also: Absynthum sal., Ley (Lye), Lixivinum, Sal. Absinth

Potation A drink, a draught. (OED)

Poterium, Poterii A drink (literally, a drinking vessel). (Estes 157)

Precordia or Præcordia The diaphragm; also, the thoracic viscera, and the epigastrium. (D 846)

Primæ viæ The first passage, i.e., the stomach and intestines. (Coxe 353)

Ptyalism, Ptyalismus A salivation or an un-natural, or copious flow of saliva. (Coxe 357) Excessive secretion of saliva frequently associated with the therapeutic use of mercury. (D 864)

Pul. or Pulv. *Pulvis.* The abbreviation for "powder." (D 2)

Pulse There are two pages about the pulse in Dunglison, and Barker describes pulse in nearly every patient: feeble, full, slow and weak, quick and weak, natural, tense (resembling a cord), wiry (like tense, but resembling a wire) etc. "In the healthy state the pulse, besides having the proper number of pulsations, is neither hard nor unusually soft; . . . In disease it wanders, more or less, from those physiological conditions. The different characters of the pulse that have been recorded are remarkably numerous. In a dictionary it is necessary to detail them, although many of them are not now regarded (1874), and some are ridiculous." (D 867–68)

Putrid Relating to a disease attributed to putrefaction of the humors or body fluids and frequently accompanied by a putrid odor; necrotizing; gangrenous. (OED)

Putrid fever Any fever thought to be caused by putrefaction or accompanied by a putrid odor. (OED) Typhus. (Coxe 360)

Putrid sore throat A severe pharyngitis; may be Streptococcus or Diphtheria. (OED)

Q. S. As much as suffices

Quassia Bark of quassy tree; a bitter tonic used to relieve fever and as an antiseptic. (Estes 160)

Quinsy Or Cynanche; generally, cynanache tonsillaris of Cullen. (Hooper) Inflammation of the upper air-passages associated with disease such as diphtheria and gangrenous tonsillitis [various causes including what would be called "Strep throat" in the twenty-first century]. (D 286–87, 882).

Resin An exudation from plants. (Coxe 368) The name given to a dry inflammable substance, not miscible in water, soluble in oils and spirits of wine, which flows in a liquid state from the trees that produce them. (Hooper) A vegetable product, commonly dry and concrete, more or less brittle. . . . Many resins are used in medicine; the greater part are purgative and irritating. Some act like acrid poisons. (D 895)

Retrocession The act of going back. A disappearance or metastasis of a tumor, eruption, &c., from the outer part of the body to the inner. (D 899) The (supposed) inward movement of a disease such as a skin disease acutely or gradually affecting internal organs. (OED)

Rhei Abbreviation of *Radix Rhei*, Chinese rhubarb, a mild cathartic, astringent, tonic, stomachic, and antiemetic. It causes stomach pain with excessive stimulation of intestinal activity. (Estes 164)

Rickets Rachitis. A morbid enlargement of the head, extremities, of bones, and belly, with much debility and paleness. (Coxe 364) A disease characterized by crookedness of the long bones; swelling of their extremities; crooked spine; prominent abdomen; large head; and often precocity of intellect. Treatment is almost wholly *hygienic*. (D883) [twenty-first century: A disease of children in which there is vitamin D deficiency, causing abnormal calcium and phosphorus metabolism leading to deficient mineralization of bone and skeletal deformities. (OED)]

Rubefacient A medicine that reddens and irritates the skin. (Estes 167)

Saccharum saturni Sugar of lead . . . used in pharmacy, for the preparation of syrups, conserves, lozenges, &c. Saccharum Saturni, Plumbi superacetas. (D 913) Acetate of lead has a sweet, styptic taste, a very white color, and silky lustre. It is astringent, and in *weak* solution cooling and sedative; in *strong*, stimulant. It is given internally in visceral and other hemorrhages, combined with opium, and is used externally, in solution, in inflammation, burns, bruises, gonorrhoea, &c. (D 815–16) Sugar of lead, same as cerussa acetata or lead acetate. Used as a cooling colyrium, or internally as a styptic astringent, anti-diaphoretic, or an anti-inflammatory sedative. An oral overdose produces colic, constipation, cramps, tremors, and nerve weakness. (Estes 44, 170)

Sago A dry fecula, or starchy sediment, obtained from the pith of a species of palm . . . Sago becomes soft and transparent by boiling in water and forms a light and agreeable liquid, much recommended in febrile, phthisical, and calculous disorders, &c. (Hooper) A dry insipid white or grey colored substance obtained from the pith of the *Sagus Rumphii, Cycas circinalis, C. revoluta,* &c., growing in the Moluccas, Philippine Isles, &c., and which is brought to us in small grains. The same substance is also obtained from the West Indies, but it is inferior to that from the East. By boiling in water or milk, sago becomes soft and transparent, and forms an agreeable and nutritious food in febrile, calculous, and other disorders. It is made palatable by sugar, lemon juice, or wine, where the last is not contraindicated. (D 916)

Sal Salts—many variations listed. (D 916–17)

Sal Absinth (Lixiva) usually refers to potash or potassium carbonate but after about 1790 sometimes refers to lye or potassium hydroxide; a diaphoretic, antacid, and diuretic. (Estes 2, 117–18) See also: Absynthum sal., Ley (Lye), Lixivinum, Potassium carbonate. Unrelated to absinth proper, an alcoholic beverage that includes the oil of wormwood (absinithium), that is addicting and hallucinogenic. (Estes 1–2, Goldstein 54)

Sal ammonia Ammonium chloride, a diaphoretic, diuretic, mild cathartic, and emetic, as dose increases; also used in antiseptic and discutient fomentations or gargles. Its effects are attributable to the "coldness of the solution" and to the stimulation produced by the salt. (Estes 8–9)

Sal sodae Sodium carbonate, Na_2CO_3 or the soluble form of the sodium salt of carbonic acid. Also, Barilla or Natron, a naturally occurring form of sodium carbonate and sodium bicarbonate. (Estes 24)

Sallop Or salep, salop: roots of *Orchis* species. Because its flowers resemble the scrotum, it was associated with the priapic power of satyrs. A tonic, aphrodisiac, and antidiarrheal medication. (Estes 170, 173)

Sanies Ichor. A thin, limpid, and green discharge, at other times to a thick and bloody kind of pus. (Hooper) A thin, corrosive fluid, presenting some of the qualities of pus and blood, and commonly exhaled at the surface of ulcers. (D 921) See also: Ichor

Scammony Scammonium. The concrete gummi-resinous juice of *Convolvulus scammonia* brought from Aleppo and Smyrna, it has a rather unpleasant smell, and a bitterish, and slightly acrid taste. It is used internally as a purgative, and externally for the itch, tinea, pains, &c. (Hooper) It causes copious watery diarrhea. (D 988, 253)

Scarlatina anginosa A sore throat with a scarlet eruption on the skin. (Coxe 379) Sore throat in which the fever is severe, the throat ulcerated, the eruption later in its appearance and less extensive, often changing to a livid hue. (D 930)

Scirrhus A tumour, hard, sometimes knotty and painful, most frequently affecting glands, terminating in cancer. (Coxe 380), (D 933)

Scordium Water germander. *Teucrium scordium.* The name, *scórdo* in Greek, signifies "garlic" from similarity of smell. The plant was formerly in high estimation, but is now justly fallen into disuse, although recommended by some in antiseptic cataplasms and fomentations. (Hooper)

Scrofulous The king's evil. A disease in the class *cachexiæ* and order *impetigines of* Cullen, known by swelled lymphatic glands, thick upper lip, obstinate ulcers, redness of the ankles, indolent tumors of the joints, fair complexion, and an irritable habit. (Hooper)

Scruple　A unit of weight = 20 grains = 1.296 grams. (Duncan 102)

Scuttle　An opening in the roof, floor, wall, etc., of a building, closed with a shutter or lid; a trap-door. (OED)

Secerning　Secreting. (D 937) Separating from the blood. (OED)

Seneka　The rattlesnake-root-milkwort. *Polygala senega*. The root was formerly thought to be a specific against the poison of a rattle-snake, and as a medication to treat inflammation in pleurisy, pneumonia, &c. but is now entirely laid aside. (Hooper) Its taste is at first acrid, and afterwards very hot and pungent. It has been given also in humoral asthma, chronic rheumatism, dropsy, croup, amenorrhœa, &c. (D 831) See also: Polygalia Senega, Snakeroot

Septon　Azote. Air unfit for respiration due to lack of oxygen, variously called phlogistic air, vitiated air, &c. Barker's references to septon are the result of Mitchill's explanation of disease. (D 943, 107)

Serosity　Serum. (D 944)

Seton　An artificial ulcer made under the skin by means of an instrument called a seton needle, which carries with it a portion of thread or silk, that is moved backwards or forwards, and thus keeps up a constant irritation. (Hooper) A piece of tape or cord passed under the skin by using a seton needle generally to allow pus to drain. (OED) See also: Issue

Sinapism　A mixture of mustard and vinegar in form of poultice. (Hooper) A mustard plaster. (Coxe 386) A cataplasm, of which mustard forms the basis, which is used for exciting redness, and acting as a counterirritant. It is prepared by mixing flour of mustard and vinegar together for the due consistence. (D 949) White or black mustard seed (*Brassica alba* or *B. negra*) used to cause redness, irritation, and mild blistering; still used to make a mustard plaster. (Estes 178)

Sizy　*Corium phlogisticum*. The grayish crust or buff, varying in thickness, observed on blood drawn from a vein during the existence of violent inflammation, pregnancy, &c. It is particularly manifest in pleurisy. (D 257) See also: Buffy, Cup

Slow fever　Febris lenta, a slow fever. (Coxe 211) This may refer to what we now call typhoid fever.

Snakeroot　The root of Virginia snakeroot, *Aristolochia serpentaria* is a tonic, diuretic, diaphoretic, and antispasmodic with the side effects of colic and vomiting. (Estes 47, 176–77) Also recommended in intermittent fevers, exanthematous diseases, and as a gargle in the putrid sore throat. (Duncan 153–54) See also: Polygalia senega, Seneka, *Cimifuga* or black snakeroot. Thacher mentions a variety *Serpentaria Kennebis* termed by Dr. Daniel Coney of Augusta, Maine, and named after the Kennebec River. (Thacher 83–84)

Snuff, Spanish　Finely pulverized and drawn into the nostrils to facilitate the release of phlegm. *Nicotiana tabacum*, unsifted Havana tobacco leaves to which ground Spanish nutshells and treacle water are added. Considered a narcotic, emetic, diuretic, and diaphoretic (Estes 136–37) Powdered tobacco used as an errhine, that is, a drug to produce sneezing. (Goldstein 257, Coxe 203)

Soluble　Relaxing. Applied to the bowels when gently relaxed. (D 959) Free from constipation, relaxed. (OED)

Specific　Medications which certainly cure particular diseases. (Coxe 389) A substance to which is attributed the special property of removing some particular disease. Probably no such remedy exists. (D 965) A treatment that exerts an invariable curative action on the disease . . . regardless of the particular patient or environment. Its mode of action was obscure as opposed to laxatives and cathartics. Until the 1860s "disease specific treatment . . . was considered illegitimate." (quackery) See John Harley Warner, *The Therapeutic Perspective: Medical Practice, Knowledge, and Identity in America, 1820–85* (Cambridge, Massachusetts: Harvard University Press, 1986), 58–80.

Spermaceti Cetaceum. A fatty matter taken from the head of the whale and purified by boiling with alkali. (Coxe 389) Relaxing demulcent and emollient used in many lotions and also for catarrh and gonorrhea (i.e., spermatorrhea). (Estes 44, 181, Thacher 179)

Spirit of Mindererus *Aqua Acetitis Ammoniae*; vulgo, Spiritus Mindereri. Water of Acetite of Ammonia, commonly called Spirit of Mindererus. (Duncan 408, D 972) Introduced by Dr. Raymond Minderer of Augsburg in 1610 as a cathartic and diaphoretic. (Estes 130)

Spiritus nitri dulcis A distillation of four parts of spirit of wine and one of nitrous acid. (Coxe 391) Dulcified spirits of nitre in alcohol. Refrigerant, tonic, diaphoretic, diuretic, and antispasmodic. (Estes 71)

Spiritus salis marini Muriatic acid made by distilling sea salt and diluted vitriolic acid. (Coxe 391) Spirits of sea salt, same as Sal. Muriaticus. (Estes 123) See also: Muriatic acid

Sponge tent A conical piece of sponge or porous cloth, frequently soaked in hot wax, cooled then placed in a wound to keep it open and allow for drainage and healing from below. (D 977)

Squill Bulb of *Scilla* or sea onion, *Urginea maritima*; a diuretic, expectorant, and diaphoretic. It is an emetic and cathartic at high doses; it also contains digitalis-like glycoside. (Estes 174) *Scilla maritima* used in dropsy. (Thacher 204-205) See also: Oxymel

ss. Half of the above—thus oz. ss. = ½ oz. (Estes 127)

Stertor, Stertorous The deep snoring which accompanies inspiration in some diseases, particularly in apoplexy. (D 984)

Sthenic Active. (D 984) Thus asthenic/sthenic means inactive/active.

Stomachic Medicines to excite and strengthen the action of the stomach. (Hooper) Stomachal. That which belongs to the stomach; that which is good for the stomach; which strengthens the stomach. A medicine that gives tone to the stomach. (D 986) A medicine that warms and strengthens the stomach. (Estes 183)

Stramonium officiale Thorn apple, a poisonous plant native to America, used as a remedy in mania and melancholy. It can be taken internally or externally as an ointment from the leaves, causing external inflammations. (Duncan 217) The leaves, roots, and seeds of thorn apple, or jimson (Jamestown) weed. It has many other common names and was used in mania and as an antiepileptic. Potent narcotic, tonic, diuretic, anodyne antispasmodic, and antitussive. Used chiefly in disorders of the nervous system. (Estes 184) See also: *Datura stramonium*

Stranguria Strangury, or discharge of urine by drops. (Coxe 395) Extreme difficulty in evacuating the urine, which issues only drop by drop, and is accompanied with heat, pain, tenesmus at the neck of the bladder, &c. (D 988)

Succus A juice expressed from a plant or its fruits. (Estes 186)

Sudorific Sweating medicines. (Coxe 397) A medicine which provokes sweating. (D 997)

Sui generis Literally "of one's or its own kind," unique. (OED)

Supercarbonate of potass   Potassium bicarbonate; a solution of Lixiva (potassium carbonate) with fixed air (carbon dioxide); dissolves lithic acid (uric acid) stones. (Estes 83, 117–18, 187)

Synocha   Inflammatory fever without local inflammation. (Coxe 401) A species of continued fever, characterized by increased heat; and by quick, strong, and hard pulse; urine high-colored; disturbance of mind slight. It requires, of course, the most active treatment. (D 1010)

Syrup of Spina Cervina   Juice of buckthorn berries, bruised ginger, powdered pimento, refined sugar. Brisk cathartic but very unpleasant, occasioning a thirst and dryness of the mouth and sometimes violent gripes. (Duncan 543) Juice of buckthorn berries, cinnamon, ginger, nutmegs, and sugar. (Coxe 402) *Rhamnus catharticus*: Syrup of buckthorn. A strong cathartic, also said to be tonic, astringent and antiseptic. Side effects inlude olic, nausea, and dry mouth. (Estes 181, 164)

Tamarinds   Employed as a laxative, for abating thirst or heat, and for correcting putrid disorders, especially those of a bilious kind. (Hooper) Fruit of *Tamarindus indica*. An acid cathartic with refrigerant and thirst-quenching properties. (Estes 190)

Tartrite of Antimony, Tart antim,   Formerly Tartar Emetic. (Duncan 433) *Antimonium tartarizatum*. Tartar emetic, a diaphoretic, cathartic, and expectorant at lower doses and emetic at higher doses, the most frequently prescribed of all antimony compounds. Sedates the circulation, while it excites the secretions. (Estes 14) Antimony potassium tartrate.

Tartrite of potash   Particularly recommended as a purgative for maniacal and melancholic patients. (Thacher, *American New Dispensatory* 259)

Tenesmus   A painful, ineffectual, and repeated effort to go to stool. (Coxe 405) Frequent, vain, and painful desires to evacuate; one of the chief symptoms of inflammation of the lining membrane of the digestive tube, as of dysentery. (D 1025)

Tent   In surgery, a tent is a small roll of lint of cylindrical or pyramidal shape, introduced into a wounds and deep ulcers to prevent them from closing before they are filled up from the bottom. Sometimes made of prepared sponge, gentian root, slippery elm, &c. (D 1026)

Testaceous   A powder consisting of burnt shells. These contain carbonate of lime chiefly, and hence the term has been applied to cretaceous substance. Most seashells are predominately calcium carbonate, an antacid. (D 1028) Pulverized shells of oysters, an antacid; sometimes burned to make quicklime. (Estes 192, 143)

Thebaica Tinctura   The best quality opium came from Thebes (modern Luxor), Egypt. The tincture is made by letting 2 oz. opium stand in 2 pints proof spirit for four days, straining, and evaporating. (Estes 193)

Theca   A sheath or covering. (Coxe 408)

Tippet   A garment, usually of fur or wool, covering the shoulder or neck and shoulders; a cape or short cloak, often with hanging ends. (OED)

Tormina   Gripes; pain of any kind. (Coxe 413) Acute colicky pains. Dysentery. (D 1048)

Tow   Stupe, or fomentation; a sweating bath. (Coxe 395) Stupa, used in certain surgical apparatuses and dressings; that is, a cloth or tow used in fomentations. A flannel or other article wrung out of hot water, plain or medicated, applied to a part, is a *stupe*. (D 991)

Tubercula   Tubercles, or small suppurating tumours. (Coxe 417)

Tumefied   Swollen. From *tumefactio*, swelling. (D 1064)

Tunic A coat, a membrane. (Coxe 417) An envelope. A name given to different membranes, which envelop organs: as the tunics or coats of the eye, stomach, bladder, &c. (D 1065)

Turner's cerate Cerate of calamine. Melt the wax and lard together, and, on cooling, add the carbonate of zinc and stir till cool. (D 193) An unguent made with calamine, cera flava, ol oliva, and unsalted butter; devised by "Dr." Daniel Turner of London in the early 18th century. (Estes 197) See also: Cerate

Turpeth mineral Same as *hydrargyrus vitrialatus*, or mercuric subsulfate. The term was coined in the sixteenth century to indicate the salt's physical resemblance to turpethium or bark of root of turbith, *Ipomoea turpethium*, a vine related to jalap. Undependable and unsafe cathartic. (Estes 197–98, Duncan 470–71) See also: Argent viv., Calomel, Corrosive sublimate, Ethiops mineral, Jalap, Mercurials, Unguent, Caml

Tympany, Tympanites From *tÿmpano*, a drum in Greek. An elastic distension of the abdomen not readily yielding to pressure, and sounding like a drum, with atrophy but no fluctuation. (Hooper) This disease is a flatulent distension of the belly, and the wind is either pent up in the intestinal canal or confined between the intestines and the membranes which line the muscles of the abdomen. (Thacher, *American Modern Practice* 561)

Typhoid Appertaining to or resembling typhus. (D 1068) Can refer to typhus-like, particularly "a state of delirious stupor occurring in certain fevers." (OED)

Typhus mitior The low, or nervous fever. (Coxe, 419) A fever characterized by small, weak, and unequal, but usually frequent pulse, with great prostration of strength, and much cerebral disturbance; its duration being generally from a fortnight to three weeks or longer. It is continued fever, accompanied with great cerebral irritation and prostration. By most writers, this disease was formerly divided into two varieties—*typhus mitior* and *typhus gravior*. *Typhus mitior* is characterized by slight shiverings; heavy, vertiginous headache; great oppression, peculiar expression of anxiety, nausea, sighing, despondency, and coma or quiet delirium. (D 1068)

Typhus or Typhous fever A species of continued fever. (Hooper) Coxe lists thirteen Typhous entries, but, alone, Typhous or Typhus is defined as a contagious fever with occasional delirium and great loss of strength. It is also associated with jail and camp fever, with icterodes (jaundice or yellow fever), nervous fever, etc. (Coxe 419) Typhous and typhoid fevers had overlapping signs and symptoms and were not separated as separate diseases until the second half of the nineteenth century.

Unguent. Caml. (abbreviation of Calomel) The use of calomel or mercurous chloride as an unguent preparation; that is, as a plaster, less viscous and oilier than an ointment. Used in scaled [ringworm of similar affliction] head and other chronic cutaneous afflictions. (D 1073) See also: Argent viv., Calomel, Corrosive sublimate, Ethiops mineral, Jalap, Mercurials, Turpeth mineral

Valetudinarian Valitudinary. One subject to frequent diseases. An invalid. (D 1088) A person of a weak or sickly constitution; one whose chief concern is his or her ill health. (Webster's Dictionary)

Vamp That part of hose or stocking which covers the foot and ankle; also, a short stocking, a sock. (OED)

Varolii A part thus named in the brain. (Coxe 351) An eminence at the upper part of the medulla oblongata, first described by Varoli. It is formed by the union of the crura cerebri and the crura cerebelli [base of the brain]. (D 835)

Verdigris "Green substance from Greece;" copper acetate. A chemical that dissolves or destroys animal matter; used for skin ulcers and other skin lesions and sometimes as a potent emetic. (Estes 79, 202.)

Vesication *Vessicativum, Tinctura*: blistering tincture, usually *tinctura cantharidis*. The application of a plaster consisting of cantharides (Spanish fly) in order to produce vesication or blistering that removes fluid directly from the body, similar to laxatives and cathartics. The term counter-irritation is also used for this procedure. (Estes 36–38, 202) See also: Blistering, Cantharides

Vin. antim Antimonical wine. (Coxe 428) Vinum *Antimonii*. Dissolve the salt in the distilled water, and while hot add sufficient wine to make a pint. Each fluid ounce contains two grains of the tartrate. The ordinary *Antimonial wine* was formerly made with *Glass of antimony* [one ounce], *Sherry* [one and a half]. (D 1104) Antimony in Spanish white wine. A diuretic and cathartic at higher doses; violently emetic at yet higher doses. (Estes 13)

Virus A Latin word, which signifies poison, but which, in medicine, has a somewhat different application. A principle unknown in its nature and inappreciable by the senses, which is the agent for the transmission of infectious diseases . . . —a morbid poison. (D 1106) Any poison. (Coxe 428) A morbid principle or substance produced in the body as a result of some disease. (OED)

Vitriol; Vitriol, Elixir of A name for compounds of vitriolic acid [sulfuric acid]. (Coxe 429) *Sulphuricum acidum aromaticum*; sulfuric acid. (D 346–47) Blue vitriol is *Ferri sulphas.—Cupri sulphas*. (D 1108) *Acidum Vitrioli Aromaticum*. Aromatic acid of vitriol, made of vitriol in wine, cinnamomum, and zingiber. Tonic, astringent, and stomachic, especially when the body has been weakened by fever. (Estes 205)

Wine-whey Take of good *milk*, two-thirds of a pint, and add *water* to make a pint. Take of *sherry*, or any other good white *wine*, two glasses, and of *sugar*, a dessertspoonful. Place the milk and water in a deep pan on the fire, and the moment it boils, pour into it the wine and sugar. Stir assiduously for 12 or 15 minutes, while it boils. Lastly, strain through a sieve. It is a good mode of giving wine in adynamic states. (D 1123) *Adynamia* or adynamic refers to extreme debility, loss of motion in the vital or natural functions. (Coxe 16)

BIBLIOGRAPHY

"Achievements in Public Health, 1900–1999." *Morbidity and Mortality Weekly Report* 48, no. 29 (July 30, 1999): 621–29.

Acierno, Louis J. *The History of Cardiology.* New York: The Parthenon Publishing Group, 1994.

Ackerknecht, Erwin H. "A Plea for a 'Behaviorist Approach in Writing History of Medicine.'" *Journal of the History of Medicine and Allied Sciences,* 22, no. 3 (1967): 211–14.

Alison, W. P. "Treatment of Scrofulous Disease with a View to Their Prevention." *Medical Recorder* 7 (1824): 613–21.

Amory, Hugh. "The New England Book Trade, 1773–1790." In *The Colonial Book in the Atlantic World,* edited by Hugh Amory and David D. Hall. A History of the Book in America, xxiv. Cambridge, UK; New York; Worcester, MA: Cambridge University Press; American Antiquarian Society, 2000.

Amsterdamska, Olga, and Anja Hiddinga. "Trading Zones or Citadels? Professionalization and Intellectual Change in the History of Medicine." In *Locating Medical History: The Stories and Their Meanings,* edited by Frank Huisman and John Harley Warner, 237–61. Baltimore: The Johns Hopkins University Press, 2004.

"An Account of a Case in Which Green Hemlock Was Applied, by Mr. Josiah Colebrook." *The London Magazine,* 1764, pp: 674–676.

Boswell, James. *The London Magazine. Or, Gentleman's Monthly Intelligencer.* Edited by Isaac Kimber and Edward Kimber, printed for R[ichard]. Baldwin, jun. at the Rose in Pater-Noster-Row [1747–1783].

Anderson, Virginia DeJohn. *Creatures of Empire: How Domestic Animals Transformed Early America.* New York: Oxford University Press, 2004.

Antony, Milton. "Caries of the 5th and 6th Ribs. Disorganization of the Right Lobe of the Lungs, with a Description of an Operation [Communicated for the New England Journal of Medicine and Surgery by George Parkman, M.D.]." *New England Journal of Medicine and Surgery* 11, no. 4 (1822): 374–76.

Apel, Thomas. "The Thucydidean Moment: History, Science, and the Yellow-Fever Controversy, 1793–1805." *Journal of the Early Republic* 34, no. 3 (2014): 315–47.

Apel, Thomas A. *Feverish Bodies, Enlightened Minds: Science and the Yellow Fever Controversy in the Early American Republic.* Stanford, CA: Stanford University Press, 2016.

Armstrong, G. L., L. A. Conn, and R. W. Pinner. "Trends in Infectious Disease Mortality in the United States During the 20th Century." *Journal of the American Medical Association* 281, no. 1 (January 6, 1999): 61–66.

Armstrong, John, and John Aikin. *The Art of Preserving Health.* Philadelphia: Benjamin Johnson [etc.], 1804.

Arner, Katherine. "Making Yellow Fever American: The Early American Republic, the British Empire and the Geopolitics of Disease in the Atlantic World." *Atlantic Studies* 7, no. 4 (December 1, 2010): 447–71.

Arnold, Thomas. *Observations on the Nature, Kinds, Causes, and Prevention of Insanity, Lunancy, or Madness.* 2 vols. Leicester, London: G. Robinson, T. Cadell, 1782.

Aronowitz, R., and J. A. Greene. "Contingent Knowledge and Looping Effects—A 66-Year-Old Man with PSA-Detected Prostate Cancer and Regrets." *New England Journal of Medicine* 381, no. 12 (September 19, 2019): 1093–96.

"Art. 7. The Physicians' Case Book." *The Medical Magazine* 1 (November 1832 1833): 298–99.

"Art. II. A Review of the Improvements, Progress, and State of Medicine in the 18th Century. Read on the First Day of the 19th Century, before the Medical Society of South-Carolina, in Pursuance of Their Vote, and Published at Their Request. By David Ramsay, M.D. 8vo. Pp. 47. Charleston. Young." *Medical Repository* 4, no. 4 (1800–1801): 390–99.

"Art. III. Recherches Sur La Medecine, Ou L'application De La Chimie a La Medecine. Par Francois Blanchet. A New-York. Parisot. 8vo. Pp. 246. 1800." *Medical Repository* 4, no. 2 (1801): 172–76.

"Art. VI. An Inaugural Dissertation on the Operation of Pestilential Fluids upon the Large Intestines Termed by Nosologists Dysentery. By William Bay, Citizen of the State of New-York. New-York. T. and J. Swords. 1797. 8vo. Pp. 109." *Medical Repository* 1 (3rd ed., 1804), no. 2 (1798): 232–38.

"Article I. The Following Important Account of a New Publication in Great-Britain, by Dr. Jenner, Entitled 'a Inquiry into the Causes and Effects of the Variolae Vaccinae, or Cow Pox,' Is Extracted from the Analytical Review for July, 1798." *Medical Repository* 2, no. 2 (1798): 255–58.

"Article IX: The Pharmacopaeia of the United States of America. 1820. By the Authority of the Medical Societies and Colleges. Boston: Printed by Wells & Lilley, for Charles Ewer. Dec. 1820. 8vo. Pp. 268." *New England Journal of Medicine and Surgery* 10, no. 3 (1821): 293–310.

"Article VIII. An Inaugural Dissertation, Showing in What Manner Pestilential Vapours Acquire Their Acid Quality, and How This Is Neutralized by Alkalis, . . . By Adolph C. Lent, Citizen of the State of New York. T. and J. Swords. 1798. 8vo. Pp. 54." *Medical Repository* 2, no. 1 (1799): 96–98.

Association, Portland Medical. *Constitution of the Portland Medical Association Together with the Rules and Regulations of the Police and Practice Adopted June 28, 1833.* Edited by Portland Medical Association. Portland, Maine: J. & W. E. Edwards, 1833.

Auenbrugger, Leopold. *Inventum Novum Ex Percussione Thoracis Humani Ut Signo Abstrusos Interni Pectoris Morbos Detegendi.* Vindobonae: Typis Joannis Thomae Trattner, 1761.

Augstein, H. F. *Prichard, James Cowles (1786–1848), Physician and Ethnologist.* Oxford, UK: Oxford University Press, 2004.

Augustin, George. *History of Yellow Fever.* New Orleans: Searcy & Pfaff Ltd., 1909.

Austin, Robert B. *Early American Medical Imprints: 1668–1820.* Arlington, MA: The Printers' Devil, 1961.

Bacon, Francis, James Spedding, and Robert Leslie Ellis. *Novum Organum.* New Universal Library. London; New York: G. Routledge; E. P. Dutton, 1800.

Baillie, Mathew. "Some Observations on Paraplegia in Adults." *New England Journal of Medicine and Surgery* 10, no. 1 (January 1, 1821): 84–85.

Baillie, Matthew. "Some Observations upon Paraplegia in Adults." *Medical Transactions of the Royal College of Physicians of London* 6 (1820): 16–26.

Ballester, Luis Garcia. "Galen as a Medical Practitioner: Problems in Diagnosis." In *Galen: Problems and Prospects*, edited by V. Nutton, 13–46. London: The Wellcome Institute for the History of Medicine, 1981.

Banks, Ronald. *Maine Becomes a State*. Middletown, CT: Wesleyan University Press, 1970.

Barberis, I., N. L. Bragazzi, L. Galluzzo, and M. Martini. "The History of Tuberculosis: From the First Historical Records to the Isolation of Koch's Bacillus." *Journal of Preventive Medicine and Hygiene* 58, no. 1 (March 2017): E9–E12.

Barker, Elizabeth Frye. *Barker Genealogy*. New York: Frye Publishing Company, 1927.

Barker, Jeremiah. "1806 Casebook." Maine Historical Society, Barker Collection 13, Box 1/5. Portland, Maine, 1806.

———. "An Account of a Malignant Fever, Sporadically Formed, in Falmouth, County of Cumberland, District of Maine." *Medical Repository* New Series, 19, no. 3 (1818): 286–90.

———. "An Account of Bilious Colics, as They Appeared in Several Towns in the County of Cumberland, District of Maine, in the Months of May, June, and July, 1801; and of the Surprising Relief Obtained Therein by Alkaline Remedies. By Dr. Jeremiah Barker, of Portland." *Medical Repository* 5 (1802): 267–72.

———. "An Account of Diseases as They Appeared in Several Parts of the District of Maine, from January, 1803, to January, 1804: Communicated in a Letter from Dr. Jeremiah Barker to Dr. Mitchill." *Medical Repository* 3, 2nd hexade (1805): 132–40.

———. "An Account of Febrile Diseases, as They Appeared in Portland and Its Vicinity, in August and September, 1801. By Jeremiah Barker, M.D." *Medical Repository* 6 (1802): 18–24.

———. "An Account of Febrile Diseases, as They Have Appeared in the County of Cumberland, District of Maine, from July, 1798, to March, 1800: Communicated in a Letter from Dr. Jeremiah Barker, of Portland, to Dr. Mitchill." *Medical Repository* 3, no. 4 (1800): 364–68.

———. "An Account of the Measles, and Some Other Distempers, as They Appeared in Several Towns in the District of Maine, from January, 1802, to January, 1803. Communicated by Dr. Jeremiah Barker, of Portland." *Medical Repository* 1, 2nd hexade (1804): 125–34.

———. "An Account of the Weather and Diseases in the County of Cumberland, District of Maine, from January, 1804, to January, 1805: Communicated in a Letter from Jeremiah Barker, M.D. of Portland, to Dr. Mitchill." *Medical Repository* 4, 2nd hexade (1807): 137–40.

———. "Beneficial Effects of Alkalies in Consumption of the Lungs." *Medical Repository* 5 (1802): 220–21.

———. "Dr. Barker of Portland, in the District of Maine, Is Preparing a Work for the Press, on Consumption and Fever. In This Work the Dr. Expects to Establish the Efficacy of Alkalies, in the Cure of Yellow Fever." *Medical Repository* 1, no. 1 (1797): 114.

———. "A History of Diseases of the District of Maine Commencing in 1735 and Continuing to the Present Time . . . . To This Is Annexed an Inquiry into the Causes, Nature, Increasing Prevalency, and Treatment of Consumption." Jeremiah Barker, Collection 13, Maine Historical Society. Portland, Maine, 1831.

————. "Letter from Jeremiah Barker in Falmouth, Maine to Benjamin Rush in Philadelphia, 22 September 1806." Historical Society of Pennsylvania, Rush Manuscripts, 1806.

————. "Letter to Dr. Joseph Whipple of Boston Thanking Him for Notifying Barker of His Election a Fellow of the Massachusetts Medical-Society." 12 Jul 1803 Countway Library Archival Collection, *Barker, Jeremiah*, B MS c 75.2.

————. "Medical by Jeremiah Barker." *Portland Gazette and Maine Advertiser*, September 15 and 22, 1806.

————. "Obstinate Eruption over the Whole Surface of the Body Cured by Chalk (Alkaline Earth, or Carbonate of Lime)." *Medical Repository* 3 (1800): 412–13.

————. "On Febrifuge Virtues of Lime, Magnesia and Alkaline Salts in Dysentery, Yellow-Fever and Scarlatina Angiosa. In a Letter from Dr. Jeremiah Barker, of Portland, (Maine) Dated May 30, 1798." *Medical Repository* 2, no. 2 (1798): 147–52.

————. "Request for Thermometrical and Meteorological Observations before 1790." *Portland Gazette*, Monday, September 29, 1806.

————. "Use of Alkalies in Cancer. Extract from a Letter of Dr. J. Barker to Dr. Mitchill, Dated Portland (Maine), March 12, 1801." *Medical Repository* 4 (1801): 414–16.

Barnes, James J. *Authors, Publishers, and Politicians: The Quest for an Anglo-American Copyright Agreement, 1815–1854*. Columbus: Ohio State University Press, 1974.

Baron, John. *Illustrations of the Enquiry Respecting Tuberculous Diseases*. London: Underwood, 1822.

Barry, William David. *Maine: The Wilder Half of New England*. 1st ed. Gardiner, ME: Tilbury House, 2012.

Bartlett, Elisha. *An Essay on the Philosophy of Medical Science*. Philadelphia: Lea & Blanchard, 1844.

Bartlett, Josiah. "Article IX a Case of Calculus of the Bladder." *Medical Communications and Dissertations of the Massachusetts Medical Society* 1 (1813): 52–56.

————. *A Dissertation on the Progress of Medical Science in the Commonwealth of Massachusetts*. Boston: T. B. Wait and Co., 1810.

————. *An Historical Sketch of the Progress of Medical Science, in the Commonwealth of Massachusetts, Being the Substance of a Discourse Read at the Annual Meeting of the Medical Society, June 6, 1810, with Alterations and Additions to January 1, 1813*. Charlestown: s.n., 1813.

Barton, Benjamin Smith. *Collections for an Essay Towards a Materia Medica of the United-States*. 2nd ed. Philadelphia: Printed for the author by Robert Carr, 1801.

Barton, William P. C. *Vegetable Materia Medica of the United States, or, Medical Botany: Containing a Botanical, General, and Medical History, of Medicinal Plants Indigenous to the United States: Illustrated by Coloured Engravings, Made after Original Drawings from Nature, Done by the Author*. 2 vols. Philadelphia: Printed and published by M. Carey & Son, 1817.

Bates, Ralph Samuel. *Scientific Societies in the United States*. 3rd ed. Cambridge: M. I. T. Press, 1965.

Batschelet, Margaret. *Early American Scientific and Technical Literature: An Annotated Bibliography of Books, Pamphlets, and Broadsides*. Metuchen, NJ: Scarecrow Press, 1990.

Bean, W. B. "Landmark Perspective: Walter Reed and Yellow Fever." *Journal of the American Medical Association* 250, no. 5 (August 5, 1983): 659–62.

Beatty, William K., and Virginia L. Beatty. "Sources of Medical Information." *Journal of the American Medical Association* 236 (July 5, 1976): 78–82.

Beddoes, Thomas. *Observations on the Nature and Cure of Calculus, Sea Scurvy, Consumption, Catarrah, and Fever.* Philadelphia: T. Dobson, 1797.

Beddoes, Thomas, and James Watt. *Medical Cases and Speculations; Including Parts IV and V of Considerations on the Medicinal Power, and the Production of Factitious Airs.* 3rd ed. Vol. 2. Bristol: Bulgin & Rosser, 1796.

Bell, Madison Smartt. *Lavoisier in the Year One: The Birth of a New Science in an Age of Revolution.* 1st ed. Great Discoveries. New York: W.W. Norton, 2005.

Bell, Whitfield J. *The Colonial Physician and Other Essays.* New York: Science History Publications, 1975.

———. "Medicine in Boston and Philadelphia: Comparisons and Contrasts, 1750–1820." In *Medicine in Colonial Massachusetts 1620–1820.* Boston: The Colonial Society of Massachusetts, 1980, 157–83.

Bentivoglio, Marina, and Paolo Mazzarello. "Chapter 12: The Anatomical Foundations of Clinical Neurology." In *Handbook of Clinical Neurology*, edited by Michael J. Aminoff, François Boller, and Dick F. Swaab, 149–68. Amsterdam: Elsevier, 2009.

Bigelow, Jacob. *American Medical Botany: Being a Collection of the Native Medicinal Plants of the United States, Containing Their Botanical History and Chemical Analysis, and Properties and Uses in Medicine, Diet and the Arts, with Coloured Engravings.* 3 vols. Boston: Published by Cummings and Hilliard, at the Boston Bookstore, no. 1, Cornhill, 1817.

———. *A Discourse on Self-Limited Diseases: Delivered before the Massachusetts Medical Society, at Their Annual Meeting, May 27, 1835.* Boston: Nathan Hale, 1835.

———. *A Treatise on the Materia Medica. Intended as a Sequel to the Pharmacopoeia of the United States.* Boston: Charles Ewer, 1822.

Billings, J. S. "Literature and Institutions." In *A Century of American Medicine: 1776–1876*, edited by Edward H. Clarke. Philadelphia: Henry C. Lea, 1876, 291–366.

Black, Elias. "Consumption of the Lungs, Illustrated by Dissection and Practice. In a Memoir by Dr. Elias Black, Late House-Physician to the New-York Hospital, and Now Physician in the City of Rio Janeiro. Addressed to the Honorable Samuel L. Mitchill. Dated Nov. 1, 1808." *Medical Repository* 1, 3rd hexade, no. 2 (1809): 116–25.

Black, William. *An Arithmetical and Medical Analysis of the Diseases and Mortality of the Human Species.* 2nd ed. London: The Author etc., 1789.

Blair, Ann. "Humanist Methods in Natural Philosophy: The Commonplace Book." *Journal of the History of Ideas* 53, no. 4 (1992): 541–51.

———. "Reading Strategies for Coping with Information Overload ca. 1550–1700." *Journal of the History of Ideas* 64, no. 1 (2003): 11–28.

———. *Too Much to Know: Managing Scholarly Information before the Modern Age.* New Haven, CT: Yale University Press, 2010.

Blake, John B. *Public Health in the Town of Boston 1630–1822.* Cambridge, MA: Harvard University Press, 1959.

Blanchet, François. "Article IX. To the Editors of the Medical Repository. Gentlemen, If the Following Observations Appear to Deserve a Place in Your Repository, in Insertion of Them Will Oblige Your Most Obedient, F. Blanchet. New-York, 24th August, 1800." *Medical Repository* 4, no. 4 (1801): 369–70.

———. "Facts and Remarks on the Antiseptic Powers of Lixivial and Oleaginious Substances: Communicated by Mr. F. Blanchet, to Dr. Mitchill." *Medical Repository* 3, no. 2 (1800): 156 APS Online.

————. *Recherches Sur La Medecine, Ou L'application De La Chimie a La Medecine*. A New-York.: De l'imprimerie de Parisot, Chatham-Street, 1800. microform, xxiij, [1], 246, [2] p.; 21 cm. (8vo).

Blocker, Jack S. *American Temperance Movements: Cycles of Reform*. Boston: Twayne Publishers, 1989.

"Blood-Letting to the Amount of Fifty-Seven Pounds Troy." *Medical Repository* 2, 3rd hexade, no. 3 (1811): 295–96.

Blumberg, Mark S. "Medical Society Regulation of Fees in Boston 1780–1820." *Journal of the History of Medicine and Allied Sciences* 39, no. 3 (1984): 303–38.

Board of, Health. "Statement of Deaths, with the Diseases and Ages, in the City and Liberties of Philadelphia, from the 2d of January 1807, to the 1st of January 1809. Communicated by the Board of Health." *Transactions of the American Philosophical Society* 6 (1809): 403–407.

Boerhaave, Herman. *Boerhaave's Aphorisms: Concerning the Knowledge and Cure of Diseases Translatd from the Last Edition Printed in Latin at Leyden, 1715*. Classics of Medicine Library ed. London: R. Cowse and W. Innys in St. Paul's Church-Yard, 1715.

————. *New Method of Chemistry; Including the Theory and Practice of That Art . . . To Which Is Prefix'd a Critical History of Chemistry and Chemists . . . Translated from the Printed Edition . . . Translated By P. Shaw*. London: J. Osborn and T. Longman, 1727.

Boerhaave, Herman, and Herman Boerhaave. *Elementa Chemiae*. 2 vols. Lugduni Batavorum: apud I. Severinum, 1732.

Bos, Kirsten I., Verena J. Schuenemann, G. Brian Golding, Hernán A. Burbano, Nicholas Waglechner, Brian K. Coombes, Joseph B. McPhee, et al. "A Draft Genome of Yersinia Pestis from Victims of the Black Death." *Nature* 478 (online October 12, 2011): 506.

Boston. Transit Commission, Boston Transit Commission. *The Ferry, the Charles-River Bridge and the Charles-Town Bridge. Historical Statement Prepared for the Boston Transit Commission by Its Chairman [G. G. Crocker] and Submitted at the Opening of the New Bridge November 27, 1899*. Edited by George G. Crocker. Boston: Rockwell and Churchill Press, 1899.

Boyle, Robert. *Experiments, Notes, &C. about the Mechanical Origine or Production of Divers Particular Qualities: Among Which Is Inserted a Discourse of the Imperfection of the Chymist's Doctrine of Qualities; Together with Some Reflections upon the Hypothesis of Alcali and Acidum, Early English books, 1641–1700; 2649:2*. London: Printed and sold by Sam. Smith at the Prince's Arms in St. Paul's Church-yard, 1690. [581] p. in various pagings.

Boylston, Zabdiel. *An Historical Account of the Small-Pox Inoculated in New England, upon All Sorts of Persons, Etc*. London: S. Chandler, 1726.

Brandish, Joseph. *Observations on the Use of Caustic Alkali, in Scrofula, and Other Chronic Diseases*. London: T. Reynolds & Son; J. Murray; J. Callow, 1811.

Brandt, Allan M. "Emerging Themes in the History of Medicine." *Millbank Quarterly* 69, no. 2 (1991): 199–214.

Bres, P. L. J. "A Century of Progress in Combating Yellow Fever." *Bulletin of the World Health Organization* 64 (1986): 775–86.

Brevaglieri, Sabina. "Science, Books and Censorship in the Academy of the Lincei: Johannes Faber as Cultural Mediator." In *Conflicting Duties: Science, Medicine and Religion in Rome, 1550–1750*, edited by Maria Pia Donato, Jill Kraye, and Institute Warburg, 133–57. London: Warburg Institute, 2009.

Brickell, John. "Theory of Puerperal Fever. Communicated in a Letter to the Editors of the Medical Repository, by Dr. John Brickell, of Savannah." *Medical Repository* 2, no. 1 (1799): 15–23.

Brock, C. Helen. "The Influence of Europe on Colonial Massachusetts Medicine." In *Medicine in Colonial Massachusetts 1620–1820*, edited by J. Worth Estes, Cash, Philip, and Christianson, Eric H., 101–43. Boston: The Colonial Society of Massachusetts distributed by the University of Virginia Press, 1980.

Brock, Helen. "North America, a Western Outpost of European Medicine." In *The Medical Enlightenment of the Eighteenth Century*, edited by Andrew Cunningham and Roger French. New York: Cambridge University Press, 1990, 194–216.

Brookes, R. *The General Practice of Physic: Extracted Chiefly from the Writings of the Most Celebrated Practical Physicians, and the Medical Essays, Transactions, Journals, and Literary Correspondence of the Learned Societies in Europe: To Which Is Prefixed, an Introduction, Containing the Distinction of Similar Diseases, the Use of the Non-Naturals, an Account of the Pulse, the Consent of the Nervous Parts, and a Sketch of the Animal Œconomy*. London: Printed for J. Newbery, 1765.

———. *A History of the Most Remarkable Pestilential Distempers That Have Appeared in Europe for Three Hundred Years Last Past: With What Proved Successful or Hurtful in Their Cure. Together with the Method of Prevention and Cure of the Plague. Founded upon the Experience of Those Who Were Practitioners When It Raged. Laid Down in Such a Manner That the Generality of People May Be Able to Manage Themselves. By R. Brookes M.D.* London, 1721.

Brooks, Geraldine. *Year of Wonders: A Novel of the Plague*. New York: Viking, 2001.

Broussais, F. J. V., and Thomas Cooper. *On Irritation and Insanity: A Work, Wherein the Relations of the Physical with the Moral Conditions of Man Are Established on the Basis of Physiological Medicine*. Columbia, SC: Printed by S. J. M'Morris, 1831.

Brown, John. *The Elements of Medicine; or a Translation of the Elementa Medicinae Brunonis*. London: J. Johnson, 1788.

Brown, Richard D. "The Healing Arts in Colonial and Revolutionary Massachusetts: The Context for Scientific Medicine." In *Medicine in Colonial Massachusetts, 1620–1820: A Conference Held 25 & 26 1978*, edited by Philip Cash, Eric H. Christianson, and J. Worth Estes. Boston: The Colonial Society of Massachusetts, 1980.

Bryan, C. S., S. W. Moss, and R. J. Kahn. "Yellow Fever in the Americas." *Infectious Disease Clinics North America* 18, no. 2 (June 2004): 275–92.

Bryan, Charles S., and Scott H. Podolsky. "Dr. Holmes at 200—the Spirit of Skepticism." *New England Journal of Medicine* 361, no. 9 (2009): 846–47.

Buchan, William M. D. *Domestic Medicine; or, the Family Physician . . . Chiefly Calculated to Recommend a Proper Attention to Regimen and Simple Medicines*. Edinburgh: Balfour, Auld & Smellie, 1769.

Burnham, John C. *What Is Medical History?* Cambridge, UK; Malden, MA: Polity, 2005.

Burrage, Walter L. *A History of the Massachusetts Medical Society*. Norwood, MA: Plimpton Press, 1923.

Burton, Robert. "An Account of a Case of Hydrophobia Successfully Treated by Copious Bleeding and Mercury. In Two Letters, from Dr Robert Burton, of Bent (Creek), in the State of Virginia, to Dr Benjamin Rush, of Philadelphia. Dated Bent-Creek (Virginia) August 21, 1803 and Sept. 18, 1803." *Medical Repository* 2, 2nd hexade, no. 8 (1805): 15–18.

Butterfield, Herbert. *The Whig Interpretation of History*. London: G. Bell & Sons, 1931.

Bynum, Helen. *Spitting Blood: The History of Tuberculosis*. Oxford: Oxford University Press, 2012.

Bynum, W. F. "Cullen and the Study of Fevers in Britain, 1760–1820." In *Theories of Fever from Antiquity to the Enlightenment*, edited by W. F. Bynum and V. Nutton, 135–47. London: Wellcome Institute for the History of Medicine; Medical History, Supplement No. 1, 1981.

———. "Cullen and the Study of Fevers in Britain, 1760–1820." *Medical History* 25, no. S1 (1981): 135–47.

———. "Health, Disease and Medical Care." In *The Ferment of Knowledge: Studies in the Historiography of Eighteenth-Century Science*, edited by G. S. Rousseau and Roy Porter, 211–53. Cambridge: Cambridge University Press, 1980.

———. *Science and the Practice of Medicine in the Nineteenth Century*. Cambridge History of Medicine. Cambridge; New York: Cambridge University Press, 1994.

Cabot, Richard C. *Differential Diagnosis*. v. 1. 4th ed. Philadelphia and London: W. B. Saunders Company, 1919.

Candage, Rufus George Frederick, and Bluehill Historical Society. *Historical Sketch of Bluehill, Maine*. Ellsworth, ME: Hancock County Publishing Company, 1905.

Carey, Mathew. *A Short Account of the Malignant Fever, Lately Prevalent in Philadelphia: With a Statement of the Proceedings That Took Place on the Subject in Different Parts of the United States*. Second ed. Philadelphia: Mathew Carey, 1793.

Carlson, E. T. "The Unfortunate Dr. Parkman." *American Journal of Psychiatry* 123, no. 6 (December 1966): 724–8.

Carpenter, George Rice, ed. *Daniel Defoe's Journal of the Plague Year*. Vol. 4, Longmans' English Classics. New York: Longmans, Green, and Co., 1895.

Carpenter, Peter, K. "Thomas Arnold: A Provincial Psychiatrist in Georgian England." *Medical History* 33 (1989): 199–216.

Cash, Philip. *Dr. Benjamin Waterhouse: A Life in Medicine and Public Service (1754–1846)*. Sagamore Beach, MA, USA: Science History Publications/USA, 2006.

———. "Professionalization of Boston Medicine, 1760–1803." In *Medicine in Colonial Massachusetts, 1620–1820*, edited by Philip Cash, Eric H. Christianson and J. Worth Estes, 69–100. Boston: The Colonial Society of Massachusetts, 1980.

Cassedy, James H. *American Medicine and Statistical Thinking, 1800–1860*. Cambridge, MA: Harvard University Press, 1984.

———. *Demography in Early America: Beginnings of the Statistical Mind, 1600–1800*. Cambridge: Harvard University Press, 1969.

Castiglioni, Arturo. *A History of Medicine*. 2nd ed. New York: Alfred A. Knopf, 1947.

Caulfield, Ernest. *A True History of the Terrible Epidemic Vulgarly Called the Throat Distemper, Which Occurred in His Majesty's New England Colonies between the Years 1735 and 1740*. New Haven: Yale Journal of Biology & Medicine for the Beaumont Medical Club, 1939.

Census, Bureau of the United States. *Heads of Families at the First Census of the United States Taken in the Year 1790: Maine*. Spartansburg, SC: The Reprint Company, originally printed by the Government Printing Office, Washington, 1908, 1978.

Chalmers, Lionel. *An Account of the Weather and Diseases of South-Carolina*. 2 vols. London: Edward and Charles Dilly, 1776.

Channing, Walter. "Practical Remarks on Some of the Predisposing Causes, and Prevention, of Puerperal Fever, with Cases." *New England Journal of Medicine and Surgery* 6, no. 2 (April 1, 1817): 157–69.

Chapman, George T. *Sketches of the Alumni of Dartmouth College, from the First Graduation in 1771 to the Present Time, with a Brief History of the Institution.* Cambridge, Massachusetts: Riverside Press, 1867.

———. *Sketches of the Alumni of Dartmouth College.* Riverside Press, p://www.dartmouth.edu/~speccoll/chapman/chapman_introduction.html.

Charon, Rita. *Narrative Medicine: Honoring the Stories of Illness.* Oxford; New York: Oxford University Press, 2006.

Chavigny, Katherine. "Reforming Drunkards in Nineteenth-Century America." In *Altering American Consciousness: The History of Alcohol and Drug Use in the United States, 1800–2000,* edited by Sarah W. Tracy, Acker, Caroline Jean, 108–23. Amherst: University of Massachusetts Press, 2004.

Cheyne, George. *The English Malady: Or a Treatise of Nervous Diseases of All Kinds.* London: G. Strahan, 1733.

———. *An Essay of Health and Long Life.* London: George Strahan etc., 1724.

———. *An Essay on Regimen. Together with Five Discourses, Medical, Moral, and Philosophical.* London: C. Rivington, 1740.

———. *Observations Concerning the Nature and Due Method of Treating the Gout.* London: G. Strahan, 1720.

Chisholm, Colin. *An Essay on the Malignant Pestilential Fever, Introduced into the West Indian Islands from Boullam, on the Coast of Guinea, as It Appeared in 1793, 1794, 1795, and 1796. Interspersed with Observations and Facts, Tending to Prove That the Epidemic Existing at Philadelphia, New-York, &C. Was the Same Fever Introduced by Infection Imported from the West Indian Islands: And Illustrated by Evidences Found on the State of Those Islands, and Information of the Most Eminent Practitioners Residing on Them.* 2nd ed. 2 vols. Vol. 1. London: Mawman, 1801.

———. "Intelligence from Dr. Chisholm since the Publication of the Second Edition of His Work on Fever." *Medical Repository* 5, no. 2 (1805): 228–34.

"Circular Address." *Medical Repository* 1, no. 1 (1797): vii–xii.

Clark, Charles E. *Maine: A Bicentennial History.* The States and the Nation Series. New York: Norton, 1977.

Clifton, Francis. *The State of Physick, Ancient and Modern, Briefly Consider'd: With a Plan for the Improvement of It.* London: J. Nourse, 1732.

———. *Tabular Observations Recommended, as the Plainest and Surest Way of Practising and Improving Physick; in a Letter to a Friend.* London: Printed for J. Brindley, and sold by the booksellers of London and Westminster, 1731.

Coffin, Nathaniel, Jeremiah Barker, Shirley Ervin, Dudley Folsom, Stephen Thomas, Aaron Kinsman. "Letter to the Massachusetts Medical-Society Requesting Permission to Allow a District of Maine Medical Society." In *Coffin, Nathaniel,* B MS c 75.2 Archives at Countway Library, Harvard, Portland, Maine, June 30, 1804.

Cohen, I. Bernard. *Science and the Founding Fathers: Science in the Political Thought of Jefferson, Franklin, Adams and Madison.* 1st ed. New York: W.W. Norton, 1995.

Colbatch, John. "A Physico Medical Essay Concerning Alkaly and Acid so Far as They Have Relation to the Cause or Cure of Distempers: Wherein Is Endeavoured to Be Proved That Acids Are Not (as Is Generally and Erroneously Supposed) the Cause of All or Most Distempers, but That Alkalies Are: Together with an Account of Some Distempers and the Medicines with Their Preparations Proper to Be Used in the Cure of Them: As Also a Short Digression Concerning Specifick Remedies."

Printed for Dan. Browne, http://gateway.proquest.com/openurl?ctx_ver=Z39.88-2003&res_id=xri:eebo&rft_val_fmt=&rft_id=xri:eebo:image:42743 Online book

Coleman, William. *Yellow Fever in the North: The Methods of Early Epidemiology*. Madison: University of Wisconsin Press, 1987.

Colgrove, James. "The Mckeown Thesis: A Historical Controversy and Its Enduring Influence." *American Journal of Public Health* 92, no. 5 (2002): 725–29.

The Compact Edition of the Oxford English Dictionary: Complete Text Reproduced Micrographically. Oxford: Oxford University Press, 1971.

Conrad, Lawrence I., and Wellcome Institute for the History of Medicine. *The Western Medical Tradition: 800 BC to Ad 1800*. Cambridge, UK; New York: Cambridge University Press, 1995.

The Constitution of the Humane Society of the State of New-York: To Which Are Subjoined the Address of the Medical Counsellors to the Citizens. New-York: Printed by J. Buel, 1795.

"[Controversy between Dr. Barker of Gorham and Dr. Nathaniel Coffin of Portland on the Prevention and Cure of Puerperal Fever]." *The Falmouth Gazette and Weekly Advertiser*, February 12, 19, 26, and March 5, 12, 1785.

Cook, H. J. "Sir John Colbatch and Augustan Medicine: Experimentalism, Character and Entrepreneurialism." *Annals of Science* 47, no. 5 (September1990): 475–505.

Cooley, Arnold James. *A Cyclopaedia of Practical Receipts, and Collateral Information in the Arts, Manufactures, and Trades, Including Medicine, Pharmacy, and Domestic Economy*. London: J. Churchill, 1845.

Coss, Stephen. *The Fever of 1721*. First Simon & Schuster hardcover ed. New York: Simon & Schuster, 2016.

Cowen, David L. *America's Pre-Pharmacopoeial Literature*. Madison, WI: American Institute of the History of Pharmacy, 1961.

———. *The Edinburgh Dispensatories*. [s.l.]: Bibliographical Society of America, 1951.

———. *Pharmacopoeias and Related Literature in Britain and America, 1618–1847*. Burlington, VT: Ashgate, 2001.

Coxe, John Redman. *The American Dispensatory . . . Illustrated and Explained, According to the Principles of Modern Chemistry: Comprehending Improvements on Dr. Duncan's Second Edition*. Philadelphia: Thomas Dobson, 1806.

———. *The Philadelphia Medical Dictionary*. 2nd ed. Philadelphia: Thomas Dobson, 1817.

Craig, William. *On the Influence of Electric Tension as a Remote Cause of Epidemic and Other Diseases*. London: John Churchill, 1859.

Crell, F. L. F. "Some Experiments on Putrefaction: By F.L.F. Crell, M.D. And Professor of Chemistry at Brunswick." *Philosophical Transactions (1683–1775)* 61 (1771): 332–44.

Cronin, J. E. *The Diary of Elihu Hubbard Smith (1771–1798)*. Philadelphia: American Philosophical Society, 1973.

Crosland, Maurice. "Chemistry and the Chemical Revolution." In *The Ferment of Knowledge: Studies in the Historiography of Eighteenth-Century Science*, edited by G. S. Rousseau and Roy Porter, 389–416. New York: Cambridge University Press, 1980.

Cullen, William. *First Lines of the Practice of Physic with Supplementary Notes, Including More Recent Improvements in the Practice of Medicine by Peter Reid*. Two volumes in one. Brookfield: E. Mirriam & Co. for Isaiah Thomas, 1807.

Cumberland Association of Congregational, Ministers. *The Centennial of the Cumberland Association of Congregational Ministers, at the Second Parish Church in Portland, Maine*. Portland ME: B. Thurston, 1888.

Cunha, B. A. "Smallpox and Measles: Historical Aspects and Clinical Differentiation." *Infectious Disease Clinics of North America* 18, no. 1 (March 2004): 79–100.

Currie, James. *Medical Reports, on the Effects of Water, Cold and Warm, as a Remedy in Fever, and Febrile Diseases; Whether Applied to the Surface of the Body, or Used as a Drink: With Observations on the Nature of Fever; and on the Effects of Opium, Alcohol, and Inanition.* Liverpool: Printed by J. M'Creery, for Cadell and Davies, London, 1797.

Currie, James, and Benjamin Vaughan. *An Abridgment of the Second Edition of a Work, Written by Dr. Currie, of Liverpool in England: On the Use of Water, in Diseases of the Human Frame; and on Fever, Opium, Strong Drink, Abstinence from Food, and the Passages through the Human Skin: With Occasional Remarks.* [Augusta, ME] and by the Booksellers of Boston, New-York, and Philadelphia: Printed by Peter Edes; sold by Mr. Edes of Augusta, and Mr. Bass of Hallowell, 1799.

Currie, William. "An Enquiry into the Causes of the Insalubrity of Flat and Marshy Situations." *Transactions of the American Philosophical Society* 4 (1799): 127–42.

———. *An Historical Account of the Climates and Diseases of the United States of America and of the Remedies and Methods of Treatment, Which Have Been Found Most Useful and Efficacious, Particularly in Those Diseases Which Depend on Climate and Situation.* Reprint ed. Arno Press, New York, 1972. Philadelphia: T. Dobson., 1792.

———. *A Sketch of the Rise and Progress of the Yellow Fever, and the Proceedings of the Board of Health, in Philadelphia, in the Year 1799: To Which Is Added, a Collection of Facts and Observations Respecting the Origin of Yellow Fever in This Country; and a Review of the Different Modes of Treating It.* Philadelphia: Budd and Bartram, 1800.

Dacome, Lucia. "Noting the Mind: Commonplace Books and Pursuit of Self in Eighteenth-Century Britain." *Journal of the History of Ideas* 65, no. 4 (2004): 603–25.

Dain, Norman. *Concepts of Insanity in the United States, 1789–1865.* New Brunswick, NJ: Rutgers University Press, 1964.

Dartmouth College and Associated Schools General Catalogue 1769–1940. Hanover NH: Dartmouth College Publications, 1940.

Darwin, Erasmus. *The Botanic Garden. A Poem, in Two Parts. Part I. Containing the Economy of Vegetation. Part II. The Loves of the Plants. With Philosophical Notes.* 3d ed. London: J. Johnson, 1795.

———. *Zoonomia, or the Laws of Organic Life.* Vol. 1. New York: T. and J. Swords, 1796.

Daston, Lorraine. "The History of Science and the History of Knowledge." *KNOW: A Journal on the Formation of Knowledge* 1, no. 1 (2017): 131–54.

Davis, Audrey B., and Jon B. Ecklund. "Magnesia Alba before Black." *Pharmacy in History* 14, no. 4 (1972): 139–46.

Davis, Joseph E. "Reductionist Medicine and Its Cultural Authority." In *To Fix or to Heal: Patient Care, Public Health, and the Limits of Biomedicine,* edited by Joseph E. Davis and Ana Marta Gonzalez, 33–62. New York: New York University Press, 2016.

Davis, Joseph E., and Ana Marta Gonzalez, eds. *To Fix or to Heal: Patient Care, Public Health, and the Limits of Biomedicine.* New York: New York University Press, 2016.

Davy, Humphry. *Researches, Chemical and Philosophical: Chiefly Concerning Nitrous Oxide, or Diphlogisticated Nitrous Air, and Its Respiration.* London: Printed for J. Johnson . . . by Biggs and Cottle, Bristol., 1800.

Deane, Samuel. *History of Scituate, Massachusetts, from Its First Settlement to 1831.* Boston: J. Loring, 1831.

"Deaths in Portland during the Year 1830." *Eastern Argus,* January 25, 1831.

Debus, Allen G. *The Chemical Promise: Experiment and Mysticism in the Chemical Philosophy, 1550–1800: Selected Essays of Allen G. Debus.* Sagamore Beach, MA: Science History Publications, 2006.

———. *Chemistry and Medical Debate: Van Helmont to Boerhaave*. Canton, MA: Science History, 2001.

Denman, Thomas. *Essays on Puerperal Fever, and on Puerperal Convulsions*. London: J. Walter, 1768.

———. *Introduction to the Practice of Midwifery*. London, 1782.

DeWees, William P. "Art. 4. An Abridgment of Mr. Heath's Translation of Baudelocque's Midwifery with Notes by William P. Dewees, Md. Lecturer on Midwifery in Philadelphia. 8vo. Pp.685. Philadelphia. Bertram and Reynolds. 1807." *Medical Repository* 5 (January 1, 1808): 291–96.

Dover, Thomas, and Augustin Belloste. *The Ancient Physician's Legacy to His Country: Being What He Has Collected Himself in Forty-Nine Years Practice, or, an Account of the Several Diseases Incident to Mankind . . . Design'd for the Use of All Private Families*. London: Printed for the relict of the late R. Bradly, 1733.

Dovovan, Arthur. *Antoine Lavoisier: Science, Administration, and Revolution*. Oxford: Blackwell, 1993.

Dow, Neal. *The Reminiscences of Neal Dow: Recollections of Eighty Years*. Portland, ME: The Evening Express Publishing Company, 1898.

Dubernard, Mr. "Use of Volatile Alkali as a Counter-Poison (from the Paris Journal De Commerce, Aug. 7, 1805)." *The Medical Repository (and review of American publications on medicine)* 3, 2nd hexade (1806): 423–24.

Duffin, J. "A Hippocratic Triangle: History, Clinician-Historians, and Future Doctors." In *Locating Medical History: The Stories and Their Meanings*, edited by Frank Huisman and John Harley Warner, 432–49. Baltimore: Johns Hopkins University Press, 2004.

Duffin, Jacalyn. *History of Medicine: A Scandalously Short Introduction*. Toronto: University of Toronto Press, 1999.

———. *Langstaff: A Nineteenth-Century Medical Life*. Toronto; Buffalo: University of Toronto Press, 1993.

———. *To See with a Better Eye: A Life of R.T.H. Laennec*. Princeton, NJ: Princeton University Press, 1998.

Duffy, John. *Epidemics in Colonial America*. Baton Rouge: Louisiana State University Press, 1953.

———. *The Healers: A History of American Medicine*. Illini books ed. Urbana: University of Illinois Press, 1979.

———. *A History of Public Health in New York City 1625–1868*. New York: Russel Sage Foundation, 1968.

———. *The Sanitarians: A History of American Public Health*. Chicago: University of Illinois Press, 1992.

Duncan, Andrew. *The Edinburgh New Dispensatory*. First Worcester ed. Worcester: Press of Isaiah Thomas, 1805.

Dunglison, Robley. *A Dictionary of Medical Science*. Philadelphia: Henry C. Lea, 1874.

Duveen, D., and H. Klickstein. "The Introduction of Lavoisier's Chemical Nomenclature into America." *Isis* 45 (1954): 278–92.

Duveen, Dennis, and Herbert S. Klickstein. "The Introduction of Lavoisier's Chemical Nomenclature into America: Part 2." *Isis* 45, no. 4 (December 1954): 368–82.

Eastburn, James. *A Catalogue of Books for 1818*. New York, 1819.

Ebert, M. "The Rise and Development of the American Medical Periodical 1797–1850." *Bulletin of the Medical Library Association* 40, no. 3 (July 1952): 243–76.

Ecklund, Jon B., and Audrey B. Davis. "Joseph Black Matriculates: Medicine and Magnesia Alba." *Journal of the History of Medicine and Allied Sciences* 27, no. 4 (1972): 396–417.

Eklund, J.B., and A. B. Davis. "Some Thoughts on the Influence of British Medicine on American Medicine in the 18th Century." *Proceedings XXIII Congress of the History of Medicine* (1972): 825–31.

Emerson, Charles Franklin. *General Catalogue of Dartmouth College and the Associated Schools 1769–1910, Including a Historical Sketch of the College.* Hanover, NH: Printed for the college, 1911.

Engs, Ruth Clifford. *Clean Living Movements: American Cycles of Health Reform.* Westport, CT: Praeger, 2000.

Estes, J. Worth. *The Changing Humors of Portsmouth: The Medical Biography of an American Town, 1623–1983.* Boston: The Francis A. Countway Library of Medicine, 1986.

———. *Dictionary of Protopharmacology.* Canton, MA: Science History Publications, 1990.

———. *Hall Jackson and the Purple Foxglove.* Hanover: University Press of New England, 1979.

———. "Introduction: The Yellow Fever Syndrome and Its Treatment in Philadelphia, 1793." In *A Melancholy Scene of Devastation: The Public Response to the 1793 Philadelphia Yellow Fever Epidemic,* edited by J. Worth Estes and Billy G. Smith, 1–17. Canton, MA, USA: Science History Publications, 1997.

———. "Lyman Spalding." In *Dictionary of American Medical Biography,* edited by Martin Kaufman, Stuart Galishoff and Todd L. Savitt. Westport, CT: Greenwood Press, 1984.

———. "Therapeutic Practice in Colonial New England." In *Medicine in Colonial Massachusetts, 1620–1820: A Conference Held 25 & 26 May 1978,* edited by Frederick S. Allis, 289–383. Boston: The Colonial Society of Massachusetts, 1980.

Estes, J. Worth, and Billy G. Smith, eds. *A Melancholy Scene of Devastation: The Public Response to the 1793 Philadelphia Yellow Fever Epidemic.* Canton, MA: Science History Publications/USA, 1997.

Fåhraeus, Robin. "The Suspension Stability of the Blood." *Physiological Reviews* 9, no. 2 (1929): 241–74.

———. *The Suspension-Stability of the Blood.* Stockholm: Norstedt, 1921.

Farren, Donald. "Subscription: A Study of the Eighteenth-Century American Trade." Doctor of Library Science, Columbia University, 1982.

Feldman, Michal, Michaela Harbeck, Marcel Keller, Maria A. Spyrou, Andreas Rott, Bernd Trautmann, Holger C. Scholz, et al. "A High-Coverage Yersinia Pestis Genome from a Sixth-Century Justinianic Plague Victim." *Molecular Biology and Evolution* 33, no. 11 (2016): 2911–23.

Ferretti, J., and W. Kohler. "History of Streptococcal Research." In *Streptococcus Pyogenes: Basic Biology to Clinical Manifestations,* edited by J. J. Ferretti, D. L. Stevens and V. A. Fischetti. University of Oklahoma Health Sciences Center: Oklahoma City, OK, 2016, 1–26.

Ferriar, John. *Medical Histories and Reflections.* 1st American ed. Philadelphia: Published by Thomas Dobson, at the Stone House, no. 41 William Fry, 1816.

Finger, Stanley. "Chapter 10: The Birth of Localization Theory." In *Handbook of Clinical Neurology,* edited by Michael J. Aminoff, François Boller, and Dick F. Swaab, 117–28. Amsterdam: Elsevier, 2009.

Fissell, Mary E. "The Marketplace of Print." In *Medicine and the Market in England and Its Colonies, C.1450–C.1850*, edited by Mark S. R. Dr Jenner and Patrick Dr Wallis, 108–32. Basingstoke, UK: Palgrave Macmillan, 2007.

Fleming, James Roger. *Meteorology in America, 1800–1870*. Baltimore: Johns Hopkins University Press, 1990.

Floyer, John. *The Physician's Pulse-Watch; or, an Essay to Explain the Old Art of Feeling the Pulse, and to Improve It by the Help of a Pulse-Watch. In Three Parts. I. The Old Galenic Art of Feeling the Pulse Is Describ'd, and Many of Its Errors Corrected: The True Use of the Pulses, and Their Causes, Differences and Prognostications by Them, Are Fully Explain'd, and Directions Given for Feeling the Pulse by the Pulse-Watch, or Minute-Glass. II. A New Mechanical Method Is Propos'd for Preserving Health, and Prolonging Life, and for Curing Diseases by the Help of the Pulse-Watch, Which Shews the Pulses When They Exceed or Are Deficient from the Natural. III. The Chinese Art of Feeling the Pulse Is Describ'd; and the Imitation of Their Practice of Physick, Which Is Grounded on the Observation of the Pulse, Is Recommended. To Which Is Added, an Extract out of Andrew Cleyer, Concerning the Chinese Art of Feeling the Pulse. By Sir John Floyer, Knight*. [in English] London: printed for Sam. Smith and Benj. Walford, at the Prince's-Arms in St. Paul's Church-Yard, 1707.

Folsom, George. *History of Saco and Biddeford*. Somersworth Portland: New Hampshire Pub. Co. Maine Historical Society, 1975.

Fothergill, John. *An Account of the Sore Throat Attended with Ulcers*. London: C. Davis, 1748.

Freeman, Samuel. *Extracts from the Journals Kept by the Reverend Thos Smith from the Year 1720 to the Year 1788, with an Appendix Containing a Variety of Other Matter Selected by Samuel Freeman*. Portland: T. Todd & Co., 1821.

Frieden, Thomas R. "A Framework for Public Health Action: The Health Impact Pyramid." *American Journal of Public Health* 100, no. 4 (2010): 590–95.

Fuller, J. "Universal Etiology, Multifactorial Diseases and the Constitutive Model of Disease Classification." *Studies in History and Philosophy of Biological and Biomedical Sciences* 67 (February 2018): 8–15.

Furdell, Elizabeth Lane. *Publishing and Medicine in Early Modern England*. Rochester, NY: University of Rochester Press; Woodbridge: Boydell & Brewer, 2002.

Fye, W. Bruce. "Ernest Henry Starling." *Clinical Cardiology* 29, no. 4 (2006): 181–82.

Gaitskell, William. "Five Cases of Puerperal Fever Successfully Treated, with Remarks." *The London Medical Repository* 3, no. 17 (1815): 365–71.

Gallup, Joseph A. *Sketches of Epidemic Diseases in the State of Vermont*. Boston: T. B. Wait & Sons, 1815.

———. "Treatment of Persons Who Have Been Bitten by Mad Dogs." *Medical Repository* 4, 2nd hexade (1807): 199–200.

Gamage, W. J. *Some Account of the Fever Which Existed in Boston during the Autumn and Winter of 1817–18. With a Few Remarks on Typhus*. Boston: Wells & Lilly, 1818.

Gamage, William. "Cases of Croup." *The New England Journal of Medicine, Surgery and Collateral Branches of Science* 6, no. 1 (1817): 24–29.

———. "On the Hooping Cough." *New England Journal of Medicine and Surgery* 6, no. 3 (July 1817): 213–28.

Garland, Joseph E. *The Centennial History of the Boston Medical Library, 1875–1975*. Boston: Boston Medical Library in the Francis A. Countway Library of Medicine, 1975.

————. "Medical Journalism in New England 1788–1924." *Boston Medical and Surgical Journal* 190 (1924): 865–79.

Garraty, John A., and Mark C. Carnes. *American National Biography*. New York: Oxford University Press, 1999.

Garrison, Fielding H. *An Introduction to the History of Medicine*. 4th, reprinted ed. Philadelphia: W. B. Saunders, 1929.

Garrison, Fielding H., and Lawrence C. McHenry. *History of Neurology. Rev. and Enl. with a Bibliography of Classical, Original and Standard Works in Neurology, by Lawrence C. Mchenry, Jr*. Springfield, IL: Thomas, 1969.

Gauchat, Gordon. "The Cultural Authority of Science: Public Trust and Acceptance of Organized Science." *Public Understanding of Science* 20, no. 6 (2011): 751–70.

The Genuine Works of Hippocrates. Edited by Francis Adams. Baltimore: Williams and Wilkins, 1939.

Gibbs, F. W. *Joseph Priestley: Adventurer in Science and Champion of Truth*. London: Thomas Nelson and Sons Ltd., 1965.

Glasse, Hannah, L. Wangford, Wine American Institute of, and Food. *The Art of Cookery, Made Plain and Easy: Which Far Exceeds Any Thing of the Kind yet Published, Containing . . . To Which Are Added, One Hundred and Fifty New and Useful Receipts, and a Copious Index*. London: Printed for a Company of Booksellers, and sold by L. Wangford, in Fleet-Street, and all other booksellers in Great Britain and Ireland . . . 1770.

Golinski, Jan. *Science as a Public Culture: Chemistry and Enlightenment in Britain, 1760–1820*. New York: Cambridge University Press, 1992.

Gordon, Alexander. *A Treatise on the Epidemic Fever of Aberdeen*. London: G. G. and J. Robinson, 1795.

Oxford Dictionary of National Biography. Oxford: Oxford University Press, 2018.

"Grand Surgical Operation." *Boston Recorder*, December 16, 1820, 204.

Grange, Kathleen M. "Dr. Samuel Johnson's Account of a Schizophrenic Illness in Rasselas (1759)." *Medical History* 6, no. 2 (1962): 162–68.

Graunt, John. *Natural and Political Observations Mentioned in a Following Index, and Made Upon the Bills of Mortality*. 3rd ed. London: John Martyn and James Allestry, Printers to the Royal Society, 1665.

Gray, Ruth, Alice MacDonald Long, Joseph C. Anderson, Lois Ware Thurston, and Society Maine Genealogical. *Maine Families in 1790*. Camden: Maine Genealogical Society, 1988.

Green, James N. "The Rise of Book Publishing." In *An Extensive Republic: Print, Culture, and Society in the New Nation, 1790–1840*, edited by Robert A. Gross and Mary Kelley, 75–127. Chapel Hill: Published in association with the American Antiquarian Society by the University of North Carolina Press, 2010.

Greene, Jeremy A. "Therapeutic Proofs and Medical Truths: The Enduring Legacy of Early Modern Drug Trials." *Bulletin of the History of Medicine* 91, no. 2 (2017): 420–29.

Greene, John C. "The Boston Medical Community and Emerging Science, 1780–1820." In *Medicine in Colonial Massachusetts 1620–1820*, 187–97. Boston: The Colonial Society of Massachusetts, 1980.

Greenleaf, Moses. *A Survey of the State of Maine in Reference to Its Geographical Features, Statistics and Political Economy*. 1970 Maine State Museum reprint ed. Portland: Shirley & Hyde, 1829.

Griffin, Simon Goodell, Octavius Applegate, and Frank H. Whitcomb. *A History of the Town of Keene from 1732, When the Township Was Granted by Massachusetts, to 1874, When It Became a City*. Keene, NH: Sentinel Print. Co., 1904.

Grob, Gerald N. *The Mad among Us: A History of the Care of America's Mentally Ill*. New York, Toronto: Free Press, Maxwell Macmillan Canada, 1994.

Gross, Robert A. "Introduction" in *An Extensive Republic: Print, Culture, and Society in the New Nation, 1790–1840*, edited by Robert A. Gross and Mary Kelley, 1–50. Chapel Hill: Published in association with the American Antiquarian Society by the University of North Carolina Press, 2010.

Growoll, Adolph. *Book-Trade Bibliography in the United States in the XIXth Century: To Which Is Added a Catalogue of All the Books Printed in the United States with Prices, and Places Where Published, Annexed Published by the Booksellers in Boston, January, 1804*. New York: Reprinted by Burt Franklin in 1939, 1898.

Guyton de Morveau, Louis Bernard, Antoine Laurent Lavoisier, Claude-Louis Berthollet, Antoine François de Fourcroy, J. H. Hassenfratz, and Pierre-Auguste Adet. *Méthode De Nomenclature Chimique*. A Paris: Chez Cuchet, libraire, rue & hôtel Serpente, 1787.

Hacker, J. David. "Decennial Life Tables for the White Population of the United States, 1790–1900." *Historical Methods* 43, no. 2 (2010): 45–79.

Hall, A. R. "On Whiggism." *History of Science* 21, no. 51 Pt 1 (March 1983): 45–59.

Hall, Courtney Robert. *A Scientist in the Early Republic: Samuel Latham Mitchill, 1764–1831*. New York: Columbia University Press, 1934.

Halle. "Observations on a Means for Preventing Cancerous Degeneration in Schirrous Congestion in the Breast." *The New England Journal of Medicine, Surgery and Collateral Branches of Science* 9, no. 1 (1820): 89–91.

Hallett, Christine. "The Attempt to Understand Puerperal Fever in the Eighteenth and Early Nineteenth Centuries: The Influence of the Inflammation Theory." *Medical History* 49 (2005): 1–28.

Hamilton, Alexander. *A Treatise on the Management of Female Complaints, and of Children in Early Infancy*. 8th ed., revised and enlarged; with hints for the treatment of the principal diseases of infants and children. Edited by Dr. James Hamilton, Junior. Edinburgh: Edinburgh, Printed for Peter Hill & Company; and sold by Longman, Hurst, Rees, Orme, and Brown, and T. & G. Underwood, London, 1821.

Hamilton, David. *The Healers: A History of Medicine in Scotland*. Edinburgh: Canongate, 1981.

Hamilton, James, and Ansel W. Ives. *Observations on the Use and Abuse of Mercurial Medicines in Various Diseases and an Appendix by Ansel W. Ives*. New York: Bliss & White, 1821.

Hamlin, Christopher. *More Than Hot: A Short History of Fever*. Johns Hopkins Biographies of Disease. Baltimore: Johns Hopkins University Press, 2014.

Hampton, J. R., M. J. Harrison, J. R. Mitchell, J. S. Prichard, and C. Seymour. "Relative Contributions of History-Taking, Physical Examination, and Laboratory Investigation to Diagnosis and Management of Medical Outpatients." *British Medical Journal* 2, no. 5969 (May 31, 1975): 486–89.

Harris, Dr. "History of a Fatal Case of Hydrocephalus. By Dr. Harris, of Kingston, Jamaica, in a Letter to Dr. Farquhar, Dated July 30th, 1805." *Medical Museum* 2, no. 1 (1806): 384–91.

Harris, H.F. "Slow Fever." *Journal of the American Medical Association* 49 (1907): 406–11.

Harris, William. "Case of Phthsis Pulmonalis, Cured by Mercury." *Philadelphia Medical Museum* 3 (1807): 119–20.

Harrison, Mark. *Contagion: How Commerce Has Spread Disease.* New Haven: Yale University Press, 2012.

Hartley, David, and Fr Sandys. "VI. Another Case of a Person Bit by a Mad-Dog, Drawn up by David Hartley, M. A. And Mr. Fr. Sandys, Communicated to the Royal Society by Francis Wollaston, Esq; F. R. S." *Philosophical Transactions* 40, no. 448 (January 1, 1738): 274–76.

Harvey, Gideon. *Morbus Anglicus, or, a Theoretick and Practical Discourse of Consumptions, and Hypochondriak Melancholy: Comprizing Their Nature, Subject, Kinds, Causes, Signs, Prognosticks, and Cures: Likewise a Discourse of Spitting of Blood, Its Differences, Causes, Signs, Prognosticks, and Cure.* London: William Thackeray, 1672.

Hatch, S. "Uncertainty in Medicine." *British Medical Journal* 357 (May 11, 2017): j2180.

Hawes, Lloyd E., and J. Worth Estes. *Benjamin Waterhouse, Md; First Professor of the Theory and Practice of Physics at Harvard and Introducer of Cowpox Vaccination into America . . . Including a Concordance of Dr. Waterhouse's Hortus Siccus.* Boston Medical Library Studies, 1. Boston: Francis A. Countway Library of Medicine, 1974.

Hawkins, Dr. Bisset. "From the Med. Gazette. Abstract of Lectures on Medical Statistics, Delivered at the College of Physicians." *Boston Medical and Surgical Journal* 1 (1828): 418–26.

Hayward, George. "Some Observations on Dr. Rush's Work on 'the Diseases of the Mind.' With Remarks on the Nature and Treatment of Insanity." *New England Journal of Medicine and Surgery* 7, no. 1 (January 1818): 18–34.

———. "Some Remarks on Delerium Vigilans; Commonly Called 'Delerium Tremens,' Mania a Potu,' 'Mania a Temulentia.'" *New England Journal of Medicine and Surgery* 11 (July 1, 1822): 235–43.

Hayward, Oliver S., and Constance A. Putnam, eds. *Improve, Perfect, & Perpetuate: Nathan Smith and Early American Medical Education.* Hanover: University Press of New England, 1998.

Hazeltine, Richard. "Observations on the Efficacy of Bloodletting in Hemoptysis." *New England Journal of Medicine and Surgery* 11, no. 4 (1822): 43–351.

Henry, Alexander. *Travels and Adventures in Canada and the Indian Territories between the Years 1760–1776.* New York: I. Riley, 1809.

Hess, Volker, and J. Andrew Mendelsohn. "Case and Series: Medical Knowledge and Paper Technology, 1600–1900." *History of Science* 48 (2010): 287–312.

Heustis, J. W. "Art. II. Remark on the Endemic Diseases of Alabama." *The American Journal of the Medical Sciences (1827–1924)* 2, no. 3 (May 25, 1828): 26.

Heustis, Jabez Wiggins. *Physical Observations, and Medical Tracts and Researches, on the Topography and Diseases of Louisiana.* Edited by T. and printer J. Swords. New York, 1817.

Hindle, Brooke. *The Pursuit of Science in Revolutionary America 1735–1789.* Chapel Hill: The University of North Carolina Press, 1956.

Historical Catalogue of Brown University. Providence: Brown University, 1905.

"Historical Outline of the Progress of Medical Science during the Past Three Years." *New England Journal of Medicine and Surgery* 2, no. 1 (1813): 1–5.

"History of Disease in Maine." *Christian Mirror,* February 22, 1828, 3.

Hoffmann, Roald. "Mme. Lavoisier." *American Scientist* 90, no. 1 (2002): 22.

Holmes, Frederic H. *Antoine Lavoisier: Or the Sources of His Quantitative Method in Chemistry.* Princeton: Princeton University Press, 1998.

—————. "The 'Revolution in Chemistry and Physics'" *Isis* 91, no. 4 (December 2000): 735–53.

Holmes, Oliver Wendell. *The Autocrat of the Breakfast Table.* Boston: Houghton, Mifflin, 1881.

—————. "Currents and Counter-Currents." In *Medical Essays: 1842–1882*, edited by Oliver Wendell Holmes, 172–208. Boston: Houghton Mifflin Company, 1911.

Holy Bible: The Washburn College Bible, Oxford Edition, King James Text, Modern Phrased Version. Oxford: Oxford University Press, 1980.

Holyoke, Edward Augustus. "A Letter to Dr. —; in Answer to His Quiries Respecting the Introduction of the Mercurial Practice in the Vicinity of Boston, Mass. Salem, Mass, Dec. 1797." *Medical Repository* 1, no. 4 (1798): 500–503.

Hooper, Robert. *A Compendious Medical Dictionary: Containing an Explaination of the Terms in Anatomy, Physiology, Surgery, Materia Medica, Chemistry, and Practice of Physic: Collected from the Most Approved Authors.* London: Printed for Murray and Highley, 1799.

Hornsby, Stephen J., and Richard William Judd. "Historical Atlas of Maine." Orono: University of Maine Press, 2015.

Horrocks, Thomas A. "Miller, Edward (1760–1812), Physician and Teacher." In *American National Biography*: Oxford: Oxford University Press, 2000.

—————. *Popular Print and Popular Medicine: Almanacs and Health Advice in Early America.* Amherst: University of Massachusetts Press, 2008.

Hosack, David. "Dr. Hosack Writes Warmly in Favour of Lime-Water." *Medical Repository* 3 (1800): 404–406.

—————. *The Modern Practice of Physic, Exhibiting the Characters, Causes, Symptoms, Prognostics, Morbid Appearances, and Improved Method of Treating the Diseases of All Climates.* The 4th American from the 5th London ed. New York: Collins & Company, 1817.

Howell, Joel D. *Technology and American Medical Practice, 1880–1930: An Anthology of Sources.* Medical Care in the United States. New York: Garland Pub., 1988.

Hruschka, John. *How Books Came to America: The Rise of the American Book Trade.* University Park: The Pennsylvania State University Press, 2012.

Hudson, Robert. *Disease and Its Control.* Westport, CT: Greenwood Press, 1983.

Huisman, Frank, and John Harley Warner, eds. *Locating Medical History: The Stories and Their Meanings.* Baltimore: Johns Hopkins University Press, 2004.

Humphreys, Margaret. "Appendix II: Yellow Fever since 1793: History and Historiography." In *A Melancholy Scene of Devastation: The Public Response to the 1793 Philadelphia Yellow Fever Epidemic*, edited by J. Worth Estes and Billy G. Smith, 183–98. Canton, MA: Science History Publications/USA, 1997.

—————. *Yellow Fever and the South.* Baltimore: The Johns Hopkins University Press, 1992.

Hunter, Henry. *Sacred Biography—or, the History of the Patriarchs to Which Is Added the History of Deborah, Ruth & Hannah Being a Course of Lectures Delivered at the Seots [Scotch, Scotts, Scots] Church.* Boston: J. White, Thomas & Andrews &c., 1794.

Hunter, John. *A Treatise on the Blood, Inflammation, and Gun-Shot Wounds.* 2 vols. Philadelphia: Thomas Bradford, 1796.

Hunter, Kathryn Montgomery. *Doctors' Stories: The Narrative Structure of Medical Knowledge.* Princeton, NJ: Princeton University Press, 1991.

Hurd, D. Hamilton. *History of Middlesex County, Massachusetts, with Biographical Sketches of Many of Its Pioneers and Prominent Men.* 3 vols. Philadelphia: J. W. Lewis & Co., 1890.

Huxham, John. *A Dissertation on the Malignant, Ulcerous Sore-Throat.* London: J. Hinton, 1757.

———. *An Essay on Fevers with Introduction by Saul Jarcho.* Canton, MA: Science History Publications (reprint 1988), 1757.

Innes, John. "An Inflammation of the Stomach, with Hydrophobia, and Other Uncommon Symptoms; by Dr. John Innes, Fellow of the College of Physicians, and Professor of Medicine in the University of Edinburgh." *Medical Essays and Observations* 1 (1752): 227–32.

"Intelligence: Revue Médicale Historique et Philosophique; Par MM. V. Bally, Bellanger, F. Bérard, Bestieu, Bousquet, Delpeon, Desportes, Double, Dunal, Esquirol, Gasc, Girandy, Jadioux, Laurent, Nicod. Prunelle, Rouzet. Ire Année (1820)—Ire Livraison. Janvier." *New England Journal of Medicine and Surgery* 10, no. 3 (1821): 311–15.

Jackson, A. C. "Recovery from Rabies." *New England Journal of Medicine* 352, no. 24 (June 16, 2005): 2549–50.

Jackson, J. "On Croup." *New England Journal of Medicine and Surgery* 1 (October 1, 1812): 383–84.

Jenner, Edward, Edward Pearce, and William Skelton. *An Inquiry into the Causes and Effects of the Variolae Vaccinae: A Disease Discovered in Some of the Western Counties of England, Particularly Gloucestershire, and Known by the Name of the Cow Pox.* London: Printed, for the author, by Sampson Low, no. 7, Berwick Street, Soho: and sold by Law, Ave-Maria Lane; and Murray and Highley, Fleet Street, 1798.

Jennings, Samuel K. "An Account of the Effects of Labor in the Cure of Pulmonary Consumption in a Letter from the Rev. Samuel K. Jennings, of Bedford County, Virginia, to Dr. Benjamin Rush." *The Philadelphia Medical Museum* 1, no. 2 (1805): 194–97.

Jewett, Nathaniel G. *The Portland Directory and Register.* Portland: Todd and Smith, 1823.

Johnson, Alfred. "Hon. James Phinney Baxter, A.M., Litt.D." *The New England Historical and Genealogical Register* 75 (July 1921): 163–74.

Johnston, Ian. *Galen on Diseases and Symptoms.* Cambridge, New York: Cambridge University Press, 2006.

Jones, Calvin. *A Treatise on the Scarlatina Anginosa: Or What Is Vulgarly Called the Scarlet Fever, or Canker-Rash. Replete with Every Thing Necessary to the Pathology and Practice, Deduced from Actual Experience and Observation.* Catskill, NY: M. Crosswell & Co, 1794.

Jones, D. S., J. A. Greene, J. Duffin, and J. Harley Warner. "Making the Case for History in Medical Education." *Journal of the History of Medicine and Allied Sciences* (November 13, 2014): 623–52.

Jordan, William B. *A History of Cape Elizabeth, Maine.* Portland, ME: House of Falmouth, Inc., 1955.

Judd, Richard William, Edwin A. Churchill, and Joel W. Eastman. *Maine: The Pine Tree State from Prehistory to the Present.* 1st ed. Orono: University of Maine Press, 1995.

Jütte, Robert, and Institut für Geschichte der Medizin Robert Bosch Stiftung. *Medical Pluralism: Past, Present, Future.* Stuttgart: Franz Steiner Verlag, 2013.

Kahn, R. J., and P. G. Kahn. "The Medical Repository—the First U. S. Medical Journal (1797–1824)." *New England Journal of Medicine* 337 (1997): 1926–30.

Kahn, Richard. "Barker, Jeremiah (1752–1835), Physician." In *American National Biography*, edited by John A. Garraty. Mark C. Carnes, 158–59. Oxford, UK: Oxford University Press for the American Council of Learned Societies, 1999.

Kaplan, Catherine O'Donnell. *Men of Letters in the Early Republic Cultivating Forums of Citizenship*. Chapel Hill, NC: Published for the Omohundro Institute of Early American History and Culture, Williamsburg, Virginia, by the University of North Carolina Press, 2008.

Karenberg, A. "Retrospective Diagnosis: Use and Abuse in Medical Historiography." *Prague Medical Report* 110, no. 2 (2009): 140–5.

Kassell, Lauren. "Casebooks in Early Modern England: Medicine, Astrology, and Written Records." *Bulletin of the History of Medicine* 88, no. 4 (2014): 595–625.

Kassirer, J. P. "Our Stubborn Quest for Diagnostic Certainty. A Cause of Excessive Testing." *New England Journal of Medicine* 320, no. 22 (June 1, 1989): 1489–91.

Kaufman, Martin, Stuart Galishoff, and Todd Lee Savitt. *Dictionary of American Medical Biography*. 2 vols. Westport, CT: Greenwood Press, 1984.

Kelly, Howard A., and Walter L. Burrage. *American Medical Biographies*. Baltimore: The Norman, Remington Company, 1920.

Kielbowicz, Richard B. "Mere Merchandise or Vessels of Culture? Books in the Mail, 1792–1942." *Papers of the Bibliographical Society of America* 82, no. 2 (June 1988): 169–200.

King, Lester S. *Medical Thinking: A Historical Preface*. Princeton, NJ: Princeton University Press, 1982.

———. *The Medical World of the Eighteenth Century*. Huntington, NY: Robert E. Krieger Publishing Co. Inc. (reprint 1971), 1958.

———. *The Philosophy of Medicine: The Early Eighteenth Century*. Cambridge, MA: Harvard University Press, 1978.

———. *The Road to Medical Enlightenment, 1650–1695*. History of Science Library (Cambridge). London: MacDonald, 1970.

———. *Transformations in American Medicine: From Benjamin Rush to William Osler*. Baltimore: Johns Hopkins University Press, 1991.

Kiple, Kenneth F. *The Cambridge World History of Human Disease*. Cambridge; New York: Cambridge University Press, 1993.

Knight, Thomas Andrew, Esq. F.R.S. "An Account of a New Mode of Preserving an Equable and Salutary Temperature of the Air of Rooms for Consumptive Patients." *The London Medical and Physical Journal* 46 (1821): 115–16.

Kuhn, Thomas S. *The Structure of Scientific Revolutions*. 3rd ed. Chicago: The University of Chicago Press, 1996.

Kuntz, Andrew. "The Fiddler's Companion: A Descriptive Index of North American and British Isles Music for the Folk Violin and Other Instruments." http://www.ibiblio.org/fiddlers/BLACK.htm#BLACK_JOKE_[1].

Kunze, H. C. "Experiments Proving the Acid Quality of the Pus, or Matter Formed on the Surface of Veneral and Cancerous Ulcers." *Medical Repository* 4, no. 3 (1800–1801): 297–98.

La Terriere, Pierre de Sales. *A Dissertation on the Puerperal Fever*. Boston: Samuel Hall, 1789.

Lach, Edward L. "Smith, Samuel Stanhope (1751–1819), Clergyman and College President." Oxford, UK: Oxford University Press, 2000.

Laennec, R. T. H. *De L'auscultation Médiate, Ou, Traité Du Diagnostic Des Maladies Des Poumons et Du Coeur: Fondé Principalement Sur Ce Nouveau Moyen D'exploration*. Paris: Chez J.-A. Brosson et J.-S. Chaudé, Libraires, 1819.

Lavoisier, Antoine. *Elements of Chemistry in a New Systematic Order, Containing All the Modern Discoveries.* Translated by Robert Kerr. New York: Dover, 1965. Edinburgh: William Creech, 1790.

———. *Traité Élémentaire De Chimie.* Paris: Gaspard-Joseph Cuchet, 1789.

Lawrence, Charles. *History of the Philadelphia Almshouses and Hospitals from the Beginning of the Eighteenth to the Ending of the Nineteenth Centuries . . . : Showing the Mode of Distributing Public Relief through the Management of the Boards of Overseers of the Poor, Guardians of the Poor and the Directors of the Department of Charities and Correction.* Philadelphia: Charles Laurence, Superintendent, 1905.

Leake, John. *Practical Observations on the Child-Bed Fever.* London: J. Walter, 1772.

Leamon, James S. "Maine in the American Revolution, 1763–1787." Chap. 7 In *Maine: The Pine Tree State from Prehistory to the Present,* edited by Richard William Judd, Edwin A. Churchill, and Joel W. Eastman, 143–68. Orono: University of Maine Press, 1995.

———. *Revolution Downeast: The War for American Independence in Maine.* Amherst: University of Massachusetts Press, 1993.

Leigh, Julian M. "Early Treatment with Oxygen: The Pneumatic Institute and Panaceal Literature of the Nineteenth Century." *Anesthesia* 29, no. 2 (1974): 194–208.

Leong, E., and A. Rankin. "Testing Drugs and Trying Cures: Experiment and Medicine in Medieval and Early Modern Europe." *Bulletin of the History of Medicine* 91, no. 2 (2017): 157–82.

Lepore, Jill. *The Name of War: King Philip's War and the Origins of American Identity.* 1st ed. New York: Knopf, 1998.

Lind, James. *Essay on Diseases Incidental to Europeans in Hot Climates with the Method of Preventing Their Fatal Consequences.* 5th ed. London: J. Murray, 1792.

———. *A Treatise on the Putrid and Remitting Marsh Fever, Which Raged at Bengal.* C. Elliot: Edinburgh, 1776.

Lindeboom, Gerrit Arie. *Herman Boerhaave: The Man and His Work.* London: Methuen, 1968.

———. "Medical Education in the Netherlands 1575–1750." In *The History of Medical Education: An International Symposium Held February 5–9, 1968,* edited by C. D. O'Malley, 201–16. Los Angeles: University of California Press, 1970.

Loison, L. "Forms of Presentism in the History of Science. Rethinking the Project of Historical Epistemology." *Studies in History and Philosophy of Science* Part A 60 (December 2016): 29–37.

Loudon, Irvine. *The Tragedy of Childbed Fever.* Oxford ; New York: Oxford University Press, 2000.

Louis, P. C. A. "Memoir on the Proper Method of Examining a Patient, and of Arriving at Facts of a General Nature." Translated by Henry I. Bowditch. In *Dunglison's American Medical Library: Medical and Surgical Monographs,* edited by Robley Dunglison and G. Andral, 149–87. Philadelphia: Waldie, 1838.

———. *Recherches Anatomico-Pathologiques Sur La Phthisie.* Paris: Gabon, 1825.

———. *Researches on the Effects of Bloodletting in Some Inflammatory Diseases, and on the Influence of Tartarized Antimony and Vesication in Pneumonitis with Preface and Appendix by James Jackson, Md.* Translated by C. G. Putnam. Recherches Sur Les Effets De La Saignée Dans Quelques Maladies Inflammatoires. English. Boston: Hilliard, Gray & Company, 1836.

Louis, P. C. A., Henry I. Bowditch, and Charles Cowan. *Pathological Researches on Phthisis*. Boston: Hilliard, Gray, 1836.

Louis, P. C. A., and Peter Martin. *An Essay on Clinical Instruction*. London: published by S. Highley, 32, Fleet Street, 1834.

Lovejoy, M. K., E. G. Shettleworth, and W. D. Barry. *This Was Stroudwater: 1727–1860*. National Society of Colonial Dames of America in the State of Maine, 1985.

Ludmerer, Kenneth M. *Learning to Heal: The Development of American Medical Education*. New York: Basic Books, 1985.

Lyman, Eliphalet. "Case of Recovery from Apparent Consumption." *The Medical and Agricultural Register, for the Years 1806 and 1807*, Boston: Manning and Loring 1807, 196–97.

Mackowiak, Philip A. "History of Clinical Thermometry." In *Fever: Basic Mechanisms and Management*, edited by Philip A. Mackowiak, xvii, 506. Philadelphia: Lippincott-Raven Publishers, 1997.

Mann, James. *A Dissertation upon the Cholera Infantum; to Which Are Added, Rules and Regulations, as Preventive Means of the Autumnal Diseases of Children; Which Gained the Boylstonian Prize for the Year 1803*. Boston: Young & Minns, 1804.

———. *Medical Sketches of the Campaigns of 1812, 13, 14. To Which Are Added, Surgical Cases; Observations on Medical Hospitals; and Flying Hospitals Attached to a Moving Army. Also, an Appendix, Compromising a Dissertation on Dysentery*. Dedham , MA: H. Mann and Co., 1816.

Massachusetts, and Carroll Davidson Wright. *Comparative Wages, Prices, and Cost of Living: (from the Sixteenth Annual Report of the Massachusetts Bureau of Statistics of Labor, for 1885)*. Boston: Wright & Potter Printing Co., 1889.

"Massachusetts Medical Society Report of Annual Meeting of the Society, Holden, June 6th, 1821." *New England Journal of Medicine and Surgery* 10, no. 3 (1821): 316–17.

Mather, Cotton, and Society American Antiquarian. *The Angel of Bethesda*. Barre, MA: American Antiquarian Society and Barre Publishers, 1972.

Matthew, H. C. G., and Brian Harrison. *Oxford Dictionary of National Biography: In Association with the British Academy: From the Earliest Times to the Year 2000*. New ed. Oxford: Oxford University Press, 2004.

Maulitz, Russel C. "Pathology." In *The Education of American Physicians: Historical Essays*, edited by Ronald L. Numbers, 122–42. Berkeley: University of California Press, 1980.

Mauskopf, Seymour. "Richard Kirwan's Phlogiston Theory: Its Success and Fate." *Ambix* 49, Part 3 (November 2002): 185–205.

Mc Lellan, Hugh D. *History of Gorham, Maine*. Portland: Smith and Sale, 1903.

McCormick, Richard P. *Rutgers: A Bicentennial History*. New Brunswick: Rutgers University Press, 1966.

McKeown, Thomas. *The Modern Rise of Population*. New York: Academic Press, 1976.

McKie, Douglas. *Antoine Lavoisier: Scientist, Economist, Social Reformer*. London: Constable, 1952.

———. "Introduction to the Dover Edition." In *Elements of Chemistry by Antoine Lavoisier; Translated by Robert Kerr*, v–xxxi. New York: Dover Publications, 1965.

McKusick, Victor A. *Cardiovascular Sound in Health and Disease*. Baltimore: Williams & Wilkins, 1958.

Mead, Richard. *A Mechanical Account of Poisons*. Dublin: S. Powell, 1736.

———. *The Medical Works of Richard Mead*. Dublin: Printed for Thomas Ewing, 1767.

"Medical and Philosophical News. Domestic. Progress of Pneumatic Medicine." *Medical Repository* 4, no. 2 (1800–1801): 183–89.

Medicine, Institute of. *Leadership Commitments to Improve Value in Healthcare: Finding Common Ground: Workshop Summary*. The National Academies Collection: Reports Funded by National Institutes of Health. Washington, DC, 2009.

Mendelsohn, J. Andrew, and Annemarie Kinzelbach. "Common Knowledge: Bodies, Evidence, and Expertise in Early Modern Germany." *Isis* 108, no. 2 (2017): 259–79.

Mettler, Cecilia Charlotte, and Fred A. Mettler. *History of Medicine; a Correlative Text, Arranged According to Subjects*. Philadelphia: Blakiston, 1947.

Micklethwait, David. *Noah Webster and the American Dictionary*. Jefferson, NC: McFarland & Company, Inc., 2000.

Miller, Genevieve. *The Adoption of Inoculation for Smallpox in England and France*. Philadelphia: University of Pennsylvania Press, 1957.

Mitchill, Samuel. "Affinities of Septic Fluids to Other Bodies. Affinities and Relations of Septic (Nitric) or Pestilential Fluids to Other Bodies. In a Letter from Dr. Mitchill, F.R.S.E. Professor of Chemistry, Agriculture and Medicine, in the College of New-York, to Sir John Sinclair, Bart. M.P. President of the Board of Agriculture, Etc. Dated New-York, the 28th of November, 1796. Intended as an Additional Article Proposed Report of the British Board of Agriculture on the Subject of Manures." *The New York Magazine, or Literary Repository*, January 1797: 9–17.

———. "An Attempt to Accommodate the Dispute among the Chemists Concerning Phlogiston. In a Letter from Dr. Mitchill to Dr. Priestley, Dated 14th Nov. 1797." *Medical Repository* 1, no. 4 (1798): 504–11.

———. "Concerning the Use of Alkaline Remedies in Fevers, and the Analogy between Septic Acid and Other Poisons; in a Letter to Thomas Percival M. D. &C of Manchester, from Dr. Mitchill, Dated New-York, January 17, 1797." *The New York Magazine, or Literary Repository*, April 1797: 180–90.

———. "Operations of Septon on Plants and Animals for the 'New-York Magazine.' On Septon (Azote) and Its Compounds, as the Operate on Plants as Food, and Animals as Poison: Intended as a Supplement to Mr. Kirwin's 'Pamphlet on Manures.' In a Letter to the Rev. Dr. Henry Muhlenberg, of Lancaster, Pennsylvania from Mr. Mitchill, on New-York, Dated October 24, 1796." *The New York Magazine, or Literary Repository*, November 1796: 569–75.

———. "Outlines of Medical Geography." *Medical Repository* 2, no. 1 (1798): 39–47.

———. *The Present State of Medical Learning in the City of New York*. New York: T. and J. Swords, 1797.

———. "Remarks on Manures: Wherein, by an Inquiry into the Nature of Septon, (Azote) and Its Relations to Other Bodies, It Will Be Seen How Nearly Physic and Farming Are A'lied to Each Other. Intended as a Sequel to Judge Peter's Agricultural Inquiries on Plaister of Paris." *Medical (The) Repository* 1(3rd ed., 1804), no. 1 (1797): 32–55.

Mitchill, Samuel L. "Article IX. Arrangement of Facts Concerning Ulcers, Sores and Tetters; Showing How Agreeably These and Similar Affections of the Skin Are Healed, in Many Cases, by Alkaline Applications: In a Letter to Thomas Trotter, M.D. Physician to the British Fleet, Etc Dated New-York, September 20, 1800." *Medical Repository* 4, no. 2 (1801): 149–54.

———. "Concerning the Use of Alkaline Remedies in Fevers, and the Analogy between Septic Acid and Other Poisons; in a Letter to Thomas Percival M. D. &C

of Manchester, from Dr. Mitchill, Dated New-York, January 17, 1797." *Medical Repository* 1 (3rd ed.), no. 2 (1798): 253–78.

———. *Explanation of the Synopsis of Chemical Nomenclature and Arrangement: Containing Several Important Alterations of the Plan Originally Reported by French Academicians.* New York: T. and J. Swords, 1801.

———. "Further Facts Tending toward an Explanation of the True Operation of Alkalis and Lime upon Other Substances. In a Letter from Dr. Mitchill to Thomas Beddoes, M.D., September 15, 1797." *Medical Repository* 1, no. 2 (1797): 185–93.

———. *Nomenclature of the New Chemistry.* New-York: T. and J. Swords, 1794. microform.

———. *The Present State of Learning in the College of New York (Columbia).* New York: T. and J. Swords, 1794.

———. *Remarks on the Gaseous Oxyd of Azote or of Nitrogene, and on the Effects It Produces When Generated in the Stomach, Inhaled into the Lungs, and Applied to the Skin: Being an Attempt to Ascertain the True Nature of Contagion, and to Explain Thereupon the Phenomena of Fever. / by Samuel Latham Mitchell, M.D. F.R.S.E. Professor of Chemistry, Natural History and Agriculture in the College of New-York.* New York: T. and J. Swords, 1795.

Mohr, James C. *Licensed to Practice: The Supreme Court Defines the American Medical Profession.* Baltimore: Johns Hopkins University Press, 2013.

Monro, Donald. *An Essay on the Dropsy.* London: E. Wilson & T. Durham, 1755.

Moore, John. *Medical Sketches: In Two Parts.* London: A. Strahan and T. Cadell, 1786.

Moore, John, Caspar Wistar, John Wilson, Andrew Way, and Joseph Groff. "An Inaugural Dissertation on Digitalis Purpurea, or Fox-Glove: And Its Use in Some Diseases: Submitted to the Examination of the Rev. John Ewing, S.T.P. Provost; the Trustees & Medical Faculty, of the University of Pennsylvania, on the Thirty-First of May 1800, for the Degree of Doctor of Medicine." Philadelphia: University of Pennsylvania, 1800.

Moran, Bruce T. *Distilling Knowledge: Alchemy, Chemistry, and the Scientific Revolution.* Cambridge, MA: Harvard University Press, 2005.

Moro-Abadía, Oscar. "Thinking about 'Presentism' from a Historian's Perspective: Herbert Butterfield and Hélène Metzger." *History of Science* 47, no. 1 (March 1, 2009): 55–77.

Morton, Leslie T. *A Medical Bibliography (Garrison and Morton).* 4th ed. Aldershot, NH: Gower Publishing Company, 1983.

Morton, Thomas G., Frank Woodbury, and Pennsylvania Hospital. *The History of the Pennsylvania Hospital, 1751–1895.* Philadelphia: Times Printing House, 1895.

Mudge, John. *A Radical and Expeditious Cure for a Recent Catarrhous Cough: Preceded by Some Observations on Respiration, with Occasional and Practical Remarks on Some Other Diseases of the Lungs; to Which Is Added a Chapter on the Vis Vitae, So Far as It Is Concerned in Preserving and Reinstanting the Health of an Animal; Accompanied with Some Strictures on the Treatment of Compound Fractures.* Edited by Edmund Allen. Real Colegio de Cirugía de San Carlos, 1779.

Mukherjee, Siddhartha. *The Emperor of All Maladies: A Biography of Cancer.* 1st Scribner hardcover ed. New York: Scribner, 2010.

Murray, John F. "A Century of Tuberculosis." *American Journal of Respiratory and Critical Care Medicine* 169, no. 11 (2004): 1181–86.

Mutschler, Ben. "Illness in the 'Social Credit' and 'Money' Economies of Eighteenth-Century New England." In *Medicine and the Market in England and Its Colonies,*

C.1450–C.1850, edited by Mark S. R. Dr Jenner and Patrick Dr Wallis, 175–95. Basingstoke, UK: Palgrave Macmillan, 2007.

Nathan, L., and K. J. Leveno. "Group A Streptococcal Puerperal Sepsis: Historical Review and 1990s Resurgence." *Infectious Diseases Obstetrics and Gynecology* 1, no. 5 (1994): 252–55.

Newhall, Barker. *The Barker Family of Plymouth Colony and County.* Cleveland: F.W. Roberts, 1900.

Noyes, Nathan. "Bill of Mortality for Newburyport, Massachusetts, for A.D. 1809, the Facts Collected and Arranged by Nathan Noyes, M.B." *Newburyport Herald*, January 16, 1810.

Numbers, Ronald L. "Do-It-Yourself the Sectarian Way." In *Medicine without Doctors: Home Health Care in American History*, edited by Judith Walzer Leavitt, Ronald L. Numbers, and Guenter B. Risse, 49–72. New York: Science History Publications, 1977.

———. *The Education of American Physicians: Historical Essays.* Berkeley: University of California Press, 1980.

Nutton, V. "Medicine in the Greek World, 800–50 BC." In *The Western Medical Tradition: 800 BC–1800 AD*, edited by Lawrence I. Conrad and Wellcome Institute for the History of Medicine, xiv. Cambridge, UK; New York: Cambridge University Press, 1995.

"Obituary." [In English]. *The Medical Repository of Original Essays and Intelligence, Relative to Physic, Surgery, Chemistry, and Natural History* 2 (November 1804–January 1805): 340.

Olef, Isadore. "Chlorosis." *New England Journal of Medicine* 225, no. 10 (1941): 258–65.

Opinel, Annick, Ulrich Tröhler, Christian Gluud, Gabriel Gachelin, George Davey Smith, Scott Harris Podolsky, and Iain Chalmers. "Commentary: The Evolution of Methods to Assess the Effects of Treatments, Illustrated by the Development of Treatments for Diphtheria, 1825–1918." *International Journal of Epidemiology* 42, no. 3 (2013): 662–76.

Outwin, Charles P. M. "Thriving and Elegant Town: Eighteenth-Century Portland as a Commercial Center." Chap. 2 In *Creating Portland: History and Place in Northern New England*, edited by Joseph A. Conforti, 20–43. Hanover, NH: University Press of New England, 2005.

———. "Thriving and Elegant, Flourishing and Populous: Falmouth in Casco Bay, 1760–1775." University of Maine, unpublished PhD dissertation, 2009.

Oxford English Dictionary. 2nd ed. Online. Oxford University Press.

Packard, Francis R. *Some Account of the Pennsylvania Hospital from Its First Rise to the Beginning of the Year 1938.* Philadelphia: Engle Press, 1938.

Packard, R. M. "The Fielding H. Garrison Lecture: 'Break-Bone' Fever in Philadelphia, 1780: Reflections on the History of Disease." *Bulletin of the History of Medicine* 90, no. 2 (2016): 193–221.

Parkman, George. *Management of Lunatics: With Illustrations of Insanity.* Boston: John Eliot, 1817.

———. *Proposals for Establishing a Retreat for the Insane.* Boston: Printed by J. Eliot, 1814.

———. "Remarks on Insanity." *New England Journal of Medicine and Surgery* 7, no. 1 (1818): 117–30.

Partington, J. R. *A History of Chemistry.* 3 vols. London: MacMillan & Co. LTD, 1964.

Pascalis, Felix. "Observations on the Ulcerated Tonsils of Children." *Medical Repository* 1, 3rd hexade, no. 1 (1809): 19–25.

Patterson, K. David. "Yellow Fever Epidemics and Mortality in the United States, 1693–1905." *Social Science and Medicine* 34, no. 8 (1992): 855–65.

Peisse, J. L. H. *Sketches of the Character and Writing of Eminent Living Surgeons and Physicians of Paris.* Translated by Elijah Bartlett. Boston: Carter, Hendee and Babcock, 1831.

Peitzman, Steven J. *Dropsy, Dialysis, Transplant: A Short History of Failing Kidneys.* Johns Hopkins Biographies of Disease. Baltimore: Johns Hopkins University Press, 2007.

Pender, Stephen. "Examples and Experience: On the Uncertainty of Medicine." *British Journal for the History of Science* 39, no. 1 (2006): 1–28.

Percival, Thomas. *Essays Medical and Experimental.* 4th ed. Warrington, 1788.

———. *Experiments on the Peruvian Bark.* London: L. Davis & C. Reymers, 1768.

Percival, Thomas, and Joseph Meredith Toner Collection (Library of Congress). *Extracts from the Medical Ethics of Dr. Percival.* Philadelphia: Clark & Raser, printers, 1823.

Pernick, Martin S. "Politics, Parties, and Pestilence: Epidemic Yellow Fever in Philadelphia and the Rise of the First Party System." In *A Melancholy Scene of Devastation: The Public Response to the 1793 Philadelphia Yellow Fever Epidemic*, edited by J. Worth Estes and Billy G. Smith, 119–46. Canton, MA: Science History Publications/USA, 1997.

Pescosolido, B. A., and J. K. Martin. "Cultural Authority and the Sovereignty of American Medicine: The Role of Networks, Class, and Community." *Journal of Health Politics, Policy and Law* 29, no. 4–5 (August–October 2004): 735–56; discussion 1005–19.

Peterson, M. C., J. H. Holbrook, D. Von Hales, N. L. Smith, and L. V. Staker. "Contributions of the History, Physical Examination, and Laboratory Investigation in Making Medical Diagnoses." *Western Journal of Medicine* 156, no. 2 (February 1992): 163–65.

Physick, Philip Syng. "Case of Hydrophobia: Communicated by Dr. Philip Syng Physick of Philadelphia to Dr. Miller." *Medical Repository and Review of American Publications* 5, no. 1 (1802): 1–5.

Pinel, Philippe. *Traité Médico-Philosophique Sur L'aliénation Mentale: Ou La Manie.* Paris: Chez Richard, Caille et Ravier, 1801.

Pinel, Philippe, and David Daniel Davis. *A Treatise on Insanity, in Which Are Contained the Principles of a New and More Practical Nosology of Maniacal Disorders Than Has yet Been Offered to the Public: Exemplified by Numerous and Accurate Historical Relations of Cases from the Author's Public and Private Practice: With Plates Illustrative of the Craniology of Maniacs and Ideots.* Sheffield: printed by W. Todd, for Messrs. Cadell and Davies, Strand, London, 1806.

Portal, Antoine, Gaspare Federigo, and Georg Friedrich Mühry. *Observations Sur La Nature et Le Traitement De La Phthisie Pulmonaire. Ed. rev. et augm. par l'auteur, avec des observations et des remarques par Murhy sic . . . qui a traduit cet ouvrage en allemand, et avec celles de Gaspard Fédérigo . . . qui l'a traduit en italien.* 2 vols. Paris: Collin, 1809.

Porter, Roy. "The Eighteenth Century." In *The Western Medical Tradition: 800 B.C.– 1800 A.D*, edited by Lawrence I. Conrad and Wellcome Institute for the History of Medicine, 371–475. Cambridge; New York: Cambridge University Press, 1995.

———. *The Greatest Benefit to Mankind: A Medical History of Humanity.* New York: W. W. Norton & Company, 1997.

Porter, Theodore M. *The Rise of Statistical Thinking 1820–1900*. Princeton: Princeton University Press, 1986.

Powell, J. H. *Bring Out Your Dead*. Reprint ed. Philadelphia: University of Pennsylvania Press, 1993.

———. *Bring Out Your Dead: The Great Plague of Yellow Fever in Philadelphia in 1793*. Studies in Health, Illness, and Caregiving. Philadelphia: University of Pennsylvania Press, 1993.

Prichard, J. C. "Cases of Typhus Fever, with Observations on the Nature and Treatment of the Disease." *Edinburgh Medical and Surgical Journal* 13 (1817): 413–27.

Priestley, Joseph. "A Letter to Dr. Mitchill, in Reply to the Preceding [Mitchill's Letter Attempting to Accomodate the Dispute on Phogiston], by Joseph Priestley." *Medical (The) Repository* 1, no. 4 (1798): 511–12.

Pringle, John. "A Continuation of the Experiments on Substances Resisting Putrefacton." *Philosophical Transactions (1683–1775)* 46 (1749–1750): 525–34.

———. "Further Experiments on Substances Resisting Putrefaction; with Experiments Upon the Means of Hastening and Promoting It." *Philosophical Transactions (1683–1775)* 46 (1749–50): 550–58.

———. "Some Experiments on Substances Resisting Putrefaction." *Philosophical Transactions (1683–1775)* 46 (1749–50): 480–88.

"Proposal for Publishing a History of Disease of the District of Maine with Endorsement by J. G. Coffin." *Eastern Argus*, January 18, 1820, 3 col 2.

"Proposal for Publishing by Subscription the History of Epidemic and Pestilential Diseases by Noah Webster, Ll.D." *Connecticut Herald*, July 10, 1832, 4.

"Puerperal Fever." *The New England Journal of Medicine, Surgery and Collateral Branches of Science* 4, no. 4 (1815): 397–98.

Ragland, Evan R. "Experimental Clinical Medicine and Drug Action in Mid-Seventeenth-Century Leiden." *Bulletin of the History of Medicine* 91, no. 2 (2017): 331–61.

Ramsay, David. *A Review of the Improvements, Progress and State of Medicine in the XVIII Century: Read on the First Day of the XIXth Century, before the Medical Society of South-Carolina, and in Pursuance of Their Vote, and Published at Their Request*. Charleston: W. P. Young, 1801.

Rand, Isaac. *Observations on Phthisis Pulmonalis, and the Use of the Digitalis Purpurea in the Treatment of That Disease: With Practical Remarks on the Use of the Tepid Bath. Read at the Request of the Massachusetts Medical Society, June 6, 1804*. Boston: Printed at the Repertory office, 1804.

Raoult, D., T. Woodward, and J. S. Dumler. "The History of Epidemic Typhus." *Infectious Disease Clinics of North America* 18, no. 1 (March 2004): 127–40.

Recamier, Joseph-Claude-Anthelme. "New Treatment of Croup." *London Medical and Physical Journal* 1 (July to December 1823): 258.

Recamier, Professor. "New Treatment of Croup." *New England Journal of Medicine and Surgery* 13 (January 1, 1824): 103.

Reece, Richard. "Croup . . . Dr. R. Reddelin of Wismar." *The Monthly Gazette of Health* 7 (4th ed.) (1822): 274.

Rees, Abraham. *The Cyclopædia, or, Universal Dictionary of Arts, Sciences, and Literature*. Philadelphia: Published by Samuel F. Bradford and Murray, Fairman and Co., 1805.

Reid, John. *A Treatise on the Origin, Progress, Prevention, and Treatment, of Consumption*. London: Phillips, 1806.

Reid, Thomas. *An Essay on the Nature and Cure of the Phthisis Pulmonalis. By T. Reid, M.D.* London: printed for T. Cadell, 1782.

Reiser, S. J. "The Clinical Record in Medicine. Part 1: Learning from Cases." *Annals of Internal Medicine* 114, no. 10 (May 15, 1991): 902–907.

Reiser, Stanley Joel. *Medicine and the Reign of Technology.* Cambridge; New York: Cambridge University Press, 1978.

"Remarks on the Treatmant of Consumption by Joseph Comstock." *Rhode-Island American, published as Rhode-Island American, and General Advertiser,* January 24, 1817.

"Reports of Cases in Private Practice." *Boston Medical and Surgical Journal* 1 (August 9, 1828): 426–29.

"Review of Saltonstall's 'Dissertation on Septon, Azote, or Nitrogene.'" *The New-York Magazine, of Literary Repository,* March 1797: 143–46.

"Review, Article III: Laennec, R. T. H. De L'auscultation Médiate, Volume One. 1819." *New England Journal of Medicine and Surgery* 10, no. 2 (1821): 132–56.

"Review, Article VIII [Concluded from Page 156.] De L'auscultation Mediate Ou Traité Du Diagnostic Des Maladies Des Poumons et Du Coeur, Fondé Principalement Sur Ce Nouveau Moyen D'exploration. Par R. T. H. Laennec, D. M. P. Médecin De L'hôpital Necker, Médecin Honoraire Des Dispensaires, Membre De La Société De La Faculté De Médecine De Paris, et De Plusieurs Autres Sociétés Nationales et Étrangères. Tome Second. A Paris, Ches J. A. Brosson et S. J. S. Chaudé, Libraires. 1819." *New England Journal of Medicine and Surgery* 10, no. 3 (1821): 265–93.

"Review. Sketches of Epidemic Diseases in the State of Vermont, from Its First Settlement to the Year 1815; with a Consideration of Their Causes, Phenomena, and Treatment. To Which Is Added, Remarks on Pulmonary Consumption. By Joseph A. Gallup, M.D. 1 Vol. 8vo. Boston, T. B. Wait & Sons, 1815." *New England Journal of Medicine and Surgery* 4 (1815): 357–72.

Richerand, M. Le Chevalier. *Account of a Resection of the Ribs and Pleura Read before the Royal Academy of Sciences of the Institute of France, April 27, 1818 . . . Translated by Thomas Wilson.* Philadelphia: Thomas Town, 1818.

———. "Richerand's Operation of Cutting into the Pleura." *The London Medical Repository, Monthly Journal, and Review* 10 (July to December, 1818): 228–36.

Riesman, David. *Thomas Sydenham, Clinician.* New York: P. B. Hoeber, Inc., 1926.

Riley, Henry T. *Dictionary of Latin Quotations, Proverbs, Maxims, and Mottos, Classical and Mediaeval: Including Law Terms and Phrases: With a Selection of Greek Quotations.* H. G. Bohn: London,1859.

Riley, James C. *The Eighteenth-Century Campaign to Avoid Disease.* New York: St. Martin's Press, 1987.

Risse, G. B. "The Quest for Certainty in Medicine: John Brown's System of Medicine in France." *Bulletin of the History of Medicine* 45, no. 1 (January–February 1971): 1–12.

Risse, G. B., and J. H. Warner. "Reconstructing Clinical Activities: Patient Records in Medical History." *Social History of Medicine* 5, no. 2 (August 1992): 183–205.

Risse, Guenter B. *Hospital Life in Enlightenment Scotland: Care and Teaching at the Royal Infirmary of Edinburgh.* Cambridge: Cambridge University Press, 1986.

———. "Introduction." In *Medicine without Doctors: Home Health Care in American History,* edited by Judith Walzer Leavitt, Ronald L. Numbers and Guenter B. Risse, 1–8. New York: Science History Publications, 1977.

———. "The Renaissance of Bloodletting: A Chapter in Modern Therapeutics." *Journal of the History of Medicine and Allied Sciences* 34, no. 1 (1979): 3–22.

Riznik, B. "The Professional Lives of Early Nineteenth-Century New England Doctors." *Journal of the History of Medicine and Allied Sciences* 19 (1964): 1.

Roberts, Lissa. "Eudiometer." In *Instruments of Science: An Historical Encyclopedia*, edited by Robert Bud and Deborah Jean Warner, 232–34. New York: The Science Museum, London and the National Museum of American History, Smithsonian Institution in assoc. with Garland Publishing, Inc., 1998.

Robinson, Victor. "The Early Medical Journals of America Founded During the Quarter Century 1797–1822." *Medical Life* 36, no. 11 (1929): 533–88.

Rolde, Neil. *The Baxters of Maine*. Gardiner, ME: Tilsbury House, 1997.

Rosen, G. "The Place of History in Medical Education." *Bulletin of the History of Medicine* 22 (September1948): 594–629.

Rosen, George. *A History of Public Health*. Baltimore: The Johns Hopkins University Press, 1958 (1993 ed.).

———. "Noah Webster—Historical Epidemiologist." *Journal of the History of Medicine and Allied Sciences* 65 (1965): 97–114.

Rosenberg, Charles E. *The Cholera Years: The United States in 1832. 1849, and 1866*. reprint, 1987 ed. Chicago: The University of Chicago Press, 1962.

———. *Explaining Epidemics and Other Studies in the History of Medicine*. New York: Cambridge University Press, 1992.

———. *No Other Gods: On Science and American Social Thought*. Baltimore: The Johns Hopkins University Press, 1997.

———. "The Therapeutic Revolution: Medicine, Meaning, and Social Change in Nineteenth-Century America." *Perspectives in Biology and Medicine* 20, no. 4 (1977): 485–506.

Rosenberg, Charles E., Janet Lynne Golden, and Francis Clark Wood Institute for the History of Medicine. *Framing Disease: Studies in Cultural History*. Health and Medicine in American Society. New Brunswick, NJ: Rutgers University Press, 1997.

Rothman, David J., Steven Marcus, and Stephanie A. Kiceluk. *Medicine and Western Civilization*. New Brunswick, NJ: Rutgers University Press, 1995.

Rothman, Sheila M. *Living in the Shadow of Death: Tuberculosis and the Social Experience of Illness in American History*. New York: BasicBooks, 1994.

Rothstein, William G. *American Medical Schools and the Practice of Medicine: A History*. New York: Oxford University Press, 1987.

———. *American Physicians in the Nineteenth Century; from Sects to Science*. Baltimore: Johns Hopkins University Press, 1972.

Rowe, William Hutchinson. *Ancient North Yarmouth and Yarmouth, Maine, 1636–1936*. Southworth-Anthoensen Press: Yarmouth, ME, 1937.

Rush, Benjamin. "An Account of the Examination of the Body of a Little Boy Who Died of Hydrophobia; Intended to Show the Probable Success of Dr. Physic's Proposal for Preventing Death by Making an Artificial Opening into the Windpipe." *Medical Repository* 1, 2nd hexade, no. 2 (August, September, October, 1803 1804): 105–09.

———. "An Account of the Salutary Effects of a Salivation, and Tonic Remedies, in Pulmonary Consumption: In Three Letters to Dr. Edward Miller, by Benjamin Rush, M.D., Professor of the Institutes of Medicine and of Clinical Practice in the University of Pennsylvania." *Medical Repository* 5 (1802): 5–10.

———. "An Account of the Successful Use of Opium, Cordial Drinks, and Animal Food, in Two Cases of Pulmonary Consumption." *Philadelphia Medical Museum* 1 (1805): 318–22.

———. *Letters*. Edited by L. H. Butterfield. 2 vols. Princeton: Princeton University Press, 1951.

————. *Medical Inquiries and Observations.* 2nd ed. 4 vols. Philadelphia: J. Conrad & Co., 1805.

————. *Medical Inquiries and Observations.* 4th ed. 4 vols. Philadelphia: Johnson & Warner, 1815.

————. *Medical Inquiries and Observations, Upon the Diseases of the Mind.* Philadelphia: Kimber & Richardson, no. 237, Market street. Merritt, printer, no. 9, Watkin's Alley, 1812.

Rutherford, Phillip R. *The Dictionary of Maine Place-Names.* Freeport, ME: Bond, Wheelwright Co, 1971.

Saltonstall, Winthrop, and Samuel L. Mitchill. *An Inaugural Dissertation on the Chemical and Medical History of Septon, Azote, or Nitrogene: And Its Combinations with the Matter of Heat and the Principle of Acidity.* New-York: T. and J. Swords, 1796.

Santayana, George. *Scepticism and Animal Faith; Introduction to a System of Philosophy.* New York: C. Scribner's Sons, 1929.

Schaffer, Simon. "Measuring Virtue: Eudiometry, Enlightenment and Pneumatic Medicine." In *The Medical Enlightenment of the Eighteenth Century*, edited by Andrew Cunningham and Roger French. New York: Cambridge University Press, 1990.

Schenck von Grafenberg, Johannes. *Paratereseon, Sive Observationum Medicarum, Rararum, Novarum, Admirabilium, &Amp; Monstrosarum, Volumen, Tomis Septem De Toto Homine Institutum. In Quo, Quae Medici . . . Abdita, Vulgo Incognita, Gravia, Periculosaáque, Circa Humani Corporis Anatomen & Fabricam, Ejusdemáue Morborum Causas, Signa, Eventus, & Curationes Accidere Comperêrunt, Exemplis Ut Plurimum & Historiis Proposita Exhibentur.* Edited by Johann Georg Schenck. Francofurti: Hoffmann, 1609.

Sears, Donald A. "Folk Poetry in Longfellow's Boyhood." *The New England Quarterly* 45, no. 1 (1972): 96–105.

Severinghaus, J. W. "Fire-Air and Dephlogistication. Revisionisms of Oxygen's Discovery." *Advances in Experimental Medicine and Biology* 543 (2003): 7–19.

Seybert, Adam. *An Inaugural Dissertation: Being an Attempt to Disprove the Doctrine of the Putrefaction of the Blood of Living Animals . . . .* Philadelphia: T. Dobson, 1793.

Shapin, Steven. "Trusting George Cheyne: Scientific Expertise, Common Sense, and Moral Authority in Early Eighteenth-Century Dietetic Medicine." *Bulletin of the History of Medicine* 77 (2003): 263–97.

Shapin, Steven, and Arnold Thackray. "Prosopography as a Research Tool in History of Science: The British Scientific Community 1700–1900." *History of Science* 12 (1974): 1–28.

Shaw, W. C. "Folklore Surrounding Facial Deformity and the Origins of Facial Prejudice." *British Journal of Plastic Surgery* 34, no. 3 (July 1981): 237–46.

Sherrill, Hunting. "An Account of the Efficacy of Blood-Letting and Cathartics in the Cure of Palsey, with Observations on That Disease; Communicated by Dr. Hunting Sherill, of Clinton, Duchess County, (N.Y.) Formerly a Resident in the New-York Almshouse, to Edward Miller, Professor of the Practice of Physic in the University of New-York. Dated June 30th, 1810." *Medical Repository Comprehending Original Essays and Intelligence* 2, 3rd hexade, no. 1 (May, June, July, 1810): 35–42.

Shipton, Clifford. *Biographical Sketches of Those Who Attended Harvard College; Sibley's Harvard Graduates, Vol. 14: 1756–1760.* Boston: Massachusetts Historical Society, 1968.

Shipton, Clifford K. *Biographical Sketches of Those Who Attended Harvard College in the Classes 1726–30; Sibley's Harvard Graduates.* Vol. 8. Boston: Massachusetts Historical Society, 1951.

————. *Biographical Sketches of Those Who Attended Harvard College in the Classes 1751–1755; Sibley's Harvard Graduates*. Vol. 13. Boston: Massachusetts Historical Society, 1965.

Shortt, S. E. D. "Physicians, Science, and Status: Issues in the Professionalization of Anglo-American Medicine in the Nineteenth Century." *Medical History* 27, no. 1 (1983): 51–68.

Shryock, Richard Harrison. *Medical Licensing in America, 1650–1965*. Baltimore: Johns Hopkins Press, 1967.

Siegfried, Robert. "An Attempt in the United States to Resolve the Differences between the Oxygen and Phlogiston Theories." *Isis* 46, no. 4 (December 1955): 327–36.

————. "The Chemical Revolution in the History of Chemistry." *Osiris* 2nd Series, Vol. 4 (1988): 34–50.

Sigerist, Henry E. *A History of Medicine*. 2 vols. Vol. 1. New York: Oxford University Press, 1967. New York: Oxford University Press, 1951.

————. *A History of Medicine: Vol. 2: Early Greek, Hindu, and Persian Medicine*. New York: Oxford University Press, 1961.

Silbey, Joel H. "Ritchie, Thomas (1778–1854), Newspaper Editor and Democratic Party Activist." Oxford, UK: Oxford University Press, 2000.

Silver, Rollo G. *The American Printer, 1787–825*. Charlottesville: Published for the Bibliographical Society of the University of Virginia by the University Press of Virginia, 1967.

Skeel, Emily Ellsworth Ford. *A Bibliography of the Writings of Noah Webster*. Edited by Edwin H. Carpenter, Jr., New York: The New York Public Library, 1958.

Skinner, Henry Alan. *The Origin of Medical Terms*. 2nd ed. Baltimore: The Williams & Wilkins Company, 1961.

Smith, Anson. "Case of Hemoptysis; to Which Is Subjoined Some Sketches Respecting the Use of Digitalis in Haemorrhagic Affections." *Medical Repository* 2, 3rd hexade, no. 3 (1811): 223–26.

Smith, Christopher U. M. "Chapter 9: Understanding the Nervous System in the 18th Century." In *Handbook of Clinical Neurology*, edited by Michael J. Aminoff, François Boller, and Dick F. Swaab, 107–14. Amsterdam: Elsevier, 2009.

Smith, Dale C. "Medical Science, Medical Practice, and the Emerging Concept of Typhus in Mid-Eighteenth Century Britain." In *Theories of Fever from Antiquity to the Enlightenment*, edited by W. F. Bynum and V. Nutton, 121–34. London: Wellcome Institute for the History of Medicine; Medical History, Supplement No. 1, 1981.

Smith, E. H. "Article VI Case of Mania Successfully Treated by Mercury." *Medical Repository* 1, no. 2 (1797): 181–84.

Smith, Elihu Hubbard, Samuel L. Mitchill, and Edward Miller. "List of Subscribers." *Medical Repository* 2, no.1, 1798: unpaginated, "accompanies the present number."

Smith, Samuel S. "An Account of the Good Effects of Copious Blood-Letting in the Cure of an Hemorrhage from the Lungs; in a Letter from the Rev. Dr. Samuel S. Smith, Prefident of the College of New Jersey, to Dr. Benjamin Rush." *The Philadelphia Medical Museum, Conducted by John Redman Coxe, M.D. (1805–1810)*, February 1, 1806: 1.

Smith, Thomas Laurens. *History of the Town of Windham*. Portland ME: Hoyt & Fogg, 1873.

Society, Cumberland District Medical. *Bylaws of the System of Police of the Cumberland District Medical Society*. Cumberland District Medical Society, 18. Portland, Maine: Arthur Shirley, printer, 1832.

"Some Account of the Disease, Which Was Epidemic in Some Parts of New-York and New-England, in the Winter of 1812–13." *The New England Journal of Medicine, Surgery and Collateral Branches of Science* 2, no. 3 (1813): 241–52.

"Some Historical Account of the Progress of Medical Science during the Last Year." *New England Journal of Medicine and Surgery* 3, no. 1 (1814): 5–11.

Sonnedecker, Glenn. "The Founding Period of the U.S. Pharmacopeia: III. The First Edition." *Pharmacy in History* 36, no. 3 (1994): 103–22.

Spalding, James Alfred. "After Consulting Hours: Jeremiah Barker, M.D., Gorham and Falmouth, Maine, 1752–1835." *Bulletin of the American Academy of Medicine* 10 (1909): 242–65.

———. *Dr. Lyman Spalding.* Boston: W. M. Leonard, 1916.

———. *Jeremiah Barker, M.D., Gorham and Falmouth, Maine, 1752–1835.* Portland, ME: s.n., 1909.

———. *Maine Physicians of 1820; a Record of the Members of the Massachusetts Medical Society Practicing in the District of Maine at the Date of Separation.* Lewiston: Lewiston Print Shop, 1928.

———. *Spalding Collection 1487.* Maine Historical Society. Unpublished, 1846–1938.

Spalding, Lyman. *A New Nomenclature of Chemistry Proposed by De Morveau, Lavoisier, Bertholet and Fourcroy.* Hanover, NH: Moses Davis, 1799.

Spalding, Lyman (1775–1821) Papers, 1798–1912 (inclusive), 1798–*c.* 1820 (bulk). Spalding, Lyman, 1775–1821, Cases of supposed incipient phthisis pulmonalis, cured by sulphate of copper and ipecacuanha, A.MS.s.; 3 sides (9 pages), circa 1818. B MS c2 Box 2, Folder 10, Countway Library of Medicine; Harvard University. Accessed February 18, 2019.

Spalding, Lyman, Barker, Jeremiah. "Beneficial Effects of Alkalis in Consumption of the Lungs." *Medical Repository* 5, no. 2 (1802): 220–21.

Spector, Benjamin. "Noah Webster: Letters on Yellow Fever Addressed to Dr. William Currie. An Introductory Essay." In *Supplements to the Bulletin of the History of Medicine (No. 9),* edited by Henry E. Siegerist and Genevieve Miller, 1–17. Baltimore: The Johns Hopkins Press, 1947.

Spence, John. "A Case of Pulmonary Consumption Cured by the Use of Digitalis Purpura: In a Letter from John Spence, M.D. Of Dumfries (Virg.) to Dr. Mitchill and Dated January 26, 1801." *Medical Repository* 5 (1802): 17–21.

Spence, John. "History of a Case of Mania, Successfully Treated, in a Series of Letters between Dr. John Spence and Dr. Benjamin Rush. Communicated to the Editor by Dr. Spence." *The Philadelphia Medical Museum* 4, no. 3 (1808): 129–48.

Spon, Charles, and Hippocrates. *C. Sponii . . . Sibylla Medica: Hippocratis Libellum Prognosticon Heroico Carmine Latine Exprimens.* Lugduni, 1661.

Stahl, Georg Ernst. *Medicinae Dogmatico-Systematicae Partis Theoreticae Sectio I [& II].* Halae 1707.

Stahl, Jasper Jacob. *History of Old Broad Bay and Waldoboro.* 2 vols. Portland, ME: Bond Wheelwright Co., 1956.

Starr, Paul. *The Social Transformation of American Medicine.* New York: Basic Books, 1982.

Stephanson, R., and D. N. Wagner. *The Secrets of Generation: Reproduction in the Long Eighteenth Century.* Toronto: University of Toronto Press, 2015.

Stern, Heinrich. *Theory and Practice of Bloodletting.* New York: Rebman Company, 1915.

Stevensen, Lloyd G. "Putting Disease on the Map: The Early Use of Spot Maps in the Study of Yellow Fever." *Journal of the History of Medicine and Allied Sciences* 20 (1965): 226–61.

Steward, William. *The Healing Art, or Art of Healing Disclosed, by a Professed Botanist. Being Alphabetically Arranged, It May Be Termed a Botanical Dictionary . . .* Ballston Spa, NY: James Comstock, 1812.

———. *The Healing Art, or, Art of Healing Disclosed by a Professed Botanist [Microform] Being Alphabetically Arranged, It May Be Termed a Botanical Dictionary by William Steward, Jun.* 1812.

Stiles, Ezra. *A Discourse on the Christian Union: The Substance of Which Was Delivered before the Reverend Convention of the Congregational Clergy in the Colony of Rhode-Island Assembled at Bristol. April 23, 1760. By Ezra Stiles, A.M. Pastor of the Second Congregational Church in Newport. [Six Lines of Quotations].* Edited by Dan Merriam, Ebenezer Merriam, Bristol Convention of the Congregational Clergy in the Colony of Rhode-Island and Rhode-Island Convention of the Congregational Clergy in the Colony of Brookfield 1799.

Stoll, Maximilian. *Rationis Medendi in Nosocomio Practico Vindobenensi.* Vienna: August Bernardi, 1777.

Straub, Wolfgang. "The Ophthalmology of Fabricius Hildanus in the 17th Century." *Documenta Ophthalmologica* 74 (1990): 21–29.

Sullivan, James. *The History of the District of Maine.* Boston: Printed by I. Thomas and E.T. Andrews, 1795.

Sweetser, William. *Dissertations on Cynache Trachealis or Croup and on the Functions of the Extreme Capillary Vessels in Health and Disease; to Which Were Awarded the Boylston Premiums for the Years 1820 and 1823.* Boston: Cummins, Hilliard & Co., 1823.

———. *A Treatise on Consumption.* Boston: T. H. Carter, 1836.

Swieten, Gehard Van. *An Abridgement of Baron Van Swieten's Commentaries Upon the Aphorisms Of . . . Herman Boerhaave . . . : Concerning the Knowledge and Cure of Diseases / by Colin Hossac. . . . In Five Volumes.* Vol. 3, London: Printed for Robert Horsfield and Thomas Longman 1774.

Swieten, Gerard, and Herman Boerhaave. *Commentaries upon Boerhaave's Aphorisms Concerning the Knowledge and Cure of Diseases. By Baron Van Swieten, Counsellor and First Physician to Their Majesties the Emperor and Empress of Germany; Perpetual President of the College of Physicians in Vienna; Member of the Royal Academy of Sciences and Surgery at Paris; H. Fellow of the Royal College of Physicians at Edinburgh; &C. &C. &C. Translated from the Latin.* Vol. 1 [in English], Vol. 11. Edinburgh: printed for Charles Elliot, Parliament Square. Sold by J. Murray, Fleet Street, London, 1776. Monograph.

Sydenham, Thomas, Samuel Johnson, and John Swan. *The Entire Works of Dr. Thomas Sydenham, Newly Made English from the Originals: Wherein the History of Acute and Chronic Diseases, and the Safest and Most Effectual Methods of Treating Them, Are Faithfully, Clearly, and Accurately Delivered. To Which Are Added, Explanatory and Practical Notes, from the Best Medicinal Writers.* London: Printed for Edward Cave, at St. John's Gate, 1742.

Talbott, John H. *A Biographical History of Medicine.* New York: Grune & Stratton, 1970.

Taylor, Alan. *Liberty Men and Great Proprietors: The Revolutionary Settlement on the Maine Frontier, 1760–1820.* Chapel Hill: Published for the Institute of Early American History and Culture, Williamsburg, Virginia, by University of North Carolina Press, 1990.

Thacher, James. *American Medical Biography: Or Memoirs of Eminent Physicians Who Have Flourished in America. To Which Is Prefixed a Succinct History of Medical Science in the United States, from the First Settlement of the Country.* Boston: Richardson & Lord and Cottons & Barnard, 1828.

———. *American Modern Practice.* Boston: Ezra Read, 1817.

———. *The American New Dispensatory Containing General Principles of Pharmaceutic Chemistry. . . . The Whole Compiled from the Most Approved Authors, Both European and American.* Boston: T. B. Wait and Co., 1810.

———. *The American New Dispensatory Containing General Principles of Pharmaceutic Chemistry. . . . With an Appendix, Containing an Account of Mineral Waters . . . And the Method of Preparing Opium. . . . The Whole Compiled from the Most Approved Authors, Both European and American.* 3rd ed. Boston: Thomas B. Wait, 1817.

Thayer, William Sydney, and William Osler. *Osler and Other Papers.* Baltimore: Johns Hopkins University Press; London: H. Milford; Oxford University Press, 1931.

To the Public with a View of Promoting the Interests of Humanity, a Number of Respectable Citizens Have Associated under the Name of "the Humane Society of the State of New-York," and Have Agreed to the Following Constitution. Variation: Early American Imprints.; 1st Series; No. 47079. References: Bristol; B8701; Shipton & Mooney; 47079. s.n.; United States; New York., 1794. Book; Internet Resource.

Toner, Joseph M. *Contributions to the Annals of Medical Progress and Medical Education in the United States before and during the War of Independence.* Washington: Government Printing Office, 1874.

Tournefort, Joseph Pitton De. *Relation D'un Voyage Du Levant, Fait Par Ordre Du Roy, Contenant L'histoire Ancienne & Moderne De Plusieurs Isles De L'archipel, De Constantinople, Des Côtes De La Mer Noire, De L'arménie, De La Georgie, Des Frontières De Perse & De L'asie Mineure.* Paris: De L'Imprimerie Royale, 1717.

Tourtelle, Etienne. *The Principles of Health (Elements of Hygiene) . . . From the Second French Ed.; Translated by G. Williamson.* Baltimore: John D. Toy, 1819.

Tracy, Dr. "Remarkable Case of Phthisis Pulmonalis, Wherein a Profuse Spontaneous Hemorrhage Seemed to Be Useful: In a Letter from Dr. Tracy, of Norwich, (Connecticut) to Dr. Mitchill, Dated July 16, 1802." *Medical Repository* 6 (1803): 256–58.

Trayser, Donald G. *Barnstable; Three Centuries of a Cape Cod Town.* Hyannis, MA: F.B. & F.P. Goss, 1939.

"'A Treatise on the Puerperal Fever Illustrated by Cases, Which Occurred in Leeds and Its Vicinity in the Years 1809–1812' by William Hey, Jr., London 1815." *New England Journal of Medicine and Surgery* 5 (1816): 85–98.

Tröhler, Ulrich. "The Introduction of Numerical Methods to Assess the Effects of Medical Interventions During the 18th Century: A Brief History." *Journal of the Royal Society of Medicine* 104, no. 11 (November 2011): 465–74.

Tryon, Warren Stenson, and William Charvat. *The Cost Books of Ticknor and Fields, and Their Predecessors, 1832–1858.* Bibliographical Society of America Monograph Series. New York: Bibliographical Society of America, 1949.

Tuchman, Barbara W. *Practicing History: Selected Essays.* 1st ed. New York: Knopf, 1981.

Ulrich, Laurel Thatcher. "'The Living Mother of a Living Child': Midwifery and Mortality in Post-Revolutionary New England." *The William and Mary Quarterly* 46, no. 1 (1989): 27–48.

———. *A Midwife's Tale: The Life of Martha Ballard, Based on Her Diary, 1785–1812.* New York City: Alfred A. Knopf, 1990.

Underwood, Edgar Ashworth. *Boerhaave's Men at Leyden and After.* Edinburgh: Edinburgh University Press, 1977.

Valencius, Bolton Conevery, David I. Spanagel, Emily Pawley, Sara Stidstone Gronim, and Paul Lucier. "Science in Early America: Print Culture and the Sciences of Territoriality." *Journal of the Early Republic* 36, no. 1 (2016): 73–123.

Vaughan, Benjamin. "Letter from Benjamin Vaughn to Benjamin Rush." In *Manuscript Correspondence of Benjamin Rush UV18*, edited by Historical Society of Pennsylvania, 1799.

———. "Letter from Benjamin Vaughn to Benjamin Rush, 21 June 1801." In *Manuscript Correspondence of Benjamin Rush UV 18, MSS 55*. Edited by Historical Society of Pennsylvania, 1801.

"A View of Mercurial Practice in Febrile Diseases. By John Warren, M.D, President of the Massachusetts Medical Society and Professor of Anatomy and Surgery in the University of Cambridge. Boston, T.B. Wait & Co. 8vo. Pp. 195, 1813." *New England Journal of Medicine and Surgery* 4 (1815): 175–81.

Wagener, Damianus Johannes Theodorus. *The History of Oncology.* Houten: Springer, 2009.

Waite, Frederick Clayton. *The Story of a Country Medical College: A History of the Clinical School of Medicine and Vermont Medical College, Woodstock, Vermont 1827–56.* Montpelier: Vermont Historical Society, 1945.

Wallace, James W. "An Account of Two Cases of Dropsy, Cured by the Loss of Blood, Extracted from a Letter from Dr. James W. Wallace of Faquier County, in Virginia, to Dr. Benjamin Rush. Dated December 16th, 1805." *Philadelphia Medical Museum* 2, no. 4 (1806): 401–403.

Ware, John. *Medical Dissertations on Hemoptysis or the Spitting of Blood, and on Suppuration, Which Obtained the Boylston Premiums for the Years 1818 & 1820.* Boston: Cummings and Hilliard, 1820.

Warner, John Harley. *Against the Spirit of System: The French Impulse in Nineteenth-Century American Medicine.* Princeton, NJ: Princeton University Press, 1998.

———. "Grand Narrative and Its Discontents: Medical History and the Social Transformation of American Medicine." *Journal of Health Politics, Policy and Law* 29, no. 4 (2004): 757–80.

———. *The Therapeutic Perspective: Medical Practice, Knowledge, and Identity in America, 1820–85.* Cambridge, MA: Harvard University Press, 1986.

Warren, John. *View of the Mercurial Practice in Febrile Diseases.* Boston: T. D. Wait & Co., 1813.

Warren, John C. "Cases of Apoplexy, with Dissections." *New England Journal of Medicine and Surgery* 1 (1812): 34–41, 154–59.

Watson, Patricia A. *The Angelical Conjunction: The Preacher-Physicians of Colonial New England.* Knoxville: The University of Tennessee Press, 1991.

Watson, William. "History of Several Cases of Phthisis Pulmonalis Treated with Mercury." *Philadelphia Medical Museum* 2, no. 1 (1806): 6–15.

Watt, Robert E. *Treatise on the History, Nature, and Treatment of Chincough: Including a Variety of Cases and Dissections. To Which Is Subjoined and Inquiry into the Relative Mortality of the Principal Diseases of Children, and the Numbers Who Have Died under Ten Years of Age, in Glasgow, during the Last Thirty Years.* Glasgow: John Smith & Son, 1813.

Wear, Andrew. "Medicine in Early Modern Europe, 1500–1700." In *The Western Medical Tradition: 800 B.C.–1800 A.D.*, edited by Lawrence I. Conrad and Wellcome Institute for the History of Medicine., xiv, 556. Cambridge; New York: Cambridge University Press, 1995.

Webster, Noah. *An American Dictionary of the English Language. With an Introd. by Mario Pei.* Reprint of 1828 Published by S. Converse ed. 2 vols. New York and London: Johnson Reprint Corporation, 1970.

———. *A Brief History of Epidemic and Pestilential Diseases with the Principal Phenomena of the Physical World Which Precede and Accompany Them and Observations Deduced from Facts Stated.* 2 vols. Hartford: Hudson and Goodwin, 1799.

———. *A Collection of Papers on the Subject of Bilious Fevers Prevalent in the United States for a Few Years Past.* New York: Hopkins, Webb & Co., 1796.

———. *Dissertations on the English Language: With Notes, Historical and Critical to Which Is Added by Way of an Appendix, an Essay on a Reformed Mode of Spelling, with Dr. Franklin's Arguments on That Subject.* Boston: Isaiah Thomas and Company, 1789.

Weston, Issac. *Our Pastor: Or, Reminiscences of Rev. Edward Payson, D.D., Pastor of the Second Congregational Church in Portland, Me.* Boston: Tappan & Whittemore, 1855.

Wheeler, George Augustus, and Henry Warren Wheeler. *History of Brunswick, Topsham, and Harpswell, Maine Including the Ancient Territory Known as Pejepscot.* Boston, MA: Alfred Mudge & son, printers, 1878.

White, Paul Dudley. *Heart Disease.* Macmillan Medical Monographs. New York: The Macmillan Company, 1931.

Whorton, James. "Chemistry." In *The Education of American Physicians: Historical Essays*, edited by Ronald Numbers, 72–94. Berkley: University of California Press, 1980.

Williams, R. P. & C. "Catalogue of Medical, Botanical, and Chemical Books for Sale by R. P. & C. Williams." Boston: R. P. & C. Williams, 1818.

Williams, Stephen W. *American Medical Biography; or, Memoirs of Eminent Physicians, Embracing Principally Those Who Have Died since the Publication of Dr. Thacher's Work on the Same Subject.* Greenfield, MA, 1845. Reprint, Millford House, 1967.

Williamson, William. *The History of the State of Maine: From Its First Discovery, A.D. 1602 to the Separation, A.D. 1820, Inclusive.* Hallowell, ME: Glazier, Masters & Co., 1832.

Willis, William. *The History of Portland, Facsimile Ed. 1972.* New Hampshire Publishing Company and Maine Historical Society ed. Portland: Bailely & Noyes, 1865.

———. *Journals of the Rev. Thomas Smith and the Rev. Samuel Deane . . . with Notes and Biographical Notices and a Summary History of Portland.* Portland: Joseph S. Bailey, 1849.

Willoughby, R. E., Jr., K. S. Tieves, G. M. Hoffman, N. S. Ghanayem, C. M. Amlie-Lefond, M. J. Schwabe, M. J. Chusid, and C. E. Rupprecht. "Survival after Treatment of Rabies with Induction of Coma." *New England Journal of Medicine* 352, no. 24 (June 16, 2005): 2508–14.

Willoughby, Westell. "A Case of Hydrophobia, Successfully Treated by Mercury; Communicated to the Medical Society of the State of New York, by Dr Westell Willoughby, of Hermiker County; and Transmitted to the Editors, by Nicholas Romayne, M.D. &C President of That Society." *Medical Repository* 6, 2nd hexade, no. 2 (August, September, and October, 1808–1809): 135–37.

Wilson, Adrian, and T. G. Ashplant. "Whig History and Present-Centred History." *The Historical Journal* 31, no. 1 (1988): 1–16.

Wilson, C. Anne. *Food and Drink in Britain: From the Stone Age to the 19th Century.* Edited by C. Anne Wilson. Chicago: 1991.

Winslow, C. E. *The Conquest of Epidemic Disease: A Chapter in the History of Ideas.* University of Wisconsin Reprint (1980) ed. Princeton: Princeton University Press, 1943.

Winslow, C. E. A. "The Epidemiology of Noah Webster." *Transactions of the Connecticut Academy of Arts and Sciences* 32 (1934): 21–109.

Winsor, Mary P. "The Practitioner of Science: Everyone Her Own Historian." *Journal of the History of Biology* 34, no. 2 (June 1, 2001): 229–45.

Wintrobe, Maxwell M. *Blood, Pure and Eloquent: A Story of Discovery, of People, and of Ideas.* New York: McGraw-Hill, 1980.

Withering, William. *An Account of the Foxglove, and Some of Its Medical Uses: With Practical Remarks on Dropsy, and Other Diseases.* Birmingham: M. Swinney for G, GJ, and J Robinson, London, 1785.

———. *An Account of the Scarlet Fever and Sore Throat, or Scarlatina Anginosa; Particularly as It Appeared at Birmingham in the Year 1778.* London: T. Cadell &c., 1779.

Worboys, Michael. *Spreading Germs: Disease Theories and Medical Practice in Britain, 1865–1900.* Cambridge, UK; New York: Cambridge University Press, 2000.

Worcester, Samuel T. *History of the Town of Hollis, New Hampshire, from Its First Settlement to the Year 1879.* Boston: A. Williams & Co., 1879.

Wright, W. F., and P. A. Mackowiak. "Origin, Evolution and Clinical Application of the Thermometer." *American Journal of the Medical Sciences* 351, no. 5 (May 2016): 526–34.

Wright, William F. "Early Evolution of the Thermometer and Application to Clinical Medicine." *Journal of Thermal Biology* 56 (2016): 18–30.

Wunderlich, C. A. *Das Verhalten Der Eigenwärme in Krankheiten (the Course of Temperature in Diseases).* Leipzig: Wigand, 1868.

"Yellow Fever Vaccine." *Morbidity and Mortality Weekly Report* 39, no. RR-6 (1990): 1–6.

Young, Joseph. "Observations on Phthisis Pulmonalis, or Consumption of the Lungs.". *The Medical Repository of Original Essays and Intelligence, Relative to Physic, Surgery, Chemistry, and Natural History* 6 (1809): 241–46.

Young, Thomas. *An Introduction to Medical Literature, Including a System of Practical Nosology . . . Together with Detached Essays, on the Study of Physic, on Classification, on Chemical Affinities, on Animal Chemistry, on the Blood, and on the Medical Effects of Climates.* London: Underwood and Blacks, 1813.

———. *A Practical and Historical Treatise on Consumptive Diseases, Deduced from Original Observations, and Collected from Authors of All Ages.* London: Underwood, 1815.

Author Index

Footnotes are indicated by n following the page numbers.

Subject Index

Footnotes are indicated by n following the page number. Illustrations are indicated by *italic* page numbers. Pages from the transcription of the Barker manuscript are indicated by **bold italics**.

A., Miss L., *333–334*
A., Mrs., *389–390*
accommodation stages, 20
accouchement, *441*
accouchers or accoucheurs, *352*, *441*
acetite of lead, *193*
acid/alkali theory, 90–91,
    100n53, 104n66
acrid bile, 51
Adams, Daniel, *366*, 367n5
Adams, Isaac, 44
Adams, Joseph, 76, *164*
adhesive plaisters, *417*
aethiops mineral. *See* ethiops mineral
agarics, *441*
ague, 1, *174*, *441*
ail, 174n21, *441*
air
    azotic, 99–100, *443*
    fixed, *206*, *448*
    salubrious, *165*, *347*
alcohol, 72–74, *166*, *395–404*
    ardent spirits, *141*, *262–65*
    articles published by Barker on, 29

Alexander, Dr., *201*
alienists, 147n24
alkaline therapy, xx, 26, 43–44, 87–117,
    209n2, *288*
    articles by Barker on, *27*, 28–29, 88,
        114–15, *291*, *292*
    Barker's use of, 100–110, 113–14, 125–26,
        195, 211n4, *212*, *217*, *289–91*, *292*
    for consumption, 88, *347*, *349*, *352–53*
    debate over, 90–95
    for fever, 51, *288–90*, *348–49*
    for mad dog poisoning, *251–52*
    for scarlatina anginosa, *209–10*,
        291, *292*
    for throat distemper, *217*, *219–20*
Allen, Elmore, *433–35*
Allen & Ticknor, 70, 81n122
aloes, *151*, *395*, *442*
aloetic pills, *388*, *442*
alphabetization, 68
alteratives, *238*, *324*, *326*, *442*
alum, *410*, *442*
amanuenses, 34n4
American Philosophical Society, 111

Watson, Susanna, *264*

Watson, William, *406–11*

Watt, James, 109–10

Watt, Robert E., *221*

Watts, Edward, *166*, *184*, *276*

Watts, Isaac, *327*, *340*

Watts, Samuel, 166n8

Webber, President Samuel, *243–44*

Webster, John, 76n102

Webster, Noah, 26, 37–38, 80–86, 174n22, 175n24, *273*

Weed, Lawrence, 70

Wells, Eleanor, *355–56*

Wheaton, Levi, 78

Wheelock, Eleazar, 328n6

whiggish or whig history, 118–19

White, Esther, *279–80*

Whitney, Samuel, *424–25*

Whitney, Sarah, 232n5

whooping cough, *221–28*

William Hyde Booksellers, 44

Williams, John, Sr., 3

Williams, Mary, 10

Williams-Barker House, *3*

Willis, Francis, *143*, 143–44n17

Willis, Thomas, 233n7

Willoughby, Westell, *258–60*

Wilson, Alexander Philip, 421n6

Wilson, Dr., *356*

Wilson, Mark, *264–65*

wine, antimonial *(vinum antimonii)*, *378*, 460

wine-whey, 460

Withering, William, *199*, 263n6

Witherspoon, Ann, 374n12

women, 439

breast cancer, *281–83*

childbed (puerperal) fever, 42–43, *183–94*, 210n2, *288*

consumption in, *302–7*, *323–46*, *390*, *392*

deaths of Barker's wives, *323–46*

healers, 56–57

ladies' dresses, *389–90*

ovarian tumors, 263n6

preeclampsia, 265n13

Woodbury, Hugh, *311*

Woodhouse, James, 94n29, 96n39

Woodville, Dr., 35n9

Worcester State Hospital, 139n11

worms, *175*

wounds, trivial: deaths following, *183–93*

yellow fever, 29–32, 84, *208*, 286n22, *287*

alkaline therapy for, 88, 102–3, 106–8

articles published by Barker on, 27, 28, 106, *291*, *292*

contagionist explanation of, 110–12

symptoms of, 123

York Retreat, 146n22

Young, John R., *383–85*

Young, Thomas, *297–98*, *306*, *352–53*, *389–90*, *395*